ATTENTION DEFICIT HYPERACTIVITY DISORDER

Contemporary *Clinical* Neuroscience

Series Editors:
Ralph Lydic and
Helen A. Baghdoyan

Attention Deficit Hyperactivity Disorder: *From Genes to Patients,* edited by *David Gozal and Dennis L. Molfese*, 2005

The Orexin/Hypocretin System: *Physiology and Pathophysiology,* edited by *Seiji Nishino and Takeshi Sakurai,* 2005

The G Protein-Coupled Receptors Handbook, edited by *Lakshmi A. Devi,* 2005

Genetics and Genomics of Neurobehavioral Disorders, edited by *Gene S. Fisch,* 2003

Sedation and Analgesia for Diagnostic and Therapeutic Procedures, edited by *Shobha Malviya, Norah N. Naughton, and Kevin K. Tremper,* 2003

Neural Mechanisms of Anesthesia, edited by *Joseph F. Antognini, Earl E. Carstens, and Douglas E. Raines,* 2002

Glutamate and Addiction, edited by *Barbara Herman,* 2002

Molecular Mechanisms of Neurodegenerative Diseases, edited by *Marie-Françoise Chesselet,* 2000

Contemporary Clinical Neuroscience

Attention Deficit Hyperactivity Disorder

From Genes to Patients

Edited by

David Gozal, MD

Kosair Children's Hospital, Research Institute, Departments of Pediatrics, Pharmacology, and Toxicology, University of Louisville, Louisville, KY

Dennis L. Molfese, PhD

Department of Psychological and Brain Sciences, University of Louisville, Louisville, KY

Humana Press Totowa, New Jersey

999 Riverview Drive, Suite 208
Totowa, New Jersey 07512

humanapress.com

Production Editor: Amy Thau

Cover design by Patricia F. Cleary

For additional copies, pricing for bulk purchases, and/or information about other Humana titles, contact Humana at the above address or at any of the following numbers: Tel.: 973-256-1699; Fax: 973-256-8341; E-mail: orders@humanapr.com or visit our website at www.humanapress.com

This publication is printed on acid-free paper. ∞
ANSI Z39.48-1984 (American National Standards Institute) Permanence of Paper for Printed Library Materials.

Printed in the United States of America. 10 9 8 7 6 5 4 3 2 1

e-ISBN: 1-59259-891-9

Library of Congress Cataloging-in-Publication Data

Attention deficit hyperactivity disorder : from genes to patients / editedby David Gozal and Dennis L. Molfese.

p. cm. -- (Contemporary clinical neuroscience)

Includes bibliographical references and index.

ISBN 1-58829-312-2 (alk. paper)

1. Attention-deficit hyperactivity disorder. I. Gozal, David. II.

Molfese, Dennis L. III. Series.

RJ506.H9A932 2005

618.92'8589--dc22

2005001924

Dedication

This book is dedicated to all the children with attention deficit hyperactivity disorder and their parents who look to us to provide a better tomorrow.

Preface

Attention deficit hyperactivity disorder (ADHD) is a common neurobehavioral disorder affecting 5–10% of children and adolescents and 3% of adults. *Attention Deficit Hyperactivity Disorder: From Genes to Patients* aims to provide a comprehensive, state-of-the-art overview of the critical aspects of ADHD, and hopefully will serve as a quick and up-to-date reference source for professionals with an interest in ADHD.

The book is divided into three major areas that follow an historical survey. The first group of chapters deals with current theories on the pathophysiology of ADHD, and focuses on neurotransmitters and the contributions and validity of animal models. The second section emphasizes the evaluation and treatment of patients with ADHD, from the day-to-day approach by the clinical psychologist to the more sophisticated anatomical and functional imaging strategies that have emerged in the last decade. In addition, chapters dealing with specific impairments, such as those pertaining to reading, social interaction, and working memory, are also included for more detailed analysis of these important aspects and their respective contributions to global functioning. The third and final section provides an expanded review on the pharmacotherapy of ADHD and the appropriate methods for selection of specific drugs for individual patients based on drug kinetics and gene expression.

David Gozal, MD
Dennis L. Molfese, PhD

Contents

Contributors

Tuija Aro, PhD • *Niilo Maki Institute, University of Jyväskylä, Jyväskylä, Finland*
Dean W. Beebe, PhD • *Psychology Division, Cincinnati Children's Hospital Medical Center, Cincinnati, OH*
Juliana S. Bloom, MEd • *Center for Clinical and Developmental Neuropsychology, The University of Georgia, Athens, GA*
Kimberly Brodsky, BA • *Department of Psychology, University of Colorado, Boulder, CO*
Nomita Chhabildas, PhD • *Department of Rehabilitation Medicine, The Children's Hospital, Denver, CO*
Daniel F. Connor, MD • *Department of Psychiatry, Division of Child and Adolescent Psychiatry, University of Massachusetts Medical School, Worcester, MA*
Melissa DelBello, MD • *Bipolar and Psychotic Disorders Research Program, Department of Psychiatry, University of Cincinnati College of Medicine, Cincinnati, OH*
Martha Bridge Denckla, MD • *Developmental Cognitive Neurology, Kennedy Krieger Institute, Professor, Neurology, Pediatrics, Psychiatry, John Hopkins University School of Medicine, Baltimore, MD*
Roscoe A. Dykman, PhD • *Arkansas Children's Nutrition Center, Arkansas Children's Hospital, Department of Psychiatry, University of Arkansas Medical Center, Little Rock, AR*
Melissa Ferguson, BA • *Department of Psychological and Brain Sciences, University of Louisville, Louisville, KY*
Alexandra P. Fonaryova-Key, PhD • *Department of Psychological and Brain Sciences, University of Louisville, Louisville, KY*
Mauricio A. Garcia, BS • *Center for Clinical and Developmental Neuropsychology, The University of Georgia, Athens, GA*
David Gozal, MD • *Kosair Children's Hospital, Research Institute, Departments of Pediatrics, Pharmacology and Toxicology, University of Louisville School of Medicine, Louisville, KY*
Scott Holland, PhD • *Imaging Research Center, Children's Hospital Medical Center, University of Cincinnati, Cincinnati, OH*
Stephen R. Hooper, PhD • *Department of Psychiatry and The Clinical Center for the Study of Development and Learning, The University of North Carolina at Chapel Hill School of Medicine, Chapel Hill, NC*
George W. Hynd, EDd • *School of Education, Purdue University, West Lafayette, IN*
Lisa M. Jonkman, PhD • *Universiteit Maastricht, Faculty of Psychology, Department of Neurocognition, Maastricht, The Netherlands*
Aiveen Kirley, MD, MRCPsych • *Department of Psychiatry, Trinity College, Dublin, Ireland*
Anne-Mari Lapveteläinen, MA • *Department of Special Education, Department of Psychology and Child Research Center, University of Jyväskylä, Jyväskylä, Finland*
Heikki Lyytinen, PhD • *Department of Psychology and Child Research Center, University of Jyväskylä, Jyväskylä, Finland*

John S. Markowitz, PharmD • *Department of Pharmaceutical Sciences, College of Pharmacy, Medical University of South Carolina, Charleston, SC*
Carlin J. Miller, PhD • *Department of Psychology, Queens College, City University of New York, Flushing, NY*
Dennis L. Molfese, PhD • *Department of Psychological and Brain Sciences, University of Louisville, Louisville, KY*
Robert D. Oades, PhD • *BioPsychology Research, The University of Duisburg-Essen Clinic for Child and Adolescent Psychiatry and Psychotherapy, Essen, Germany*
Louise M. O'Brien, PhD • *Kosair Children's Hospital Sleep Medicine and Apnea Center, Division of Pediatric Sleep Medicine, Department of Pediatrics, University of Louisville School of Medicine, Louisville, KY*
Kennerly S. Patrick, PhD • *Department of Pharmaceutical Sciences, College of Pharmacy, Medical University of South Carolina, Charleston, SC*
Bruce F. Pennington, PhD • *Department of Psychology, University of Denver, Denver, CO*
Jonathan C. Pfeifer, MD • *Department of Psychiatry, University of Cincinnati College of Medicine, Cincinnati, OH*
Barry W. Row, PhD • *Kosair Children's Hospital Research Institute, Department of Pediatrics, University of Louisville, Louisville, KY*
Lucia A. Ruocco, DR • *Department of Experimental Medicine, Second University of Naples, Naples, Italy*
Vivienne Ann Russell, PhD • *Department of Human Biology, Faculty of Health Sciences, University of Cape Town, Cape Town, South Africa*
Adolfo G. Sadile, MD • *Department of Experimental Medicine, Second University of Naples, Naples, Italy*
Ashley Scott, BA • *Department of Psychology, University of Denver, Denver, CO*
Margaret Semrud-Clikeman, PhD • *Department of Educational Psychology, University of Texas-Austin, Austin TX*
Michelle Shanahan, BA • *Department of Psychology, University of Denver, Denver, CO*
Jack Stevens, PhD • *Columbus Children's Hospital, Department of Pediatrics, Ohio State University, Columbus, OH*
Hana Tur-Kaspa, PhD • *Constantiner School of Education, Tel Aviv University, Tel Aviv, Israel*
Daniela Vallone, MD • *Department of Experimental Medicine, Second University of Naples, Naples, Italy*
Jaap van der Meere, PhD • *Laboratory of Developmental and Experimental Clinical Psychology, University of Groningen, Groningen, The Netherlands*
Davide Viggiano, MD, PhD • *Department of Experimental Medicine, Second University of Naples, Naples, Italy*
Lisa Lee Weyandt, PhD • *Department of Psychology, Central Washington University, Ellensburg, WA*
Erik G. Willcutt, PhD • *Department of Psychology, University of Colorado, Boulder, CO*
Emily A. Williams, BA • *School of Education, The University of North Carolina at Chapel Hill, Chapel Hill, NC*
Benjamin Yerys, MA • *Department of Psychology, University of Denver, Denver, CO*

1

Historical Aspects of Attention Deficit Hyperactivity Disorder

Roscoe A. Dykman*

1. INTRODUCTION

It would be impossible to cover in this book the thousands of articles that have been written on the subject of hyperactivity and related disorders over the last 50 to 60 yr. This chapter focuses on the early history, giving enough recent history to track major ideas and relations as the author sees them. But even here, there are problems. If one looks at the reference lists in books on this subject, it becomes immediately obvious that the lists are quite different, with each writer paying attention to his or her particular interests. Current research reports and hundreds of reviews of attention deficit hyperactivity disorder (ADHD) suffer from an immense historical amnesia. Concepts change, and many of the historical ideas are revisited and passed on cloaked in new terminology. The criteria now used to identify these children compared with those used some 50 yr ago, although more refined and less inclusive, are not all that different. You see a child in the cafeteria who is overly active, impulsive, and inattentive (three items); he will likely satisfy the current ADHD criteria. However, what was once largely speculation regarding a neurological basis and related genetic basis for ADHD is now supported by a large number of very good studies, which will be discussed in the subsequent chapters of this book. Much has happened in the last 10 yr. And yet, there remains much to do for those of us who love unresolved issues.

1.1. *What Is in a Name?*

One of the earliest descriptions of what we now recognize as ADHD appeared in a nursery rhyme written by Heinrich Hoffman in 1863 *(1)*.

"Phil, stop acting like a worm,
The table is no place to squirm."
Thus speaks the father to his son,
severely says it, not in fun.
Mother frowns and looks around
although she doesn't make a sound.
But Phillip will not take advise,
he'll have his way at any price.

*Dr. Dykman is a Professor Emeritus in the Department of Psychiatry, University of Arkansas for Medical Sciences and a Professor of Research in the Arkansas Children's Nutrition Center, 1212 Marshall Street, Little Rock, Arkansas, 72202.

From: *Attention Deficit Hyperactivity Disorder: From Genes to Patients*
Edited by: D. Gozal and D. L. Molfese © Humana Press Inc., Totowa, NJ

He turns,
and churns,
he wiggles
and jiggles
Here and there on the chair;
Phil, these twists I cannot bear.

There have been many other names in addition to Fidgety Phil, including brain damage syndrome *(2)*, organic driveness *(3)*, organic behavior syndrome *(4)*, minimal brain damage syndrome *(5)*, hyperkinetic impulse disorder *(6)*, cerebro-asthenic syndrome *(7,8)*, minimal brain dysfunction (MBD) *(9)*, hyperactivity *(10)*, hyperkinetic syndrome *(11)*, attention deficit syndrome *(12)*, hyperactive child syndrome *(13)*, intention disorder *(14,15)*, attention deficit disorder (ADD) (American Psychiatric Association [APA] *[14]*), and ADHD *(15)*.

We were the first *(12)* to suggest that the term MBD be replaced by an attentional definition. The cerebro-asthenic term of Luria *(7,8)* described two types of children—an excitatory distractible type, and an inhibitory–inattentive type with a low threshold for fatigue. Luria was greatly influenced by Pavlov *(18,19)*, who put the concept of behavioral inhibition on the map; Pavlov, in turn, was affected by Sherrington *(20,21)*, who described both inhibitory and excitatory reflex pathways. Pavlov was the first to study behavioral inhibition in a systematic way, a concept now referred to by Barkley *(22)* as response inhibition. The concept of inhibition is pervasive in the classical conditioning literature, affording an explanation for the differentiation of conditional stimuli, the restriction of generalization gradients so that stimuli can be more specific in generating responses, the extinction of responses by withdrawal of reinforcement, and the spontaneous restoration (disinhibition) of once-extinguished responses.

As is evident, a large number of writers have cast their nets into the field of diagnosis with no substantial agreement even to this day. Ross and Ross *(23)* traced the concept of minimal brain damage back to neurological papers by Still *(2)* and Tredgold *(24)*. Still *(2)* described children who exhibited violent outbursts, wanton mischievousness, destructiveness, a lack of responsiveness to punishment, and an abnormal incapacity for sustained attention. These severe symptoms are more like those of children we now recognize under the terms conduct disorder (CD) and oppositional/defiant disorder (ODD). It is important to note that Still and Tredgold wrote about minimal brain damage, which is related to minimal brain dysfunction but is not the same construct. MBD as conceived in the 1960s had more to do with subtle nonorganic differences in the "wiring" of neuronal connections and associated neurotransmitter deficiencies than with structural damage to the brain.

To answer the question raised by heading of this section, one could say that children identified as having this heterogenous disorder may differ depending on the diagnostic name used. The name MBD included children that were both hyperactive (HY) and learning disabled (LD) or both. LD is completely ignored in the definition of ADHD, but ADHD children can be classified as LD by another diagnostic definition *(25)*. However, the net effect is that much of the published literature ignores the comorbid nature of ADHD and LD. It is also obvious that some of the other definitions—indeed, the meaning of the term "hyperkinesis" as originally used—referred to children with a more severe pathology than our garden-variety ADHD child.

2. THE MBD AND EARLY ADD PERIOD

The MBD label became popular with the publication of a paper by Clements and Peters *(9)* and even more so via a book written by Paul Wender *(26)*. Clements and Peters were greatly influenced by a number of writers: the pioneering work of Strauss and Lehtinen *(27)*, who enumerated the characteristics of children with known brain damage; the study of Bradley *(28)* showing that Benzedrine reduced hyperactivity; the published work on perinatal risk factors (e.g., bleeding in pregnancy, low birth weight) in causing behavior and learning problems; and a variety of other papers suggesting that neurological impairment results in behavioral and emotional symptomatology *(6,29–34)*. The MBD term as used by Clements and Peters designated children who were HY, LD, or both. It included one or more of the following signs: specific learning deficits, perceptual-motor deficits, general coordination deficits, hyperkinesis (extreme overactivity), impulsivity, emotional lability, short attention span and/or distractibility, "equivocal" neurological signs, and borderline abnormal or abnormal electroencephalogram (EEG). Clements and Peters gave a description of MBD that could be used to describe ADD/ADHD today:

> It is important to emphasize that a given child may not have symptoms in all or even many of these areas; each child has his own particular cluster of symptoms. The level of his intelligence and the nature of his underlying temperament determine the form and the excellence of his maneuvers to compensate for the deficits or deviations.
>
> It is probable that certain general principles underlie the above symptoms. For example, most may be due to perceptual defects having to do with the capacity to receive, hold, scan, and selectively screen out stimuli in a sequential order; to sustain a repertoire of background gestalten as compared to foreground gestalten; to perceive the subtle and often abstract behavior gestalten, which allow proper socialization to take place. Proprioception may be one of the perceptual areas at fault in some of these children, i.e., manifesting as a deficiency in the ability to perceive, discriminate between, and retain images of sequential body movements in space. It may be that there is a deficiency in inhibitory functions having to do with checking and suspending verbal or motor activity until the incoming sensory stimuli are compared with stored information. When the fantastic complexity of the brain is considered, with its myriad interlocking circuits and groupings of circuits, it is not surprising that in the presence of any disordering of stimuli-monitoring that each child should manifest a unique cluster of symptoms, and that he should be handicapped in learning and adaptive behavior if the environment is sufficiently trying relative to the magnitude of the defect.

This paper received some 20,000 requests for reprints, but is seldom mentioned in current texts. It is clear, as suggested above, that Clements and Peters were writing about issues that later became translated into ADD or ADHD, namely problems of attention, impulsivity, hyperactivity, and working memory (incoming stimuli compared with stored information).

A study by Peters et al. *(35)* indicated that MBD children have many "suspect" soft and hard neurological signs and that many of these tend to disappear as these children age. Peters had developed a neurological examination that he used routinely in testing all children he saw in his clinic long before the paper just cited was written. The consistency of findings of suspect signs is what led him to conclude that there must be a neurological basis for the disorder.

The MBD label excluded children with other serious psychiatric problems—autism, schizophrenia, and mental retardation. It was argued that for a child to receive the MBD label, he or she must be near average, average, or above average in intelligence. It was generally felt that the IQ cutoff should be 85 to 90.

Dykman and colleagues published a number of studies bearing on the issue of the validation of the MBD diagnosis. In one early laboratory study *(36)*, it was found that MBD children do not get as aroused to respond as easily as controls judging by their heart rate and skin

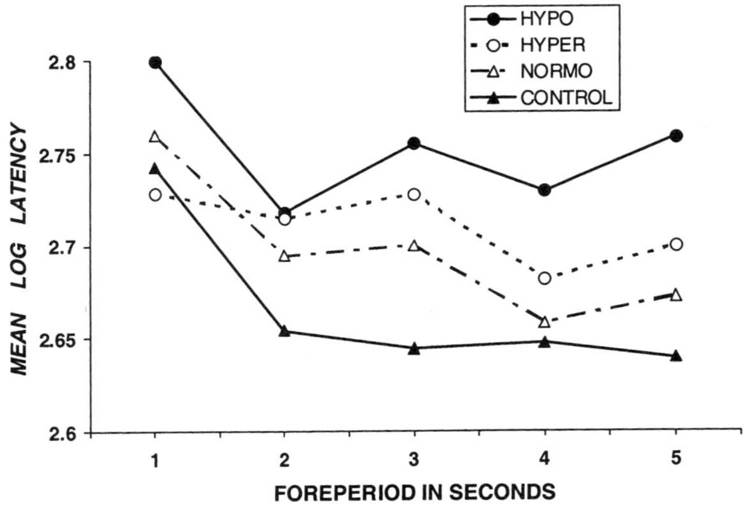

Fig. 1. Mean log latencies in relation to foreperiod: the time from onset of the get-ready stimulus (colored light) to onset of imperative stimulus (white light). *See* text for discussion.

conductance responses in a learning situation in which money was earned for correct responses and lost for incorrect responses. The MBD children (most both LD and HY) made many more mistakes than controls both in failing to respond to the appropriate cues or responding to cues inappropriately. This was the first study to show the autonomic underarousal of MBD children, and it was something not expected from what we knew about the restlessness of most of them. This was strictly tied to performance; baseline levels did not differ in controls and MBD subjects.

These studies were followed by others examining conditioning and reaction times (RTs) in a variety of go/no-go tasks *(37–39)*. In one of these go/no-go paradigms *(38)*, we used a reversal task and tested readiness to respond over a period of 5 s. After subjects had been trained to respond to a red light and not to a green light, the conditions were reversed, and they were told now to respond to the green light and not the red light. They were instructed to watch the lights and press a reaction time key as soon as a white light followed the green light in the reversal task (red light was not reinforced). The mean log latency of foreperiod RTs differed with hypoactive subjects least able to maintain a readiness to respond (*see* Fig. 1). Of course, there is no way to know whether the decrement seen in maintaining a readiness to respond is attributable to reduced inhibition, increased excitation, or both in some way. All we know from these results for sure is that in maintaining a readiness to press an RT key, groups from worst to best were; hypoactive, HY, normoactive, and control.

In thinking about hypothesized states of nervous system, we thought of reciprocal relations; i.e., if attention is directed to one place or topic then attention to other places or topics are automatically partially inhibited. This does not mean that background stimuli are ignored by the nervous system. Indeed, we know from event-related potential studies that these stimuli do register, but normally not with sufficient strength to enter our awareness or as something to which we should or must attend *(40,41)*. We know from the classic work of Darrow *(42)* and Lacey et al. *(43,44)* that when attention turns in—as when solving a problem in mental arithmetic—heart rate (HR) increases, but if attention turns to the outer environment, such as occurs when one gets ready to respond to a forthcoming event, and hence must pay close attention, HR decreases. This turning of attention in or out may occur very rapidly, and the speed of switching is important. We have speculated that this depends on some kind of switch, possibly in the diencephalon *(45)*, which is quickly and automatically activated by connections from the frontal lobes *(12)*. But the point here is that the focus of attention taking place in a few milliseconds can change the occurrence of the next beat of the heart.

It should be obvious from what was said above that the MBD term had been dropped by us by this time in favor of terms, such as LD subtyped into three categories (hyper-, hypo-, and normoactive), and, in some cases, looking at children in these same categories who were not LD. In our 1971 paper *(12)*, we suggested that MBD be replaced by what these children, whatever subtype, have in common: namely, problems of inattention. Attention was treated as a unitary trait consisting of four interrelated components: alertness, stimulus selection, focusing, and vigilance.

During this same period we became involved in medication studies, thinking that these might provide clues as to subtypes as well as improved treatments. In the first study, we contrasted a new drug (at the time), pemoline (Cylert®), with methylphenidate *(46)*. The study was double-blind ($n = 99$ MBD children ages 6–12). Dosages of pemoline and methylphenidate, assumed a priori to be equally effective, were compared over a period of 8 wk with each other and with a placebo. Ratings of symptoms (Conners scales, which can now be found in almost any book marketing psychological tests and software) were available from four sources—physician, parent, teacher, and child—and obtained at 4 and 8 wk. The percentages of cases improved on methylphenidate at wk 8 relative to placebo were 73.3 for physician ratings and 78.6% ($p < 0.05$) for teacher ratings ($p < 0.01$). The corresponding physician and teacher ratings for pemoline were 66.7 and 53.1 (not significant). However, the same ratings by psychologist favored pemoline (81.8% vs 73.7%), with both gains significant ($p < 0.01$). The average nonresponder varied with the type of rating scale and was in excess of 19% on all ratings (about one-fifth of all subjects). This suggested the existence of subtypes not identified by the MBD label, and this issue remains unresolved today for children with the newer label of ADHD as well.

We also had available continuous performance data (AX paradigm). It was found that methylphenidate speeded RT to target stimuli (child pressed a RT key whenever an *X* occurred but only if the preceding letter was an *A*). However, performance on pemoline was no better than that on placebo.

The teacher rating scale (Conners' 33-item teacher rating scale) was subdivided into five factors (aggressive–antisocial, restless–hyperactivity, emotionalism, distractibility, and immaturity). Methylphenidate significantly improved scores on all factors except immaturity. In contrast, pemoline improved scores on only three factors (restless–hyperactivity, emotionalism, and distractibility).

A second study (the company funding pemoline research lost interest in the contrast of the competing drug) looked at only pemoline vs placebo at 3, 6, and 9 wk, but it had only 18 subjects. Pemoline was found to improve scores on factors of emotionalism, aggressive-antisocial behavior, and restlessness. Pemoline is an effective treatment, and is one worth trying in cases that fail on methylphenidate *(47)*. Its side effects may be a bit more dangerous: two of our subjects showed elevated liver enzymes. However, there are many choices of drugs now that were not available at this earlier time. One of the more interesting findings never further researched was that pemoline had a staggering effect in improving scores on the nonverbal part of the Wechsler Intelligence Scale for Children (WISC).

2.1. *Our Early Neurological Speculation*

On the basis of this research cited above, we engaged in a bit of neurologizing, which in retrospect seemed reasonably decent and anticipated much of what came later. The following comes from the Dykman et al. 1971 paper *(12)*:

> Organically based deficiencies in attention explain, we believe, the poorer performance, the slower reaction times, the lower amplitude contingent negative variation wave (expectancy wave) and the decreased physiological reactivity of learning disabled in learning situations.

The following structures were identified as playing an important role in the regulation of attention:

1. The descending fibers from the cortex to the reticular formation, as well as ascending fibers from the reticular formation to the cortex (feedback loop), with the former system being most important.
2. A forebrain inhibitory system described by Clemente *(48)* capable of inhibiting both somatic and visceral responses.

Electrical stimulation of the Clemente system had been shown in animals to suppress movement, synchronize electrical cortical activity, and produce sleep. This inhibitory effect is proportional to the degree of stimulation: a weak stimulus slows but does not halt ongoing behavior. It is not difficult to imagine a child whose inhibitory system, via conditioning, is turned on to some degree every time he enters the classroom.

A third mechanism was postulated, namely one located in the diencephalon that controls the switching of attention in or out or from one stimulus to another *(45)*. We followed William James in saying that it is necessary to reciprocally inhibit one activity when focus is turned to another activity. Russian investigators have talked about this same concept in a more behavioral way under the construct of mobility of nervous processes. Most important, we postulated that HY children are weak in inhibitory control (cortex to downstream arousal centers) because they habituate slowly to novel stimuli and they manifest considerable recovery or restoration of extinguished responses. Hypoactive children were assumed to be opposite in these characteristics. We also assumed, following Luria *(7,8)*, that either deficit, too much or too little inhibition, produced failure in the classroom—one from not being able to pay attention in, for example, solving a problem in mental arithmetic, and the other from not attending sufficiently to understand the problem.

Ackerman et al. *(49)* did a follow-up study on 23 HY, LD boys, first studied in grade school and reevaluated at age 14. These boys were contrasted with two other LD groups, 25 normoactives and 14 hypoactives, including 31 controls. Controls had no problems when first seen in grade school, but the LD children had either failed a grade or were near failure despite average or better intellectual endowment and normal advantage. At follow-up, all three groups remained significantly disadvantaged in relation to controls in academic and cognitive measures and in complex RT (the conditioning task described above). Half the hyperactives had experienced major conflicts with authority, and more than one third of hypoactives exhibited psychologically disturbing behaviors (Minnesota Counseling Inventory). Not surprisingly, HY subjects were found to be most open and hypoactive subjects most closed. Mental health of normoactives appeared comparable to controls. In studying heart rate changes, it was found that the heart rates of hypoactive children did not decelerate immediately on tone onset (a get-ready-to-respond signal). This slowness differentiated hypoactive children from other groups. In any case, none of this early research had much of an impact in sustaining the life of MBD.

By 1976 we felt that the attentional approach did not provide a sufficient causal explanation *(14,15)* for MBD, and proposed an information-processing model. At this time, we became concerned with the role of intention as the mechanism controlling attention and other important mediating processes. We wrote as follows *(12)*:

> Occam's Razor says that we should move from the simple to the complex in experimentation and interpretation. We should not look for a higher level of explanation when a lower level explanation suffices. From this standpoint the most parsimonious approach is to consider arousal as the basic defect for MBD. We have been down this road before, and for various reasons, which will become clear as we go along, it has not proved satisfactory. In 1971, we turned to attention as the next elementary phenomenon. Still dissatisfied, we now move to a considerable elaboration, adding intention and other psychological processes *(50)*. There are significant differences between the concepts of attention and intention, at least as we define them. Attention relates to the adequacy of one's informational gathering ability, focusing and stimulus selection (sampling environment). Intention has more do with the utilization of information, its implications and consequences. In a broader philosophical sense, intention connotes attitudes, values, will power, or sustained attention *(51)*. The philosophical and neurophysiological question is the same: Is it that the MBD child cannot sustain his attention or will not?
>
> … Two kinds of behavioral/deficiencies produced by injuries of the frontolimbic areas and associated cortex *(52)* are very similar to those seen in MBD children—hyperactivity, impulsiveness, perseveration or inability to switch from one action to another, dissociation of action and verbalization, and disregard for rules and consequences. Clearly these behaviors tend to be associated more with intention than attention, if there is a difference. Perhaps, we are talking about two aspects of faulty attention—one a defect in the primary sensory pathways having to do with the reception and storage of information and the other with inattentiveness (intention) as a personality trait.

In commenting on the MBD concept some 30 yr later, Barkley *(53)* stated:

> The concept of MBD died a slow death as it became recognized as vague, overinclusive, with little or no prescriptive value, and without much neurological evidence *(54)*. Its value remained in its emphasis on neurological mechanisms over the often excessive, pedantic, and convoluted environmental ones proposed at that time. This was particularly true of those etiological hypotheses stemming from psychoanalytic theory, which blamed parental and family factors entirely for these problems.

It is interesting that so much of what goes around comes around again and again. Barkley now has his own neurological theory, although he might protest labeling it as such. His latest theory of response inhibition is based on much of what we have learned about the frontal lobes in the last 50 yr and to its credit it is carefully formulated in terms of testable hypotheses.

Taylor *(55)* described MBD as an unsavory neurological construct. He cites Bax and MacKeith *(56)* who say that the vagaries of MBD are not only a barrier to communication but can also do harm by making physicians think they have done something useful in applying the label MBD. Yet Taylor states that it may be useful for clinicians to use the term MBD in advising parents or teachers, when the intent is to explain that an individual child's problems might be caused by cerebral pathology. So whereas Taylor does not like the term as a diagnostic label, he is apparently not opposed to its use in communicating to parents the causes of a child's problems. Taylor is wrong, however, when he says that MBD implies a single cause for many forms of LD. As may be seen by the aforementioned quote from Clements and Peters, MBD refers to a variety of different cerebral dysfunctions, but one can only guess which ones from knowing the symptoms of a given child.

Although we played a role in the demise of the MBD concept by suggesting the substitute term attentional deficit syndrome *(12)*, we have never understood the harsh criticisms MBD received. A neurological colleague once said MBD is a term developed by persons with minimal brains. But there are many good and logical reasons to believe that LD and ADD involve deficits of the central nervous system (*see* Chapters 2,3,5,8,9 and 17). The operant zeitgeist that pervaded both psychology and psychiatry during the "MBD era" attributed too much to environment and too little to genetics, and was strongly opposed to the biological causality explicit in the term MBD.

Is the MBD concept dead? Not quite; at least for learning disabilities it is alive in some circles. The National Joint Committee on Learning Disabilities (NJCLD) *(57)* defined learning disabilities in terms of MBD. This definition has gained wide acceptance according to Bigler *(58)*; it states that learning disabilities are "intrinsic to the individual, presumed to be a result of CNS [central nervous system] dysfunction, and may occur across the life span" *(57)*. This assumes that learning disabilities have neurological causes and may be permanent.

It is perhaps important to note that a number of pediatricians still use the MBD conceptualization in describing children. One of our clinician physicians at Arkansas Children's Hospital, Dr. Mark Swanson outlined eight ways in which LD and ADHD are similar and, by inference, belong under one diagnostic label (personal communication).

1. Both have a presumed, if not precisely identified, underlying abnormal anatomic or physiologic brain process.
2. Both are disorders on a continuum, from mild to severe, leading to a certain arbitrariness about who "has" the condition.
3. Both have been functionally, or operationally, defined as a series of clinical behaviors.
4. Both are clinically diagnosed, with no unequivocal physiological tests available to the physician to aid in diagnosis.
5. Both are likely present but unexpressed at birth (i.e., often children with these conditions are not identified until school age and only retrospectively are some subtle indicators apparent in the preschool years).
6. Both have clinical manifestations that vary greatly with environmental factors, especially those at home and in school.
7. Both require input and assessment from nonmedical professionals.
8. Both have interventions that are largely derived from collective wisdom and experience, rather than from unequivocal scientific studies.

3. IMPORTANT EARLY WORK OF OTHERS

Virginia Douglas, writing in this same period, did much to change the MBD concept to ADD with her presidential address to the Canadian Psychological Association in 1972. The subsequent paper, entitled "Stop, Look, and Listen," has been cited more often than any other early paper. She presented evidence suggesting that the problems of inattention and impulsivity were more important defining characteristics than hyperactivity *(59)*. The research of Douglas and collaborators indicated that sustained attention was a major problem for HY children and that these children's problems of sustaining attention could occur in situations in which there were no significant distractions *(60–64)*. This research pointed to the following four major deficits:

1. Inability to inhibit impulsive responses.
2. Inability to modulate arousal levels.
3. An inordinate need to seek immediate reinforcement.
4. Most importantly, deficits in the regulation of attention and effort (our intention notion).

Colleagues of Douglas at McGill University have contributed much to our understanding of ADD. Particularly important has been the research of Weiss and associates, who followed the development of HY children into adolescence and adulthood *(65–68)*. Weiss et al. *(68)* note that although the excessive motor activity of these children is often diminished by adolescence, their problems with sustained attention and impulsivity persist. There are many additional studies indicating that hyperactivity may result in appreciable problems in later life *(49,53,69–71)*.

In terms of the evolution of diagnostic criteria, Keith Conners was by far the most important contributor. He developed the first rating forms useful in assessing hyperactivity, impulsivity, and inattention *(72)*. He was the first to recognize the need to quantify measures of inattention and impulsivity as the major problems of these children. Conners' impact on the field of disruptive behavior disorders continues to this day. He has done as much to stimulate the development of rating scales assessing child psychopathology than any other person, and his well-known scales have been, and are currently, among the rating scales of choice.

In 1981, Barkley and others began to question the concept of attention deficit as the defining characteristic for ADD/ADHD *(73–75)*. It was recognized that children in many psychiatric diagnostic categories were overactive and inattentive, and it was noted that the excessive activity and inattention of the children who were labeled ADD tended to be situational in nature and did not occur in all conditions *(11,76)*. This, of course, was what we were struggling with in our paper on intention.

There were other changes occurring in this period that brought about needs for a greater clarity in diagnosis and treatment. There was a tremendous outcry about the number of these children who were placed on drugs—stimulant medication in particular. It was claimed that the medications prescribed for these children would stunt their growth, and respectable investigators were accused of being paid off by the drug companies. It was so bad that the Food and Drug Administration began an investigation of some of the researchers who were involved in drug studies. It was stated that hyperactivity results from such factors as poor nutrition *(54)*, rapid cultural changes *(78)*, or food allergies *(79)*, or that hyperactivity is a "myth" created by poor teachers and parents *(80,81)*. But none of these claims were supported by any reasonable scientific evidence *(53,82,83)*.

In his generally excellent book, Barkley *(53)* states that one of the most exciting developments of the 1980s was the notion that ADD is a motivational disorder and not an attention disorder, which goes back to the inclusion of intention in the MBD era. In discussing this "newer" movement, Barkley writes:

> As more rigorous and technical studies of attention in ADHD children appeared in the 1980s, an increasing number failed to find evidence of problems with sustained attention under some experimental conditions while observing them under others *(62,74,75,84–87)*. These findings, coupled with the realization that both instructional and motivational factors played a strong role in determining the presence of ADHD symptoms, led some investigators to hypothesize that motivation may be a better model for explaining the deficits seen in ADHD children *(88,89)*. Following this line of reasoning, others pursued a functional analysis of these symptoms; they hypothesized deficits in the stimulus control over behavior, particularly by rules and instructions *(73,90)*.

Barkley later added to a rule-based deficit the notion that responses to behavioral consequence might also be impaired *(53,74)*. This same idea or notion was advocated by other writers *(75,91–93)*. The basic notion is that ADHD arises out of insensitivity to consequences—i.e., reinforcement or punishment. This same idea had been put forth earlier by Wender *(26)* in his classic book on MBD and in our papers on intention. Lou et al. *(94,95)* suggest that ADHD children exhibit deficits in brain-reward centers and their cortical regulating limbic circuits. In several papers, we described these same circuits as accounting for the difficulty of MBD children *(12,14,38)*.

Studies using both school-based and clinic-referred samples have consistently shown HY/ADD children to be rated more adversely on impulsivity and aggressive/defiant symptomatology than nonhyperactive ADD children, whereas nonhyperactive ADD children are rated more adversely on internalizing symptomatology, such as anxiety and withdrawal or shyness *(53,96–100)*.

Both types of ADD children exhibit more difficulties in academic areas than controls, but neither group has been consistently found to have greater problems than the other *(101,102)*. Studies contrasting HY and nonhyperactive ADD children on cognitive neuropsychological measures have provided mixed results. Of those reviewed by Lahey and Carlson *(102)*, half found few or no differences. Sergeant and Scholten *(103,104)* studied two small ($n = 8$) groups of ADD children with hyperactivity and ADD children without hyperactivity in a visual search task where speed and accuracy were compared. Compared with controls, both groups were significantly slower but only the ADHD children were less accurate. Sergeant and Scholten *(104)* also concluded that hyperactive children with attention problems show deficits in resource allocation, as they are less able than the solely inattentive type to meet task demands. The HY group's latencies were inconsistently related to accuracy, whereas the other groups exhibited the oft-reported speed–accuracy trade-off. Frank and Ben-Nun *(105)* found HY-inattentive children ($n = 21$) to show significantly greater abnormalities than non-HY inattentive ADD children ($n = 11$) in visual perception, visual sequential memory, and writing performance. The HY group also showed significantly greater abnormality on "soft" neurological signs.

Larger samples of HY ($n = 42$) and non-HY ($n = 48$) ADD children were contrasted by Barkley et al. *(53)*. In addition to comprehensive ratings obtained from parents and teachers, the investigators analyzed performance on the WISC-R and Wide Range Achievement Test-R (WRAT-R) and on several laboratory tasks. They also made behavioral observations as the children performed on selected tasks. The HY/ADD but not the non-HY ADD group had significantly poorer scores than controls on the arithmetic subtest of the WISC-R. The nonhyperactive group was significantly poorer on the coding subtest than both the HY group and controls. These two ADD groups did not differ, however, on any of the WRAT-R subtests or in the percentage identified as having specific learning disabilities. On a continuous performance task (CPT), the HY/ADD group made more errors of omission than the control group but the two ADD subgroups did not differ. Neither did they differ in errors of commission even though the mean of the HY/ADD group was double that of the nonhyperactive ADD group (scores were highly variable, however).

Jensen et al. *(106)* related the severity of ADHD to the presence of co-occurring disorders. It is suggested that a child with ADHD plus an anxiety disorder might do equally well with medication, behavioral therapy, or both. On the other hand, he states that a child with only ADHD or ADHD plus ODD and/or CD is likely to do best with medication. The combination of both behavioral therapy and medication is likely to be best if anxiety is added to the mixture of ADHD and other disruptive behavior symptoms. Unlike the majority of ADHD children, there are many who do not respond to medication. Also, ADHD children who fail to respond to one medication often respond well to another *(107)*. This suggests additional subtypes based on neuropharmacological differences. We really need more treatment studies that will provide clues as to the causes of these differences in subtypes. In a preliminary pilot study *(108)*, we found that a nutritional supplement containing certain saccharides known to be important in cell communication were about as good as methylphenidate in improving behavior at home. ADHD children are known to be fussy eaters, and there have been no rigorous studies of the influences of different nutrients in these children.

A number of authors have questioned the notion that the central problem of HY children is a defect in sustained attention *(87,109–111)*. Douglas *(84)* used a large battery of tests designed to measure attention, and concluded that the basic information processing capabilities of ADHD children are intact. She attributed their defects to faulty self-regulation. Sergeant *(75)* concluded that ADHD children do not have problems of either selective or sustained attention. His basic conclusion was much the same as that of Douglas, namely that the problems of ADHD children are more in the area of modulating attention or in the allocation of resources. Swanson et al. *(112)* reported that there is, in fact, a subgroup of ADD/ADHD children who do have attentional problems. This subgroup satisfied rigorous diagnostic criteria, which excludes many children currently labeled as ADD/ADHD in research studies. It may be circular to say that self-regulation explains the attentional defects seen in ADHD children, inasmuch as inattention to environmental cues could explain deficiencies in self-regulation.

Van der Meere et al. *(113)* used a self-paced paper-and-pencil cancellation test to study sustained attention in HY children. This was a follow-up on the earlier work of Sykes et al. *(111)* showing that the sustained attention deficit of HY children occurs in experimenter-paced but not in self-paced tasks. Van der Meere et al. argued that if a self-paced task were divided into blocks, attention would have to wane as a function of the number of blocks. It was argued that the slope for HY children over time would have to exhibit a significantly steeper descent than that of controls to prove that HY children have a sustained attention deficit. They found that although HY subjects perform more poorly than controls over all time periods, the slopes for the two groups were equal, leading to a conclusion that the deficit was not in sustained attention.

4. ADDITIONAL STUDIES FROM OUR LABORATORY

4.1. Pribram Task

We proposed, on the basis of our earlier work and that of others *(72,114,115)*, that attention deficits characterize LD, as well as HY, children. Like Douglas in her classic 1972 *(50)* paper "Stop, Look and Listen," we argued that attentional deficits rather than motoric restlessness should be of central research interest. Even though the majority of LD children exhibit ADD symptoms, ADD cannot be said to be the sole or major cause of a learning disability, because many ADD children, even HY ones, learn to read and spell at an age-appropriate rate. This observation led us to believe that the major problem for LD children might be in the area of selective attention and for HY children in the area of sustained attention. Moreover, we theorized, as stated above, that the failure of HY children to sustain attention was the result of a lack of will to do so *(15)*. Here we moved toward what William James *(51)* termed intention. We further speculated that intention reflects frontal lobe action whereas selective attention, especially as used in reading, reflects temporal lobe involvement.

To test this theory, we modified a paradigm that Karl Pribram *(116)* had used to assess frontal and temporal lobe functioning in monkeys *(117,118)*. The child was asked to scan a visual field, discover the target symbol, learn to stay with the target for five trials, search for a new target, and so on. He began with a visual field size of only two symbols, but the field size was increased by steps up to 12 symbols. Symbol presentation was under computer control, and any given symbol could occur in any one of 12 windows on a given trial. There were two kinds of trials: search trials, which involved finding the to-be-rewarded stimulus, and after-search reward trials, which involved staying with the correct object until it was no longer rewarded (five trials). The child received one penny for each correct response. Total earnings were continually updated by a computer and displayed on a screen. Failures to choose the target consistently after discovery were not rewarded and were considered after-search lapses. In Pribram's monkeys, after-search lapses were increased by frontal lobe damage and search trials by temporal lobe damage.

Subjects consisted of 20 HY boys, each with scores of 15 or higher on the 10 items of the Conners, hyperkinesis index, and scores above 90 on both the WRAT-R and the Gray Oral Test; 20 LD boys with average reading scores on both reading tests below 90, and the hyperkinesis index under 15; and 20 adequate students with reading scores above 90 on both reading tests, and hyperkinesis scores below 15.

Unfortunately for the specifics of the theory, the reading-disabled (RD) group did not differ from HY children in the number of search trials, after-search lapses, or RT. Both clinical groups were, however, inferior to controls. When we later studied mixed HY–RD subjects, they, too, were inferior to controls but not distinguishable from the "pure" clinical groups on Pribram performance measures. This research suggests that both HY and RD children have deficiencies in behaviors mediated by the frontal and temporal lobes.

Half the HY children told us they had become tired and wanted to quit the Pribram task. The RD children, though tired, did not want to quit, yet they became inattentive as the difficulty of the task increased. The HY boys were more attracted to novelty than were the RD children. In the early trials of one procedural condition where the new symbol added to the visual field was always the one to be chosen for reward, HY children tended to choose the novel stimulus immediately, whereas RD children did not *(117)*. This attractiveness to novelty points to deficiencies in behavioral inhibition that are insufficient to counteract the excitatory tendencies to respond. It may not be just too little inhibition or too much excitation, but the absence of a balance between the reciprocal neural connections between these two processes.

In another sample of ADD (inattentive type), HY, and RD boys, the majority, when unmedicated, exhibited lapses of attention and extraneous responding (key play) in the intertrial intervals of the Pribram task *(118)*. As with the first sample, the HY boys were far more deviant in extraneous responding than were the RD subjects. Methylphenidate dramatically decreased extraneous responding, particularly in HY subjects, and also improved about equally the accuracy of all clinical groups *(118)*. Interestingly, the drug had a greater effect in decreasing after-search errors than in decreasing search trials; i.e., it improved sustained, more than selective, attention (or memory).

Electrocortical data, obtained from 1 s before and 1 s after each display of stimuli at electrode sites C3, C4, P3, and P4 (areas we thought were most important at that time) were Fourier-transformed and subjected to a principal components analysis. Four components were extracted, accounting for 87% of the variance. The first component had strong loadings between 16 and 20 Hz and weaker loadings between 8 and 10 Hz. The RD children had significantly lower scores on this component than the controls, with the HY boys intermediate; however, the mixed HY–RD group, which was expected to be the most impaired, was, in fact, the least impaired of the clinical groups by this measure. We have no good explanation of this finding. It may be that the combination HY–RD is compensating in some degree as regards arousal, e.g., RD children try harder whereas HY children are more easily aroused than pure RD children. These electrocortical results show that controls exhibited superior task specific arousal (i.e., more β and α activity) to the clinical groups.

In sum, the RD children did not differ from HY children as predicted on the Pribram task, but the study did yield evidence to suggest their deficits in certain regions of the frontal, central, and parietal lobes contribute to difficulties in learning and behavioral control: the assertiveness of HY and the passivity of RD children, the excessive key play of the HY boys and their attraction to novelty; and the inferior search-and-hold performance of all clinical groups. However, the fact that there were no differences in search and perseverance errors and reaction times suggests that the major problems of these clinical groups are in the domain of attention and in the regulation of motor responses.

4.2. Nervous System Sensitivity

A new variable related to attention was added to our studies, which we termed sensitivity of the CNS. Russian investigators place this presumably innate response bent along a weak-strong continuum, and Western biologically oriented psychologists such as Buchsbaum *(119–121)*, Eysenck *(122)*, Fowles *(123)*, Gray *(124,125)*, and Zuckerman et al. *(126,127)* believe this response propensity to be an important dimension of personality or cognitive style. As RD and HY children differ along a dimension of passivity and assertiveness, it was hypothesized that these traits might have an underlying physiological basis in CNS sensitivity. According to the Russian literature *(128,129)*, a person with a strong nervous system responds to increases in stimulus intensity with an orderly increase in physiological activity and an orderly decrease in reaction times (RTs). In contrast, the sensitive type shows an orderly increase up to a point and then responds less vigorously (i.e., exhibits protective inhibition). Buchsbaum *(119)* used the terms "augmentation" and "reduction" to describe such gradients obtained from electrocortical evoked potentials. He reasoned, vis-à-vis the Russian experiments, that strong types augment and weak types reduce.

Four subtypes of children were studied: HY, LD, HY + LD, and inattentive but not HY. Vasilev *(129)* had subtyped subjects on the basis of differences in press-and-release RTs with tones ranging in intensity from soft to very loud. With some subjects both RTs were linear, with the difference between press and release more or less constant across intensities, and with others the lines crossed at the higher levels of intensity. Vasilev described the type with parallel slopes as strong (insensitive) and those with nonparallel slopes as weak (sensitive), and following Buchsbaum, strong was equated with augmenting and weak with reducing. Each child heard a tone at four intensities (55, 70, 85, and 100 dB), and was told after a warning light to press a reaction-time key when a 250-ms tone occurred (4 s interval from warning lights to tones), and release the key as quickly as possible when the tone ended. A strength of nervous system ratio was computed for each child by first determining the line of best fit across the four tones *(130–132)*. The fitted press latency to the 100-dB tone was divided by the fitted release latency to that tone (release times were faster than press times).

There were three conditions: baseline in which subjects received no reward; high-gain–low-frustration, in which subjects received four pennies for each correct response and lost two pennies for a slow response with a payoff ratio of 4:1; and a low-gain–high-frustration condition with a payoff ratio of 1:2. In the latter subjects lost as much as they gained. The presentation of stimuli was controlled by computer; with thresholds for payoff continuously upgraded every 12 trials, keeping the payoff ratios close to the values just described. The strong types maintained a more or less parallel separation of the two reaction times at all conditions whereas the weak types showed a convergence of the two latencies at the higher intensity levels in all conditions. The high-gain–low-frustration condition yielded the fastest RTs.

Contrary to expectation, girls did not have weaker or more sensitive nervous systems than boys, although girls rated themselves as less tolerant of intense stimuli. The boys (because there were more of them) were enrolled in a blinded crossover study contrasting methylphenidate and placebo. The prescribing physician, who was not informed of the subtype of the child, adjusted dosage levels. It was found out when the code was broken that children typed as weak (predominantly HY) received higher doses of methylphenidate than those typed strong. Gray's *(133)* theory suggests an explanation of this paradox; namely, a weak nervous system requires more intense stimuli than a strong to reach the threshold of concentration (or focused attention). Also, following Gray, one could reason that children with attention disorders who have strong nervous systems would be able to concentrate attention and effort better with low to moderate doses of stimulant medications. These predictions fit the facts, as we know them today, reasonably well.

Using the Buchsbaum measure (N1–P2 wave of the event-related potential [ERP]), Dykman et al. *(134)* found, as Buchsbaum did, that children diagnosed as HY had more augmenting ERP slopes to tones ranging from soft to loud than did non-HY ADD or RD children *(134)* but there was considerable overlap. More HY subjects than those in other groups were classified as weak or sensitive on the RT measure *(135,136)*. Non-HY ADD children typed strongest on the RT measure. There was little relation, however, between the ERP measure of augmentation and the RT measure of CNS strength. On theoretical grounds, the ERP measure should be a better measure of strength than RT, because it represents CNS activity in the first 200 to 300 ms of information processing.

HR generally decelerates as a person prepares to respond and then accelerates with the response (*see* Fig. 2). As may be seen, whereas ADD and RD groups exhibited less marked anticipatory response than controls, no systematic differences were found among the clinical groups *(137)*. But with clinical diagnosis ignored, HR levels were consistently higher in ERP reducers than augmenters, and reducers switched more quickly from HR deceleration to acceleration.

Dykman et al. *(134)* suggested that the higher tonic levels of the HY boys could reflect their irritation with this rather boring task, whereas their less marked phasic reactivity to the warning and imperative stimuli could mirror inattentiveness and/or lack of involvement. This interpretation is compatible with the findings of Zahn et al. *(138)*, who reported higher HR levels in externalizing boys (HY, aggressive, or both) than controls as the subjects

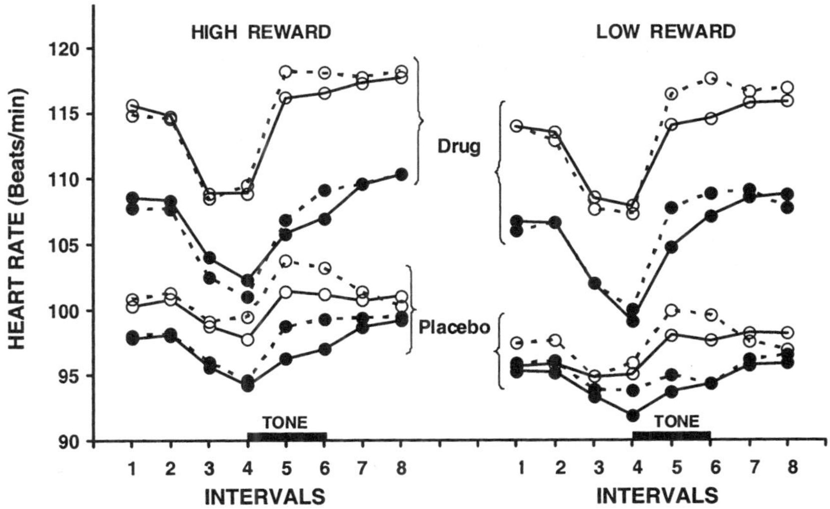

Fig. 2. Mean heart rate (HR) levels for 8 contiguous 1-s intervals from warning light to tone (imperative stimulus). *See* text for discussion.

participated in orienting and reaction time RT tasks. However, the Dykman et al. experiment featured reward and the Zahn et al. study did not. These results can also be interpreted as supporting the Gray–Fowles–Quay model of activation, which predicts greater HR increases to reward in antisocial than in prosocial persons. This research also showed a strong relationship between augmentation–reduction and drug–dose and drug–response *(132)*. Relative to reducers, augmenters received smaller doses and had a superior drug response as judged by teacher ratings ($p < 0.02$).

Figure 3 shows the major relations between experimental variables in the pretreatment session of the sensitivity study and the subsequent clinically titrated methylphenidate doses. Our intent was to determine whether we could predict these carefully titrated dose levels from the pretreatment data. This analysis showed that many of the predictor variables were related at a low level, and that their conjoint effect was highly significant (multiple $R = 0.892$, $p < 0.001$). In this figure, type refers to the RT measure of weak-strong and slope to the ERP measure of augmentation–reduction. In general, we found a highly significant relation between augmentation–reduction and drug–dose and drug–response *(132)*. Relative to reducers, augmenters received smaller doses and had a superior drug response as judged by teacher ratings ($p < 0.01$).

In sum, the most significant findings were the relation of drug titration and response to sensitivity variables as assessed from RT and ERP slopes to tones ranging from soft to very loud. Augmenters were blindly clinically titrated at significantly lower doses of methylphenidate than reducers and they had a much better medication response than reducers. This could mean that ADD reducers (more HY children in this category) need medication other than methylphenidate, need no medication at all, or that increasing doses of drug are really not beneficial. Nearly all children, regardless of diagnostic label, improved in their classroom ratings with the clinically titrated drug dose, and all became more rapid in RT. Most important, the CNS dimension of sensitivity was a better predictor of drug efficacy than the diagnostic label given a child: HY, LD, etc.

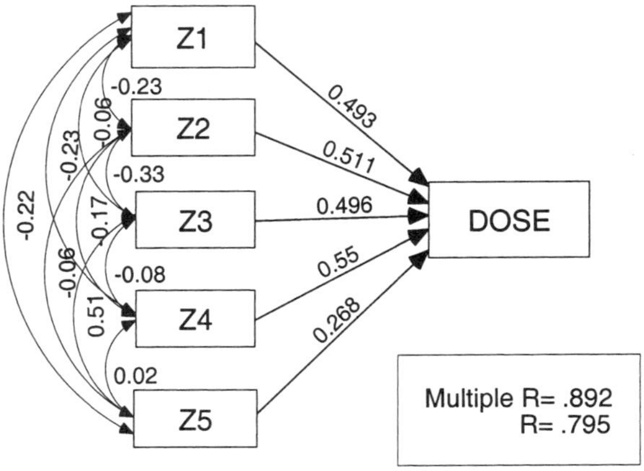

Fig. 3. Multiple regression analysis predicting methylphenidate dosage levels from five sets of variables. Z1 = age + weight, Z2 = ERP type-reaction time (RT) slope, Z3 = press RT low reward-press RT no reward, Z4 = 3 × heart rate (HR) high reward + HR low reward-2 × HR no reward, Z5 = skin conductance counts low reward-2 × SC counts high reward. *See* text for discussion.

4.3. *Sternberg Task*

In this experiment, subjects were shown a set of one to three letters on a screen for a brief time followed by the removal of the letters (blank screen). A probe (letter in or not in the set) was given and subjects indicated whether the probe was or was not in the set by pressing either a "yes" RT key or a "no" RT key. In different experiments the size of the memory set is varied, generally from one to five stimuli. Sternberg *(139)* had found that the searching task was serial; i.e., searching continued one stimulus at a time until the whole set was searched even though the matching object had already been found. Obviously, this rarely happens in real-life situations. Most importantly, Sternberg adduced evidence showing that the zero intercept estimated by the slope of RT on the *Y*-axis plotted against the memory set size on the *X*-axis represented the accumulated time for encoding (storing in memory), decision to respond, and response execution time. The slope of the function was assumed to assess the scanning operation (retrieval time and comparison process).

Sergeant *(140)* used two versions of this task, hoping to show that attention deficits in HY children show up in the scanning operation (the slope of the memory set function). Although HY subjects had slower RTs, the difference in RTs did not interact with set size (zero intercept difference in controls and clinical subjects). This indicated that the differences were in the earlier stages of processing (encoding and response organization). In a second experiment, Sergeant *(103,104,140)* found that the severity of hyperactivity was not indexed by any of the Sternberg variables.

Holcomb et al. *(141)* studied reading-disabled subjects and controls (24 in each group). The subjects had no co-occurring diagnoses except for inattention without hyperactivity. In this experiment, set sizes of 1, 3, and 5 consonants in the English language were varied from trial to trial. This was an ERP study focusing on the relation of RT to P3 amplitude and latency (time for P3 to attain peak maximum). P3 amplitudes had been shown to be inversely related to the amount of information to be processed, and P3 latency to the timing of processes related to stimulus evaluation or decision time *(142)*. It was also known at this time that P3 latency decreases as children age *(143,144)*. Certain age differences arose in the analyses of the data, so subjects were divided into two age groups (8–9 vs 10–11 yr of age).

The RT slopes (RT on set size) was quadratic with a bigger timing loss from set size 1 to set size 3 than from set size 3 to set size 5. This indicated that serial search was not used by many subjects. P3 latencies showed no significant age effect; but the age separation was not as great as in the studies reported by Courchesne *(143)*, who had shown that P3 latency decreases from childhood to adolescence. Unlike RT, P3 latencies (at Cz and Oz) significantly separated the two groups, but only in the interaction with response type (yes or no). P3 latencies increased significantly with increases in set size for both "no" and "yes" responses. However, for "no" responses the P3 latency of RDs decreased from set size 3 to set size 5, suggesting a breakdown in the timing of decisional processes with increasing cognitive load.

There was a huge gap between the peak P3 response and RT: P3 was 672 ms earlier than RT at set size 1, 1918 ms at set size 2, and 1039 ms at set size 5. The reported findings for adult studies are about half of these values *(145)*. McCarthy and Donchin *(146)* theorized that the response/selection processes are manifest in RT but not in P3 latency. If the present data have any validity, it is very unlikely that response variables could account for as much of the time as all the preceding stages together. Holcomb et al. *(141)* suggested that P3 latency might index an early decisional process on which subjects are unwilling to base a response.

The task proved too difficult for the younger RD subjects, and an analysis of errors suggested a good deal of impulsive responding in this group, which was most evident at set size 5. The two groups did not differ in scanning rate, possibly because of the large number errors made in deciding whether the probe was in or not in the set. The Sternberg task is thought not to be reliable when error rates exceed 10%, and in this study the error rate for younger subjects was 16.6%. Controls had significantly earlier P3 peaks than the RD subjects; this suggests differences in encoding, although the possibility of differences in mechanisms controlling response cannot be ruled out since they also influence the zero intercept. P3 amplitudes at the larger memory loads required by the larger sets was more of a problem for RDs than for controls. RD subjects made more errors at all set sizes than did controls, and the percentage of correct responses was greater in controls than in RDs for both "no" and "yes" responses.

4.4. Dykman et al. Three-Subtype Theory

This research *(147–150)* was based on the work of Loney and Milich *(151)*, and was published three years before the Diagnostic and Statistical Manual of Mental Disorders, 4th edition (DSM-IV) was published. For a relatively large ADD sample (159 boys meeting DSM-III criteria for ADD with and without hyperactivity disorder), we performed a K-means cluster analysis of the scores from the two Iowa factors and from our own ADD index (composed of 10 attention items from DSM-III). We closely adhered to the recommendations of Skinner *(152)*, who said that (1) cluster analysis should be based on a theory of the nature of the disorder, which implied that the theory specify the number of groups to be derived in advance, and (2) the clusters should be subjected to close scrutiny for internal consistency and validity and external validity. External validity has to do with whether the groups differ significantly on outcome measures not used in the original cluster analysis. Internal validity refers to the internal consistency of the clusters and to whether the clusters can also be derived by different cluster methods. We derived three subtypes: pure ADD, not hyperactive (n = 49), ADDH (n = 63 boys, ADD and hyperactive), and ADDHA (n = 47 boys, ADDH and aggressive). About half of the subjects in each subtype were LD. This cluster analysis was based entirely on white males; there were insufficient subjects to look at sex and race differences. We further divided the subjects into those who did and did not satisfy criteria for LD and found that the percentage of LD children in each of the three groups was similar (about half in each group by our criteria). It is important for the reader to bear in mind that our study was based on children referred to our clinics for evaluation and treatment; it was not an epidemiological sample where the overlap with LD and other psychiatric disorders is less than in referred groups.

We had a variety of measures supporting the external validity of the three groups. The three groups were significantly separated by teacher ratings other than those used to perform the cluster analysis. The ADDHA group differed from the ADD only (without hyperactivity and aggression) in socialization skills, impulsivity, and the impatient/aggressive traits associated with the type A personality *(153)*. Parents rated the ADDHA group higher on the externalizing scale of the Child Behavior Checklist *(154)*, but the groups did not differ on the internalizing scale. Nor did the groups differ on self-ratings on the Junior Personality Inventory *(155)*. However, physiological data supports the existence of the three subtypes (*see* Section 6).

There are studies other than those of Loney and associates that suggest the validity of an aggressive subtype of ADHD *(156–160)*. Pelham and Bender *(161)* noted that more than half of ADHD children have significant problems in relating to peers, which may be owing, in part, to aggressiveness. Also, aggression is more often a characteristic of male than female hyperactive subjects, and ADHD symptoms are relatively common in mentally retarded children *(161,162)*.

4.5. Categorical vs Dimensional Classification

Dykman and Ackerman *(149)* attempted to tackle the problem of dimensional vs categorical analysis in the diagnosis of ADHD. We adhered to a schema that Fletcher and colleagues *(163–166)* had used in some of their studies of LD *(167)*. These authors closely followed the recommendations of Skinner *(153,168)* described in the report above.

The analyses in our paper were based on 182 children evaluated in our clinic for school-related problems. All children were administered the Diagnostic Interview for Children and Adolescents (DICA), developed by Herjanic and Reich *(169)*. Those admitted to the study met the criteria for ADD based on the DICA attention items endorsed by the child's caretaker. As the child rated himself or herself, parents were asked to agree of disagree with each answer. All subjects were between 7 and 11 years old with a full-scale IQ greater than 85, were of good health, and had a normal educational experience. Controls were 33 males and 19 females, all Caucasian except for one African American male. In addition to the WISC-R, children were administered the WRAT-R and several rating scales. Teachers were paid $10 to fill out three forms: our expanded Conners questionnaire (which includes 10 items assessing the ADD symptoms listed in DSM-III); the Mathews Youth Test for Health (MYTH) *(153)*, which assesses two components of type A behavior (competitiveness and aggressiveness-irritability); and the Yale Psychoeducational Questionnaire *(170)*, which was factor-analyzed for research purposes. This analysis yielded five factors: sustained attention (SATT); academic aptitude (ACAP); hyperactivity (HYP); impulsivity (IMP); and socialization (SOC). Caregivers filled out the Achenbach and Edelbrock *(154)* Child Behavior Checklist (CBCL), an instrument often used to assess childhood psychopathology.

On the day of the laboratory visit the child was administered two self-rating scales, the Junior Personality Inventory *(155)* and the Arkansas Thrill Seeking Scale, modified after the Sensation Seeking Scale developed by Zuckerman *(171,172)* to make the items easier for children to understand. Subjects were also given Gordon's *(173)* test of Differential Reinforcement of Low Response Rates (DRL), a task that purports to measure IMP (inability to inhibit responses); the Trail Making Test (parts A and B), presumably sensitive to brain dysfunction *(174)*; a 10-min coding task; an expanded symbol inverted version of the WISC-R subtest, believed by us to be a very good measure of sustained attention; and a timed arithmetic task (20 simple addition and subtraction problems).

The project psychiatrist decided whether a given diagnosis was possible on the basis of scores for each diagnostic category on the DICA. Following Skinner *(152)*, three major subtypes of ADHD were hypothesized: ADD only (inattentive), ADDH (inattentive and HY), and ADDHA (inattentive, HY, and aggressive). The DICA simply classifies children as ADHD and groups together symptoms of HYP, inattention, and impulsiveness.

To test the theory, a K-means cluster analysis was computed using three teacher-rated behavior scales: the Loney and Milich *(151)* Iowa hyperactivity (IHY), the Iowa aggression (IAGG) factors (derived from the Conners rating scale), and the Arkansas ADD index, which incorporated the DSM-III ADD items. The three-factor cluster solution supported our *a priori* hypothesis by correctly assigning the majority of subjects to one of three groups, but many subjects were placed in two classes. The Iowa scale was used to establish cut points, and the scores replicated with few exceptions the results of the cluster analysis. Subjects were classified as ADD if IHY scores of 8 or less and IAGG scores of 6 or less, as ADDH if IHY scores greater than 8 and IAGG scores of 6 or less, and ADDHA if IHY scores greater than 8 and IAGG scores greater than 6.

LD—in this case reading disability—was determined by the method of discrepancy scores, i.e., standardized achievement scores in reading and spelling at least 10 points lower than the WISC-R full-scale IQ. Eighty-two (74 boys and 8 girls) met criteria for dyslexia; no subgroup of ADHD had a significantly higher number of RD subjects than any other. The ADD-not-RD group did not differ from controls in IQ or achievement measures, with the exception of lower spelling scores, as expected. Both the control and the ADD-not-RD group scored higher on cognitive measures than did the RD groups.

As for other DICA diagnoses, the ADDHA group had the highest rate of diagnoses per child (0.94), with ADD next (0.90) and ADDH last (0.75). There was significant tendency for more ADDHA boys to have a diagnosis of CD, but no other differences in rates of disorder were found. It was found that the solely RD children had a significantly higher rate of separation anxiety than other groups.

The paper presents external validation data supporting the three basic ADHD subtypes for teacher data, parent data, child self-report data, and performance data (all tests and rating scales listed above that were not used in assigning subjects to groups). By univariate analysis, the following variables were significant in discriminating the three groups: MYTH aggression (MYA), Yale sustained attention, and Yale SOC. A discriminant analysis yielded three Yale factors in the following order of importance: Yale HYP, Yale SOC, and Yale IMP. MYA dropped out because it correlated substantially with all three Yale factors.

Like others, we found that behavior ratings from different sources do not always agree *(151)*. Different groups make different interpretations of the same items, which is a bit surprising when the items are so simply stated. In a univariate test, two scales of the parent ratings were significant in discriminating groups: parent HYP ratings and externalizing score on the CBCL. A stepwise discriminant analysis of all parent ratings (Conners HYP and attention

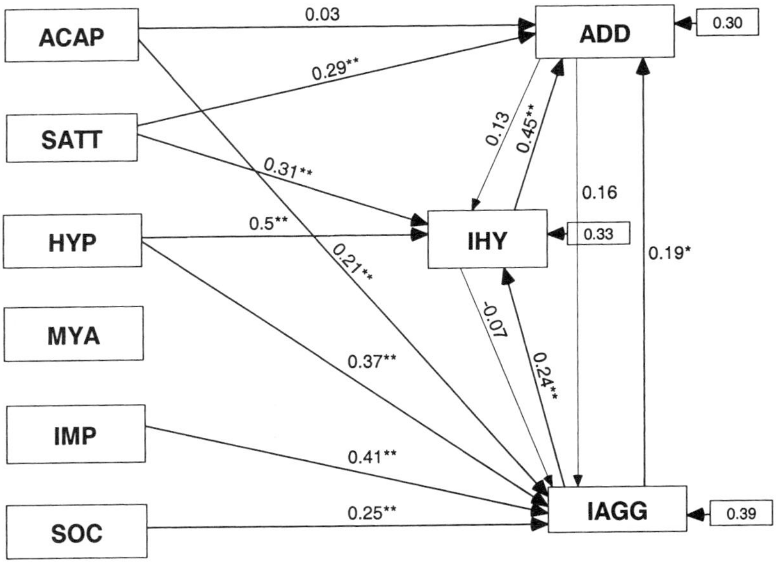

Fig. 4. This standardized path diagram shows teacher ratings with Yale factors on the left prediction Iowa tests on the right. *See* text for explanation. $*p < 0.05$ $**p < 0.01$.

scores, internalizing and externalizing scores from the CBCL) used only the Conners measures of inattention and hyperactivity. Parent ratings were not as good as the teacher ratings in demarcating groups.

The second part of this paper, the dimensional part, performed analyses in two different ways, first by canonical correlations and then by path analysis (the LISREL program). These analyses used teacher ratings first and parent ratings second as the basic data. The LISREL SIMPLIS results *(175)* and the canonical analyses were concordant overall, and the path analysis of the teacher ratings are shown in Fig. 4. These are ratings by teachers, and Yale factors on the left are used to predict the Iowa factors on the right. The exogenous variables on the right are academic achievement (ACAP), Yale SATT scores, Yale HYP scores, MYA scores, Yale IMP scores, and Yale SOC scores. The significant paths are darker lines ($p < 0.05$); lighter lines are not significant. The proportion of variance explained by all the variables, which include minimal contributions from paths not shown, was 0.64 (64%). The corresponding percentages for IHY and IAGG were 67% and 60%, respectively. It will be noted that IHY is related to only two variables: SATT and HYP on the Yale. ADD is also related to only two variables, but IAGG is related to four variables.

This model shows that the ADD factor (inattentiveness) increases with increases of HYP as assessed by the Iowa rating scale, i.e., HYP is more likely to elevate inattention symptoms than the reverse (the path with the darker line is significant at $p < 0.01$). An increase in IAGG elevates IHY ($p < 0.01$ for the path with the darker line) but the reverse path; HYP to aggression is not significant. The two paths leading from ADD to other variables are not significant. It can also be seen that IHYP is related to only two Yale variables, HYP and SATT; ADD is also related to only two Yale variables, academic achievement and SATT; but aggression is related to four variables, Yale hyperkinesis, IMP, and SOC, and MYA.

Figure 5 shows the LISREL model relating parent data to teacher data. Parent HY and ADD ratings come from the Conners scales, and externalizing and internalizing from the

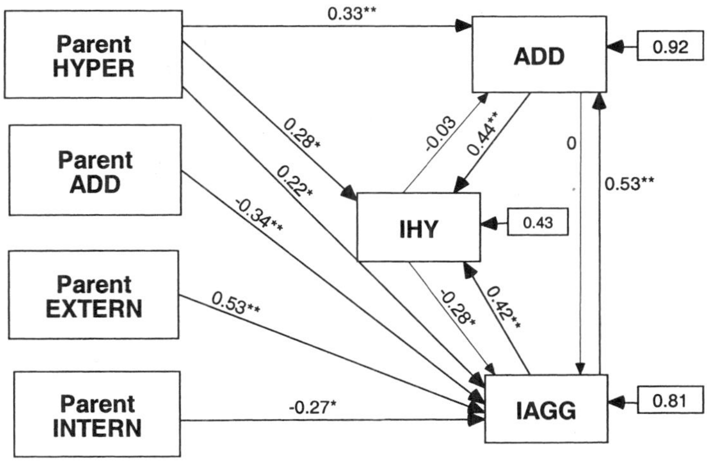

Fig. 5. Path diagram standardized for the prediction of teacher ratings from parent ratings. *See* text for explanation. * *p*, 0.05, ** *p*, 0.01.

CBCL *(154)*. The scores on the right are the ratings from the three Iowa scales (ADD, HY, and Aggression). The dominant pathways from IAGG to HY (0.42) and from ADD to IHY are logical. Note that ADD has little effect on IAGG but that IAGG has a sizable effect on ADD, again a logical connection. We conclude from the path coefficients that parents do not discriminate the behavioral groups as well as teachers do.

These models are entirely different types than those obtained by categorical analyses. There are no discrete subtypes, just the interplay of continuous variables, and no rules for assigning ADHD children to subtypes, but they could be derived. It was clear that the clusters derived from even our best rating scales, i.e., teacher ratings, were not homogenous. Any one of the three groups had individuals located in the space of the other groups. The dimensional analysis is superior to the categorical results in showing the structural relations of variables.

5. ASCENDING DSMS AND RELATED RESEARCH ON DIAGNOSIS

ADD in various versions of the American Psychiatric Association diagnostic manuals *(16,17,25,176)* has gradually changed. In DSM-II, the "hyperkinetic" definition was restricted to youths with maladaptive levels of inattention, impulsiveness (IMP), and motor restlessness. DSM-III took a categorical approach with diagnosis based on the number of items entered on three separate lists of items, measuring inattention, IMP, and motoric activity. DSM-III was much more specific than DSM-II in definitions of ADD, and placed a greater emphasis on inattention and IMP than on HYP. It also described a subtype referred to as ADD/WO (inattention without hyperactivity). DSM-III-R took a dimensional approach in which 8 of 14 symptoms had to be present (some of the items were composites of inattention and hyperactivity). DSM-III-R did not include items enabling one to make a reliable diagnosis of the inattentive, non-HY child, and this manual substituted ADHD for the ADD of earlier versions.

Although the dimensional approach of DSM-III-R resulted in considerable criticism, it stimulated a large amount of research, which for the most part favored categorical classification *(102,177)*. The most significant advances in diagnosis have been attributed by many to Lahey and associates. Lahey and Carlson (as cited in ref. *170*) write as follows in describing subtypes:

> To date, the experimental literature on ADD/WO [what is now called the inattention type of ADHD, author's insert] strongly suggests three conclusions. First, factor analytic studies consistently indicate that covariation among the symptoms of ADD [another term used frequently then and to some extent even now for ADHD and/or just the inattentive type, author's insert] reflect two largely independent dimensions. One dimension consists of symptoms descriptive of motor hyperactivity and impulsive behavior, whereas the second dimension consists of symptoms describing inattention, disorganization, and difficulty in completing tasks. Second, it no longer seems doubtful that ADD/WO exists as a clinical entity. As in the case of ADD/H [the HY-impulsive subtype, author's insert] approximately half of the clinic referred children with ADD/WO also qualify for other DSM-III diagnoses. Third, the description of children with ADD/WO yielded by these studies differs from ADD/H in important ways—ADD/WO are characterized by fewer serious conduct problems, less impulsivity, greater sluggishness, greater anxiety, and greater depressed mood. Children with ADD/WO tend to be unpopular with their peers, are often perceived as socially withdrawn, but are less likely to be actively rejected than children with ADD/H.

The definition of ADHD in DSM-IV was formulated through extensive field trials *(178,179)*. The field trials were based on 380 children identified by parents and teachers as HY and/or inattentive. It was somewhat disturbing that a study of this magnitude could not have obtained teacher ratings on more subjects because they seem to a better indicator of problems than parent ratings. The Diagnostic Interview Schedules for children *(180–183)*, parents, and teachers were used, but as indicated the three ratings were not available for all youths. The net effect of all this elaborate research was to come up with three subtypes of ADHD: an inattentive type not HY, a HY–impulsive type, and a combined type possessing symptoms of both types.

Subsequently, Barkley *(184)*, although admitting improvement in the diagnosis of ADHD in the new manual, came down almost as hard on the revised criteria as he had done earlier in discussing the death of MBD. He states that the empirically based ADHD diagnosis in DSM-IV is the most advanced of all the DSMs. He gives Lahey credit for his role as head of the field trial data analyses. But this is the end of the praise. First, he recognizes, as have others, the problems with the inattentive type of ADHD, suggesting that it may not be a subtype of ADHD. These children differ from the HY–impulsive type being less attentive and having more school problems. Second, he is also concerned that the combined type may not be different form the HY–impulsive type, just a later stage of development of the same condition. He says if the HY–impulsive type eventually moves into the combined type there is no need for a separate category for the latter. Judging by the literature, the combined type would in fact appear to capture the greatest number of children. Third, he notes that the field trial was based on children aged 4–16, and that the diagnostic items may be inappropriate for children out of this age range. It is suggested that this might result in the over inclusion of children below the age of 4 and the under inclusion of late adolescents and adults. Fourth, he mentions possible gender bias, i.e., whether the symptom lists are equally appropriate for boys and girls and whether the cut scores for diagnosis should be the same in the two groups. Fifth, he thinks the pervasive criteria create a problem (must be observable at home and school and for adults at home and at work). He cites research showing low levels of agreement between ratings of teachers and parents. The insistence on the double criteria reduces the number of youth who will receive a diagnosis of ADHD, and he argues that the disorder may be more evident in one situation than another. He says that parents are more likely to see their children as ODD rather than ADHD, whereas teachers are likely to see them as ADHD rather than ODD. It would seem obvious, as is stated in the article, that the combined type may have a more severe form of ADHD than the other types. These seem to be the main points, but he is also concerned with other problems, such as the criteria for onset and persistence, (7 yr of age and 6 mo persistence) in DSM-IV. It is clear that these are issues that will have to be revisited in any revision of DSM-IV.

6. RESEARCH DIAGNOSTIC CRITERIA

One of the most important relatively recent innovations is the development of strict research diagnostic criteria (RDC). These were proposed by Bloomingdale and Sergeant *(185)*, because DSM-III-R definitions resulted in an inordinately high prevalence rate. The RDC criteria included suggestions made by Taylor and colleagues *(55,186,187)* and are in line with the criteria of the International Classification of Diseases (ICD), Version 9 *(188,189)* or Version 10 *(190)*. The specific recommendations follow:

1) A stringent severity criterion is recommended. The cutoff value (expressed in terms of symptoms required) is higher than the cutoff value specified in DSM-III or DSM-III-R; the percentage required for a RDC diagnosis is 75% (6 out of 8), compared to 50% for DSM-III (8 out of 16) and 57% for DSM-III-R (8 out of 14).

2) Concurrent validation by standardized parent and teacher rating scales is required. The requirement of a "statistically abnormal" score on a standardized rating scale should exclude all but a specified small percentage (e.g., 3% to 5%) of the children in the population defined by age and sex norms.

3) The temporal course of symptoms is specified. Early onset (before age 7 years) and duration (at least 2 years) are required to ensure that fluctuations in attention due to stress would not lead to a diagnosis.

4) The presence of symptoms in at least two of three settings (home, school, and clinic) are required. Due to the low correlation between sources, this should reduce the prevalence of the disorder for any given level of severity.

Swanson et al. *(112)* add further restrictions to the definition, increasing the homogeneity of children satisfying the aforementioned restrictive criteria. It is important to remember that this is for the stated purpose of obtaining a homogenous group of ADD/ADHD subjects. These are as follows:

1) If the ADD/ADHD symptoms have an early onset and are expressed (perhaps in different but age expected forms) across developmental periods before another disorder is manifested, we recommend that the ADHD symptoms be considered primary.

2) If the symptoms of the other disorder appear first, or if the presence of ADD/ADHD symptoms varies with the waxing and waning of the other disorder or specified environmental conditions, we recommend that the ADD/ADHD symptoms be considered secondary.

3) We propose that a diagnosis of ADD/ADHD be made only on the basis of primary symptoms.

Swanson et al. were concerned, as we have been, with the overlap of ADHD and LD. The California studies *(191)* indicate very little overlap when a 1.5-standard-deviation discrepancy score between performance on standardized achievement and intelligence tests is used to define LD. Surprising, not a single one of their ADD/ADHD children qualified for LD when this discrepancy score was used. About 10% qualify for LD when a 1-standard-deviation discrepancy score is used, and this agrees with results reported in the Connecticut longitudinal study *(192)* and the findings of a study in the Netherlands *(86)*. Swanson et al.

believe that the overlap with other disorders, including LD, is minimal when the criteria outlined above are imposed. However, they recognize that these children may have various degrees of activity including passivity and aggressiveness. Using their more restricted definition, Swanson et al. were able to say that the term "attention deficit" is warranted. A possible limitation of the Swanson data is that they may not be representative of sex, age, race, and social class, factors that would markedly affect the LD and ADD/ADHD overlap. It would appear that the children Swanson recruits were mainly from mid- to upper social stratification levels.

7. EPIDEMIOLOGY

In the introduction to their book, Shaywitz and Shaywitz *(193)* say that ADD is now recognized as the most common neurobehavioral disorder of children. It affects children from earliest infancy through school and into adult life. According to this article, estimates for ADD with or without HYP range from 10 to 20% *(194)*. DSM-IV estimates the prevalence of ADHD to be much lower (3–5% in school-age children). Shekim et al. *(195)* report that symptoms of ADD/ADHD persist into adulthood in one-third to one half of subjects who receive this diagnosis in childhood, and that the overwhelming majority of adult subjects have other co-occurring diagnoses.

A problem that Barkley *(184)* pointed out in discussing the limitations of DSM-IV was that of diagnosing ADD/ADHD reliably in the preschool years. However, Palfrey et al. *(196)* had earlier evaluated children at eight checkpoints between birth and age four, and the writers report that 13% of the children met criteria for possible ADD/ADHD at one or more checkpoints. However, only 5% of the group evidenced definite symptoms that persisted into kindergarten. The peak age for the identification of symptoms was 3.5 yr. It is obviously dangerous to make a diagnosis of ADD/ADHD in the preschool years, because many young children demonstrate behaviors associated with this condition, which is in fact normal for their age. We simply do not have reliable information on the prevalence of ADD/ADHD in preschool children.

It is clear that prevalence can be made very low by imposing restrictive criteria, but if this were done it might exclude many children who need help. There is an inverse relation between prevalence and the severity of restrictive diagnostic criteria. Moreover, the identification of ADHD or LD in families living in poverty or near poverty is problematic. Symptoms of restlessness and inattentiveness could occur in children who are not adequately prepared for school, particularly if they have been reared in an environment in which the importance of learning has not been emphasized.

8. ETIOLOGY: POSSIBLE CAUSES AND MODIFIERS

Some of the presumed causes of ADHD are no longer discussed, and the remaining chapters of the book will bring the readers up to date on important new developments. Conclusions from myriad studies suggest the following:

1. Lead and related issues are rarely a cause *(197)*.
2. Food additives (salicylates, food dyes, and preservatives), have a trivial effect at best *(82,198,199)*.
3. Sugars desserts, and candy bars appear to have little or no effect in exaggerating ADHD symptoms *(177,200,201)*.
4. Alcohol can be a cause but certainly but explains only a minority of cases *(202,203)*.

5. Parental conflict, common in families with ADHD children does not cause ADHD but can certainly exaggerate the severity of symptoms *(204–213)*.
6. Genetic factors appear to be more important than all others as a cause of both ADHD and LD.

8.1. Genetic Research

Of the many studies in this area, among the best are those by John DeFries, Bruce Pennington, and colleagues at the University of Colorado and those of Jim Stevenson and associates in England. Gillis et al. *(214)* used a sophisticated regression model developed by DeFries and Fulker *(215,216)* to estimate the heritability of ADHD. Subjects were 37 pairs of monozygotic (MZ) and 37 pairs of dizygotic (DZ) twins. At least one member of each pair of twins had a reading disability and at least one member of each pair, not necessarily the one with a reading disability, satisfied criteria for ADD as diagnosed by the parent form of the DICA-P developed by Herjanic and Reich *(169)*. Proband-wise concordance rates for ADHD were 79% for MZ and 32% for DZ twins. Age was not a significant predictor of DICA-P scores; i.e., the heritability (h^2) of ADD as diagnosed by the DICA did not vary with age. The h^2 coefficient was very high (0.98); i.e., nearly all the variance in DICA-P scores was attributed to heredity (coefficient varies from 0 to 1). It was concluded that HYP symptoms as expressed by the DICA are highly heritable.

Stevenson et al. *(217)* reported results from two twin samples, one from London (n = 190 pairs) and one from Colorado (n = 260 pairs). The proportion of ADHD probands that also had a spelling disability was 24% and the proportion of spelling probands that were ADHD was 30%. It was estimated that about 75% of the co-occurrence of these two conditions was a result of shared genetic influences. The differences between these two estimates were not statistically significant, which lends credence to the supposition of a subgroup of children in which both spelling and ADHD are influenced by a common gene or genes. The almost equal two-way percentages in this study are contradictory to the general impression that while ADHD can "cause" LD, the reverse is less likely *(218)*.

There are a number of other studies pointing to the importance of heredity. Familial risk for ADD/ADHD and antisocial behaviors is higher among the relatives of children who have a conjoint diagnosis of both ADD/ADHD and CD than among the relatives of children who are only ADD/ADHD *(219–225)*. Faraone et al. *(222)* found that the family members of probands with ADHD and ODD had a higher risk for ADHD and CD than the family members of probands with ADHD alone. However, the risk was lower for "familial spread" than in a group who were comorbid for both ADD/ADHD and CD. Biederman et al. *(226)* report significant prevalence of mood, anxiety, and antisocial disorders in the first-degree relatives of ADHD children. Elsewhere, Biederman et al. *(227)* report an association between anxiety disorders and ADD/ADHD, with the risk of anxiety disorders among the relatives of ADD/ADHD children higher than that for the relatives of normal children *(220,227)*.

9. BIOLOGICAL STUDIES AND THEORIES OF ADD/ADHD

9.1. Quay and Gray

Quay *(92)* speculates that ADHD, CD, and anxiety/withdrawal (AW) disorder can be differentiated in terms of Gray's *(124)* theory of two important control systems: a behavioral inhibition system (BIS) and a behavioral reward system (REW). In Gray's theory, increases in responding brought about by positive reinforcement ("hope") and by both active avoidance and escape paradigms (reward is escape from punishment, or "relief") are under the control of REW. Reductions in responding that occur in extinction procedures and passive avoidance are under the control of BIS. Anxiety is activity in the BIS that is cued by conditioned stimuli that signal fear or frustration. Predatory aggression, on the other hand, is under the control of REW. Gray has postulated anatomic loci for these two systems: the reward system corresponds to the catecholaminergic structures mediating the rewarding effects of self-stimulation of the brain *(228)*. The BIS, a supposed noradrenergic system, is localized in the lateral and medial septal areas and in the connections of these to the hippocampus.

Stimulant drugs enhance the activity of both REW and BIS. Quay speculates that there is a relatively greater enhancement of BIS than of REW in ADHD children given stimulant medication, thus bringing the two systems into balance. He concludes that ADHD children have a deficiency in the BIS system, noting that antianxiety medications tend to affect them adversely. Again and again, deficiencies in inhibition are emphasized, beginning with the early papers of Luria *(7)*. Because amphetamine improves passive avoidance but does not improve CD, and because catecholamine antagonists (haloperidol and propranolol) appear to decrease CD, Quay suggests that CD seems most related to oversensitivity to reward. He attributes anxiety/withdrawal disorders to an overactive BIS. Gray's two systems are supported by a considerable amount of experimental evidence and the extrapolations of Quay appear to be very reasonable. In particular, autonomic studies of heart rate and skin conductance reactivity suggest that HY children are more difficult to arouse than normal children, which supports Quay's notion of an underactive BIS.

9.2. Barkley's Theory of Response Inhibition

Judging by recent reports on ADHD children it appears that Barkley's theory is slowly but surely becoming the preferred theory for most writers. He is concerned only with the HY–impulsive type and mainly with the explanation of IMP. Barkley *(22)* defines response or behavioral inhibition as consisting of three interrelated components:

1. Inhibiting the initial prepotent response to an event.
2. Stopping an ongoing response or response pattern, thereby permitting a delay in the decision to respond or continue responding.
3. Protecting this period of delay and the self-directed responses that occur within in it from disruption by competing responses (interference control).

Barkley ties self-regulation to response inhibition and interference control, saying that "there can be no actions taken toward the self aimed at modifying a future consequence related to an event if the individual has already responded to that event." This appears to mean that any opportunities to modify an outcome must occur in the period of inhibition (delay) of the prepotent response, including the timing of when it is to be executed. Inhibition protects the self-directed and often covert actions to the self that occur in the delay period, protects the prepotent responses that are about to be executed, and protects against extraneous sources on interference.

According to Barkley, executive function (EF) and self-regulation depend on response inhibition, and the problems of ADHD children, particularly their impulsiveness, result in deficiencies in EF and the psychosocial processes they control, e.g., time estimation and inner speech. In an article in which Barkley *(229)* responds to criticism of his theory, he says, "Nevertheless, unlike other views of EF and ADHD, the model I have set forth though certainly imperfect, is far more specific about the origins and nature of EF and more closely aligned with an evolutionary perspective than any view yet proposed of either of these domains." He claims that the deficits in EF are devastating and that they are far more important in understanding the problems of ADHD children than their trivial impairment in capacity to pay attention. I would not disagree with the impairment in EF as being important, but would only add that perhaps the most important EF is the capacity to focus attention and ignore distracting thoughts and stimuli. It is also obvious that there are many different EFs and control mechanisms involving relations of frontal lobes with other structures in the brain, and even variations in control of different types of attention (sustained, selective). So it is somewhat of a misnomer to speak as though there is only one EF. Barkley, however, is apparently talking about only those EF functions that are affected by or related to ADHD, but it is difficult to know where these leave off and others begin.

9.3. *Pavlov's Ignored Contributions*

Many of these concepts discussed above have a counterpart in the writings of Pavlov *(18,19)* in providing insights into the nature of inhibition that are not generally known. A prepotent response for Barkley is a conditional response (CR) for Pavlov, and it can be negative (inhibitory) or positive (excitatory). This definition could be expanded a bit to include any kind of instrumental learning, including operant responses. Most psychologists have finally discovered that you cannot teach a rabbit to swim like a duck *(230)*. So all learning depends on some inherent biological structure, whether a fear of snakes or the learning of a language. In simple differential conditioning there are two stimuli, one that is reinforced (more accurately paired in the case of Pavlovian conditioning) and one that is not reinforced *(231)*. The negative conditional stimulus (CS) never reinforced produces responses of some kind (no zero level attained) in the conditioning of heart rate, blood pressure, or urinary retention. However, more precise and less generalized systems, such as salivation in anticipation of food and motor actions to avoid noxious stimuli, do attain a no-appearance (zero) level with repeated nonreinforcements. However, in neither case does the level of response measure the depth of inhibition. Pavlov showed in a variety of experiments that the inhibitory state deepens with additional pairings and this does not show up in the negative CR being partial or completely absent. The number of trials it takes to convert a negative CS to a positive CS increases as a function of the number of presentations of the negative CS.

Pavlov also showed that the elaboration of a trace CR (CS terminates before unconditioned stimulus [US] onset) or delayed CR (US overlaps the CS but there is a delay of 5–60 s or more between the onset of CS and US) is associated with a period of inhibition known as the "inhibition of delay". The period of inhibition, which can be interrupted by distracting stimuli (disinhibition) but less so the better established the response (the greater the number of reinforcements). This would seem to be akin to the protective delay of Barkley. Pavlov was insistent that inhibition of the type described here was mediated by the cortex; he referred to it as internal inhibition, in contrast to the type of direct inhibition seen in antagonistic muscular responses or reflexes. I would argue that dogs must also be capable of self-regulation to some extent if they can refrain from making premature responses and resist the onslaughts of distracting stimuli. However, Pavlov recognized an excitable type of dog, not unlike ADHD children in temperament, that had great difficulty in developing delayed or trace CRs. In one series of very interesting experiments, Pavlov's group found that if a delay interval—say, of 15–20 s—is firmly established, it is very difficult and some instances impossible to change to a shorter interval. Even if the CS–US interval is shortened, the CR may continue to occur at the previously established delay interval.

These early findings seem to us to support many of the conjectures of Barkley, including those mentioned by the prominent writers he references *(232–234)*. Pavlov and his associates studied individual animals intensively over long periods of time. His null or no hypothesis was not a statistic but an experimental manipulation to prove a point. It is a shame that the books that do mention his work do so in such a cavalier and superficial manner.

10. CONCLUSION

The reader can judge for himself or herself whether the label ADHD is better than MBD in terms of the accuracy of diagnosis in terms of characterizing the problems of these children. The former is descriptive, whereas the latter implies a neurological etiology. The symptoms now used to identify ADHD children are the same as in the days of MBD, with changes in wording and in the groupings of symptoms. The gain, not to be overlooked, is that the definition of ADHD is less inclusive than the definition of MBD. To make a statement that will appear even more ludicrous to those working on classification, I believe that one might do almost as well in categorizing ADHD by using only one or two items in each category of DSM-IV (inattention, HYP, and IMP). Each item selected would be rated for severity on some 4–5-point Likert scale, e.g., "often fails to give close attention to details" or "makes careless mistakes in schoolwork or other activities," is often "on the go" or "often acts as if driven by a motor, often has difficulty awaiting turn." The first mentioned item may not be a pure item in that it appears to also involve impulsive behavior. Nonetheless, a limited set of items might do the job about as well as all items now used, as none of these requires a severity rating.

Whether the basic deficits in ADHD children are in the areas of attention, self-regulation, EF, or some other process continue to be hotly debated issues. The boundaries among inattention/ attention, working memory, arousal, EF, and effort are more than just somewhat obscure. One could, for example, substitute terms like the following for ADHD: intention disorder *(14,15)*, inhibition disorder *(12,22,50,234)*, motivation disorder *(53,62,75,88,235)*, short-term memory disorder *(140,141)*, rule-based disorder *(74,84,93)*, or even MBD if we remove LD from the definition. Almost any label would be acceptable, if truly descriptive or better explanatory of the symptoms of these children.

The problem with MBD is that it is an onerous term that is less attractive to parents and teachers than ADHD. In any case, the label ADHD should be replaced if a better descriptor can be found. ADHD children differ from normal controls in having deficits in functioning or structure of many parts of the brain and not just the frontal lobes (*see* ref. *236* for latest ERP studies; *237* for neural substrates involved; *238* and *239* for gene research; *240* for corpus callosum; *241* for temporal and parietal lobes; and *242* for caudate nucleus; *See also* Chapter 6). In addition to involvement of cortical areas, there is also evidence for differences in ADHD children and controls at the level of the control centers regulating spinal reflexes *(243–246)*.

Is inattention a trivial problem, as Barkley *(229)* suggests? I think not. It is one of the most important executive functions. Research on this measure should go beyond the usual topics of sustained and selected attention. Most important is the quick shifting of attention between within and without. This occurs within a few milliseconds and has an immediate effect on directional changes in heart rate *(43,44,247)*. The approach by Posner et al. *(248,249)* is basic to this issue, although I found in unpublished work that Posner's paradigms are often too difficult for children.

We now know with reasonable certainty that the most important factor predisposing to ADHD is inheritance from a long line of ancestors (*see* Subheading 8.1, genetic causes and later chapters in this book). The environmental influences most important in accounting for some ADHD cases, probably not the common variety seen every day in clinics, would include such factors as inadequate nutrition, intrauterine growth problems, developmental deficits leading to brain injury, accidents injuring the brain, lead poisoning, and fetal alcohol syndrome (*see* Section 8.). Also, it is clear from our work and others *(15,22,93)* that rewards, as well as stimulant medication, have the effect of normalizing the performance of ADHD or MBD children in situations demanding close attention and effort.

Another issue of importance is that of categorical vs dimensional analysis. Research is scant in this area and more is needed. Our research reported above *(149)* favors dimensional analysis. New research should utilize ratings that are comprehensive enough to cover the major dimensions of ADHD including aggression, modeled after the research that has been done on the mmpi to identify important combinations of disorders. Some combination of the Achenbach CBCL, the long-form Conners Rating Scales, and other relevant items from structured interviews should be used. Separate scales should be constructed for parents and teachers. Teacher ratings are better than parent ratings for purposes of identifying children deviant from their normal age-matched controls. Teacher and parent ratings are poorly correlated even when the same items are being rated, and factor analyses of ratings that include both teachers and parents segregate more by who does the rating than by the nature of the item *(149)*.

Turning to the merits of categorical analysis, DSM-IV provides the possibility of classifying subjects in any one category into a large number of other co-occurring categories. The problem is that most research, which targets any one diagnostic category, tends to ignore the co-occurring disorders, and in ADHD the most frequent ones are learning disabilities and ODDs. The latter identifies the type of HY child that Dykman et al. *(147)* referred to as the ADDHA. Of course, it would not be necessary in future modifications of DSM-IV to include LD or aggression as a part of the definition of ADHD, if investigators were more rigorous in defining co-occurring disorders and not treating LD or ADHD as pure categories unless children with only one disorder were recruited. Pure types, however, are difficult to find.

Finally, would it be possible, with some combination of tests or rating forms now on the market plus laboratory tests, to develop a classification system that is realistic both in subtyping and in identifying the underlying problems of ADHD and LD children? For LD, phonetic abilities should be assessed because this is the problem for many of them *(250)*. This assessment should include standardized tests of reading, spelling, and arithmetic, including verbal and performance IQ. Laboratory tests that would seem to be of value in pinpointing the underlying defects are the go/no-go tests, readiness to respond tests with different delays, the continuous performance task, and the distraction tasks used in our early MBD studies (*see* Section 2.), the stop task *(234)*, and conditioning tests involving frustrative reward and relatively long delay intervals before reinforcement. The behavioral part of the test battery should assess HYP, impulsiveness, inattention, learning problems, and aggression (e.g., frustrative nonreward). Paradigms should be designed to allow for autonomic and brain function measures to be taken in the laboratory while subjects are performing the behavioral tests. Once worked out, software could be developed and marketed for use by clinicians with perhaps just behavioral measures and reaction times. This suggested approach calls for some consideration of reversing the usual course of external validation, going from tests to diagnosis rather than from diagnosis to tests, and a greater inclusion of what we have learned about the relationships between behavior and brain function in the diagnosis and treatment of the disorder.

ACKNOWLEDGMENTS

The preparation of this chapter was supported in part by funds from USDA CRIS 6251-51000-002-03S. The writer wishes to express his appreciation for the editorial help of RT (Terry) Pivik, a research collaborator and a good friend, and to Lisa Witcher, research technologist, who made sure that the reference list was complete and helped in the final preparation of the chapter.

REFERENCES

1. Conners CK, Wells KC. Hyperkinetic children: A neuropsychosocial approach. In: Kazdin AE, ed. Developmental clinical psychology and psychiatry, vol. 7. Beverly Hills, CA: SAGE Publications, 1986:1–160.
2. Still GF. The Coulstonian Lectures on some abnormal psychical conditions in children. Lancet 1902;1:1008, 1077, 1163–1012, 1082, 1168.
3. Kahn E, Cohen LH. Organic driveness: A brain stem syndrome and one experience. N Eng J Med 1934;210:748–756.
4. Bradley C, Bowen M. School performance of children receiving amphetamine (Benzedrine) sulfate. Am J Psychiatry 1941;97:91–103.
5. Strauss AA, Kephart NC, Lethihen LE, Foldenherg S. Psychopathology and education of the brain injured child, vol. 2. Progress in theory and clinic. New York: Grune & Stratton, 1947.
6. Laufer MW, Denhoff E, Solomons G. Hyperkinetic impulse disorder in children's behavior problems. Psychosom Med 1957;19:38.
7. Luria AR. The role of speech in the regulation of normal and abnormal behavior. New York: Liveright, 1961.
8. Luria AR. Frontal lobe syndrome. In: Vinken PJ, Brown GW, ed. Handbook of clinical neurology. Amsterdam; North-Holland, 1969;725–757.
9. Clements SD, Peters JE. Minimal brain dysfunction in the school-age child. Arch Gen Psychiatry 1962;6(185):197.
10. Werry JS. Studies of the peractive child IV: An empirical analysis of the minimal brain syndrome. Arch Gen Psychiatry 1968;19:9–16.
11. Rutter M, Graham P, Yule W. A neuropsychiatric study in childhood. Clinics in developmental medicine. London: S.I.M.P. with Heihemann, 1970;35–36.
12. Dykman RA, Ackerman PT, Clemente C, Peters JE. Specific learning disabilities: an attentional deficit syndrome. In: Mykelbust H, ed. Progress in learning disabilities. New York: Grune & Stratton, 1971.
13. Cantwell DP. Genetics of hyperactivity. Journal of Child Psychology in Psychiatry 1975;16:261–264.
14. Dykman RA, Ackerman PT. An information processing model of minimal brain dysfunction. In: Sankarn DV, ed. Mental health in children. Westbury, NY: PJD Publications, 1976:375–409.
15. Dykman RA, Ackerman PT. The MBD problem: Attention, intention and information processing. In: Anderson RP, Holcomb CG, eds. Learning disability/minimal brain dysfunction. Springfield, IL: Charles C. Thomas, 1976.
16. American Psychiatric Association. Diagnostic and statistical manual of mental disorders. 3rd ed. Washington, DC: APA, 1980.
17. American Psychiatric Association. Diagnostic and statistical manual of mental disorders. 3rd ed. rev. Washington, DC: APA, 1987.
18. Pavlov IP. Conditioned reflexes. (Anrep GV, trans.). London: Oxford University Press, 1927.
19. Pavlov IP. Lectures on conditioned reflexes. New York: International Publishers, 1928.
20. Sherrington CS. Integrative action of the nervous system. New Haven, CT; Yale University Press, 1906.
21. Sherrington CS. Man on his nature. New York: Doubleday, 1953.

22. Barkley RA. Response inhibition in attention-deficit hyperactivity disorder. Ment Retard Dev Dis Res Rev 1999;5:177–184.
23. Ross DM, Ross SA. Hyperactivity: research, theory and action. New York: Wiley, 1976.
24. Tredgold AF. Mental deficiency (amentia). New York: W. Wood, 1908.
25. American Psychiatric Association. Diagnostic and statistical manual of mental disorders. 4th ed. Washington, DC: APA, 1994.
26. Wender PH. Minimal brain dysfunction in children. New York: Wiley, 1971.
27. Strauss AA, Lehtinen LE. Psychopathology and education of the brain-injured child. New York: Grune & Stratton, 1947.
28. Bradley C. The behavior of children receiving Benzedrine. Am J Psychiatry 1937;94:577.
29. Bender MB. Disorders in perception. Springfield, IL: Charles C. Thomas, 1952.
30. Burks HF. The hyperkinetic child. Exceptional Child 1960;27:18–26.
31. Eisenberg L. Psychiatric implications of brain damage in children. Psychiatr Q 1957;31:72.
32. Gerstmann J. Syndrome of finger agnosia, disorientation for right and left, agraphia, and acalculia: Local diagnostic value. Arch Neurol Psychiatry 1940;44:398.
33. Hallgren B. Specific dyslexia: A clinical and genetic study. Acta Psychiatrica Scandinavia 1950;Suppl. 65.
34. Lawrence MM. Minimal brain injury in child psychiatry. Compr Psychiatry 1960;1:360.
35. Peters JE, Dykman RA, Ackerman PT, Romine JS. The special neurological examination of children with learning disabilities. (minimal brain dysfunction). Dev Med Child Neurol 1975;17:63–78.
36. Boydstun JA, Ackerman PT, Stevens DA, Clements SD, Peters JE, Dykman RA. Physiologic and motor conditioning and generalization in children with minimal brain dysfunction. Conditioned Reflex 1968;3(2):81–104.
37. Ackerman PT, Peters JE, Dykman RA. Children with learning disabilities: WISC profiles. J Learning Disabilities 1971;4:150–166.
38. Dykman RA, Walls RC, Suzuki T, Ackerman PT, Peters JE. Children with learning disabilities: V. conditioning, differentiation and the effect of distraction. Am J Orthopsychiatry 1970;40(766):782.
39. Stevens DA, Boydstun JA, Dykman RA, Peters JA, Sinton DW. Presumed minimal brain dysfunction in children. Relationship to performance on selected behavioral tests. Arch Gen Psychiatry 1967;16(3):281–285.
40. Giard MH, Lavikainen J, Reinikainen R, Perrin F, Bertrand O, Pernier J, et al. Separate representations of stimulus frequency, intensity, and duration in auditory sensory memory: An event-related potential and dipole-model analysis. J Cogn Neurosci 1995;13–135.
41. Naatanen R. Processing negativity: An evoked potential reflection of selective attention. Psychol Bull 1992;92:605–640.
42. Darrow CW. Differences in physiological reactions to sensory and ideightonal stimuli. Psychol Bull 1929;26:185–201.
43. Lacey JI. Psychophysiological approaches to the evaluation of psychotherapeutic process and outcome. Research in psychotherapy. Washington, DC: American Psychological Association, 1959;160–208.
44. Lacey JI, Lacey B. Some autonomic central nervous system interrelationships. In: Black P, ed. Physiological correlates of emotion. New York: Academic Press, 1970:205–227.
45. Penfield W. Consciousness, memory and man's conditional reflexes. In: Kagen J, Pribram K, eds. On the biology of learning. New York: Harcourt, Brace & World, 1969:127–168.
46. Dykman RA, McGrew J, Harris TS, Peters JE, Ackerman PT. Two blinded studies of the effects of stimulant drugs on children: Pemoline, methylphenidate, and placebo. In: Anderson RP, Halcomb CG, eds. Learning Disability/Minimal Brain Dysfunction Syndrome. Springfield, IL: Charles C. Thomas, 1976:217–235.
47. Page JG, Bernstein JE, Janicki RS, Michelli FA. A multi-clinic trial of pemoline in childhood hyperkinesis. In: Conners CK, ed. Clinical use of stimulant drugs in children. Amsterdam: Excerpta Medica, 1974:98–124.

48. Clemente C. Forebrain mechanisms related to internal inhibition and sleep. Conditional Reflex 1968;3:145–174.
49 Ackerman PT, Dykman RA, Peters JE. Teenage status of hyperactive and non-hyperactive learning disabled boys. Am J Orthopsychiatry 1977;45:577–596.
50. Douglas VI. The problem of sustained attention and impulse control in hyperactive and normal children. Can J Behav Sci 1972;4:259–282.
51. James W. The principles of psychology. London: Dover, 1890.
52. Milner B. Effects of different brain lesions on card sorting. Arch Neurol 1963;9:90–100.
53. Barkley RA. Attention-deficit hyperactivity disorder: A handbook for diagnosis and treatment. New York, Guilford Press, 1990.
54. Kirk SA Behavioral diagnoses and remediation of learning disabilities. In: Proceedings of the annual meeting: Conference on exploration into the problems of the perceptually handicapped child, vol. 1. Evanston, IL, 1963:1–7.
55. Taylor EA. The overactive child. Spastics international medical publications. Oxford: Blackwell Scientific Publications, 1986.
56. Bax M, MacKeith R. Minimal cerebral dysfunction. Little club clinics in developmental medicine. London: Spastics Society with Heinemann, 1963.
57. National Joint Committee on Learning Disabilities. Letter from the NJCLD to member organizations, 1989.
58. Bigler ED. The neurobiology and neuropsychology of adult learning disorders. J Learning Disabilities 1992;25(8):488–506.
59. Campbell SB, Douglas VI, Morganstern G. Cognitive styles in hyperactive children and the effect of methylphenidate. J Child Psychol Psychiatry, 1971;12:55–67.
60. Douglas VI. Higher mental processes in hyperactive children: implications for training. In: Knights R, Bakker D, eds. Treatment of hyperactive and learning disordered children. Baltimore, MD: University Park Press, 1980: 65–92.
61. Douglas VI. Treatment and training approaches to hyperactivity: Establishing internal or external control. In: Whalen C, Henker B, eds. Hyperactive children: the social ecology of identification and treatment. New York: Academic Press, 1980:283–318.
62. Douglas VI. Attentional and cognitive problems. In: Rutter M, ed. Developmental neuropsychiatry. New York: Guilford Press, 1983.
63. Freibergs V, Douglas VI. Concept learning in hyperactive and normal children. J Abnorm Psychol 1969;74:388–395.
64. Parry, P. The effect of reward on the performance of hyperactive children. Unpublished, 1973.
65. Hechtman L, Weiss G. Controlled prospective fifteen year follow-up of hyperactives as adults: Non-medical drug and alcohol use and ant-social behaviour. Can J Psychiatry 1986;31(6):557–567.
66. Hechtman L, Weiss G, Perlman T. Hyperactives as young adults: past and current substance abuse and antisocial behavior. Am J Orthopsychiatry 1984;54(3):415–425.
67. Hechtman L, Weiss G, Perlman T. Young adult outcome of hyperactive children who received long term stimulant treatment. J Am Acad Child Adolesc Psychiatry 1984;27:261–269.
68. Weiss G, Hechtman L. Hyperactive children grown up. New York: Guilford Press, 1986.
69. Gittleman R, Mannuzza S, Shenker R, Bonagura N. Hyperactive boys almost grown up: I. Psychiatric status. Arch Gen Psychiatry 1985;42(10):937–947.
70. Mendelson W, Hohnston N, Stewart MA. Hyperactive children as teenagers: A follow-up study. J Nerv Mental Dis 1971;153:273–279.
71. Satterfield JH, Satterfield B, Schell AM, Hoppe CM. Psychosocial effects on delinquency rates in ADD youths and control subjects: an eight-year prospective study. In: Bloomingdale LM, ed. Attention deficit disorder, vol. 3: new research in attention, treatment, and psychopharmacology. Oxford, England: Pergamon Press, 1988:1–19.
72. Conners CK. A teacher rating scale for use in drug studies with children. Am J Psychiatry 1969;126:884–888.

73. Barkley RA. Hyperactive children: A handbook for diagnosis and treatment. New York: Guilford Press, 1981.
74. Barkley RA. Do as we say not as we do: The problem of stimulus control and rule-governed behavior in children with attention deficit disorder with hyperactivity. Paper presented at the High Point Conference, Toronto, Canada, 1984.
75. Sergeant, J. From DSM-III attentional deficit disorder to functional defects. In: Bloomingdale LM, Sergeant J, eds. Attention deficit disorder: criteria, cognition, and intervention. New York: Pergamon Press, 1988:183–198.
76. Rutter M. Attention deficit disorder/hyperkinetic syndrome: Conceptual and research issues regarding diagnosis and classification. In: Sagvoldenand T, Archer T, eds. Attention deficit disorder: clinical and basic research. Hillsdale, NJ: Erlbaum, 1989.
77. Milich R, Pelham WE. Effects of sugar ingestion on the classroom and playgroup behavior of attention deficit disordered boys. J Consult Clin Psychol 1986;54(5):714–718.
78. Block GH. Hyperactivity: A cultural perspective. J Learning Disabilities 1977;110(236):240.
79. Feingold B. Why is your child hyperactive? New York: Random House, 1975.
80. Conrad P. The discovery of hyperkinesis: notes on the medicalization of deviant behavior. Social Problems 1975;23:12–21.
81. Schrag P, Divoky D. The myth of the hyperactive child. New York: Pantheon, 1975.
82. Conners CK. Food additives and hyperactive children. New York: Plenum Press, 1980.
83. Ross DM, Ross SA. Hyperactivity: current issues, research and theory (2nd ed.). New York: Wiley, 1982.
84. Douglas VI. Cognitive deficits in children with attention deficit disorder with hyperactivity. In: Bloomingdale LM, Sergeant J, eds. Attention deficit disorder: Criteria cognition intervention. New York: Pergamon Press, 1988:65–82.
85. Sergeant J, Van der Meere J. The diagnostic significance of attentional processing: its significance for ADDH classification: a future DSM. In: Sagvolden T, Archer T, eds. Attention deficit disorder: clinical and basic research. Hillsdale, NJ: Erlbaum, 1987:151–166.
86. Van der Meere J, Sergeant J. Controlled processing and vigilance in hyperactivity: time will tell. J Abnorm Child Psychol 1988;16(6):641–655.
87. Van der Meere J, Sergeant J. Focused attention in pervasively hyperactive children. J Abnorm Psychol 1988;16(6):627–639.
88. Rosenthal RH, Allen TW. An examination of attention, arousal, and learning dysfunctions of hyperkinetic children. Psychol Bull 1978;85:689–715.
89. Sroufe LA, Sonies BC, West WD, Wright FS. Anticipatory heart rate deceleration and reaction time in children with and without referral for learning disability. Child Dev 1973;44:267–273.
90. Willis TJ, Lovaas I. A behavioral approach treating hyperactive children. In: Millichap JG, ed. Learning disabilities and related behavior. Chicago: Year Book of Medical Publications, 1977:119–140.
91. Beninger RJ. Dopamine and learning: Implications for attention deficit disorder and hyperkinetic syndrome. In: Sagvoldenand T, Archer T, eds. Attention deficit disorder: Clinical and basic research. Hillsdale, NJ: Erlbaum, 1989:323–338.
92. Quay HC. Attention deficit disorder and the behavioral inhibition system: the relevance of the neuropsychological theory of Jeffrey A. Gray. In: Bloomingdale LM, Sergeant J, eds. Attention deficit disorder: criteria, cognition, and intervention. New York, NY: Pergamon Press, 1988:117–126.
93. Quay HC. The behavioral reward and inhibition system in childhood behavior discrder. In: Bloomingdale LM, ed. Attention deficit disorder, vol. 3: New research in attention, treatment, and psychopharmacology. Oxford, England: Pergamon Press, 1988:176–186.
94. Lou HC, Henriksen L, Bruhn P. Focal cerebral hypoperfusion in children with dysphasia and/or attention deficit disorder. Arch Neurol 1984;41(8):825–829.
95. Lou HC, Henriksen L, Bruhn P, Borner H, Nielsen JB. Striatal dysfunction in attention deficit and hyperkinetic disorder. Arch Neurol 1989;46(1):48–52.

96. Berry CA, Shaywitz SE, Shaywitz BA. Girls with attention deficit disorder: a silent minority? A report on behavioral and cognitive characteristics. Pediatrics 1985;76(5):801–809.
97. Cantwell DP, Baker L. Attention deficit disorder with and without hyperactivity: a review and comparison of matched groups. J Am Acad Child Adolesc Psychiatry 1992;31(3):432–438.
98. Edelbrock C, Costello AJ, Kessler MD. Empirical corroboration of attention deficit disorder. J Am Acad Child Adolesc Psychiatry 1984;23(3):285–290.
99. Lahey BB, Schaughency EA, Strauss CC, Frame CL. Are attention deficit disorders with and without hyperactivity similar or dissimilar disorders? J Am Acad Child Adolesc Psychiatry 1984;23(3):302–309.
100. Shaywitz SE. Early recognition of vulnerability-EREV. Technical report of Connecticut State Department of Education. Hartford, CT: State Department of Education, 1986.
101. Carlson CL, Lahey BB, Neeper R. Direct assessment of the cognitive correlates of attention deficit disorders with and without hyperactivity. J Psychopathol Behav Assess 1986;8(1): 69–86.
102. Lahey BB, Carlson CL. Validity of the diagnostic category of attention deficit disorder without hyperactivity: A review of the literature. J Learning Disabilities 1991;24(2):110–120.
103. Sergeant JA, Scholten CA. On resource strategy limitations in hyperactivity: cognitive impulsivity reconsidered. J Child Psychol Psychiatry 1985;26(1):97–109.
104. Sergeant JA, Scholten CA. On data limitations in hyperactivity. J Child Psychol Psychiatry 1985;26(1):111–124.
105. Frank Y, Ben-Nun Y. Toward a clinical subgrouping of hyperactive and non-hyperactive attention deficit disorder: results of a comprehensive neurological and neuropsychological assessment. J Diseases of Children 1988;142:153–155.
106. Jensen PS, Hinshaw SP, Kraemer HC, Lenora N, Newcorn JH, Abikoff HB et al. ADHD comorbidity findings from the MTA study: comparing comorbid subgroups. J Am Acad Child Adolesc Psychiatry 2001;40(2):147–158.
107. Vitiello B, Severe JB, Grenhill LL, Arnold LE, Abikoff HB, Bukstein OG, et al. Methylphenidate dosage for children with ADHD over time under controlled conditions: lessons from the MTA. J Am Acad Child Adolesc Psychiatry 2001;40(2):188–196.
108. Dykman RA, Dykman KD. The effects of nutritional supplements on attentional-deficit hyperactivity disorder. Integrative Physiol Behav Sci 1998;33:49–60.
109. O'Dougherty M, Nuechterlein KH, Drew B. Hyperactive and hypoxic children: signal detection, sustained attention, and behavior. J Abnorm Psychol 1984;93:178–191.
110. Schachar R, Logan G, Wachsmuth R, Chajczyk D. Attaining and maintaining preparation: a comparison of attention in hyperactive, normal, and disturbed control children. J Abnorm Child Psychol 1988;16(4):361–378.
111. Sykes DH, Douglas VI, Morgenstern G. Sustained attention in hyperactive children. J Child Psychol Psychiatry 1973;14:213–220.
112. Swanson JM, Shea C, McBurnett K, Potkin SG, Fiore C, Crinella F. Attention and hyperactivity. In: Ennis JT, ed. The development of attention: research and theory. North-Holland: Elsevier Science Publishers, 1990.
113. Van der Meere J, Wekking E, Sergeant J. Sustained attention and pervasive hyperactivity. J Child Psychol Psychiatry Allied Disciplines 1991;32(2):275–284.
114. Conners CK. Symptom patterns in hyperkinetic, neurotic and normal children. Child Dev 1970;41:667–682.
115. Sprague RL, Barnes KR, Werry JS. Methylphenidate and thioridazine: learning, reaction time, activity and classroom behavior in disturbed children. Am J Orthopsychiatry 1970;40:615–628.
116. Pribram KH. Memory and the organization of attention. In: Lindsey D, Lumsdaine A, eds. Brain function and learning. Press of California University; Berkeley 1967:79–122.
117. Dykman RA, Ackerman PT, Oglesby DM. Selective and sustained attention in hyperactive, learning-disabled and normal boys. J Nerv Mental Disord 1979;167(5):288–297.

118. Dykman RA, Ackerman PT, McCray DS. Effects of methylphenidate on selective and sustained attention in hyperactive, reading-disabled, and presumably attention-disordered boys. J Nerv Ment Disord 1980;168(12):745–752.
119. Buchsbaum MS. Self-regulation of stimulus intensity: augmenting/reducing and the average evoked response. In: Schwartz GE, Shapiro D, eds. Consciousness and self-regulation. New York: Plenum Publishing, 1976.
120. Buchsbaum MS, Wender P. Average evoked responses in normal and minimally brain dysfunctioned children treated with amphetamine. Arch Gen Psychiatry 1973;29:764–770.
121. Buchsbaum MS. Neurophysiological studies of augmenting and reducing. In: Petrie A, ed. Individuality in pain and suffering, vol. 2. Chicago: University of Chicago Press, 1978.
122. Eysenck MW. Learning, memory, and personality. In: Eysenck HJ, ed. A model of personality. New York: Springer, 1981:169–209.
123. Fowles DC. The three arousal model: Implications of Gray's two factor learning theory for heart rate, electrodermal activity, and psychopath. Psychophysiol 1980;17:87–104.
124. Gray JA. Elements of a two-process theory of learning. New York: Academic Press, 1975.
125. Gray JA. A critique of Eysenck's theory of personality. In: Eysenck HJ, ed. A model for personality. New York: Springer, 1981:246–276.
126. Zuckerman M, Murtaugh TM, Siegel J. Sensation seeking and cortical augmenting-reducing. Psychophysiol 1974;11:535–542.
127. Zuckerman M, Buchsbaum M, Murphy DL. Sensation seeking and its biological correlates. Psychol Bull 1980;88:187–214.
128. Nebylitsyn VD. Fundamental properties of the human nervous system. New York: Plenum, 1972.
129. Vasilev AN. The relation between reaction time to the onset and termination of signal as an inde of strength of the nervous system. Voprosy Psikhologii 1960;6:113–122.
130. Ackerman PT, Dykman RA. Automatic and effortful information-processing deficits in children with learning and attention disorders. Topics in Learning and Learning Disabilities 1982;2(2):12–22.
131. Ackerman PT, Dykman RA, Holcomb PJ, McCray DS. Methylphenidate effects on cognitive style and reaction time in four groups of children. Psychiatry Res 1982;7(2):199–213.
132. Dykman RA, Ackerman PT, Clements SD, Peters JA. Physiological manifestations of learning disability. J Learning Disabilities 1983;16(1):45–53.
133. Gray JA. Strength of the nervous system as a dimension of personality in man: a review of work from the laboratory of B.M. Teplov. In: Gray JA, ed. Pavlov's typology. New York: Macmillan, 1964:157–287.
134. Dykman RA, Holcomb PJ, Ackerman PT, McCray DS. Auditory ERP augmentation-reduction and methylphenidate dosage needs in attention and reading disabled children. Psychiatry Res 1983;9:255–269.
135. Ackerman PT, Holcomb PJ, McCray DS, Dykman RA. Studies of nervous system sensitivity in children with learning and attention disorders. Pavlovian J Biol Sci 1982;17(1):30–41.
136. Ackerman PT, Dykman RA, Oglesby DM. Sex and group differences in reading and attention disordered children with and without hyperkinesis. J Learning Disabilities 1983;16(7):407–415.
137. Ackerman PT, Holcomb PJ, Dykman RA. Effects of reward and methylphenidate on heart rate response morphology of augmenting and reducing children. Int J Psychophysiol 1984;1:301–316.
138. Zahn TP, Kruesi M, Rapoport J. Autonomic activity in boys with externalizing disorders. Psychophysiol 1989;26:67.
139. Sternberg S. Discovery of processing stages: extensions of Donder's method. In: Koster WG, ed. Attention and performance II. Amsterdam: Noord-Holland, 1969.
140. Sergeant, JA. Attentional studies in hyperactivity. Unpublished doctoral dissertation. Rijksuniversiteit te Groningen. Lennoxtown, Holland, 1981.
141. Holcomb PJ, Ackerman PT, Dykman RA. Cognitive event-related brain potentials in children with attention and reading deficits. Psychophysiol 1985;22(6):656–667.

142. Donchin E, Heffley EF. The independence of the P300 and the CNV reviewed: A reply to Wastell. Biol Psychol 1979;9(3):177–188.
143. Courchesne E. Neurophysiological correlates of cognitive development: Changes in long-latency event-related potentials from childhood to adulthood. Electroencephalogr Clini Neurophysiol 1978;45:468–482.
144. Courchesne E. Cognitive components of the event-related brain potential: Changes associated with development. In: Gaillard AWK, Ritter W, ed. Tutorials in ERP research: Endogenous components. Amsterdam: North Holland, 1983:329–344.
145. Ford J, Roth W, Mohs R, Hopkins W, Kopell B. Event-related potentials from young and old adults during a memory retrieval task. Electroencephalogr Clin Neurophysiol 1979;47:450–459.
146. McCarthy G, Donchin E. A metric for thought: A comparison of P300 latency and reaction time. Science 1980;211:77–80.
147. Dykman RA, Ackerman PT. Attention deficit disorder and specific reading disability: Separate but often overlapping disorders. J Learning Disabilities 1991;24:96–103.
148. Dykman RA, Ackerman PT. Diagnosing dyslexia: IQ regression plus cut-points. J Learning Disabilities 1992;25(9):574–576.
149. Dykman RA, Ackerman PT. Cluster versus dimensional analysis of attention deficit disorders. In: Matson J, ed. Handbook of hyperactivity in children. Needham Heights, MA: Allyn & Bacon, 1993:11–34.
150. Livingston RL, Dykman RA, Ackerman PT. The frequency and significance of additional self-reported psychiatric diagnoses in children with attention deficit disorder. J Abnorm Child Psychol 1990;18(5):465–478.
151. Loney J, Milich R. Hyperactivity, inattention, and aggression in clinical practice. In: Wolraich M, Routh DK, ed. Advances in developmental and behavioral pediatrics. Greenwich, CT: JAI Press, 1982:2113–2147.
152. Skinner HA. Toward the integration of classification theory and methods. Abnorm Psychol 1981;90:68–87.
153. Matthews KA, Angulo J. Cardiovascular responses of boys exhibiting the type A behavior pattern in children: Assessment of children's competitiveness, impatience-anger, and aggression. Child Dev 1980;51:466–475.
154. Achenbach TM, Edelbrock C. Manual for the child behavior checklist and revised child behavior profile. Burlington, VT: University of Vermont Department of Psychiatry, 1983.
155. Eysenck HJ, Eastings MS, Eysenck SBG. Personality measurement in children: A dimensional approach. J Special Education 1970;4:261–277.
156. Atkins MS, Pelham WE, Licht MH. The differential validity of teacher ratings of inattention/overactivity and aggression. J Abnorm Child Psychol 1989;17(4):423–435.
157. Campbell SB, Paulauskas S. Peer relations in hyperactive children. J Child Psychol Psychiatry 1979;20:233–246.
158. Johnston C, Pelham WE. Teacher rating predict peer ratings of aggression at 3-year follow-up in boys with attention deficit disorder with hyperactivity. J Consult Clin Psychol 1986;54(4):571–572.
159. Pope AW, Bierman KL, Mumma GH. Relations between hyperactive and aggressive behavior and peer relations at three elementary grade levels. J Abnorm Child Psychol 1989;17:253–267.
160. Whalen CK, Henker B, Collins BE, Finck D, Dotemoto S. A social ecology of hyperactive boys: Medication effects in structured environments. J Appl Behav Analysis 1979;12:65–81.
161. Pelham WE, Bender MB. Peer relationships in hyperactive children: Description and treatment. In: Gadow KD, Bialer I, eds. Advances in learning and behavioral disabilities, vol. 1. Greenwich, CT: JAI Press, 1982.
162. Landau S, Milich R. Social communication patterns of attention-deficit-disordered boys. J Abnorm Child Psychol 1988;16(1):69–81.

163. Fletcher JM. External validation of learning disability typologies. In: Rourke BP, ed. Neuropsychology of learning disabilities: Essentials of subtype analysis. New York: Guilford Press, 1985:187–211.
164. Fletcher JM, Morris R. Classification of disabled learners: Beyond exclusionary definitions. In: Ceci SJ, ed. Handbook of cognitive, social, and neuropsychological aspects of learning disabilities. Hillsdale, NJ: Lawrence Erlbaum Associates, 1986:55–80.
165. Fletcher JM, Francis DJ, Morris RD. Methodological issues in neuropsychology: Classification, measurement and the comparison of non-equivalent groups. In: Boller F, Grafman J, eds. Handbook of neuropsychology vol. 1. Amsterdam: Elsevier, 1988:83–110
166. Fletcher JM, Morris RD, Francis DJ. Methodological issues in the classification of attention-related disorders. In: Shaywitz SE, Shaywitz BA, ed. Attention deficit disorder comes of age. Austin, TX: Pre-ed, 1992:13–24.
167. Hooper SR. The classification of developmental disorders: An overview. In: Hooper SR, Hynd GW, Mattison RE, eds. Developmental disorders: diagnostic criteria and clinical assessment. Hillsdale, NJ: Lawrence Erlbaum Associates Publishers, 1992:1–21.
168. Skinner HA. Construct validation approach to psychiatric classification. In: Klerman GL, ed. Contemporary directions in psychopathology. New York: Guilford, 1986:307–330.
169. Herjanic B, Reich W. Development of a structured psychiatric interview for children: Agreement between child and parent on individual symptoms. J Abnorm Child Psychol 1982;10(3):307–324.
170. Shaywitz SE. Yale neuropsychoeducational assessment scales. New Haven, CT: Yale University Press, 1979.
171. Zuckerman M. Sensation seeking: beyond the optimal level of arousal. Hillsdale, NJ: Lawrence Erlbaum Associates, 1979.
172. Zuckerman M. A biological theory of sensation seeking. In: Zuckerman M, ed. Biological bases of sensation seeking, impulsivity, and anxiety. Hillsdale, NJ: Lawrence Erlbaum Associates, 1983.
173. Gordon M. The assessment of impulsivity and mediating behaviors in hyperactive and non-hyperactive boys. J Abnorm Child Psychol 1979;6:221–236.
174. Reitan RM. The Halstead-Reitan Neuropsychological test battery. Tucson, AZ: Neuropsychol Press, 1985.
175. Joreskog KG, Sorbom D. LISREL 8 structural equation modeling with SMPLIS command language. Hillsdale, NJ: Lawrence Erlbaum Associates Publishers, 1993.
176. American Psychiatric Association. Diagnostic and statistical manual of mental disorders, 2nd ed. Washington, DC: APA, 1968.
177. Lahey BB, Pelham WE, Schaughency EA, Atkins MS, Murphy HA, Hynd G et al. Dimensions and types of attention deficit disorder. J Am Acad Child and Adolescence Psychiatry 1988;27(3):330–335.
178. Lahey BB, Applegate B, McBurnett K, Biederman J, Greenhill L, Hynd GW et al. DSM-IV field trials for attention deficit/hyperactivity disorder in children and adolescents. Am J Psychiatry 1994;151:1673–1685.
179. Applegate B, Lahey BB, Hart EL, Biederman J, Hynd GW, Barkley RA et al. Validity of the age-of-onset criteria for ADHD: A report from the DSM-IV field trials. J Am Acad Child and Adolescence Psychiatry 1997;36:1211–1221.
180. Edelbrock C, Costello AJ. Structured psychiatric interviews for children. In: Rutter M, Tuma AH, Lann IS, eds. Assessment and diagnosis in child psychopathology. New York: Guilford Press, 1988:87–112.
181. Shaffer D, Fisher P, Piacentini J, Schwab-Stone M, Wicks J. NIMH diagnostic interview schedule for children-version 2.3. New York: New York State Psychiatric Institute, 1991.
182. Shaffer D, Schwab-Stone M, Fisher P, Cohen P, Piacentini J, Davies M, et al. The diagnostic interview schedule for children-revised version (DISC-R): I. Preparation, field testing, interrater reliability and acceptability. Journal of the American Academy

183. Shaffer D, Fisher P, Dulcan MK, Piacentini J, Schwab-Stone M, Lahey BB et al. The second version of the NIMH Diagnostic interview schedule for children (DISC-2). J Am Acad Child Adolesc Psychiatry 1996;35:865–877.
184. Barkley RA. A closer look at the DSM-IV criteria for ADHD: some unresolved issues. ADHD Reports 1995;3(3):1–6.
185. Bloomingdale LM, Sergeant J. Attention deficit disorder: criteria, cognition, intervention. New York: Pergamon Press, 1988.
186. Taylor EA, Everitt B, Thorley G, Schachar R, Rutter M, Wieselberg M. Conduct disorder and hyperactivity: II A cluster analytic approach to the identification of a behavioral syndrome. Br J Psychiatry 1986;149:768–777.
187. Taylor EA. Attention deficit and conduct disorder syndromes. In: Rutter M, Tuma AH, Lann IS, eds. Assessment and diagnosis in child psychopathology. New York: Guilford Press, 1988:377–407.
188. World Health Organization. International Classification of Diseases, 9th ed. Geneva, 1978.
189. Rutter M. Diagnostic validity in child psychiatry. Adv in Biological Psychiatry 1978;2:2–22.
190. World Health Organization. International Classification of Diseases, 10th ed. Geneva, 1990.
191. Forness SR, Cantwell DP, Swanson JM, Hanna GL, Youpa D. Differential effects of stimulant medication on reading performance of boys with hyperactivity with and without conduct disorder. J Learning Disabilities 1991;24(5):304–10.
192. Shaywitz SE, Shaywitz BA. Attention deficit disorder: current perspectives. Pediatr Neurol 1987;3(3):129–135.
193. Shaywitz SE, Shaywitz BA. Attention deficit disorder comes of age. Austin, TX: PRO-ED, 1992.
194. Shaywitz SE, Shaywitz BA. Attention deficit disorder: Current perspectives. In: Kavanagh JF, Truss TJ, eds. Learning disabilities: Proceedings of the national conference. Parkton, MD: York Press, 1988.
195. Shekim WO, Asarnow RF, Hess E, Zaucha K, Wheeler N. A clinical and demographic profile of sample of adults with attention deficit hyperactivity disorder, residual state. Compr Psychiatry 1990;31(5):416–425.
196. Palfrey JS, Levine MD, Walker DK, Sullivan M. The emergence of attention deficits in early childhood: a prospective study. Dev Behav Pediatr 1985;6:339–348.
197. Fergusson DM, Fergusson JE, Horwood LJ, Kinzett NG. A longitudinal study of dentine lead levels, intelligence, school performance and behaviour: III. Dentine lead levels and attention/activity. J Child Psychol Psychiatry Allied Disciplines 1988;29(6):811–824.
198. Kavale KA, Forness SR. Hyperactivity and diet treatment: A meta-analysis of the Feingold hypothesis. J Learning Disabilities 1983;16(6):324–330.
199. Taylor JF. The hyperactive child and the family. New York: Random House, 1980.
200. Gross MD. Effects of sucrose on hyperactive children. Pediatrics 1984;74:876–878.
201. Wolraich M, Milich JR, Stumbo P, Schultz F. The effects of sucrose ingestion on the behavior of hyperactive boys. Pediatrics 1985;106:675–82.
202. Alterman AI, Tarter RE, Baughman TG, Bober BA, Fabian SA. Differentiation of alcoholics high and low in childhood hyperactivity. Drug and Alcohol Dependence 1985;15(1–2): 111–121.
203. Alterman AI, Petrarulo E, Tarter RE, McGowan JR. Hyperactivity and alchoholism: familial and behavioral correlates. Addictive Behaviors 1982;7(4):413–421.
204. Barkley RA, DuPaul GJ, McMurray MB. Attention deficit disorder with and without hyperactivity: clinical response to three dose levels of methylphenidate. Pediatrics 1991;87(4):519–531.
205. Beck SJ, Young GH, Tarnowski KJ. Maternal characteristics and perceptions of pervasive and situational hyperactive and normal controls. J Amer Acad Child Adolesc Psychiatry 1990;29(4): 558–565.
206. Campbell SB, Breaux AM, Ewing LJ, Szumowski EK, Pierce EW. Parent-identified problem preschoolers: mother-child interaction during play at intake and 1-year follow-up. J Abnorm Child Psychol 1986;14(3):425–440.
207. Cantwell DP. Families with attention deficit disordered children and others at risk. J Chem Dependency Treatment 1988;1(2):163–186.

208. Danforth JS, Barkley RA, Stokes TF. observations of parent-child interactions with hyperactive children: Research and clinical implications. Clin Psychol Review 1991;11(6):703–727.
209. Lambert NM. Adolescent outcomes of hyperactive children-perspectives on general and specific patterns of childhood risk for adolescent educational, social, and mental health problems. Paper presented at the Annual Convention of the American Psychological Association, New York, 1987.
210. Marshall VG, Longwell L, Goldstein MJ, Swanson JM. Family factors associated with aggressive symptomatology in boys with attention deficit hyperactivity disorder: a research note. J Child Psychol Psychiatry Allied Disciplines 1990;31(4):6.
211. Schachar R, Wachsmuth R. Hyperactivity and parental psychopathology. J Child Psychol Psychiatry Allied Disciplines, 1990;31(3):381–392.
212. Schachar R, Wachsmuth R. Family dysfunction and psychosocial adversity: comparison of attention deficit disorder, conduct disorder, normal and clinical controls. Special issue: Childhood disorders in the context of the family. Can J Behav Sci 1991;23(3):332–348.
213. Talmadge J, Barkley RA. The interactions of hyperactive and normal boys with their fathers and mothers. J Abnorm Child Psychol 1983;11(4):565–579.
214. Gillis JJ, Gilger JW, Pennington BF, DeFries JC. Attention deficit disorder in reading-disabled twins: Evidence for a genetic etiology. J Abnorm Child Psychol 1992;20(3):303–315.
215. DeFries JC, Fulker DW. multiple regression analysis of twin data. Behav Genetics 1985;15:467–473.
216. DeFries JC, Fulker DW. Multiple regression of twin data: Etiology of deviant scores versus individual differences. Acta Geneticae Medicae et Gemellogie 1988;37:205–216.
217. Stevenson J, Pennington BF, Gilger JW, DeFries JC, Gillis JJ. Hyperactivity and spelling disability: testing for shared genetic aetiology. J Child Psychol Psychiatry 1993;34(7):1137–1152.
218. McGee R, Williams S, Moffitt T, Anderson J. A comparison of 13-year-old boys with attention deficit and /or reading disorder on neuropsychological measures. J Abnorm Child Psychol 1989;17(1):37–53.
219. Biederman J, Munir K, Knee D. Conduct and oppositional disorder in clinically referred children with attention deficit disorder: A controlled family study. J Am Acad Child and Adolesc Psychiatry 1987;26(5):724–727.
220. Biederman J, Munir K, Knee D, Armentano M, Autor S, Waternaux C et al. High rate of affective disorders in probands with attention deficit disorder and in their relatives: a controlled family study. Am J Psychiatry 1987;114(3):330–333.
221. Faraone SV, Biederman J, Keenan K, Tsuang M. A family-genetic study of girls with DSM-III attention deficit disorder. Am J Psychiatry 1991;148(1):112–117.
222. Faraone SV, Biederman J, Keenan K, Tsuang M. Separation of DSM-III attention deficit disorder and conduct disorder: Evidence from a family-genetic study of American child psychiatric patients. Psychol Med 1991;21(1):109–121.
223. Sandberg ST, Rutter M, Taylor E. Hyperkinetic disorder in psychiatric clinic attenders. Dev Med Child Neurol 1978;20:279–299.
224. Singer SM, Stewart MA, Pulaski L. Minimal brain dysfunction: differences in cognitive organization in two groups of index cases and their references. J Learning Disabilities 1981;14:470–473.
225. Stewart MA, DeBlois CS. Psychiatric disorder in the parents of hyperactive boys and those with conduct disorder. J Child Psychol Psychiatry 3 A.D.;21:283–292.
226. Biederman J, Faraone SV, Keenan K, Knee D, Tsuang M. Family-genetic and psychosocial risk factors in DSM-III attention deficit disorder. J Am Acad Child Adolesc Psychiatry 1990;29(4):526–533.
227. Biederman J, Faraone SV, Keenan K, Steingard R, Tsuang M. Familial association between attention deficit disorder and anxiety disorders. Am J Psychiatry 1991;148(2):251–256.
228. Olds ME, Fobes JC. The central basis of motivation: intracranial self-stimulation studies. Palo Alto, CA: Annual Reviews, 1981.
229. Barkley RA. The executive functions and self-regulation: An evolutionary neuropsychological perspective. Neuropsychol Rev 2001;11(1):1–29.

230. Breland K, Breland M. The misbehavior of organisms. American Psychol 1961;16:681–684.
231. Dykman RA, Gantt WH, Whitehorn JC. Conditioning as emotional sensitization and differentiation. Psychol Monogr 1956;7(15):27–35.
232. Dennis M. Frontal love function in childhood and adolescence: A heuristic for assessing attention regulation, executive control, and the international states important for social discourse. Dev Neuropsychol 1991;7(3):327–358.
233. Dennis M, Barnes MA, Donnelly RE, Wilkinson M, Humphreys RP. Appraising and managing knowledge: Metacognitive skills after childhood head injury. Dev Neruopsychol 1996;12(1):77–103.
234. Schachar R, Tannock R, Marriott M, Logan G. Deficient inhibitory control in attention deficit hyperactivity disorder. J Abnorm Child Psychol 1995;23(4):411–437.
235. McInerney R, Kerns K. Time reproduction in children with ADHD: motivation matters. Child Neuropsychol 2003;9(2):91–108.
236. Barry RJ, de Pascalis V, Hodder D, Clarke AR, Johnstone SJ. Preferred EEG brain states at stimulus onset in a fixed interstimulus interval auditory oddball task and their effects on ERP components. Int J Psychophysiol 2003;47(3):187.
237. Ernst M, Kimes AS, London ED, Matochik JA, Eldreth D, Tata S et al. Neural substrates of decision making in adults with attention deficit hyperactivity disorder. Am J Psychiatry 2003;160(6):1061–1070.
238. Healey EC, Reid R. ADHD and stuttering: a tutorial. J Fluency Disorders 2003;28(2):79–92, quiz 93.
239. Roman T, Schmitz M, Polanczyk GV, Eizirik M, Rohde LA, Hutz MH. Is the alpha-2A adrenergic receptor gene (ADRA2A) associated with attention-deficit/hyperactivity disorder? Am J Med Genetics 2003;120B(1):116–120.
240. Hynd GW, Semrud-Clikeman M, Lorys AR, Novey ES. Corpus callosum morphology in attention deficit-hyperactivity disorder: morphometric analysis of MRI. Special series: Attention deficit disorder. J Learning Disabilities 1991;24(3):141–146.
241. Leonard CM, Voeller KS, Lombardino LJ, Morris MK, Hynd GW, Alexander AW, et al. Anomalous cerebral structure in dyslexia revealed with magnetic resonance imaging. Arch Neurol 1993;50:461–469.
242. Pineda DA, Restrepo MA, Sarmiento RJ, Gutierrez JE, Vargas SA, Quiroz YT, et al. Statistical analyses of structural magnetic resonance imaging of the head of the caudate nucleus in Colombian children with attention-deficit hyperactivity disorder. 2002.
243. Mercier L, Pivik RT. Spinal motoneuronal excitability during wakefulness and non REM sleep in hyperkinesis. J Clin Neuropsychol 1983;5:321–336.
244. Pivik RT, Bylsma FW. Spinal motoneuronal excitability in hyperkinesis: Effects of the jendrassik manoeurvre. Int J Psychophysiol 1990;9:85–89.
245. Pivik RT, Mercier L. Spinal motoneuronal excitability in hyperkinesis: H-reflex recovery function and homosynaptic depression during wakefulness. J Clin Neuropsychol 1981;3:215–236.
246. Pivik RT, Bylsma FW, Margittai K. Abnormal motoneuronal excitability in hyperkinetic children. Psychophysiology 1986;23:146–155.
247. Lacey JI, Kagan J, Lacey BC, Moss HR. The visceral level: Situational determinants and behavioral correlates of autonomic response patterns. In: Knapp PH, ed. Expression of the emotions in man. New York: International University Press, 1963: 161–196.
248. Posner MI, Cohen Y, Rafal RD. Neural systems and the control of spatial orienting. Philosophical Transactions of the Royal Society of London (Biology) 1982;187–198.
249. Posner MI, Walker JA, Friedrich FJ, Rafal RD. Effects of parietal injury on covert orienting of attention. J Neuroscience 1984;4:1863–1874.
250. Wagner RK, Torgesen JK. The nature of phonological processing and its causal role in the acquisition of reading skills. Psychol Bull 1987;101:192–212.

2
Scanning the Genome for Attention Deficit Hyperactivity Disorder

Aiveen Kirley

1. INTRODUCTION

In the past decade, there have been exciting developments in the understanding of the genetic basis of susceptibility to attention deficit hyperactivity disorder (ADHD). This chapter reviews the genetic epidemiology (family, twin, and adoption studies) of ADHD and summarizes the neurobiological evidence (pharmacology, animal models, and neuroimaging studies) that points to particular candidate genes. Relevant findings from genetic studies of dopaminergic, serotonergic, and noradrenergic candidate genes are provided. New directions in the field are discussed briefly, such as the move to characterize endophenotypes, meta-analyses of association studies, and emerging genetic linkage studies.

2. GENETIC EPIDEMIOLOGY OF ADHD

Evidence reviewed in the preceeding chapter suggests that ADHD is a heterogeneous condition that has many causes, and is considered as a final common pathway for a variety of complex brain developmental processes *(1)*. The exact etiology of ADHD is unknown, but a substantial genetic element has been implicated from family, twin, and adoption studies.

2.1. *Family Studies in ADHD*

Family studies investigate the degree of familial clustering of a disorder. Thapar and Scourfield *(2)* summarize family, twin, and adoption studies in ADHD. Family studies have shown an increased risk of ADHD in the families of children with ADHD (whether defined using the *Diagnostic and Statistical Manual of Mental Disorders*, 3rd edition (DSM-III) or DSM-III-R diagnostic criteria) with reported relative risks (λ) of between 4 and 5.4 for first-degree relatives *(3,4)*.

2.2. *Twin Studies in ADHD*

A drawback of family studies is that they cannot disentangle genetic from environmental sources of transmission. Twin and adoption studies assist in doing so. The occurrence of twinning creates a natural experiment in psychiatric genetics *(5)*. If a disorder is strongly influenced by genetic factors then the risk to co-twins of ill probands should be greatest when the twins are monozygotic. The risk to dizygotic twins should exceed the risk to controls but

From: *Attention Deficit Hyperactivity Disorder: From Genes to Patients*
Edited by: D. Gozal and D. L. Molfese © Humana Press Inc., Totowa, NJ

should not be greater than the risk to siblings. Twin data are used to estimate heritability (h^2), which measures the degree to which a disorder is influenced by genetic factors. Twin studies *(2)* have consistently shown the importance of genetic influences on ADHD, whether defined as a categorical diagnosis (i.e., as defined by DSM) or as a quantitative measure of symptomatology, with reported h^2 estimates of between 0.39 and 0.91.

2.3. *Adoption Studies in ADHD*

As with twinning, the occurrence of adoption provides another useful experiment for psychiatric genetics *(5)*. Whereas parents can confer a disease risk to their biological children via both biological and environmental pathways, they can confer risk to adoptive children only via an environmental pathway. Thus by examining both the adoptive and the biological relatives of ill probands, genetic and environmental sources of familial transmission can be disentangled. Thapar and Scourfield *(2)* provide an overview of adoption studies in ADHD. Although published adoption studies of ADHD are much less recent than the twin studies and have some methodological drawbacks, such as small sample size, nonsystematic ascertainment, or the failure to use standardized measures or diagnostic criteria, overall the findings have been consistent in showing the importance of genetic factors. Biological parents of hyperactive children appear to show higher rates of hyperactivity and ADHD *(4,6,7)*, and poorer performance on cognitive measures of attention *(8)* than adoptive relatives. Similarly in a study of separately fostered siblings, in accordance with expectations of a genetic etiology, hyperactive children showed greater concordance with their biological siblings than their half-siblings *(9)*.

2.4. *Mode of Genetic Transmission of ADHD*

The exact mode of transmission for genes underlying ADHD remains unknown. Segregation analyses *(6,10–12)* have proposed models of inheritance from major gene effects through oligogenic to polygenic and multifactorial models, but the differences in statistical "fit" between multifactorial genetic models and single-gene inheritance is modest. It appears more likely that several interacting genes of modest effect cause ADHD. This multifactorial concept is consistent with ADHD's high population prevalence (2–7%) and high concordance in monozygotic twins (68–81%), but modest recurrence risks to first-degree relatives.

3. NEUROBIOLOGICAL THEORIES OF ADHD

The overall pattern of neuropsychological, neuroimaging, and neurotransmitter-related findings in ADHD is consistent with the hypothesis that ADHD is associated with dysfunction in the frontosubcortical pathways mediated by catecholamine neurotransmission, which control attention and motor behavior. Dopaminergic, serotonergic, and noradrenergic systems have come under close scrutiny and each has contributed candidate genes for genetic analysis.

3.1. *Dopaminergic Theories of ADHD*

Evidence to support dopaminergic dysfunction in ADHD derives from the neuropharmacology of stimulant medication, the behavior and biochemistry of animal models, and neuroimaging studies.

3.1.1. Neuropharmacological Evidence

The mainstay of treatment for ADHD is methylphenidate and other psychostimulant medications (dextroamphetamine, pemoline), which are known to inhibit the dopamine transporter *(13)*, thus increasing the availability of dopamine in the synaptic cleft. Knowledge of the mechanism of action for methylphenidate and its possible inhibitory cortical effects via dopaminergic and/or noradrenergic pathways *(14)* strongly support a theory of dopaminergic dysfunction in ADHD.

3.1.2. Animal Studies

Animal models also support a dopaminergic hypothesis in ADHD. Mice without a functioning dopamine transporter (DAT1 knockout [KO] mice) have high extracellular striatal dopamine levels, a doubling of the rate of dopamine synthesis *(15)*, decreased dopamine and tyrosine hydroxylase in striatum *(16)*, and a nearly complete loss of functioning of dopamine autoreceptors *(17)*. They display markedly increased locomotor and stereotypic activity compared to normal (wild-type) mice *(15,18)*. The reduced striatal dopamine may be most relevant to a hypodopaminergic theory of ADHD. Also, selective destruction of dopamine neurons by 6-hydroxydopamine results in hyperactivity and learning difficulties in mice *(19)*. The spontaneously hypertensive rat (SHR) has also been used as an animal model of ADHD because of the SHR's locomotor hyperactivity and impaired discriminative performance. Russell *(20)* showed that the altered presynaptic regulation of dopamine in SHR led to the downregulation of the dopamine system. The authors hypothesized that this may have occurred early in development as a compensatory response to abnormally high dopamine concentrations. The coloboma mouse mutant exhibits a behavioral phenotype similar to that of ADHD. It is characterized by spontaneous motor hyperactivity, head-bobbing, and ocular dystrophy. The phenotype of this model has been shown to be the result of a deletion of the Synaptosomal-associated protein 25 (*SNAP-25*) gene (located in mouse chromosome 2) *(21)*. *SNAP-25* is a presynaptic plasma membrane protein that is expressed highly and specifically in the nerve cells. The gene encodes a protein essential for synaptic vesicle fusion and neurotransmitter release. Interestingly, it is possible to treat the hyperactivity of this mouse with D-amphetamine and it can be genetically "rescued" by a transgene-encoding *SNAP-25* inserted within the Cm deletion.

3.1.3. Neuroimaging Studies

Structural brain imaging studies *(22)* have shown abnormalities in the frontal lobe and subcortical structures (globus pallidus, caudate, corpus callosum), regions known to be rich in dopamine neurotransmission and important in the control of attention and response to organization *(23–25)*. The most consistent findings are hypoactivity of frontal cortex and subcortical structures, usually on the right side. Functional imaging has shown that dopamine transporter density is increased in ADHD patients compared with controls *(26–29)*, and that administration of methylphenidate reduces transporter density to near-normal levels in ADHD patients *(27,28)*. These findings lend further support to dopaminergic dysfunction in ADHD.

3.2. Serotonergic Theories of ADHD

As reviewed by Manor et al. *(30)* and Quist et al. *(31)*, evidence from human and animal studies suggests that serotonergic system genes should also be considered as likely candidates genes in ADHD. For example, whole blood, serum, and platelet serotonin concentrations have been noted as decreased in children with ADHD *(32–34)*. Selective serotonin reuptake inhibitors are moderately efficacious in the treatment of ADHD *(35)*. Animal studies indicate that both frontal cortex dopamine and serotonin play important roles in the modulation of attention and response control *(36,37)*. Disruption of the dopamine transporter in mice (DAT-KO mice) results in a phenotype that resembles human ADHD, a marked hyperactivity apparently resulting from high extracellular dopamine levels in the absence of the dopamine transporter *(18)*. Treatment of these mice with both psychostimulants and serotonergic drugs produced a paradoxical calming effect that was independent of any changes of extracellular levels of dopamine in the striatum. These results suggested that a different mechanism must be involved in DAT-KO mice. The hypothesis was that serotonin neurotransmission mediated motor activity alterations in the mice, whereas extracellular dopamine concentrations remained unchanged *(15)*.

3.3. *Noradrenergic Theories of ADHD*

Recent work in human and animal studies also suggests the involvement of the adrenergic system in ADHD. In rodents, norepinephrine (NE) depletion results in increased distractibility and motor hyperactivity *(38)*, and in nonhuman primates, stimulation of the noradrenergic system has been shown to improve cognitive function and distractibility *(39)*. Noradrenergic projections are particularly dense in the frontal cortex and cingulate gyrus. These regions are involved in mood stabilization and sleep regulation, as well as attention and alertness *(40,41)*. Animals and humans with lesions in the prefrontal cortex show poor attention regulation and disorganized, impulsive, and hyperactive behaviors, similar to those observed in ADHD. Pharmacological studies have demonstrated the clinical usefulness of NE inhibitors (such as desipramine, nortriptyline, and atomoxetine) in the treatment of ADHD *(42,43)*. The mode of action of these antidepressants is to block the reuptake of dopamine and norepinephrine and consequently increase the release of the monoamines into the extraneuronal space. The improvement in ADHD symptoms with tricyclic antidepressants has been attributed to the actions of these drugs in the reuptake of NE *(44)*.

4. FINDINGS FROM GENETIC STUDIES IN ADHD

Having reviewed the evidence for involvement of catecholamine dysregulation in ADHD, molecular genetic studies of candidate genes from these systems are summarized. To date, most reported findings relate to dopaminergic system genes, but emerging evidence also implicates serotonergic and noradrenergic system genes.

4.1. *Dopaminergic System Genes*

Molecular genetic studies have produced strong evidence for dopaminergic involvement in ADHD. The gene encoding the dopamine transporter, *DAT1*, was the initial candidate gene studied. This gene is of particular interest as the transporter is the principal target for methylphenidate and other psychostimulant medication used to treat patients with ADHD *(45,46)*. The polymorphism of interest is a 40-bp sequence of a variable number tandem repeat (VNTR) located in the 3′ untranslated region of the *DAT1* gene, which maps to chromosome 5p15.3 *(47,48)*. Ten different alleles can be found, according to the presence of 3 to 13 copies of this 40-bp repeat, the most prevalent allele being the 10-repeat (or 480-bp) allele *(49)*. Cook et al. *(50)* first reported association between the 480-bp *DAT1* allele and ADHD. Since then, this finding has been replicated by some groups *(51–56)*, but not by others *(57–64)*.

The reported odds ratios for the *DAT1* 480-bp allele from the above studies range from 1.38 to 2.67 and suggest that *DAT1* is a gene of small effect in ADHD. Conflicting results may be owing to many factors, such as the lack of statistical power, in individual samples, to find genes of small effect, differences in the diagnostic definition of ADHD, hidden population stratification, genetic heterogeneity, and a variation between samples of linkage disequilibrium with a nearby "causal" variant. A meta-analysis by Maher et al. *(65)*, in which eleven studies were included, yielded a marginally nonsignificant pooled odds ratio estimate of 1.27 (95% CI 0.99–1.63, $p = 0.06$).

DRD4, the gene encoding the dopamine D4 receptor, has also attracted interest as a candidate gene. The dopamine D4 receptor mediates the postsynaptic action of dopamine. There have been several studies examining for association between the 7 repeat (148-bp) allele of the 40-bp VNTR in exon 3 of the *DRD4* gene and ADHD with positive results in many *(66–76)* but not all *(77–82)* studies. A recent meta-analysis of *DRD4* by Faraone et al. *(83)* supported an overall association with a small odds ratio between *DRD4* and ADHD. Case-control studies were more strongly significant (OR = 1.9, $p = 0.00000008$) than family-based studies (OR = 1.4, $p = 0.02$).

Other dopamine receptor genes have also been investigated as candidate genes in ADHD. There have been published reports of association between the 148-bp *DRD5* allele and ADHD *(52,53,75,84,85)*. Moreover, a recent joint and meta-analysis by Lowe et al. *(86)* confirms that *DRD5* is a susceptibility gene (of minor effect) for ADHD (OR = 1.25, $p = 0.00005$). Further analysis of the data suggested that *DRD5* contributes risk for the inattentive but not the hyperactive symptoms.

Other studies have focused on genes involved in regulation of dopamine synthesis and metabolism. Eisenberg et al. *(87)* reported association between a high-activity related catechol-*O*-methyltransferase (*COMT*) allele and ADHD. Other groups refuted this finding *(53,88–91)*. A number of groups *(52,53,92,93)* have reported association at the A2 allele of the TaqI polymorphism of the gene (*DBH*) encoding the enzyme dopamine β-hydroxylase.

Another candidate gene potentially related to dopamine transmission is the gene for the synaptic vesicle docking fusion protein, *SNAP-25*. As described previously, this gene has also been implicated in the etiology of ADHD based on the mouse mutant strain coloboma *(94)*. Recent studies by Barr et al. *(95)*, Brophy et al. *(96)*, and Kustanovich et al. *(97)* reported evidence for association with polymorphisms in the 3′ untranslated region of this gene. However, another study by Mill et al. *(98)* found association with variants at the opposite end of the *SNAP-25* gene (near the 5′-untranslated region).

4.2. Serotonergic System Genes

The efficiency of serotonergic signaling is controlled by the serotonin transporter 5-hydroxytryptamine transporter (*5-HTT*), which removes serotonin from the synaptic cleft. A polymorphism (44-bp insertion/deletion) located upstream of the transcriptional site of the transporter was found to influence the expression of the gene, consequently altering the levels of reuptake of dopamine. The homozygous insertion (*L/L*) yields a higher level of *5-HTT* expression than the heterozygous (L/S) or the homozygous deletion (*S/S*). An association between the *L/L 5-HTTLPR* (5-HTT promoter region) genotype and ADHD has been reported *(99–101)*. Zoroglu et al. *(102)* observed that the *5-HTTLPR S/S* genotype was significantly lower in ADHD patients than in the controls. Pharmacological studies using the 5-hydroxytryptamine 1B receptor (*5-HT1B*) agonist RU24969 suggest that the activation of the 5-HT1B receptor in mice leads to increased anxiety and locomotion in these animals. In addition,

5-HT1B knockout mice display an increased locomotor response to cocaine acquisition and alcohol intake, along with hyperactivity and aggressive behavior *(103)*. The hyperlocomotion effect of this agonist is absent in the mouse lacking 5-HT1B, indicating that the agonist effect is mediated by this receptor. Hawi et al. *(104)* and Quist et al. *(105)* reported association between a 5-HT1B polymorphism (861G-C) and ADHD. The serotonin HTR2A is a G protein-coupled receptor functioning in signal transduction. Antagonism of 5HT2A has been shown to reduce dopamine-induced hyperactivity in mice *(106,107)*. Hyperlocomotion induced by the noncompetitive *N*-methyl-D-aspartate antagonist (MK-801) in mice is attenuated by the nonselective 5-HT2A antagonist ritanserine and by the 5-HT2A selective antagonist MDL100907 *(107)*. Several recent studies have investigated 5-HT2A markers for possible association with ADHD, with association reported by Quist et al. *(106)* and Levitan et al. *(108)* but not by Hawi et al. *(104)* and Zoroglu et al. *(109)*.

4.3. Noradrenergic System Genes

Molecular genetic analysis of ADHD and noradrenergic system genes is an emerging area but there have been few findings of association to date. Barr et al. *(110)* and McEvoy et al. *(111)* found no association between polymorphisms at the norepinephrine transporter protein and ADHD. Similarly, negative findings of association have reported for the adrenergic α2A ($ADRA_{2A}$) *(112)* and α2C ($ADRA_{1C}$ and $ADRA_{2C}$) receptors *(113)*.

5. CONFLICTING FINDINGS IN GENETIC STUDIES OF ADHD

Despite compelling evidence for a genetic basis to ADHD and findings of association replicated across several studies, the findings in ADHD are, to date, not definitive. If, as hypothesized, ADHD is a complex genetic disorder, with many susceptibility genes each of small effect *(114–116)*, the pattern of results seen to date is to be expected. Other factors that might account for conflicting results include power limitations secondary to small sample size, differences between the populations of origin of the samples, differences in measuring and defining the phenotype, and clinical heterogeneity with different distributions of the subtypes between samples.

6. FUTURE DIRECTIONS IN GENETIC STUDIES OF ADHD

6.1. Endophenotypes for ADHD

Evidence is emerging in support of endophenotypes or ADHD subtypes in which genes may exert a larger effect than in the categorical diagnosis. Recent studies have examined whether specific genetic risk factors for ADHD correlate with measures of hyperactivity in population samples. Their hypothesis is that if ADHD were a continuous trait, investigation of association between genes (quantitative trait loci [QTL]) and continuous measures of the phenotype would be a more appropriate strategy in the identification of susceptibility variants. To date, there have been few QTL association studies in ADHD and findings have been mixed. In an epidemiological sample, Curran et al. *(117)* selected children on the basis of high and low scores on the five ADHD items of the Strengths and Difficulties Questionnaire and found a significant relationship between the *DRD4* 7-repeat allele and high-scoring children. However, Mill et al. *(118)* did not replicate this finding. Similarly, Todd et al. *(119)* failed to demonstrate any significant association between the *DRD4* 7-repeat allele and DSM-IV ADHD subtypes or ADHD subtypes derived by latent class analysis in an epidemiological twin sample.

Several family studies have investigated the effect of comorbid disorders on the familiality of ADHD. These studies *(4,120–130)* suggest that relatives of probands with ADHD and comorbid conduct disorder (CD) are at greater risk for ADHD than relatives of probands with ADHD alone and that ADHD and comorbid CD may represent a separate familial subtype. Data from Faraone *(129)* calculated the risk ratios (λs) of ADHD in relatives when different subtypes of ADHD are used to select families. Relative risk ratios varied from 4 to 5.4 among relatives of probands with ADHD alone but rose from 5 to 8.9 in relatives of probands with ADHD and CD or bipolar disorder. Twin studies also suggest that the genes that influence conduct disorder symptoms are the same as those that contribute to trait measures of ADHD *(125,131,132)*. Overall the evidence reviewed suggests that ADHD and certain comorbid disorders represent groups in which genes exert a greater effect and may prove useful for the identification of genetic risk factors. To date, there have been a limited number of studies investigating genetic association with clinical measures of the ADHD phenotype. Holmes et al. *(133)* reported significant association between the *DRD4* 7-repeat allele and children with ADHD and comorbid "conduct problems" in a clinical sample. Rowe et al. *(134)* examined retrospectively reported conduct disorder symptoms in parents of ADHD children and found that parents with the *DRD4* 7-repeat allele had more conduct disorder symptoms than parents possessing other genotypes. However, Tahir et al. *(75)* reported significant nontransmission of this allele to children with comorbid oppositional/defiant disorder or CD.

There has been increasing interest in investigating genes associated with neuropsychological endophenotypes of ADHD. Given the difficulty in defining the diagnostic phenotype, more objective measures of behavior are attractive. Owing to the extensive literature on neuropsychological abnormalities in ADHD, such markers may prove useful for further genetic study. This is an emerging research area, and to date, there are few consistent findings. A twin study by Goodman and Stevenson *(135)* found that measures of inattentiveness (freedom from distractibility and "E" scan attentiveness) were moderately influenced by genetic factors (32–42%). More recent twin studies found a significant genetic contribution to hyperactivity and variability of reaction times on the "stop" task *(131)* and genetic influences on Matching Familiar Figures Test-derived measures of impulsiveness *(133)*. To date, there have been few findings of association between specific candidate genes and neuropsychological measures of ADHD. Langley et al. *(136)* found that possession of the DRD4 7 repeat allele was associated with an inaccurate, impulsive response style on neuropsychological tasks that was not explained by ADHD symptom severity.

6.2. Alternative Strategies to Association Mapping and Meta-Analysis

The candidate gene approach has been reasonably successful because of the presence of *a priori* hypotheses based on animal and pharmacological studies. However, because of the increased availability of markers for study and advances in gene mapping technology, systematic genome scans will be required for the identification of further risk alleles for ADHD. Such studies are under way *(137,138)*. These might identify new genes and new neurobiological hypotheses. Future directions for studies in ADHD genetics include the use of collaboration to increase sample size and consequently power to detect association with genes of small effect. Meta-analysis of individual studies is becoming more common and will assist confirmation of candidate genes. This approach has been successful in the cases of the *DRD4 (83)* and *DRD5* genes *(86)*. Functional analysis of associated gene variants will be necessary to assist evaluation of neurobiology. For example, recent studies *(139,140)* have shown that the 10-repeat allele of the *DAT1* VNTR polymorphism increases dopamine transporter expression and work by Miller and Madras *(141)* suggests that single nucleotide polymorphisms within the *DAT1* 480-bp VNTR differentially affect dopamine transporter expression.

Finally, the importance of environmental etiological factors in ADHD should not be overlooked. Future work in ADHD would benefit from incorporating environmental measures into the study design to examine gene–environment interactions.

REFERENCES

1. Jensen PS. ADHD: Current concepts on etiology, pathophysiology and neurobiology. Child Adolesc Psychiatr Clin N Am 2000;9:557–572.
2. Thapar A, Scourfield J. Childhood disorders. In: McGuffin P, Owen MJ, Gottesman II, eds. Psychiatric genetics and genomics. Oxford University Press, 2002:154–180.
3. Biederman J, Faraone SV, Keenan K, et al. Further evidence for family-genetic risk factors in attention deficit hyperactivity disorder (ADHD): patterns of comorbidity in probands and relatives in psychiatrically and pediatrically referred samples. Arch Gen Psychiatry 1992;49:728–738.
4. Faraone SV, Biederman J, Monuteaux M. Toward guidelines for pedigree selection in genetic studies of attention deficit hyperactivity disorder. Genet Epidemiol 2000;18:1–16.
5. Faraone SV, Tsuang D, Tsuang MT. Genetics and mental disorders: a guide for students, clinicians and researchers. New York: Guilford, 1999.
6. Morrison JR, Stewart MA. The psychiatric status of the legal families of adopted hyperactive children. Arch Gen Psychiatry 1973;28:888–891.
7. Cantwell DP. Genetics of hyperactivity. J Child Psychol Psychiatry 1975;16:261–264.
8. Alberts-Corush J, Firestone P, Goodman JT. Attention and impulsivity characteristics of the biological and adoptive parents of hyperactive and normal control children. Am J Orthopsychiatry 1986;56:413–423.
9. Safer DJ. A familial factor in minimal brain dysfunction. Behav Genet 1973;3:175–186.
10. Deutsch CK, Mattyse S, Swanson JM, Farkas LG. Genetic latent structure analysis of dysmorphology in attention deficit disorder. J Am Acad Child Adolesc Psychiatry 1990;29:189–194.
11. Faraone SV, Biederman J, Chen WJ, et al. Segregation analysis of attention deficit hyperactivity disorder. Psychiatr Genet 1992;2:257–275.
12. Hess EJ, Rogan PK, Domoto M, Tinker DE, Ladda RL, Ramer JC. Absence of linkage of apparently single gene mediated ADHD with the human syntenic region of the mouse mutant coloboma. Am J Med Genet 1995;60:573–579.
13. Amara S, Kuhar M. Neurotransmitter transporters: recent progress. Ann Rev Neurosci 1993;16:73–93.
14. Zametkin AJ, Rapoport JL. Noradrenergic hypothesis of attention deficit disorder with hyperactivity: a critical review. In: Meltzer HY, ed. Psychopharmacology: the third generation of progress. New York: Raven, 1987:837–842.
15. Gainetdinov RR, Wetsel WC, Jones SR, Levin ED, Jaber M, Caron MG. Role of serotonin in the paradoxical calming effect of psychostimulants on hyperactivity. Science 1999;83:397–401.
16. Jaber M, Dumartin B, Sagne C, et al. Differential regulation of tyrosine hydroxylase in the basal ganglia of mice lacking the dopamine transporter. Eur J Neurosci 1999;11:3499–3511.
17. Jones SR, Gainetdinov RR, Hu XT, et al. Loss of autoreceptor functions in mice lacking the dopamine transporter. Nat Neurosci 1999;2:649–655.
18. Giros B, Jaber M, Jones S, Wightman RM, Caron M. Hyperlocomotion and indifference to cocaine and amphetamine in mice lacking the dopamine transporter. Nature 1996;379:606–612.
19. Garfinkel BD, Wender PH. Attention deficit hyperactivity disorder. In: Kaplan HI, Sadock BJ, eds. Comprehensive textbook of psychiatry. Baltimore: Williams and Wilkins, 1989:1831.
20. Russell VA. The nucleus accumbens motor-limbic interface of the spontaneously hypertensive rat as studied in vitro by the superfusion slice technique. Neurosci Biobehav Rev 2000;24:133–136.

21. Hess EJ, Collins KA, Wilson MC. Mouse model for hyperkinesis implicates SNAP in behavioural regulation. J Neurosci 1996;16:3104–3111.
22. Faraone SV, Doyle AE. The nature and heritability of attention-deficit/hyperactivity disorder. Child Adolesc Psychiatr Clin N Am 2001;10:299–316.
23. Lou HC, Henriksen L, Bruhn P. Focal cerebral dysfunction in developmental learning disabilities. Lancet 1990;335:8–11.
24. Zametkin AJ, Nordahl TE, Gross J, et al. Cerebral glucose metabolism in adults with hyperactivity of childhood onset. N Engl J Med 1990;323:1361–1366.
25. Rubia K, Overmeyer S, Taylor E, et al. Inhibitory control of hyperactive adolescents in fMRI. In: Toga AW, Frackowiak RSJ, Mazziotta JC, eds. Neuroimage Third International Conference on Functional Mapping of the Human Brain (May 19–23, Copenhagen, Denmark). New York: Academic Press, 1997.
26. Dougherty DD, Bonab AA, Spencer TJ, Rauch SL, Madras BK, Fischman AJ. Dopamine transporter density in patients with attention deficit hyperactivity disorder. Lancet 1999;354:9196.
27. Dresel S, Krause J, Krause K-H, LaFougere C Brinkbaumer K, Kung HF. Attention deficit hyperactivity disorder: binding of [^{99m}Tc]TRODAT-1 to the dopamine transporter before and after methylphenidate treatment. Eur J Nucl Med 2000;27:1518–1524.
28. Krause KL, Dresel SH, Krause J, Kung HF, Tatsch K. Increased striatal dopamine transporter in adult patients with attention deficit hyperactivity disorder: effects of methylphenidate as measured by single photon emission computed tomography. Neurosci Let 2000;285:107–110.
29. Cheon KA, Ryu YH, Kim YK, Namkoong K, Kim CH, Lee JD. Dopamine transporter density in the basal ganglia assessed with [(123)I]IPT SPET in children with attention deficit hyperactivity disorder. Eur J Nucl Med Mol Imaging 2003;30:306–311.
30. Manor I, Eisenberg J, Tyano S, et al. Family-based association study of the serotonin transporter promoter region polymorphism (5-HTTLPR) in attention deficit hyperactivity disorder. Am J Med Genet (Neuropsychiat Genet) 2001;105:91–95.
31. Quist JK, Barr CL, Schachar R, et al. Evidence for the serotonin HTR2A receptor gene as a susceptibility factor in attention deficit hyperactivity disorder (ADHD). Mol Psychiatry 2000; 5:537–541.
32. Bhagavan HN, Coleman M, Coursin DB. The effect of pyridoxine hydrochloride on blood serotonin and pyridoxal phosphate contents in hyperactive children. Pediatrics 1975;55:437–441.
33. Coleman M. Serotonin concentrations in whole blood of hyperactive children. J Pediatrics 1971;78:985–990.
34. Spivak B, Vered Y, Yoran-Hegesh R, et al. Circulatory levels of catacholamines, serotonin and lipids in attention deficity hyperactivity disorder. Acta Psychiatr Scand 1999;88:300–304.
35. Barrickman L, Noyes R, Kuperman S, Schumacher E, Verda M. Treatment of ADHD with fluoxetine: a preliminary trial. J Am Acad Child Adolesc Psychiatry 1991;30:762–767.
36. Ruotsalainen S, Sirvio J, Jakala P, Puumala T, MacDonald E, Riekkinen P Sr. Differential effects of three 5-HT receptor antagonists on the performance of rats in attentional and working memory tasks. Eur Neuropsychopharmacol 1997;7:99–108.
37. Puumala T, Sirvio J. Changes in activities of dopamine and serotonin systems in the frontal cortex underlie poor choice accuracy and impulsivity of rats in an attention task. Neuroscience 1998;83:489–499.
38. Barr CL, Wigg K, Zai G, et al. Attention-deficit hyperactivity disorder and the adrenergic receptors α1C and α2C. Mol Psychiatry 2001;6:334–337.
39. Arnsten AF, Steere JC, Hunt RD. The contribution of alpha 2-noradrenergic mechanisms of prefrontal cortical cognitive function. Potential significance for attention-deficit hyperactivity disorder. Arch Gen Psychiatry 1996;53:448–455.
40. Wang Y, Xu F, Gainetdinov P, Caron M. Genetic approaches to studying norepinephrine function: knockout of mouse norepinephrine transporter gene. Biol Psychiatry 1999;46:1124–1130.
41. Aston-Jones G, Rajkowski J, Cohen J. Role of locus coeruleus in attention and behavioral flexibility. Biol Psychiatry 1999;46:1309–1320.

42. Davids E, Zhang K, Kula NS, Tarazi FI, Baldessarini RJ. Effects of norepinephrine and serotonin transporter inhibitors on hyperactivity induced by neonatal 6-hydroxydopamine lesioning in rats. J Pharmacol Exp. Ther 2002;301:1097–1102.
43. Popper CW. Pharmacological alternatives to psychostimulants for the treatment of attention-deficit/hyperactivity disorder. Child Adolesc Psychiatr Clin N Am 2000;3:605–646.
44. Biederman J, Spencer T. Attention-deficit/hyperactivity disorder (ADHD) as a noradrenergic disorder. Biol Psychiatry 1999;46:1234–1242.
45. Volkow ND, Wang GJ, Fowler JS, Gatley SJ, Logan J, Ding YS. Dopamine transporter occupancies in the human brain induced by therapeutic doses of oral methylphenidate. Am J Psychiatry 1998;155:1325–1331.
46. Seeman P, Madras BK. Anti-hyperactivity medication: methylphenidate and amphetamine. Mol Psychiatry 1998;3:386–396.
47. Vandenberg DJ, Persico AM, Hawkins AL, et al. Human dopamine transporter gene (DAT1) maps to chromosome 5p15.3 and displays a VNTR. Genomics 1992;14:1104–1106.
48. Sano A, Kondoh K, Kakimoto Y, Kondo I. A 40-nucleotide repeat polymorphism in the human dopamine transporter gene. Hum Genet 1993;91:405–406.
49. Min Kang A, Palmatier MA, Kidd KK. Global variation of a 40-bp VNTR in the 3′-untranslated region of the dopamine transporter gene (SLC6A3). Biol Psychiatry 1999;46:151–160.
50. Cook EH, Stein MA, Krasowski MD, et al. Association of attention-deficit disorder and the dopamine transporter gene. Am J Hum Genet 1995;56:993–998.
51. Gill M, Daly G, Heron S, Hawi Z, Fitzgerald M. Confirmation of association between attention deficit hyperactivity disorder and a dopamine transporter polymorphism. Mol Psychiatry 1997;2:311–313.
52. Daly G, Hawi Z, Fitzgerald M, Gill M. Mapping susceptibility loci in attention deficit hyperactivity disorder: preferential transmission of parental alleles at DAT1, DBH and DRD5 to affected children. Mol Psychiatry 1999;4:192–196.
53. Kirley A, Hawi Z, Daly G, et al. Dopaminergic system genes in ADHD: towards a biological hypothesis. Neuropsychopharmacology 2002;27:607–619.
54. Waldman ID, Rowe DC, Abramowitz A, et al. Association and linkage of the dopamine transporter gene and attention-deficit hyperactivity disorder in children: Heterogeneity owing to diagnostic subtype and severity. Am J Hum Genet 1998;63:1767–1776.
55. Barr CL, Xu C, Kroft J, et al. Haplotype study of three polymorphisms at the dopamine transporter locus confirm linkage to attention-deficit/hyperactivity disorder. Biol Psychiatry 2001;49:333–339.
56. Curran S, Mill J, Tahir E, et al. Association study of a dopamine transporter polymorphism and attention deficit hyperactivity disorder in UK and Turkish samples. Mol Psychiatry 2001;6:425–428.
57. Asherson P, Virdee V, Curran S, et al. Association study of DSM IV attention deficit hyperactivity disorder (ADHD) and monoamine pathway genes. Am J Med Genet Neuropsychiatr Genet 1998;81:549.
58. Palmer CG, Bailey JN, Ramsey C, et al. No evidence of linkage or linkage disequilibrium between DAT1 and attention deficit hyperactivity disorder in a large sample. Psychiatr Genet 1999;9:157–160.
59. Holmes J, Payton A, Barrett JH, et al. Family-based and case control association study of the dopamine D4 receptor gene and dopamine transporter gene in attention deficit hyperactivity disorder. Mol Psychiatry 2000;5:523–530.
60. Swanson JM, Flodman P, Kennedy J, et al. Dopamine genes and ADHD. Neurosci Biobehav Rev 2000;24:21–25.
61. Lunetta KL, Faraone SV, Biederman J, Laird NM. Family-based tests of association and linkage that use unaffected sibs, covariates, and interactions. Am J Hum Genet 2000;66:605–614.
62. Roman T, Schmitz M, Polanczyk G, Eizirik M, Rohde LA, Hutz MH. Attention-deficit hyperactivity disorder: a study of association with both the dopamine transporter gene and the dopamine D4 receptor gene. Am J Med Genet Neuropsychiatr Genet 2001;105:471–478.

63. Todd RD, Jong YI, Lobos EA, Reich W, Heath AC, Neuman RJ. No association of the dopamine transporter gene 3′ VNTR polymorphism with ADHD subtypes in a population sample of twins. Am J Med Genet Neuropsychiatr Genet 2001;105:745–748.
64. Muglia P, Jain U, Inkster B, Kennedy J. A quantitative trait locus analysis of the dopamine transporter gene in adults with ADHD. Neuropsychopharmacology 2002;27:655–662.
65. Maher BS, Marazita ML, Ferrell RE, Vanyukov MM. Dopamine system genes and attention deficit hyperactivity disorder: a meta-analysis. Psychiatr Genet 2002;12:207–215.
66. LaHoste GL, Swanson JM, Wigal SB, et al. Dopamine D4 receptor gene polymorphism is associated with attention deficit hyperactivity disorder. Mol Psychiatry 1996;1:121–124.
67. Swanson JM, Sunohara GA, Kennedy JL, et al. Association of the dopamine receptor D4 (DRD4) gene with a refined phenotype of attention deficit hyperactivity disorder (ADHD): a family-based approach. Mol Psychiatry 1998;3:38–41.
68. Smalley SL, Bailey JN, Palmer CG, et al. Evidence that the dopamine D4 receptor is a susceptibility gene in attention deficit. Mol Psychiatry 1998;3:427–430.
69. Rowe DC, Stever C, Giendinghagen LN, et al. Dopamine DRD4 receptor polymorphism and attention deficit hyperactivity disorder. Mol Psychiatry 1998;3:419–426.
70. Faraone SV, Biederman J, Weiffenbach B, et al. Dopamine D4 gene 7-repeat allele and attention deficit hyperactivity disorder. Am J Psychiatry 1999;156:768–770.
71. Barr CL, Wigg KG, Bloom S, et al. Further evidence from haplotype analysis for linkage of the dopamine D4 receptor gene and attention deficit hyperactivity disorder. Am J Med Genet 2000; 96:262–267.
72. Muglia P, Jain U, Macciardi F, Kennedy JL. Adult attention deficit hyperactivity disorder and the dopamine D4 receptor gene. Am J Med Genet 2000;96:273–277.
73. Holmes J, Payton A, Barrett JH, et al. Family-based and case control association study of the dopamine D4 receptor gene and dopamine transporter gene in attention deficit hyperactivity disorder. Mol Psychiatry 2000;5:523–530.
74. Sunohara GA, Roberts W, Malone M, et al. Linkage of the dopamine D4 receptor gene and attention-deficit/hyperactivity disorder. J Am Acad Child Adolesc Psychiatry 2000;39:1537–1542.
75. Tahir E, Yazgan Y, Cirakoglu B, Ozbay F, Waldman I, Asherson PJ. Association and linkage of DRD4 and DRD5 with attention deficit hyperactivity disorder (ADHD) in a sample of Turkish children. Mol Psychiatry 2000;5:396–404.
76. Mill J, Curran S, Kent L, et al. Attention deficit hyperactivity disorder (ADHD) and the dopamine D4 receptor gene: evidence of association but no linkage in a UK sample. Mol Psychiatry 2001;6:440–444.
77. Castellanos FX, Lau E, Tayebi N, et al. Lack of association between a dopamine-4 receptor polymorphism and attention deficit hyperactivity disorder: genetic and brain morphometric analyses. Mol Psychiatry 1998;3:431–434.
78. Comings DE, Gonzalez N, Wu S, et al. Studies of the 48 bp repeat polymorphism of the DRD4 gene in impulsive, compulsive, addictive behaviors: Tourette syndrome, ADHD, pathological gambling, and substance abuse. Am J Med Genet Neuropsychiatr Genet 1999;20,88:358–368.
79. Eisenberg J, Zohar A, Mei-Tal G. A haplotype relative risk study of the dopamine D4 (DRD4) exon III repeat polymorphism and attention deficit hyperactivity disorder (ADHD). Am J Med Genet 2000;96:258–261.
80. Hawi Z, McCarron M, Kirley A, Fitzgerald M, Gill M. No association of the dopamine DRD4 receptor with attention deficit hyperactivity disorder (ADHD) in the Irish population. Am J Med Genet Neuropsychiatr Genet 2000;96:268–272.
81. Kotler M, Manor I, Sever Y, et al. Failure to replicate an excess of the long dopamine D4 exon III repeat polymorphism in ADHD in a family-based study. Am J Med Genet 2000;96:278–281.
82. Todd RD, Neuman RJ, Lobos EA, Jong YJ, Reich W, Heath AC. Lack of association of dopamine D4 receptor gene polymorphisms with ADHD subtypes in a population sample of twins. Am J Med Genet Neuropsychiatr Genet 2001;105:432–438.

83. Faraone SV, Doyle AE, Mick E, Biederman J. Meta-analysis of the association between the dopamine D4 7-repeat allele and attention deficit hyperactivity disorder. Am J Psychiatry 2001;158:1052–1057.
84. Barr CL, Wigg KG, Feng Y, et al. Attention-deficit hyperactivity disorder and the gene for the dopamine D5 receptor. Mol Psychiatry 2000;5:548–551.
85. Payton A, Holmes J, Barrett JH, et al. Examining for association between candidate gene polymorphisms in the dopamine pathway and attention-deficit hyperactivity disorder: a family-based study. Am J Med Genet 2001;105:464–470.
86. Lowe N, Kirley A, Hawi Z, et al. Joint analysis of DRD5 marker concludes association with ADHD confined to the predominantly inattentive and combined subtypes. Am J Hum Gen 2004;74:348–356.
87. Eisenberg J, Mei-Tal G, Steinberg A, et al. Haplotype relative risk study of catechol-O-methyltransferase (COMT) and attention deficit hyperactivity disorder (ADHD): association of the high-enzyme activity Val allele with ADHD impulsive-hyperactive phenotype. Am J Med Genet 1999;15,88:497–502.
88. Barr CL, Wigg K, Malone M, Schachar R, Tannock R, Roberts W, Kennedy JL. Linkage study of catechol-*O*-methyltransferase and attention-deficit hyperactivity disorder. Am J Med Genet Neuropsychiatr Genet 1999;88:710–713.
89. Hawi Z, Millar N, Daly G, Fitzgerald M, Gill M. No association between catechol-*O*-methyltransferase (COMT) gene polymorphism and attention deficit hyperactivity disorder (ADHD) in an Irish sample. Am J Med Genet Neuropsychiatr Genet 2000;96:282–284.
90. Tahir E, Curran S, Yazgan Y, Ozbay F, Cirakoglu B, Asherson PJ. No association between low- and high-activity catecholamine-methyl-transferase (COMT) and attention deficit hyperactivity disorder (ADHD) in a sample of Turkish children. Am J Med Genet 2000;96:285–288.
91. Manor I, Kotler M, Sever Y, et al. Failure to replicate an association between the catechol-*O*-methyltransferase polymorphism and attention deficit hyperactivity disorder in a second, independently recruited Israeli cohort. Am J Med Genet 2000;96:858–860.
92. Roman T, Schmitz M, Polanczyk GV, Eizirik M, Rohde LA, Hutz MH. Further evidence for the association between attention-deficit/hyperactivity disorder and the dopamine-α-hydroxylase gene. Am J Med Genet (Neuropsych Genet) 2002;114:154–158.
93. Wigg K, Zai G, Schachar R, et al. Attention deficit hyperactivity disorder and the gene for dopamine beta-hydroxylase. Am J Psychiatry 2002;159:1046–1048.
94. Wilson MC. Coloboma mouse mutant as an animal model of hyperkinesis and attention deficit hyperactivity disorder. Neurosci Behav Rev 2000; 24:51–55.
95. Barr CL, Feng Y, Wigg K, et al. Identification of DNA variants in the SNAP-25 gene and linkage study of these polymorphisms and attention-deficit hyperactivity disorder. Mol Psychiatry 2000;5:405–409.
96. Brophy K, Hawi Z, Kirley A, Fitzgerald M, Gill M. Synaptosomal-associated protein 25 (SNAP-25) and attention deficit hyperactivity disorder (ADHD): evidence of linkage and association in the Irish population. Mol Psychiatry 2002;7:913–917.
97. Kustanovich V, Merriman B, McGough J, McCracken JT, Smalley SL, Nelson SF. Biased paternal transmission of SNAP-25 risk alleles in attention-deficit hyperactivity disorder. Mol Psychiatry 2003;8:309–315.
98. Mill J, Curran S, Kent L, et al. Association study of a SNAP-25 microsatellite and attention deficit hyperactivity disorder. Am J Med Genet (Neuropsych Genet) 2003;114:269–271.
99. Manor I, Eisenberg J, Tyrano S, et al. Family based association study of the serotonin transporter promoter region polymorphism (5-HTTLPR) in attention deficit hyperactivity disorder. Am J Med Genet 2001;105:91–95.
100. Seeger G, Schloss P, Schmidt MH. Functional polymorphism within the promoter of the serotonin transporter gene is associated with severe hyperkinetic disorder. Mol Psychiatry 2001;6:235–238.
101. Kent L, Doerry U, Hardy E, et al. N. A family based association study of three serotonin transporter polymorphisms in attention deficit hyperactivity disorder (ADHD). Mol Psychiatry 2002;7:908–912.

102. Zoroglu SS, Erdal ME, Alasehirli, et al. Significance of serotonin transporter gene 5-HTTLPR and variable number of tandem repeat polymorphism in attention deficit hyperactivity disorder. Neuropsychobiology 2002;45:176–181.
103. Brunner D, Buhot MC, Hen R, Hofer M. Anxiety, motor activation and maternal-infant interactions in 5HT 1B knockout mice. Behav Neurosci 1999;113:587–601.
104. Hawi Z, Dring M, Kirley A. et al. Serotonergic system and attention deficit hyperactivity disorder (ADHD), a potential susceptibility locus at the 5-HT(1B) receptor gene in 273 nuclear families from a multicentre sample. Mol Psychiatry 2002;7:718–725.
105. Quist JF, Barr CL, Schachar R. et al. The serotonin 5-HT 1B receptor gene and attention deficit hyperactivity disorder. Mol Psychiatry 2003;8:98–102.
106. Quist JF, Barr CL, Schachar R. et al. Evidence for the serotonin HTR2A receptor gene as a susceptibility factor in attention deficit hyperactivity disorder (ADHD). Mol Psychiatry 2000;5:537–541.
107. O'Neill MF, Hearon-Maxwell CI, Shaw G. 5-HT2 receptor antagonism reduces hyperactivity induced by amphetamine, cocaine and MK-801 but not D1 agonist C-APB. Pharm Biochem Behav 1999;63:237–243.
108. Levitan RD, Masellis M, Basile VS. et al. Polymorphism of the serotonin-2A receptor gene (HTR2A) associated with childhood attention deficit hyperactivity disorder (ADHD) in adult women with seasonal affective disorder. J. Affect Disorder 2002;71:229–233.
109. Zoroglu SS, Erdal ME, Erdal N, Ozen S, Lashirli B, Sivasli E. No evidence for an association between the T102c and 1438 G/A polymorphisms of the serotonin 2A receptor gene in attention deficit hyperactivity disorder in a Turkish population. Neuropsychobiology 2003;47:17–20.
110. Barr CL, Kroft J, Feng Y, et al. The epinephrine transporter gene and attention-deficit hyperactivity disorder. Am J Med Genet 2002;114:255–259.
111. McEvoy B, Hawi Z, Fitzgerald M, Gill M. No evidence of linkage or association between the norepinephrine transporter (NET) gene polymorphisms and ADHD in the Irish population. Am J Med Genet 2002;114:665–666.
112. Xu C, Schachar R, Tannock R, et al. Linkage study of the α2A adrenergic receptor in attention-deficit hyperactivity disorder families. Am J Med Genet 2001;105:159–162.
113. Barr CL, Wigg K, Zai G, et al. Attention deficit hyperactivity disorder and the adrenergic receptors α1C and α2C. Mol Psychiatry 2001;6:334–337.
114. Suarez BK, Hampe CL, Van Eerdewegh P. Problems of replicating linkage claims in psychiatry. Anal Gen Data 1998;23–46.
115. Tannock R. Attention deficit hyperactivity disorder: advances in cognitive, neurobiological and genetic research. J Child Psychol Psychiatr 1998;39:65–99.
116. Faraone SV, Biederman J. Pathophysiology of ADHD. In: Davis K, Charney D, Coyle JT, Nemeroff C, eds. Psychopharmacology: the fifth generation of progress, version 2. New York: Lippincott, Williams and Wilkins 2002.
117. Curran S, Mill J, Sham P, Rijsdijk F, Marusic K, Taylor E, Asherson P. QTL association analysis of the DRD4 exon 3 VNTR polymorphism in a population sample of children screened with a parent rating scale for ADHD symptoms. Am J Med Genet Neuropsychiatr Genet 2001;105:387–393.
118. Mill J, Caspi A, McClay J, et al. The dopamine D4 receptor and the hyperactivity phenotype: a developmental-epidemiological study. Mol Psychiatry 2002;7:383–391.
119. Todd RD, Neuman RJ, Lobos EA, Jong YJ, Reich W, Heath AC. Lack of association of dopamine D4 receptor gene polymorphisms with ADHD subtypes in a population sample of twins. Am J Med Genet Neuropsychiatr Genet 2001;105:432–438.
120. Barkley RA, Fischer M, Edelbrook, C, Smallish L. The adolescent outcome of hyperactive children diagnosed by research criteria: III. Mother-child interactions, family conflicts and maternal psychopathology. J Child Psychol Psychiatry 1991;32:233–255.
121. Faraone SV, Biederman J, Keenan K, Tsuang MT. Separation of DSM-III attention deficit disorder and conduct disorder: evidence from a family-genetic study of American child psychiatric patients. Psychol Med 1991;21:109–121.

122. Frick PJ, Lahey BB, Christ MG, Green S. History of childhood behaviour problems in biological relatives of boys with attention deficit hyperactivity disorder and conduct disorder. J Clin Child Psychol 1991;20:445–451.
123. Szatmari P, Boyle M, Offord D. Familial aggregation of emotional and behavioural problems of childhood in the general population. Am J Psychiatry 1993;150:1398–1403.
124. Wosniak J, Biederman J, Mundy E, Mennin D, Faraone SV. A pilot family study of childhood-onset mania. J Am Acad Child Adolesc Psychiatry 1995;34:1577–1583.
125. Silberg J, Rutter M, Meyer J, et al. Genetic and environmental influences on the covariation between hyperactivity and conduct disturbance in juvenile twins. J Child Psychol Psychiatry 1996;37:803–816.
126. Lahey BB, Piacentini JC, McBurnett K, Stone P, Hartdagen S, Hynd G. Psychopathology in the parents of children with conduct disorder and hyperactivity. J Am Acad Child Adolesc Psychiatry 1988;27:163–170.
127. Lahey BB, Russo MF, Walker JL. Personality characteristics of the mothers of children with disruptive behaviour disorders. J Consult Clin Psychol 1989;57:512–515.
128. Faraone SV, Biederman J. Neurobiology of attention-deficit hyperactivity disorder. Biol Psychiatry 1998;44:951–958.
129. Faraone SV. Genetics of childhood disorders: XX. ADHD, part 4: Is ADHD genetically heterogeneous? J Am Acad Child Adolesc Psychiatry 2000;39:1455–1457.
130. Smalley SL, McCracken J, McGough J. Refining the ADHD phenotype using affected sibling pair families. Am J Med Genet Neuropsychiatr Genet 2001;105:31–33.
131. Kuntsi J, Stevenson J. Psychological mechanisms in hyperactivity: II. The role of genetic factors. J Child Psychol Psychiatry 2001;42:211–219.
132. Thapar A, Harrington R, McGuffin P. Examining the comorbidity of ADHD related behaviours and conduct problems using a twin study design. B J Psychiatry 2001;179:224–229.
133. Holmes J, Hever T, Hewitt L, et al. A pilot twin study of psychological measures of attention deficit hyperactivity disorder. Behaviour Genetic 2002;32:389–395.
134. Rowe DC, Stever C, Chase D, Sherman S, Abramowitz A, Waldman ID. Two dopamine genes related to reports of childhood retrospective inattention and conduct disorder symptoms. Mol Psychiatry 2001;6:429–433.
135. Goodman R, Stevenson J. A twin study of hyperactivity: II. The aetiological role of genes, family relationships and perinatal adversity. J Child Psychol Psychiatr 1989;30:691–709.
136. Langley K, Marshall L, van den Bree M, et al. Association of the dopamine D4 receptor gene 7-repeat allele with neuropsychological test performance of children with ADHD. Am J Psychiatry 2004;161:134–138.
137. Fisher SE, Francks C, McCracken JT, et al. A genomewide scan for loci involved in attention-deficit/hyperactivity disorder. Am J Hum Genet 2002;70:1183–1196.
138. Bakker SC, van der Meulen EM, Buitelaar JK, et al. A whole-genome scan in 164 Dutch sib pairs with attention-deficit/hyperactivity disorder: suggestive evidence for linkage on chromosomes 7p and 15q. Am J Hum Genet 2003;72:1251–1260.
139. Fuke S, Suo S, Takahashi N, Koike H, Sasagawa N, Ishiura S. The VNTR polymorphism of the human dopamine transporter (DAT1) gene affects gene expression. Pharmacogen Journal 2001;1:152–156.
140. Mill J, Asherson P, Browes C, D'Souza U, Craig I. Expression of the dopamine transporter gene is regulated by the 3′ UTR VNTR: evidence from brain and lymphocytes using quantitative RT-PCR. Am J Med Genet Neuropsychiatr Genet 2002;114:975–979.
141. Miller GM, Madras BK. Polymorphisms in the 3′-untranslated region of human and monkey dopamine transporter genes affect reporter gene expression. Mol Psychiatry 2002;7:44–55.

3
Dopamine Knockouts and Behavior

Davide Viggiano, Daniela Vallone, Lucia A. Ruocco, and Adolfo G. Sadile

1. INTRODUCTION

The expression of behavior is regulated by complex cortical neural networks. These interact with several telencephalic structures, such as the basal ganglia, amygdala complex, and hippocampal cortex. All these systems are modulated by subcortical influences (*see* ref. *1*), represented by cholinergic neurons of Meynert's basal nucleus, dopamine (DA) neurons in the ventral tegmental area (VTA), serotonergic neurons in the raphe nuclei, norepinephrine neurons in the locus coeruleus, and histamine neurons in the posterior hypothalamus.

Each subsystem is involved in different aspects of behavioral performance—e.g., accuracy for acetylcholine (Ach), latency for DA, impulsivity for serotonin, and distractability for norepinephrine (*2, see also* Chapter 5).

Moreover, the involvement of DA in behavior is also supported by neuropsychiatric disorders, such as schizophrenia, manic-depressive psychosis, and attention deficit hyperactivity disorder (ADHD).

2. DOPAMINE FUNCTIONS

DA is a slow-acting neurotransmitter utilized in the mammalian central nervous system. DA functions include regulation of blood pressure, movements, goal-directed behavior, cognition, attention, and reward. Dysregulation of DA systems has been associated to several neuropsychiatric disorders such as Parkinson's disease (PD), which is caused by a selective degeneration of mesostriatal (MS) DA neurons, and schizophrenia and ADHD, which are both associated with a dysfunction of mesocorticolimbic (MCL) neurons. In fact, most antipsychotic drugs used in schizophrenia act as DA receptor (DAR) antagonists, whereas ADHD symptoms are generally alleviated by drugs that regulate Dopaminergic (DAergic) transmission.

Moreover, drugs of abuse, such as cocaine, amphetamine, opiates, nicotine, and alcohol, show addictive action by modifying DA neurotransmission *(3–5)*.

Finally, DA projections to the nucleus accumbens and frontal cortex have been shown by many studies to be involved in the mediation of reward, motivation, consummatory behavior, and learning *(3,6–10)*.

From: *Attention Deficit Hyperactivity Disorder: From Genes to Patients*
Edited by: D. Gozal and D. L. Molfese © Humana Press Inc., Totowa, NJ

3. BRAIN DA SYSTEMS

The majority of the cell bodies of DA neurons are grouped in two nuclei, named substantia nigra and VTA, or numbered from A8 to A10 in the caudolateral to rostromedial direction, all of which are located in the ventroanterior midbrain *(11)*. Their axons topographically project to the caudate nucleus and putamen (dorsal striatum, CPu), to the ventral striatum including nucleus accumbens, and to most areas of the neocortex, especially the prefrontal cortex (PFC) *(12)*.

The classical description of the MS system consisted of a projection originating in the pars compacta of the substantia nigra (A9 cell group) and the retrorubral field (A8 cell group) and terminating in the CPu.

DA terminals in the CPu synapse mainly on γ-aminobutyric acid (GABA) medium spiny neurons *(11,13,14)*, which represent the major output of this system.

In this region, DA D2 receptors (D2Rs) are expressed both postsynaptically, on striatal medium spiny neurons, as well as presynaptically, on DAergic nerve terminals originating in the substantia nigra pars compacta.

Two different pathways have been described, originating from striatal neurons expressing D1 (named direct pathway) or D2 (indirect pathway) receptors. They are anatomically and functionally independent, though substantial revisions to this model have been proposed, as well as the anatomical strict segregation of the DARs.

Another level of CPu organization consists of a patch- or striosome-like nonhomogeneous DA innervation that is surrounded by a later-developing, diffuse matrix innervation.

On the other hand, DA neurons in the VTA project mainly to the ventral striatum (nucleus accumbens and olfactory tubercle complex) and to the PFC, giving rise to the mesolimbic (ML) and mesocortical branches of the MCL system.

In fact, the medial ML system is primarily derived from the A10 neurons situated in the VTA from where axons arrive to the ventral striatum and PFC *(12,15)*. However, a strict anatomical separation between ML and MS systems does not exist because DA efferents from both the substantia nigra and VTA overlap in a large ventral and medial segment of the CPu *(15)*.

The ML DA system synapses on the shafts of the dendritic spines of medium spiny GABA neurons of nucleus accumbens *(16)*, whereas glutamate inputs from a variety of cortical sources synapse on the heads of the same spines *(17)*.

An increased DA release has been shown in the nucleus accumbens during behavioral activation *(18)*; previous studies investigated the involvement of the MCL and MS DA systems in the control of activity, orienting, scanning times toward environmental stimuli, and emotional reactivity in mouse model systems.

Anatomical, functional, and neurochemical evidence all justify the division of the nucleus accumbens in a rostral area, termed pole, a dorsocaudal area (accumbens core) and a ventrocaudal component (accumbens shell).

No anatomical separation exists between the accumbens core and the CPu; they are anatomically continuous, and both show a patch–matrix organization. Conversely, the border between core and shell can be rapidly recognized using immunohistochemical markers, such as substance P (SP), calbindin, neurotensin, or enkephalin.

Moreover, the core and shell connections are very different. The core region is involved in a corticostriatal circuitry to parts of the frontal lobe, and its enkephalin-ir cells have reciprocal connections with the VTA (*see* ref. *19*).

The shell has a complex organization and could be included in a loop comprising the dorsal PFC, the lateral ventral pallidum and substantia nigra.

Mesencephalic (mes) VTA DA neurons receive glutamate inputs mainly from the frontal cortex and lead to reward effects, as demonstrated by electrical and pharmacological stimulation with phenciclidin of glutamate frontal neurons *(17,20–22)*.

Other psychostimulants, such as amphetamine and cocaine, when injected into the nucleus accumbens, are rewarding as they induce self-administration and place preference behavior by interaction with presynaptic ML DA terminals *(23–26)*. In addition, opiates are also self-rewarding into the VTA by acting on μ and Δ receptors, probably through disinhibition of GABAergic interneurons *(27–31)*.

4. ONTOGENESIS

The mesDA system is specified in the embryonic ventral midbrain around embryonic day 12 (E12) in the mouse. The specification of neurotransmitter identity and appropriate integration in the developing brain depend on molecular differentiation cascades and on the commitment of this region signals from organizers surrounding the ventral midbrain progenitor neurons *(32–34)* (for a review, *see* ref. *35*).

Early organizers of general patterning and development of the ventral midbrain require the orchestration of a number of genes, such as *Engrailed1 (36,37)*, *Engrailed2 (38)*, *Pax2 (39)*, *Pax5 (40)*, *Wnt1 (36)*, *Shh (41)*, and *Fgf8 (33,34)*. *Ptx3* and *Nurr1*, two transcription factors, are implicated in specification of the mesDA system. The homeobox gene *Ptx3*, whose expression in the brain is restricted to mesDA neurons *(42)*, and the orphan nuclear hormone receptor *Nurr1*, are in fact required for induction of the enzyme tyrosine hydroxylase, which catalyzes the initial step in DA biosynthesis *(43,44)*. Recently the LIM class homeobox gene *Lmx1b* has been shown to take part in this phenomenon *(45)*.

The projection of DA neurons to the target site and the induction of DARs on postsynaptic sites are both complex events.

The specification of dopaminergic pathways is thought to require at least the action of a class of genes, such as ephrins *(46)*. It is interesting to note that the expression of such genes continues throughout life and can change after cocaine treatment *(46)*.

On the other side, the specification of DAR subclasses appears to be at least in part independent of the synthesis of DA itself, as suggested by knockout (KO) studies (*see* Heading 7).

5. THYROSINE HYDROXYLASE

The modulating effects of DA on locomotor activity and cognitive performance have been recently studied by knocking out the thyrosine hydroxylase (*TH*) gene, the rate-limiting enzyme in catecholamine (DA and norepinephrine [NE]) synthesis, thus giving rise to DA and NE KO mice *(47,48)*. These mice survive embryogenesis, but die at 3 to 4 wk of age because of the severe hypoactivity/hypophagic behavior. However, the synthesis of NE can be normalized by transgenic expression of TH under the control of the DA-β-hydroxylase promoter. This pure DA KO mouse survives, displays normal norepinephrine synthesis, but makes no DA *(49)*. Mice lacking DA are severely hypoactive. This supports the hypothesis that activation of the DA systems influences locomotor activity *(48)*.

The same DA KO mice displayed an enhanced behavioral response to D1-like or D2-like receptor agonists owing to hypersensitive, long-loop feedback pathways. The expression of D1-like and D2-like receptors, in fact, was normal in the DA KO striatum. The observations suggest that DA is not required during embryonic and postnatal development for adequate expression of D1-like and D2-like receptors *(48)*.

6. DOPAMINE TRANSPORTER

The dopamine transporter (DAT) is a membrane transporter that clears DA from the synaptic cleft. This is also the main mechanism for clearance of released DA *(50,51)*. DAT represents the major target for amphetamine and methylphenidate, the main pharmacological treatments for ADHD *(52)*. DAT is expressed on presynaptic DA terminals, and can be used as specific marker for DA fibers.

An association between ADHD and polymorphisms in the *DAT* gene has been reported *(53–55)*.

The DAT KO displays hyperactivity *(56)*, which is likely to be owing to higher levels of brain DA, because of the absence of the clearance of DA from the synaptic cleft. Moreover, DAT KO mice reduce hyperactivity after treatment with psychostimulants, although they lack the DAergic target of psychostimulants. This suggest that psychostimulants, such as methylphenidate, could improve ADHD symptoms acting on non-DA sites, such as the serotonin (5 HT) system.

Behavioral analysis in the DAT KO is complicated by the growth-retardation phenotype *(57)*. In fact, these mice show anterior pituitary hypoplasia, dwarfism, lactation deficits, and high mortality *(57)*.

Therefore, a mutant mouse with a decreased DAT level (knockdown) has been developed *(58)*. These mice express 10% of wild-type DAT levels (DAT knockdown), and are in a chronic state of hyper-DAergic activity. Moreover, they do not display the growth-retardation phenotype.

From the behavioral point of view, DAT knockdown mice have normal basal activity but become hyperactive in novel environments. Therefore, hyperactivity may be related to increased responses to novelty *(59)*, decreased habituation *(60–63)*, and higher motivational state.

It is still highly controversial whether ADHD is characterized by a hyper-DAergic or hypo-DAergic transmission *(52)*. Consistent with the hyper-DA hypothesis, hyperactivity is usually related to a hyper-DAergic state *(64,65)*. Furthermore, recent studies in ADHD patients have found a positive correlation between high DA metabolite homovanillic acid (HVA) levels and hyperactivity *(66,67)*. DAT knockdown and KO mice *(56)* support the hyper-DA hypothesis.

The hypo-DAergic hypothesis of ADHD derives mainly from beneficial effects of psychostimulants (amphetamine and methylphenidate), which enhance DAergic transmission, in improving ADHD symptoms *(52)*. However, DAT KO mice provide potential explanations for the calming effect of psychostimulants. In DAT KO mice, psychostimulant inhibition of locomotor activity is, in fact, mediated by an increased release of serotonin *(56)*.

Moreover, all drugs (amphetamine, apomorphine, and quinpirole) that can activate DA D2 autoreceptors have a pronounced inhibitory effect on locomotor activity in DAT knockdown mice, whereas drugs that do not have an autoreceptor component (SKF-81297) have a less-pronounced stimulatory effect on locomotor activity. This suggests that the inhibitory effect of methylphenidate in ADHD may be the result of an altered balance between autoreceptor and heteroreceptor functions.

7. DA RECEPTORS

DA exerts its action on pre-, post-, and extrasynaptic receptors. Several excellent papers in the literature review the structure, function, and molecular biology of DARs (*see* ref. *68,69*). They can be subdivided into two subfamilies, the D1-like (D1 and D5 receptors [D1Rs and D5Rs]) and D2-like (D2Rs, D3, and D4 receptors [D3Rs and D4Rs]), distinguished on the basis of their structure and pharmacology *(70)*. The known DA receptors are members of the G protein-receptor family with seven hydrophobic domains, an extracellular N-terminus, and an intracellular C-terminus. In the second and third intracellular loops there are sequences for phosphorylation *(68)*.

D1-like receptors have been shown to couple the stimulation of adenylyl cyclase activity, whereas the D2-like subfamily can reduce cyclic adenosine monophosphate (cAMP) production as well as regulate the activity of various ion channels. Thus, the response to DA is mediated by the accumulation of a second messenger molecule, such as cAMP for the D1 class, which amplifies the signal by several orders of magnitude. The accumulation of cAMP regulates numerous enzymatic processes in neurons, e.g., activating protein kinase A, leading to phosphorylation and activation of calcium channels. At the moment, much evidence shows that D1Rs can also activate phospholipase C-phosphatidylinositol hydrolysis.

The D2-like class involves a different second messenger cascade. In particular, D2Rs mediate a phosphatidylinositol-linked mobilization of intracellular calcium (though differences exist between the isoforms L and S; *see* Subheading 7.2.); moreover, D2Rs are likely to regulate potassium currents by G protein mechanisms, and to increase the release of arachidonic acid.

Systemic administration of D1 but not D2 agonists induces enhanced expression of the immediate-early genes *c-fos* and *zif268* in the cerebral cortex and striatum. Concomitant D1Rs and D2Rs appear to produce a synergistic effect on *c-fos* expression. Further studies have given some insights on the mechanism of D1–D2 synergism. In fact, the D1R and D2R mRNAs have a wider distribution and are more expressed in the central nervous system (CNS) as compared with their pharmacologically related counterparts. This reflects the broader number of functions mediated by these receptors in the CNS, including the modulation of cognitive, sensorimotor, and neuroendocrine effects, as compared with more limited functions that may be mediated by the other DA receptor types.

The striatonigral GABA neurons preferentially express D1Rs, coexpress SP and dynorphin, and project to the entopeduncular nucleus and substantia nigra pars reticulata. D2Rs are, instead, segregated on GABA neurons containing enkephalin and projecting to the globus pallidus or function as autoreceptors on DA terminals (*see* Subheading 7.2. for a description of D2 isoforms). Similarly, in the accumbens D1-expressing cells are SP-positive, whereas D2-expressing ones are enkephalin- and neurotensin-positive. Therefore, segregation of D1 and D2 with different neuropeptides appears as good anatomical description, with few cells coexpressing D1Rs and D2Rs. However, D1Rs and D2Rs have recently been shown to colocalize in striatal medium spiny neurons *(71,72)*. This is in agreement with the evidence that rats do not self-administer either selective D1 or D2 agonists by themselves but do self-administer a mixture of the two *(73)*.

The DA release associated with behavioral activation *(18)* is regulated by presynaptic DA acting at D2 and D3 autoreceptors and by blockade of the firing of DA neurons in the VTA by DA D2 autoreceptors. This short-term regulation of DA release is also controlled by afferent excitatory and inhibitory inputs from a variety of different neural systems.

The D3R appears to act as inhibitor of cAMP production using a putative G_i protein. D3–D2 interactions are very complex (*see* Subheading 7.3.3. for a discussion from the behavioral point of view). For example, D3Rs in the accumbens shell activate neurotensin gene expression, whereas D2Rs in the accumbens pole inhibit neurotensin expression. Generally, D2Rs and D3Rs appear to be expressed in different locations.

D4R distribution differs markedly from that of D2 and D3. It appears to have a high affinity for clozapine, which has made its study exciting from the clinical point of view, because of clinical applications of clozapine in schizophrenic patients. The D4R has polymorphic forms in the human population, with certain polymorphisms being more represented in ADHD patients.

In the following sections, we analyze the distribution of DARs, along with functional aspects. Moreover, the problem of defining the functional role of each receptor subtype has been recently addressed using genetically altered animals lacking individual receptor subtypes. So far, mice lacking D1R, D2R, D3R, D4R, and D5Rs or some of their combinations have been produced *(74,75)*. In addition, KOs for DA transporter, thyrosine hydroxylase, and DA cyclic adenosine 3′, 5′-monophosphate–regulate phosphoprotein (DARPP32), all of which intervene in DA functions, have been created.

7.1. D1 Receptors

7.1.1. Cerebral Distribution

Numerous regions of the CNS express the D1R mRNA, such as both neocortical and palleo-cortical areas, with the highest levels of expression in the frontal, anterior cingulate, orbital, insular, piriform, and entorhinal cortex. In neocortical areas the D1R is localized predominantly in layers V and VI, which are known to be the receptive layers for DA projections. It is interesting to note here that all DA receptors are present in the PFC *(76,77)*, which receives DA projections. However, they are also expressed in other cortical areas that are apparently devoid of DA terminals, thus suggesting that other sources of DA may exist, such as norepinephrine terminals.

The D1R is also localized in the anterior olfactory nuclei, where an independent DA system has been largely described *(78,79)*.

More caudally, D1R mRNA expression is high within the rat striatum, in a subpopulation of medium spiny neurons expressing dynorphin and substance P and projecting to the substantia nigra pars reticulata *(72)*. A subpopulation of medium spiny neurons coexpresses SP, enkephalin, and both D1-type and D2-type DARs *(71,76)*; the projection of this subpopulation is not known.

Cellular expression of D1 mRNAs is also high in the accumbens shell and septal pole. Therefore, D1Rs could modulate cortical activity, providing a functional interaction between basal ganglia and the cerebral cortex *(80)*.

Cells expressing D1R mRNA are also localized in the dorsal division of the lateral septum and in the ventral hippocampus, mainly in the dentate gyrus.

D1 mRNA in the amygdaloid complex is expressed at high levels in the intercalated nuclei and at lower levels in basolateral, medial, central, and cortical nuclei. This exclusive localization might be important in alterations of motivational aspects of D1 KO mice, such as rearing frequency.

D1 is expressed widely in various thalamic (anterior dorsal, anterior ventral, centromedial, paracentral, ventromedial, ventrolateral, posterior nuclei, lateral habenula, and dorsolateral geniculate body) and hypothalamic (supraoptic, suprachiasmatic, paraventricular, and rostral arcuate) nuclei.

There are high levels of D1R binding in the substantia nigra pars reticulata, but not in the substantia nigra pars compacta or VTA. This is in agreement with the primary postsynaptic function of D1R.

In the hindbrain few nuclei express D1R, such as lateral parabrachial, facial nuclei, locus coeruleus, and dorsal raphe. The last two nuclei would suggest an involvement of D1R in the regulation of norepinephrine and serotonin systems.

Interestingly, high levels of D1 mRNA expression are observed in the granular cells of the cerebellum.

It is interesting to note that although D1Rs, D2Rs and D3Rs have been described in the rat cerebellum, no DA fibers have been detected in the same region (although a DA projection to the cerebellum has been suggested in humans). However, the cerebellum receives an important norepinephrine innervation (similarly to the cerebral cortex, *see* Subheading 7.1.1.). Moreover, alterations in cerebellar development have been suggested in ADHD children *(65)*.

7.1.2. Target Mutations

Animals lacking the D1R show an approx 30% reduced body weight and a smaller brain *(81)*. They show normal or increased locomotor activity when tested in a standard rat cage with photocells *(82–85)*. However, the rearing rate in these animals is strongly decreased *(81,84–86)*, as well as grooming sequences. The decrease in rearing frequency could indicate an alteration in motivational aspects of behavior.

Moreover, sniffing sequences did not differ from wild-type animals, in contrast with the effects of D1 anatagonists, which reduce both rearing and sniffing behaviors. Moreover, D1 agonists are known to increase locomotor activity.

There is also evidence of retarded habituation in several tasks in the same KO mice with a different genetic background, thus raising the problem of the interaction of phenotype with background genes *(84,86)*.

The effect of a different background on D1 KOs could be explained in terms of the basal state of the DA system. In fact, recent evidences show that the modulation of D1Rs using selective agonists or antagonists gives different results in normal rats and in hyper-DAergic, hyperactive rats or mice, such as the Naples High-Excitability (NHE) rats (*86a*). It is also possible that the D1 KO leads to compensatory changes or that the effects of D1Rs in the wild-type (WT) animal are interactive on a neural network basis. This issue remains to be resolved, perhaps by development of conditional postnatal D1R KO mice.

7.2. D2 Receptor

The activity of DA neurons in the midbrain is modulated by the release or exogenous DA, which interacts with a subclass of DA receptors that act as "autoreceptors" and belong to the D2R family *(87–99)*. They regulate the firing rate of DA neurons in the short term (depolarization block *[100]*).

These receptors are involved in the synthesis and release of pituitary hormones *(92,93,101)* and control of motor activity *(87–89)*.

DA D2Rs represent the major target of antipsychotic drugs and are involved in various neuropathological conditions, including PD, Tourette's syndrome, and drug addiction *(87,102,103)*.

By alternative splicing, the D2R gene encodes two molecularly distinct isoforms *(102)*, named long (D2L) and short (D2S) *(104)*. These isoforms differ by an insertion of 29 amino acids in the third intracellular loop of the D2L receptor, and are coexpressed in a ratio favoring the long isoform. D2L acts mainly at postsynaptic sites and D2S serves presynaptic autoreceptor functions *(29,98,105–107)*.

7.2.1. Cerebral Distribution

The limbic cortex (anterior cingulate, orbital, and insular) expresses high levels of D2R mRNA. Scattered positive cells are also present in layers IV–VI of the frontal, parietal, temporal, and occipital cortex.

D2 is present in the large cells of the globus pallidus and CPu. In fact, the D2-type receptors are largely restricted to a subpopulation of medium spiny neurons expressing enkephalin and projecting primarily to the pallidum *(108)*.

D2R is present from the dorsal lateral to the intermediate lateral septum, into the diagonal band of Broca, the dorsal and ventral hippocampus, lateral division of the central nucleus, and basomedial amygdala *(78)*.

Similarly, in the bed nucleus of the stria terminalis, zona incerta, the lateral preoptic area, anterior hypothalamic area, and lateral hypothalamus there is expression of D2R.

More caudally, D2R is detectable in the posterior division of the arcuate nucleus and lateral mammillary nuclei.

D2R in the midbrain and hindbrain is likely to be involved in autonomic functions and in the regulation of DA release. Here cells expressing D2R mRNA are detectable in the DAergic cells of the substantia nigra pars compacta, the VTA, and in the magnocellular cells of the red nucleus that are part of the rubrospinal pathway.

More dorsally, cells expressing D2R mRNA are localized in the intermediate and deep layers of the superior colliculus and in the periaqueductal gray, where they may be important in modulating analgesic responses. Morphine-induced analgesia could be related to D2R expressed in midbrain and pontine nuclei. In raphe nuclei D2R may serve to regulate serotonin release.

D2R mRNA is present in a number of brainstem nuclei (including the dorsal tegmental, lateral lemniscus, locus coeruleus, parabrachial, and trigeminal).

7.2.2. Target Mutations

D2L R KO *(93,98)* and the combined D2 L + S R *(88)* KO mice have been generated.

D2R-null mice (–/–) *(88,90)* have been studied in our laboratory, in collaboration with H. Westphal and E. Borrelli, in different behavioral paradigms. In particular, we have studied behavioral activation in novelty situations *(109)*.

The experimental system was a scaled-down Làt-maze (for a detailed protocol see ref. *109*). The dependent variables were the frequency of corner crossings (indexing traveled distance or locomotor activity) and the frequency and duration of rearings on hindlimbs and leanings against the walls (orienting frequency and nonselective attention).

D2R KO demonstrated fewer corner crossings than WT littermates (Fig. 1). In fact, when traveled distance was taken as the activity index, D2R mutants were less active than WT controls, in agreement with other experiences *(110,111)*.

D2R KO mice also showed a significant reduction in rearing frequency relative to the WT group.

Finally, D2R mutants increased scanning durations over time of testing, in comparison to WT controls, as assessed by regression analysis (Fig. 1). However, the heterozygotic D2R KO mice showed the highest score, and the homozygotes an intermediate score (Fig. 1), thus revealing a nonlinear relation between the number of normal alleles and the duration of rearings. Therefore, the D2R appears to be important in the modulation of the scanning phase of attention.

These data, in agreement with other findings *(88)*, suggest that D2Rs control activity, as D2R KO mice could represent an animal model of PD. The absence of depolarization block owing to the lack of mesencephalic autoreceptors in DA neurons is likely to increase DA release and subsensitivity of D1Rs. This leads to reduced firing of thalamocortical neurons. It is interesting to note that the lack of D2L as R subtype is able to reduce locomotor activity and

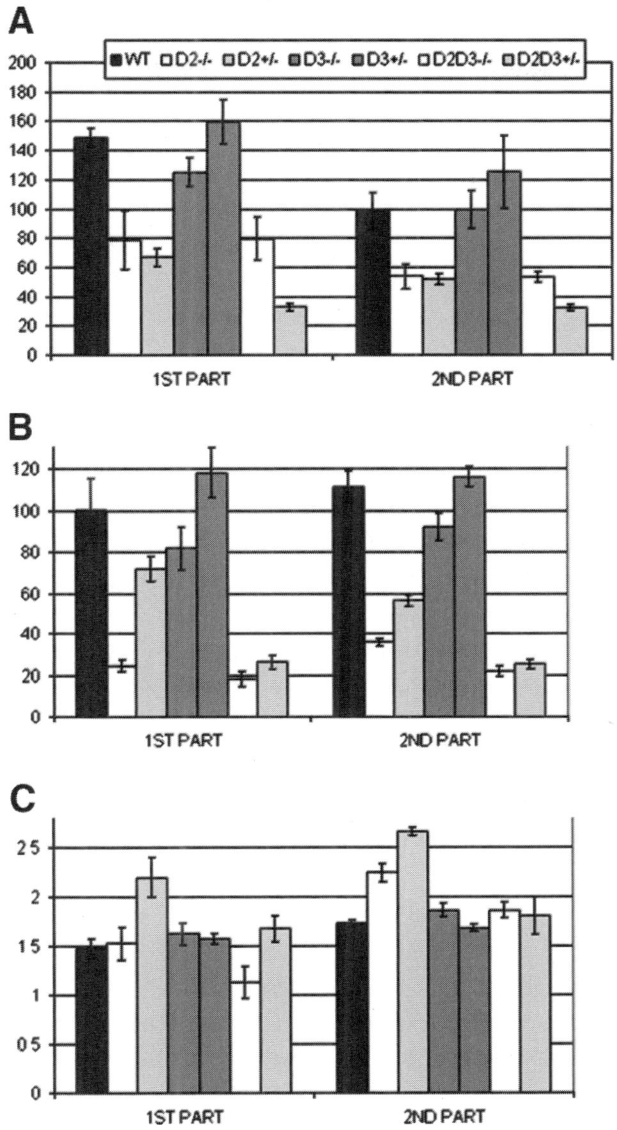

Fig. 1. Behavioral profile of D2, D3, and D2/D3 knockout (KO) mice derived from exposure to a spatial novelty. **(A)** Horizontal activity expressed as frequency of corner crossings indicating traveled distance. **(B)** Vertical activity expressed as frequency of rearing on hindlimbs, indicating orienting behavior toward environmental stimuli. **(C)** Nonselective attention indexed by the duration of individual rearing episodes that indicates scanning duration. Data are expressed as mean ± standard error of the mechanic and pertain to the first and second parts of a 30-min exposure to a Làt maze. Subjects were adult male (n = 6/group) wild-type controls, heterozygous D2± and homozygous D2–/–, heterozygous D3± and homozygous D3–/–, double heterozygous D2D3±, and double homozygous D2D3 –/– KO mice. WT, wild-type. For further details *see* ref. *(109)*, from which this figure has been elaborated.

rearings as well *(111)*. Moreover, the interaction of D2L with D1R might be selectively involved in rearing behavior, whereas D2S with D1 in stereotypic behavior *(112)*.

The interpretation of this KO mouse is complicated by a large reshaping of the DA network, as suggested by hyperDA innervation and increased DAT expression *(113)*.

7.3. D3 Receptor

7.3.1. Cerebral Distribution

Examination of the D3 receptor in the rat brain indicates that the distribution is distinct from the D2R, more localized and less expressed. It is expressed on post- and presynaptic sites, where it can function as autoreceptor, though studies on KO mice suggest that D2R is the only release-regulating autoreceptor *(94)*.

Cells expressing D3R mRNAs are not detected in either neocortical or palleocortical areas, but are predominantly in the ventral striatum, in particular in the nucleus accumbens shell and septal pole. The expression of D3R mRNA in the islands of Calleja is the highest observed in the CNS and appears to be selective for D3 (the same region displays no expression of D1Rs and D2Rs).

The localization of D3R in these regions might be responsible for the hyperactive behavior of D3 KO mice.

The medial portion of the lateral septum, the dentate gyrus of the hippocampus, and a few scattered areas in the medial amygdala also express D3R.

Geniculate bodies and various hypothalamic regions (paraventricular nucleus, centromedial, gelatinosus, ventromedial, ventrolateral nuclei, zona incerta) are positive for D3R, suggesting a role in hypothalamic regulation.

The localization of D3R mRNA in the cells of the substantia nigra is controversial *(114,115)*. Low levels of D2R mRNA expression are also seen in the inferior olive, in cerebellar lobules 9 and 10, and in the parafluculus, where it is localized in large Purkinje cells.

7.3.2. Target Mutations

D3R-null mice (–/–) *(116,117)* have been studied in different behavioral paradigms. Here we review their response to behavioral activation in novelty situations using the same experimental paradigm already described (*see* Subheading 7.2.).

The heterozygous D3 +/– demonstrated a biphasic time-dependent effect, as there was an increase in the first 15 min followed by a steep decrease in the second 15 min of the test. This contrasts with a monotonic decline in the WT group and the absence of significant habituation for the D3 –/– mutant mice, as assessed by regression analysis.

The frequency of rearings of the heterozygous and homozygous D3R groups was higher and lower respectively, as compared to WT littermate control group, during the first and the second part of the testing period. In fact, D3R +/– were more active than controls, in agreement with previous observations *(116)*. However, nonselective attention, indexed by the duration of rearing episodes, was not changed.

Post hoc, the composition of variance revealed that the D3R KO heterozygous mice had a significantly different emotionality from the control group. In fact, when the defecation score was taken to index the emotional response of the animal in Broadhurst's terms *(118)* the heterozygous D3R phenotype displayed a reduced neurovegetative response.

In summary, D3R KO heterozygous mice were more active than D3R KO homozygous and WT animals, which contrasts with previous observations *(116)* showing both mutants more active than controls. This discrepancy is likely to be of methodological origin, as activity of different nature are being monitored. In fact, Accili et al. *(116)* monitored the crossing of a square divided floor, i.e., a spontaneous activity of tonic nature. In contrast, in the Làt maze, i.e., a squared corridor, a low activity indexes a high spatial orientation, and a high exploration a low spatial orientation. In other words, D3R heterozygous mice apparently show a cognitive defect, whereas the homozygous mice are slightly better in comparison to heterozygous and control mice (see also ref. *117*).

The nonselective attention of D3R mutants, as assessed by rearing duration, was not different from WT controls, but D3 –/– showed a slightly higher duration in the second part of the test. Therefore, the D3R appears not to be involved in the modulation of scanning phase of attention.

Finally, D3Rs expressed in a single allele (KO heterozygous mice) appear to be involved in the control of emotional reactivity. Recent evidence *(119)* suggests that D3R contributes to postsynaptic negative modulation of the ML DA pathway.

7.3.3. D2/D3 and D2/D1 Interactions

The study of D1, D2, and D3 KO raise the question of the possible interaction of these receptors in modulating complex behavioral phenomena. Therefore, in our lab we have previously characterized double homozygous D2/D3 –/– (D2–/–; D3–/–) or double heterozygous D2/D3 +/– (D2+/–; D3+/–) mutants and WT (D2+/+; D3 +/+). The double-mutant mice were then tested in the Làt maze as reported in Subheading 7.2.2.

The D2/D3 –/– double mutants were less active than the WT littermate group. In particular, the activity decline was significant only between WT and double homozygous mutants D2/D3 –/– as assessed by regression analysis.

As shown in Fig. 1, only the homozygous double D2/D3 –/– mutant groups were significantly less active than WT in the first part, as well as in the second part of the testing period.

The double homozygote D2/D3 –/– mice presented a lower rearing frequency than wild-type controls over the entire testing period. Only the homozygous D2/D3 KO mice displayed significantly lower scanning times as compared with control mice in the first part of the test. In addition, the homozygous mice and the controls prolonged rearing duration in the second part as compared with the first part of the testing period.

Therefore, for the double-mutant D2R/D3R phenotype, the D2/D3 –/– were less active than WT mice. Thus, in the interaction between D2R and D3R subtypes the D2R phenotype seems predominant.

Further, the D2R/D3R –/– double-mutants demonstrated shorter scanning times compared to WT controls, but only in the first part of the test.

Third, the double D2R/D3R mutants indicate an interaction between these two receptor subtypes and a prevalence D2R on D3R gene expression.

A double KO D1/D3R has been also characterized. These mice display a summation of the behavioral profiles of D1 and D3 KO mice, e.g., increased locomotor activity (*see* D3 KO) and reduced rearing frequency (*see* D1 KO) *(120)*.

7.4. D4 Receptor

The DA D4R has recently received much attention because of reports that specific tandem repeat polymorphisms of the human *D4R* gene correlate with higher than average novelty-seeking scores on questionnaires *(121,122)*, although others have been unable to replicate these findings *(123–125)*. Moreover, specific polymorphisms of the D4 allele have been linked to ADHD (*see* Chapter 2).

7.4.1. Cerebral Distribution

D4R plays a role in modulating approach–avoidance responses in general and novelty-related exploration in particular *(126)*, as suggested in KO mice studies, and by the distribution in brain areas that could mediate the observed reductions in behavioral responses to novelty.

Glutamatergic pyramidal neurons of the frontal cortex *(76,127,128)* that project to the CPu and the substantia nigra *(129)* display high expression of D4R. This receptor in the frontal cortex is likely to be under the influence of both noradrenergic inputs and DAergic inputs. In fact, norepinephrine is only fivefold less potent at this receptor than DA *(130)*. This circuit plays an important role in regulating cognitive processes and emotional status and is in fact one of the main targets of antipsychotic drugs.

The DA D4R is not expressed on DA neurons of the substantia nigra.

7.4.2. Target Mutations

D4R KO mice *(81,126)* show reduced behavioral responses to novelty *(126)*. This is consistent with the hypothesis that a lack of D4R function may lead to decreased novelty-seeking in humans *(121,122)*. D4 KO mice show also increased locomotor response to ethanol, cocaine, and methamphetamine *(128)*. These mice also have increased DA synthesis and its conversion to DOPAC in the CPu *(128)*.

This phenotype can be explained observing that the stimulation of the MS pathway *(131)* by glutamate induces DA release *(132)*. Thus, frontal cortical D4Rs may alter the activity of MS DA neurons by modulating the release of glutamate onto these neurons.

An association between polymorphisms of the *D4R* gene and personality profile of the novelty-seeking trait *(121,122)* is in agreement with D4R role in modulating behavioral responses to novelty. Moreover, behavioral disorders, such as drug abuse *(133,134)*, pathological gambling *(135)*, and ADHD *(136,137)*, have recently been correlated to the same D4R alleles that are associated with novelty-seeking.

The behavioral effects of the full D4R KO in mice cannot be predicted in humans, wherein multiple alleles are reported *(138)*. Nevertheless, in humans 2% of the population has a null allele for the D4R *(139)*, but no behavioral reports are available.

7.5. D5 Receptor

The D5 DAR has a high affinity for DA, compared with other DARs, and has constitutive activity *(140,141)*, suggesting that the D5 DAR may be activated in the absence or presence of low concentrations of endogenous agonist. The D5 DAR is functionally coupled to the activation of adenylate cyclase, and GABA-A receptor-mediated activity through both second messenger cascades *(142)*, as well as through direct receptor–receptor interactions *(143)*. Interestingly, recent reports have suggested a possible association of the D5 *DAR* gene with schizophrenia *(144)* or substance abuse *(145)*.

The physiological and behavioral roles of the D5R have been difficult to characterize because of overlapping pharmacological properties of the D1Rs and D5Rs. There are few ligands selective for either subtype *(70)*, and DA is one, demonstrating approx 10-fold higher affinity at the D5 DAR compared with the D1. To further elucidate the physiological roles of the D5 DAR, mice lacking functional D5 DARs have been generated *(146)*.

7.5.1. Cerebral Distribution

The D5 receptor mRNA is very restricted, with the highest expression in the hippocampus and basal ganglia *(76,77)*, and to specific thalamic and hypothalamic nuclei.

In the hypothalamus, D5R may regulate circadian rhythms *(147)* and female sexual behaviors *(148,149)*.

Cells expressing D5R mRNAs are not detected in either neocortical or palleocortical areas, though immunoreactivity has been shown in various cortical regions.

There are suggestions that cells expressing D5R mRNA are also localized in the lateral mammillary nuclei *(141)*. Within the periphery, D5 DARs have been found in adrenal tissue *(150)*, kidney, and also the gastrointestinal tract, where they may exert a protective effect on the intestinal mucosa *(151)*.

7.5.2. Target Mutations

Approaches to the problem of D5R roles include the use of antisense technologies to downregulate D1 or D5 DAR expression, as well as the creation of D1 DAR-deficient mice *(74,75,146)*.

The antisense knockdown of D5R expression has suggested a role for the D5 DAR in regulating female sexual behaviors *(148,149)* and locomotor responses to DAergic agonists *(152)*.

The D5 DAR-KO mice are viable, have normal development, and are fertile *(146)*. This contrasts with antisense studies *(148,149)* that described suppression of lordosis behavior in D5 DAR knockdown-receptive females.

D5 mutant animals were hypertensive, exhibiting significantly elevated blood pressures *(146)*. This can be attributable to increased sympathetic tone, possibly of central origin. In fact, D5R deletion results in an oxytocin-dependent sensitization of V1 vasopressin and non-NMDA glutamatergic receptor-mediated pathways, potentially within the medulla, leading to increased sympathetic outflow *(146)*.

7.6. DA and Cyclic Adenosine 3′, 5′-Monophosphate-Regulated Phosphoprotein

The DARPP-32 is a phosphoprotein that plays a central role in the biology of dopaminoceptive neurons. DA and numerous other neurotransmitters may alter the phosphorylation and/or dephosphorylation of DARPP-32. In its phosphorylated state DARPP-32 is an extremely potent inhibitor of protein phosphatase-1 (PP-1), a major multifunctional serine/threonine protein phosphatase in the brain. PP-1, in turn, regulates phosphorylation and activity of many physiological effectors, such as voltage-gated ion channels and neurotransmitters. Studies of mice lacking the *DARPP-32* gene have provided convincing evidence that this protein plays an essential role in mediating the actions and interactions of DA and other neurotransmitters that act on dopaminoceptive neurons. These studies have also shown that the DARPP-32/PP-1 cascade is a major target for psychostimulants and antipsychotic drugs (for a review *see* ref. *153*).

8. BEHAVIOR AND DARs

When an animal is introduced in a nonfamiliar environment, novelty triggers an array of behavioral traits leading eventually to the mapping of the spatial context. In particular, rodents display behaviors such as walking about, rearing on the hindlimbs, leaning against walls, and sniffing (*see* ref. 154). They are all associated to hippocampal electrical activity of low frequency in the range of 3.5 to 8 Hz (RSA or "theta"; *see* ref. *155*). Walking and rearing have both spatial and non-spatial components, which are intimately interconnected. Therefore, the compound novelty-related set of stimuli activates the parallel processing of information in attentional, motivational, and emotional networks. The expression of vertical activity in the Làt maze is thought to share cognitive (spatial) and noncognitive (nonspatial) components. The latter prevails in the first part, whereas the former prevails in the second part of testing *(156)*. Moreover, walking and rearing have been genetically dissociated in mice *(157)* and rats *(158)*, suggesting that different genes control these behavioral traits.

Table 1
Summary of Behavioral Data on Dopamine Knockouts

Target	Rearing frequency	Locomotor activity	Notes
TH	L	L	
DAT	N	N	H in novel situations
D1	L *(81,84,85)*	N *(84,85)*; H *(83)*	
D2 L + S	L *(109,111)*	L *(88,109,111)*	
D3	H *(109,116,117)*	H *(109,116,117)*	
D4	N	L *(81,126)*	
D5	N *(146)*	N *(146)*	
D1 + D3	L *(120)*	H *(120)*	
D2 + D3	L *(109)*	L *(109)*	

N, normal; H, high; L, low; TH, thyrosine hydroxylase; DAT, dopamine transporter.

Recently, a series of studies has demonstrated that the duration of rearing episodes in a novelty situation index the level of nonselective attention toward environmental stimuli *(159–161)*.

Several studies have shown an increased DA release in the nucleus accumbens associated with behavioral activation *(19)*. This DA release can be controlled by the activation of presynaptic DA D2 autoreceptors and by the blockade of the firing of DA neurons in the VTA, wherein DA is also released at somatodendritic level, activating D2 autoreceptors, which hyperpolarize membrane potential. In addition, this short-term regulation of DA release is controlled by afferent excitatory and inhibitory inputs from raphe 5HT, locus coeruleus NE neurons, GABA VTA interneurons, medium spiny accumbal GABA projecting neurons, and glutamate frontal neurons in a complex network-based operational manner *(162)*.

The participation of each DAR in such processes is of interest because their selective regulation could be useful in the treatment of several psychiatric disorders. In particular, ADHD has been hypothesized to be underlined by a DA dysfunction on the bases of theoretical considerations, and experimental and clinical observations (for a review, *see* ref. *65*).

Therefore, the exact knowledge of each DAR subtype is of great clinical importance for the treatment of ADHD.

The KO technology has been useful in this direction (*see* Table 1 for a summary of KO studies). The wealth of studies reviewed here suggest that D1Rs and D4Rs could be directly involved in the pathogenesis of ADHD (*see also* Chapter 2) and that D2Rs might be important for the action of some therapeutic drugs, such as methylphenidate (*see* Chapter 22).

However, the results deriving from KO mice studies is hampered by the fact that this technique blocks the expression of a given receptor at early stages of development. In fact, DA systems that develop in absence of the deleted receptor might undergo compensatory changes, if the deletion is not lethal. An alternative strategy to overcome this problem is represented by inducible mutagenesis that allows blockage of the expression of a given protein in the adult organism. The main disadvantage of the latter is represented by tissue responsiveness as, for instance, skin responds in 100% of the cases, whereas the brain responds in only 10–15% of cases.

Recently, it has been shown that inhibitory small RNAs, conveyed to the target by viral vectors, may block the expression of specific proteins *(152,163–165)*.

Otherwise, the use of animal lines selected for specific behavioral traits might shed light on ADHD-DA-behavior relationship. In fact, a few rat lines feature the main aspects of ADHD *(166)*, i.e., the juvenile spontaneously hypertensive rat (SHR) (*167*; *see also* Chapter 4), the Wistar–Kyoto hyperactive *(168)*, and the NHE *(169)*. The juvenile SHR is used most often, because it is hyperactive and inattentive but not yet hypertensive, and it responds to psychostimulants with a paradoxical sedative effect similarly to ADHD children *(170)*. Moreover, these models are complementary as they mimic different variants of ADHD *(52)*.

Studies in genetic models of ADHD, such as the juvenile SHR and NHE rats, have shown a hyperfunctioning MCL system. This inference is based in the SHR on defective D2 autoreceptors *(171)*, an impaired inhibition of VTA neurons by accumbal neurons in the anterior portions of this structure *(172)*, and by the paradoxical reduction of DA neurons firing by low doses of psychostimulants (methylphenidate and amphetamines *[170,173]*). Reduced hyperactivity and increased attention are induced by endogenous cannabinoids *(174,175)*.

ADHD has a substantial genetic component, with a heritability of 0.75–0.91 *(58)*, and recent studies have indicated an association between a polymorphism in the human *DAT* gene and ADHD (*54,55*; *see also* ref. *65*). Taken together, results from both DA KO, DA receptor KO and the DAT KO and knockdown mice support the hyper-DAergic hypothesis for ADHD. In fact, DAT KO and knockdown mice are hyper-DAergic and hyperactive, whereas DA KO mice are severely hypoactive. Moreover, all DA receptor KO mice are hypoactive in different tasks, with the exclusion of DA D3 mice.

As previously reported, the main reason for hypothesizing a hyper-DA state in ADHD derive from the beneficial effects of psychostimulants in ADHD, which are known to increase dopamine tone.

However, DAT KO mice suggest two potential mechanisms by which psychostimulants may inhibit hyperactivity: increased serotonergic activity and/or a shift in the balance between DA autoreceptor and heteroreceptor function.

In conclusion, our working hypothesis focusing on a hyperfunctioning MCL system implies a developmental restricted period of vulnerability to DA-induced neurotoxicity. Therefore the therapeutical strategy should block the firing of DA neurons by low doses of psychostimulants acting at mesD2 autoreceptors.

ACKNOWLEDGMENTS

We are grateful to H. Westphal and E. Borrelli for scientific support with their KO mice, and Y. Bozzi, M. Pignatelli, and G. Grammatikopoulos for assistance in the conduct of the experiments. This research was supported by grants form Miur-COFIN 2001/2002 and Ministry of Health special funds.

REFERENCES

1. Robbins TW, Everitt BJ. Motivation and reward. In: Zigmond MJ, Bloom FE, Landis SC, Roberts JL, Squire LR, eds. Fundamental neuroscience. New York: Academic Press, 1999;1245–1277.
2. Robbins TW. Arousal systems and attentional processes. Biol Psychol 1997;45:57–71.
3. Wise RA, Hoffman DC. Localization of drug reward mechanisms by intracranial injections. Synapse 1992;10:247–263.
4. Wise RA. Neurobiology of addiction. Curr Opin Neurobiol 1996;6:243–251.

5. Wise RA. Brain reward circuitry: insights from unsensed incentives. Neuron 2002;36:229–240.
6. Fibiger HC, Phillips AG. Reward, motivation, cognition, psychobiology of mesotelencephalic dopamine systems. In: Bloom FE, ed. Handbook of physiology–the nervous system IV. Baltimore, MD, Williams and Wilkins, 1986.
7. Canavan AGM, Passingham RE, Marsden CD, Quinn N, Wyke M, Polkey CE. The performance on learning tasks of patients in the early stages of Parkinson's disease. Neuropsychol 27:141–156.
8. Robinson TE, Berridge KC. The neural basis for drug craving: an incentive-sensitization theory of addiction. Brain Res Rev 1993;18:247–291.
9. Knowlton BJ, Mangels JA, Squire LR. A neostriatal habit learning system in humans. Science 1996;273:1399–1402.
10. Robbins TW, Everitt BJ. Neurobehavioural mechanisms of reward and motivation. Curr Opin Neurobiol 1996;6:228–236.
11. Andeìn NE, Fuxe K, Hamberger B, Hokfelt T. A quantitative study on the nigro-neostriatal dopamine neurons. Acta Physiol Scand 1966;67:306–312.
12. Kalivas PW, Nakamura M. Neural systems for behavioral activation and reward. Curr Opin Neurobiol 1999;9:223–237.
13. Dahlstrom A, Fuxe K. Evidence for the existence of monoamine-containing neurons in the central nervous system. I. Demonstration of monoamines in cell bodies of brain stem neurons. Acta Physiol Scand 1964;62, Suppl. 232:1–55.
14. Freund TF, Powell JF, Smith AD. Tyrosine hydroxylase-immunoreactive boutons in synaptic contact with identified striatonigral neurons, with particular reference to dendritic spines. Neuroscience 1984;13:1189–1215.
15. Deutch AY, Bourdelais AJ, Zahm DS. The nucleus accumbens core and shell: accumbal compartments and their functional attributes. In: Kalivas PW, Barnes CD, eds. Limbic circuits and neuropsychiatry. CRC Press, London: 1993:45–88.
16. Bouyer JJ, Park DH, Joh TH, Pickel VM. Chemical and structural analysis of the relation between cortical inputs and tyrosine hydroxylase-containing terminals in rat neostriatum. Brain Res 1984;302:267–275.
17. Carlezon WA, Jr., Wise RA. Microinjections of phencyclidine (PCP) and related drugs into nucleus accumbens shell potentiate medial forebrain bundle brain stimulation reward. Psychopharmacology (Berl) 1996;128:413–420.
18. Zahm DS. An integrative neuroanatomical perspective on some subcortical substrates of adaptive responding with emphasis on the nucleus accumbens. Neurosci Biobehav Rev 2000;24:85–105.
19. Sellings LH, Clark PB. Segregation of amphetamine reward and locomotor stimulation between nucleus accumbens medial shell and core. J Neurosci 2003;23:6295–6303.
20. Routtenberg A. Intracranial chemical injection and behavior: A critical review. Behav Biol 1972;7:601–641.
21. Corbett D, Silva LR, Stellar JR. An investigation of the factors affecting development of frontal cortex self-stimulation. Physiol Behav 1985;34:89–95.
22. You Z-B, Tzschentke TM, Brodin E, Wise RA. Electrical stimulation of the prefrontal cortex increases cholecystokinin, glutamate, and dopamine release in the nucleus accumbens: an in vivo microdialysis study in freely moving rats. J Neurosci 1998;18:6492–6500.
23. Hoebel BG, Monaco AP, Hernandez L, Aulisi EF, Stanley BG, Lenard L. Self-injection of amphetamine directly into the brain. Psychopharmacology (Berl) 1983;81:158–163.
24. Carr GD, White NM. Conditioned place preference from intra-accumbens but not intra-caudate amphetamine injections. Life Sci 1983;33:2551–2557.
25. Carlezon WA, Jr., Devine DP, Wise RA. Habit-forming actions of nomifensine in nucleus accumbens. Psychopharmacology (Berl) 1995;122:194–197.
26. Fallon JH, Loughlin SE. Monoamine innervation of the forebrain: collateralization. Brain Res Bull 1982;9:295–307.
27. Bozarth MA, Wise RA. Intracranial self-administration of morphine into the ventral tegmental area in rats. Life Sci 1981;28:551–555.

28. Welzl H, Kuhn G, Huston JP. Self-administration of small amounts of morphine through glass micropipettes into the ventral tegmental area of the rat. Neuropharmacology 1989;28:1017–1023.
29. Devine DP, Wise RA. Self-administration of morphine, dopamine MGO, and DPDPE into the ventral tegmental area of rats. J Neurosci 1994;14:1978–1984.
30. David V, Durkin TP, Cazala P. Differential effects of the dopamine D2/D3 receptor antagonist sulpiride on self-administration of morphine into the ventral tegmental area or the nucleus accumbens. Psychopharmacology (Berl) 2002;160:307–317.
31. Johnson SW, North RA. Opioids excite dopamine neurons by hyperpolarization of local interneurons. J Neurosci 1992;12:483–488.
32. Hynes M, Rosenthal A. Specification of dopaminergic and serotonergic neurons in the vertebrate CNS. Curr Opin Neurobiol 1999;9:26–36.
33. Ye W, Shimamura K, Rubenstein JL, Hynes MA, Rosenthal A. FGF and Shh signals control dopaminergic and serotonergic cell fate in the anterior neural plate. Cell 1998;93:755–766.
34. Shamim H, Mahmood R, Logan C, Doherty P, Lumsden A, Mason I. Sequential roles for Fgf4, En1 and Fgf8 in specification and regionalisation of the midbrain. Development 1999; 126:945–959.
35. DiPorzio U, Pernas-Alonso R, Perrone-Capano C. Development of dopaminergic neurons. Austin, TX: Landes company, 1999.
36. Danielian PS, McMahon AP. Engrailed-1 as a target of the Wnt-1 signalling pathway in vertebrate midbrain development. Nature 1996;383:332–334.
37. Wurst W, Auerbach ABJAL. Multiple developmental defects in Engrailed-1 mutant mice: an early mid-hindbrain deletion and patterning defects in forelimbs and sternum. Development 1994;120:2065–2075.
38. Hanks M, Wurst W, Anson-Cartwright L, Auerbach AB, Joyner AL. Rescue of the En-1 mutant phenotype by replacement of En-1 with En-2. Science 1995;269:679–682.
39. Favor J. The mouse Pax2(1Neu) mutation is identical to a human PAX2 mutation in a family with renal-coloboma syndrome and results in developmental defects of the brain, ear, eye, and kidney. Proc Natl Acad Sci USA 1996;93:13,870–875.
40. Urbanek P, Fetka I, Meisler MH, Busslinger M. Cooperation of Pax2 and Pax5 in midbrain and cerebellum development. Proc Natl Acad Sci USA 1997;94:5703–5708.
41. Hynes M. Induction of midbrain dopaminergic neurons by Sonic hedgehog. Neuron 1995;15:35–44.
42. Smidt M. A novel homeodomain gene Ptx3 has higly restricted brain expression in mesencephalic dopaminergic neurons. Proc Natl Acad Sci USA 1997;94:13,305–13,310.
43. Zetterstrom RH, Solomin L, Jansson L, Hoffer BJ, Olson L, Perlmann T. Dopamine neuron agenesis in Nurr1-deficient mice. Science 1997;276:248–250.
44. Saucedo-Cardenas O, Quintana-Hau JD, Le WD, et al. Nurr1 is essential for the induction of the dopaminergic phenotype and the survival of ventral mesencephalic late dopaminergic precursor neurons. Proc Natl Acad Sci USA 1998;95:4013–4018.
45. Smidt MP, Asbreuk CH, Cox JJ, Chen H, Johnson RL, Burbach JP. A second independent pathway for development of mesencephalic dopaminergic neurons requires Lmx1b. Nat Neurosci 2000;3:337–341.
46. Yue Y, Widmer DA, Halladay AK, Cerretti DP, Wagner GC, Dreyer JL, Zhou R. Specification of distinct dopaminergic neural pathways: roles of the Eph family receptor EphB1 and ligand ephrin-B2. J Neurosci 1999;19:2090–2101.
47. Kobayashi K, Morita S, Sawada H, et al. Targeted disruption of the tyrosine hydroxylase locus results in severe catecholamine depletion and perinatal lethality in mice. J Biol Chem 1995;270:27,235–27,243.
48. Zhou QY, Palmiter RD. Dopamine-deficient mice are severely hypoactive, adipsic, and aphagic. Cell 1995;83:1197–1209.
49. Zhou QY, Quaife CJ, Palmiter RD. Targeted disruption of the tyrosine hydroxylase gene reveals that catecholamines are required for mouse fetal development. Nature 1995; 374:640–643.

50. Jones SR, Gainetdinov RR, Jaber M, Giros B, Wightman RM, Caron MG. Profound neuronal plasticity in response to inactivation of the dopamine transporter. Proc Natl Acad Sci USA 1998;95:4029–4034.
51. Giros B, Jaber M, Jones SR, Wightman RM, Caron MG. Hyperlocomotion and indifference to cocaine and amphetamine in mice lacking the dopamine transporter. Nature 1996;379:606–612.
52. Swanson JM, Sergeant JA, Taylor E, Sonuga-Barke EJS, Jensen PS, Cantwell DP. Attention deficit hyperactivity disorder and hyperkinetic disorder. Lancet 1998;351:329–343.
53. Cook EH, Jr., Stein MA, Krasowski MD, et al. Association of attention-deficit disorder and the dopamine transporter gene. Am J Hum Genet 1995;56:993–998.
54. Gill M, Daly G, Heron S, Hawi Z, Fitzgerald M. Confirmation of association between attention deficit hyperactivity disorder and a dopamine transporter polymorphism. Mol Psychiatry 1997;2:311–331.
55. Waldman ID, Rowe DC, Abramowitz A, et al. Association and linkage of the dopamine transporter gene and attention-deficit hyperactivity disorder in children: heterogeneity owing to diagnostic subtype and severity. Am J Hum Genet 1998;63:1767–1776.
56. Gainetdinov R, Wetsel W, Jones S, Levin E, Jaber M, Caron M. Role of serotonine in the paradoxical calming effect of psychostimulants on hyperactivity. Science 1999;283:397–401.
57. Bosse R, Fumagalli F, Jaber M, et al. Anterior pituitary hypoplasia and dwarfism in mice lacking the dopamine transporter. Neuron 1997;19:127–138.
58. Zhuang X, Oosting RS, Jones RS, et al. Hyperactivity and impaired response habituation in hyperdopaminergic mice. PNAS 2001;98:1982–1987.
59. Crabbe JC. Genetic differences in locomotor activation in mice. Pharmacol Biochem Behav 1986;25:289–292.
60. Laviola G, Renna G, Bignami G, Cuomo V. Ontogenetic and pharmacological dissociation of various components of locomotor activity and habituation in the rat. Int J Dev Neurosci 1988;6:431–438.
61. Pecina S, Cagniard B, Berridge KC, Aldrige JW, Zhuang X. Hyperdopaminergic mutant mice have higher "wanting" but not "liking" for sweet rewards. J Neurosci 2003;23:9395–9402.
62. Gimenez-Llort L, Martinez E, Ferre S. Different effects of dopamine antagonists on spontaneous and NMDA-induced motor activity in mice. Pharmacol Biochem Behav 1997; 56:549–553.
63. Gerlai R, McNamara A, Choi-Lundberg DL, et al. Impaired water maze learning performance without altered dopaminergic function in mice heterozygous for the GDNF mutation. Eur J Neurosci 2001;14:1153–1163.
64. Nestler EJ. Molecular neurobiology of drug addiction. Neuropsychopharmacology 1994;11:77–87.
65. Castellanos FX, Tannock R. Neuroscience of Attention-Deficit/Hyperactivity Disorder: the search for endophenotypes. Nature Reviews 2002;3:617–628.
66. Castellanos FX, Giedd JN, Eckburg P, et al. Quantitative morphology of the caudate nucleus in attention deficit hyperactivity disorder. Am J Psychiatry 1994;151:1791–1796.
67. Castellanos FX, Giedd JN, Marsh WL, et al. Quantitative brain magnetic resonance imaging in attention-deficit hyperactivity disorder. Arch Gen Psychiatry 1996;53:607–616.
68. Jackson DM, Westlind-Danielsson A. Dopamine receptors: molecular biology, biochemistry and behavioural aspects. Pharmacol Ther 1994;64:291–370.
69. Missale C, Nash SR, Robinson SW, Jaber M, Caron MG. Dopamine receptors: from structure to function. Physiol Rev 1998;78:189–225.
70. Neve KA, Neve RL. The dopamine receptors. Totowa NJ, Humana Press, 1997.
71. Gerfen CR. The neostriatal mosaic: multiple levels of compartmental organization. Trends Neurosci 1992;15:133–139.
72. Aizman O, Brismar H, Uhlen P, et al. Anatomical and physiological evidence for D1 and D2 dopamine receptor colocalization in neostriatal neurons. Nat Neurosci 2000;3:226–230.
73. Ikemoto S, Glazier BS, Murphy JM, McBride WJ. Role of dopamine D1 and D2 receptors in the nucleus accumbens in mediating reward. J Neurosci 1997;17:8580–8587.

74. Sibley DR. New insights into dopamine rgic receptor function using antisense and genetically altered animals. Annu Rev Pharmacol Toxicol 1999;39:313–341.
75. Glickstein SB, Schmauss C. Dopamine receptor function: lessons from knockout mice. Pharmacol Ther 2001;91:63–83.
76. Ariano MA, Wang J, Noblett KL, Larson ER, Sibley D. Cellular distribution of the rat D4 dopamine receptor protein in the CNS using anti-receptor antisera. Brain Res 1997;752:26–34.
77. Ciliax DJ, Nash N, Heilman C, et al. Dopamine D5 receptor immunolocalization in rat and monkey brain. Synapse 2000;37:125–145.
78. Weiner DM, Levey AI, Sunahara RK, et al. D1 and D2 dopamine receptor mRNA in rat brain. Proc Natl Acad Sci USA 1991;88:1859–1863.
79. di Porzio U, Pernas-Alonso R, Perrone-Capano C. Development of dopaminergic neurons. Landes, Austin, TX, 1999:1.
80. Blandini F, Fancellu R, Orzi F, et al. Selective stimulation of striatal dopamine receptors of the D1- or D2-class causes opposite changes of fos expression in the rat cerebral cortex. Eur J Neurosci 2003;17:763–770.
81. Drago J, Padungchichot P, Accili D, Fuchs S. Dopamine receptors and dopamine transporter in brain function and addictive behaviors: insight from targeted mouse mutants. Dev Neurosci 1998;20:188–203.
82. Xu M, Hu XT, Cooper DC, et al. Elimination of cocaine-induced hyperactivity and dopamine-mediated neurophysiological effects in dopamine D1 receptor mutant mice [see comments]. Cell 1994;79:945–955.
83. Xu M, Moratalla R, Gold LH, et al. Dopamine D1 receptor mutant mice are deficient in striatal expression of dynorphin and in dopamine-mediated behavioral responses. Cell 1994;79:729–742.
84. Drago J, Gerfen CR, Lachowicz JE, et al. Altered striatal function in a mutant mouse lacking D1A dopamine receptors. Proc Natl Acad Sci USA 1994;91:12,564–568.
85. Drago J, Gerfen CR, Westphal H, Steiner H. D1 dopamine receptor-deficient mouse: cocaine-induced regulation of immediate-early gene and substance P expression in the striatum. Neuroscience 1996;74:813–823.
86. McNamara FN, Clifford JJ, Tighe O, et al. Congenic D1A dopamine receptor mutants: ethologically based resolution of behavioural topography indicates genetic background as a determinant of knockout phenotype. Neuropsychopharmacology 2003;28:86–99.
86a. Viggiano D, Vallone D, Ruocco LA, Sadile AG. Behavioral pharmacological, morpho-functional molecular studies reveal a hyperfunctioning mesocortical dopamine system in an animal model of attention deficit and hyperactivity disorder. Neurosci Biobehav Rev 2003;27:683–689.
87. Jackson DJ, Westlind-Danielsson A. Dopamine receptors: Molecular biology, biochemistry and behavioural aspects. Pharmacol Ther 1994;64:291–369.
88. Baik JH, Picetti R, Saiardi A, et al. Parkinsonian-like locomotor impairment in mice lacking dopamine D2 receptors. Nature 1995;377:424–428.
89. Kelly MA, Rubinstein M, Phillips TJ, et al. Locomotor activity in D2 dopamine receptor-deficient mice is determined by gene dosage, genetic background, and developmental adaptations. J Neurosci 1998;18:3470–3479.
90. Jung MY, Skryabin BV, Arai M, et al. Potentiation of the D2 mutant motor phenotype in mice lacking dopamine D2 and D3 receptors. Neuroscience 1999;91:911–924.
91. Maldonado R, Saiardi A, Valverde O, Samad TA, Roques BP, Borrelli E. Absence of opiate rewarding effects in mice lacking dopamine D2 receptors. Nature 1997;388:586–589.
92. Saiardi A, Bozzi Y, Baik JH, Borrelli E. Antiproliferative role of dopamine: loss of D2 receptors causes hormonal dysfunction and pituitary hyperplasia. Neuron 1997;19:115–126.
93. Kelly MA, Rubinstein M, Asa SL, et al. Pituitary lactotroph hyperplasia and chronic hyperprolactinemia in dopamine D2 receptor-deficient mice. Neuron 1997;19:103–113.
94. L'hirondel M, Cheramy A, Godeheu G, et al. Lack of autoreceptor-mediated inhibitory control of dopamine release in striatal synaptosomes of D2 receptor-deficient mice. Brain Res 1998;792:253–262.

95. Mercuri NB, Saiardi A, Bonci A, et al. Loss of autoreceptor function in dopaminergic neurons from dopamine D2 receptor deficient mice. Neuroscience 1997;79:323–327.
96. Koeltzow TE, Xu M, Cooper DC, et al. Alterations in dopamine release but not dopamine autoreceptor function in dopamine D3 receptor mutant mice. J Neurosci 1998;18:2231–2238.
97. Mansour A, Meador-Woodruff JH, Bunzow JR, Civelli O, Akil H, Watson SJ. Localization of dopamine D2 receptor mRNA and D1 and D2 receptor binding in the rat brain and pituitary: an in situ hybridization-receptor autoradiographic analysis. J Neurosci 1990;10:2587–2600.
98. Usiello A, Baik JH, Rouge-Pont F, et al. Distinct functions of the two isoforms of dopamine D2 receptors. Nature 2000;408:199–203.
99. Rouge-Pont F, Usiello A, Benoit-Marand M, Gonon F, Piazza PV, Borrelli E. Changes in extracellular dopamine induced by morphine and cocaine: crucial control by D2 receptors. J Neurosci 2002;22:3293–3301.
100. Grace AA, Bunney BS, Moore H, Todd CL. Dopamine-cell depolarization block as a model for the therapeutic actions of antipsychotic drugs. Trends Neurosci 1997;20:31–37.
101. Doppler W. Regulation of gene expression by prolactin. Rev Physiol Biochem Pharmacol 1994;124:93–130.
102. Picetti R, Saiardi A, Samad TA, Bozzi Y, Baik J-H, Borrelli E. Dopamine D2 receptors in signal transduction and behavior. Crit Rev Neurobiol 1997;11:121–142.
103. Di Chiara G. The role of dopamine in drug abuse viewed from the perspective of its role in motivation. Drug Alcohol Depend 1995;38:95–137.
104. Dal Toso R, Sommer B, Ewert M, et al. The dopamine D2 receptor: two molecular forms generated by alternative splicing. EMBO J 1989;8:4025–134.
105. Kahn RA, Weinberger J, Panah M. How selective is 7-nitroindazole, an inhibitor of neuronal nitric oxide synthase? Response. Anesth Analg 1998;86:679–680.
106. Weiger TM, Holmqvist MH, Levitan IB, et al. A novel nervous system beta subunit that downregulates human large conductance calcium-dependent potassium channels. J Neurosci 2000;20:3563–3570.
107. Montmayeur J-P, Borrelli E. Transcription mediated by a cAMP-responsive promoter element is reduced upon activation of dopamine D2 receptors. Proc Natl Acad Sci USA 1991;88:3135–3139.
108. Gerfen CR. The neostriatal mosaic: multiple levels of compartmental organization. Trends Neurosci 1992;15:133–149.
109. Vallone D, Pignatelli M, Grammatikopoulus G, et al. Activity, non-selective attention and emotionally in dopamine D-2/D-3 receptor knock out mice. Behav Brain Res 2002;130:141–148.
110. Clifford JJ, Usiello A, Vallone D, Kinsella A, Borrelli E, Waddington JL. Topographical evaluation of behavioural phenotype in a line of mice with targeted gene deletion of the D2 dopamine receptor. Neuropharmacology 2000;39:382–390.
111. Wang Y, Xu R, Sasaoka T, Tonegawa S, Kung M-P, Sankoorikal E-B. Dopamine D2 long receptor-deficient mice display alterations in striatum-dependent functions. J Neurosci 2000;20:8305–8314.
112. Fetsko LA, Xu R, Wang Y. Alterations in D1/D2 synergism may account for enhanced stereotypy and reduced climbing in mice lacking dopamine D2L receptor. Brain Res 2003;967:191–200.
113. Parish CL, Finkelstein DI, Drago J, Borrelli E, Horne MK. The role of dopamine receptors in regulating the size of axonal arbors. J Neurosci 2001;21:5147–157.
114. Bouthenet ML, Souil E, Martres MP, Sokoloff P, Giros B, Schwartz JC. Localization of dopamine D3 receptor mRNA in the rat brain using in situ hybridization histochemistry: comparison with dopamine D2 receptor mRNA. Brain Res 1991;564:203–219.
115. Sokoloff P, Giros B, Martres MP, Bouthenet ML, Schwartz JC. Molecular cloning and characterization of a novel dopamine receptor (D3) as a target for neuroleptics. Nature 1990;347:146–151.
116. Accili D, Fishburn CS, Drago J, et al. A targeted mutation of the D3 dopamine receptor gene is associated with hyperactivity in mice. Proc Natl Acad Sci USA 1996;93:1945–1949.
117. Xu M, Koeltzow TE, Santiago GT, et al. Dopamine D3 receptor mutant mice exhibit increased behavioral sensitivity to concurrent stimulation of D1 and D2 receptors. Neuron 1997;19:837–848.

118. Cornett LE, Breckinridge SM, Koike TI. Induction of V2 receptors in renal medulla of homozygous Brattleboro rats by arginine vasopressin. Peptides 1989;10:985–991.
119. Narita M, Mizuo K, Mizoguchi H, et al. Molecular evidence for the functional role of dopamine D3 receptor in the morphine-induced rewarding effect and hyperlocomotion. J Neurosci 2003;23:1006–1012.
120. Wong JY, Clifford JJ, Massalas JS, Kinsella A, Waddington JL, Drago J. Essential conservation of D(1) mutant phenotype at the level of individual topographies of behaviour in mice lacking both D(1) and D(3) dopamine receptors. Psychopharmacology (Berl) 2003;167:167–173.
121. Benjamin J, Li L, Patterson C, Greenberg BD, Murphy DL, Hamer DH. Population and familial association between the D4 dopamine receptor gene and measures of novelty seeking. Nat Genet 1996;12:81–84.
122. Ebstein RP, Novick O, Umansky R, et al. Dopamine D4 receptor (D4DR) exon III polymorphism associated with the human personality trait of novelty seeking. Nat Genet 1996;12:78–80.
123. Malhotra AK, Virkkunen M, Rooney W, Eggert M, Linnoila M, Goldman D. The association between the dopamine D4 receptor (D4DR) 16 amino acid repeat polymorphism and novelty seeking. Mol Psychiatry 1996;1:388–391.
124. Vandenbergh DJ, Zonderman AB, Wang J, Uhl GR, Costa PT. No association between novelty-seeking and dopamine D4 receptor (D4DR) exon III seven repeat alleles in Baltimore Longitudinal Study of Aging participants. Mol Psychiatry 1997;2:417–419.
125. Kuhn K, Meyer K, Nothen MM, Gansicke M, Papassotiropoulos A, Maier W. Allelic variants of dopamine receptor D4 (D4DR) and serotonin receptor 5HT2c (HTR2c) and temperament factors: replication tests. Am J Med Genet 1999;88:168–172.
126. Dulawa SC, Grandy DK, Low MJ, Paulus MP, Geyer MA. Dopamine D4 receptor-knockout mice exhibit reduced exploration of novel stimuli. J Neurosci 1999;19:9550–9556.
127. Mrzljak L, Bergson C, Pappy M, Huff R, Levenson R, Goldman-Rakic PS. Localization of dopamine D4 receptors in GABAergic neurons of the primate brain. Nature 1996;381:245–248.
128. Rubinstein M, Phillips TJ, Bunzow JR, et al. Mice lacking dopamine D4 receptors are supersensitive to ethanol, cocaine, and methamphetamine. Cell 1997;90:991–1001.
129. Carter CJ. Topographical distribution of possible glutamatergic pathways from the frontal cortex to the striatum and substantia nigra in rats. Neuropharmacology 1982;21:379–383.
130. Lanau F, Zenner M, Civelli O, Hartman D. Epinephrine and norepinephrine act as potent agonists at the recombinant human dopamine D4 receptor. J Neurochem 1997;68:804–812.
131. Westerink BHC, Santiago M, De Vries JB. The release of dopamine from nerve terminals and dendrites of nigrostriatal neurons induced by excitatory amino acids in the conscious rat. Naunyn Schmiedebergs Arch Pharmacol 1992;345:523–529.
132. Overton P, Clark D. Electrophysiological evidence that intrastriatally administered N-methyl-D-aspartate augments striatal dopamine tone in the rat. J Neural Transm 1992;4:1–14.
133. Kotler M, Cohen H, Segman R, et al. Excess dopamine D4 receptor (D4DR) exon III seven repeat allele in opioid-dependent subjects. Mol Psychiatry 1997;2:251–254.
134. Shields PG, Lerman C, Audrain J, et al. Dopamine D4 receptors and the risk of cigarette smoking in African-Americans and Caucasians. Cancer Epidemiol Biomarkers Prev 1998;7:453–458.
135. de Castro PI, IA, Torres P, Saiz-Ruiz J, Fernandez-Piqueras J. Genetic association study between pathological gambling and a functional DNA polymorphism at the D4 receptor gene. Pharmacogenetics 1997;7:345–348.
136. LaHoste GJ, Swanson JM, Wigal SB, et al. Dopamine D4 receptor gene polymorphism is associated with attention deficit hyperactivity disorder. Molec Psychiatry 1996;1:121–124.
137. Faraone SV, Biederman J, Weiffenbach B, et al. Dopamine D4 gene 7-repeat allele and attention deficit hyperactivity disorder. Am J Psychiatry 1999;156:768–770.
138. Asghari V, Sanyal S, Buchwaldt S, Paterson A, Jovanovic V, Van Tol HH. Modulation of intracellular cyclic AMP levels by different human dopamine D4 receptor variants. J Neurochem 1995;65:1157–1165.

139. Nothen MM, Cichon S, Hemmer S, et al. Human dopamine D4 receptor gene: frequent occurrence of a null allele and observation of homozygosity. Hum Mol Genet 1994;3:2207.
140. Sunahara RK, Guan HC, O'Dowd BF, et al. Cloning of the gene for a human dopamine D5 receptor with higher affinity for dopamine than D1. Nature 1991;150:614–619.
141. Tiberi M, Caron MG. High agonist-independent activity is a distinguishing feature of the dopamine D1B receptor subtype. J Biol Chem 1994;269:27,925–931.
142. Yan Z, Surmeier DJ. D5 dopamine receptors regulate Zn2+-sensitive GABAA currents in striatal cholinergic interneurons through a PKA/PP1 cascade. Neuron 1997;19:1115–1126.
143. Liu F, Wan Q, Pristupa ZB, Yu XM, Wang YT, Niznik HB. Direct protein-protein coupling enables cross-talk between dopamine D5 and -aminobutyric acid A receptors. Nature 2000;403:274–280.
144. Muir WJ, Thomson ML, McKeon P, et al. Markers close to the dopamine D5 receptor gene (DRD5) show significant association with schizophrenia but not bipolar disorder. Am J Med Genet 2001;105:152–158.
145. Vanyukov MM, Moss HB, Gioio AE, Hughes HB, Kaplan BB, Tarter RE. An association between a microsatellite polymorphism at the DRD5 gene and the liability to substance abuse: pilot study. Behav Genet 1998;28:75–82.
146. Hollon TR, Bek MJ, Lachowicz JE, et al. Mice lacking D5 dopamine receptors have increased sympathetic tone and are hypertensive. J Neurosci 2002;22:10,801–811.
147. Rivkees S, Lachowicz JE. Functional D1 and D5 dopamine receptors are expressed in the suprachiasmatic, supraoptic and paraventricular nuclei of primates. Synapse 1997;26:1–10.
148. Apostolakis EM, Gara J, Fox C, et al. Dopamine rgic regulation of progesterone receptors: brain D5 dopamine receptors mediate induction of lordosis by D1-like agonists in rats. J Neurosci 1996;16:4823–4834.
149. Apostolakis EM, Garai J, O'Malley BW, Clark JH. In vivo regulation of central nervous system progesterone receptors: cocaine induces steroid-dependent behavior through dopamine transporter modulation of D5 receptors in rats. Mol Endocrinol 1996;10:1595–604.
150. Dahmer MK, Senogles SE. Dopaminergic inhibition of catecholamine secretion from chromaffin cells: evidence that inhibition is mediated by D4 and D5 dopamine receptors. J Neurochem 1996;66:222–232.
151. Mezey E, Eisenhofer G, Harta G, et al. A novel nonneuronal catecholaminergic system: exocrine pancreas synthesizes and releases dopamine. Proc Natl Acad Sci USA 1996;93:10,377–82.
152. Dziewczapolski G, Menalled LB, Garcia MC, Mora MA, Gershanik OS, Rubinstein M. Opposite roles of D1 and D5 dopamine receptors in locomotion revealed by selective antisense oligonucleotides. Neurorep 1998;9:1–5.
153. Greengard P, Allen PB, Nairn AC. Beyond the dopamine receptor: the DARPP-32/protein phosphatase-1 cascade. Neuron 1999;23:435–447.
154. Sadile AG. Long-term habituation of theta-related activity components of albino rats in the Làt-maze. In: Sanberg PR, Ossenkopp KP, Kavaliers M, eds. Motor activity and movement disorders: measurement and analysis. Totowa, NJ: Humana Press, 1996:1–54.
155. Whishaw IQ, Vanderwolf CH. Hippocampal EEG and behavior: changes in amplitude and frequency of RSA (theta rhythm) associated with spontaneous and learned movement patterns in rats and cats. Behav Biol 1973;8:461–484.
156. Pellicano MP, Siciliano F, Sadile AG. The dose and genotype-dependent effects of post-trial MK-801 and CPP on long-term habituation to novelty in rats reveal a modulatory role of NMdopamine receptors on behavioral plasticity. Neurosci Lett Suppl 1992;43:S86.
157. Van Abeelen JHF. Genetics of rearing behavior in mice. Behav Genet 1970;1:71–76.
158. Sanders DC. The Bethlem lines: genetic selection for high and low rearing activity in rats. Behav Genet 1981;11:491–503.
159. Aspide R, Fresiello A, De Filippis G, Gironi Carnevale UA, Sadile AG. Non selective attention in a rat model of hyperactivity and attention deficit: subchronic methylphenidate and nitric oxide synthesis inhibitor treatment. Neurosci Biobehav Rev 2000;24:59–71.

160. Aspide R, Gironi Carnevale UA, Sergeant JA, Sadile AG. Non-selective attention and nitric oxide in putative animal models of attention-deficit hyperactivity disorder. Behav Brain Res 1998; 95:123–133.
161. Aspide R, Gironi Carnevale UA, Sagvolden T, Sergeant JA, Sadile AG. Novelty-induced rearing duration as index of attention at low motivational levels in two animal models of ADHD in children. Proc IBNS, Cancun, Mexico, 1996;5:65.
162. Grillner P, Mercuri N. Intrinsic membrane properties and synaptic inputs regulating the firing activity of the dopamine neurons. Behav Brain Res 2002;130:149–169.
163. Chiasson BJ, Armstrong JN, Hooper ML, Murphy PR, Robertson HA. The application of antisense oligonucleotide technology to the brain: Some pitfalls. Cell Mol Neurobiol 1994;14:507–522.
164. Landgraf R, Naruo T, Vecsernyes M, Neumann I. Neuroendocrine and behavioral effects of antisense oligonucleotides. Eur J Endocrinol 1997;137:326–335.
165. Menalled LB, Dziewczapolski G, Garcia MC, Rubinstein M, Gershanik OS. D3 receptor knockdown through antisense oligonucleotide administration supports its inhibitory role in locomotion. Neurorep 1999;10:3131–3136.
166. Sadile AG, ed. Modeling ADHD in rodent mutants. Neurosci Biobehav Rev 2000;24:1–169.
167. Sagvolden T. Behavioral validation of the spontaneously hypertensive rat (SHR) as an animal model of attention-deficit hyperactivity disorder (AD/HD). Neurosci Biobehav Rev 2000;24: 31–40.
168. Moisan M, Courvoisier H, Bihoreau M, et al. A major quantitative trait locus influences hyperactivity in the WKHA rat. Nature Genet 1996;14:471–473.
169. Cerbone A, Pellicano MP, Sadile AG. Evidence for and against the Naples high- and low-excitability rats as genetic model to study hippocampal functions. Neurosci Biobehav Rev 1993;17:295–304.
170. Solanto MV. Neuropsychopharmacological mechanisms of stimulant drug action in attention-deficit hyperactivity disorder: a review and integration. Behav Brain Res 1998;94:127–152.
171. Russell VA. The nucleus accumbens motor-limbic interface of the spontaneously hypertensive rat as studied in-vitro by the superfusion slice technique. Neurosci Biobehav Rev 2000;24:133–136.
172. Sadile AG. Multiple evidence of a segmental defect in the anterior forebrain of an animal model of hyperactivity and attention deficit. Neurosci Biobehav Rev 2000;24:161–169.
173. Viggiano D, Vallone D, Sadile A. Dysfunctions of the dopamine systems and ADHD: evidence from animals and modeling. Neural Plast 2004;11:97–114.
174. Beltramo M, Rodriguez de Fonseca FR, Navarro M, et al. Reversal of dopamine D_2-receptor responses by an anandamide trasport inhibitor. J Neurosci 2000;20:3401–3407.
175. Viggiano D, Ruocco LA, Pignatelli M, Grammatikopoulos G, Sadile AG. Prenatal elevation of endocannabinoids corrects the unbalance between dopamine systems and reduces activity in the Naples high excitability rats. Neurosci Biobehav Rev 2003;27:129–139.

4

The Spontaneously Hypertensive Rat as a Model of Attention Deficit Hyperactivity Disorder

Vivienne Ann Russell

1. INTRODUCTION

Attention deficit hyperactivity disorder (ADHD) is a heterogeneous disorder with multiple contributing factors, both genetic and environmental, as evidenced by the multiple susceptibility genes that have been identified and the inconsistencies in different family studies *(1)*. Diagnosis of ADHD is based on behavioral symptoms because there is, as yet, no biological marker. Animal models of ADHD are useful because they mimic various aspects of the disorder and have the advantage of genetic homogeneity, environmental control, and the possibility of early intervention *(2)*. Animal models include exposure to neurotoxins and genetic variants. The spontaneously hypertensive rat (SHR) is the most extensively investigated genetic model and the only animal model that has been shown to demonstrate all the behavioral characteristics of ADHD, namely, hyperactivity, impulsivity, and problems with sustained attention *(2–5)*.

SHRs and their progenitors' Wistar–Kyoto (WKY) control rats, look identical and have similar body weights *(6)*. SHRs were originally bred from WKY for their hypertension *(7)*. Major differences between SHRs and WKYs are summarized in Table 1. The difference in blood pressure between SHRs and WKYs is not apparent at 2 wk of age but is seen to increase with age from 4 to 10 wk *(6,8)*. SHRs are hyperactive at 3–4 wk of age *(6)*, so for SHRs to serve as a model for ADHD, it is best to compare prehypertensive, 3- to 4-wk-old SHRs with age-matched WKYs. Unfortunately, most of the information that is available has been gathered from adult SHRs, but in many cases these findings have been replicated in juvenile, prehypertensive rats. Sagvolden and colleagues showed that SHRs are not only hyperactive in several different situations but are also impulsive and unable to sustain attention *(2–5,9,10)*. Multiple fixed-interval delay of reinforcement schedules were used to determine reactivity to reinforcers, activity, and impulsivity, while measurement of extinction of reinforced behavior provided information about sensitivity to stimulus change and sustained attention *(2)*. When their behavior was controlled by a fixed-interval operant reinforcement schedule, SHR activity was initially similar to WKY but was found to increase progressively toward the end of the session *(2)*. This was interpreted to suggest that SHRs had similar reactivity to reinforcers compared to WKYs but SHRs became overactive in the absence of novel stimuli *(2)*. Toward the end of testing, SHRs displayed bursts of responses with short interresponse intervals, which was interpreted as impulsivity *(2)*. In fact, SHRs

From: *Attention Deficit Hyperactivity Disorder: From Genes to Patients*
Edited by: D. Gozal and D. L. Molfese © Humana Press Inc., Totowa, NJ

frequently displayed short sequences of activity on tasks and rapid changes between activities, consistent with impulsivity *(2,10,11)*. During the extinction phase, SHRs did not differ from WKYs in terms of sensitivity to stimulus change; SHRs noticed when the light signaled that the schedule had changed and they ceased to respond, suggesting no obvious sensory problems *(2)*. Unlike WKYs, however, SHRs resumed lever pressing after a short while, just like ADHD children in similar signaled extinction trials, suggesting that SHRs have deficient sustained attention *(2)*. Similar to ADHD, SHR behavior was suggested to be more variable than that of controls *(2,12)*. SHRs were also suggested to display cognitive impulsivity, in that SHRs, but not WKYs, had great difficulty pressing one lever more than seven times before changing to a second lever in a task that required a certain number of presses on the first lever before switching to the second lever in order to obtain a reinforcer *(2)*.

Differences in the behavior of SHR and control WKY rats were suggested to be a result of altered reinforcement of appropriate behavior *(2,4,5)*. Reinforcers act retroactively to increase the probability of repeating a behavior that led to the reward *(2)*. The reinforcing effect is greatest when the reinforcer is delivered immediately after the appropriate behavior and becomes less effective as the delay between the behavioral response and the reinforcer increases *(2)*. SHRs have been suggested to have a steeper and shorter delay-of-reinforcement gradient than WKYs, which allows them to respond more rapidly to immediate reinforcers causing hyperactivity, and to respond less effectively to reinforcers that occur after a delay, resulting in poor stimulus control of behavior *(2–5)*. When reinforcers are infrequent, the lack of stimulus control due to the short delay-of-reinforcement gradient causes SHRs to lose their focus on the task and behave inappropriately, which is interpreted as impaired sustained attention *(2)*. The variability of behavior seen in both SHRs and ADHD children has been attributed to the fact that the behavior that is reinforced is the behavior that occurs immediately before a reinforcer is delivered *(2,4,5)*. Impulsivity, defined as responses emitted with short interresponse intervals, is observed in SHRs when reinforcers are infrequent in a familiar environment; SHRs are not hyperactive or impulsive in a novel situation where reinforcers are frequent *(2,4,5)*.

2. DOPAMINE HYPOFUNCTION HYPOTHESIS

Because the most effective treatment of ADHD involves the use of psychostimulant drugs, such as methylphenidate and D-amphetamine, which inhibit the dopamine transporter (DAT) and thereby increase the extracellular concentration of dopamine, ADHD symptoms have been suggested to result from hypoactivity of dopamine systems in the brain *(13)*. Results obtained with SHRs support this hypothesis. Low doses of D-amphetamine and methylphenidate reduced the hyperactivity of SHR and a stroke-prone substrain of SHRs *(14,15)*. In fixed-interval schedules of reinforcement of bar-presses by water, the psychomotor stimulants were shown to weaken control by immediate reinforcers and strengthen control by delayed reinforcers, thereby improving sustained attention *(4)*. Impaired function of the mesolimbic dopamine system was suggested to produce a shorter and steeper delay gradient in both SHRs and children with ADHD, giving rise to hyperactivity, motor impulsivity, and impaired sustained attention *(2,4,5,13)*. Impaired function of the mesocortical dopamine system was suggested to produce cognitive impulsiveness and impaired nigrostriatal dopamine function was suggested to cause "extrapyramidal" symptoms of ADHD *(2,4,5,13)*.

3. DOPAMINERGIC SYSTEMS

Changes that have been identified in the central nervous system of SHRs have provided insight into possible neural disturbances of ADHD. In vitro stimulation-evoked release (electrical and/or exposure to high K^+ concentration) of dopamine from terminals of mesocortical, mesolimbic, and nigrostriatal dopamine neurons of SHR is significantly less than WKY *(16–22)*. Dopamine D2 receptor-mediated inhibition of dopamine release was greater in SHR caudate-putamen and nucleus accumbens than WKY, whereas dopamine D2 receptor function was unchanged in the prefrontal cortex of SHR *(19,20)*. Increased efficacy of endogenous dopamine activation of D2 autoreceptors was suggested to account for the decreased release of dopamine in SHR striatum *(19,20)*. This downregulation of dopamine transmission was suggested to have occurred as a compensatory reaction to abnormally elevated dopamine levels at an early stage of development, perhaps as a result of exposure to stress or a genetic defect *(19)*. Consistent with decreased stimulus-evoked release of dopamine, postsynaptic D1 receptors are increased in the caudate putamen and nucleus accumbens of SHR *(23–25)*. The increase in D1 receptors is reversed by methylphenidate treatment, suggesting that psychostimulants increase dopamine activation of D1 receptors *(23–25)*. Indicative of decreased function, SHR have reduced expression of calcium/calmodulin-dependent protein kinase II and *c-fos* gene in the anterior striatum *(26–28)*. Consistent with increased DAT expression in SHR striatum, extracellular dopamine levels are decreased and D-amphetamine-stimulated release of dopamine from SHR striatal slices is greater than WKY *(16,17,22,25,29)*. D-amphetamine causes dopamine release by reversal of DAT, so increased DAT would increase dopamine release in response to D-amphetamine *(30)*. Although SHRs have increased numbers of DAT, the dopamine uptake carrier appears to function normally in the nucleus accumbens and caudate putamen of SHRs. Inhibition of uptake by low concentrations of methylphenidate or nomifensine increased the electrically stimulated release of dopamine to the same extent in SHRs and WKYs *(18,22)*. Vesicle storage of dopamine was suggested to be impaired in SHRs, as SHRs released less dopamine from vesicle stores in response to membrane depolarization and more dopamine from cytoplasmic stores in response to D-amphetamine when compared with WKYs *(19)*. Although SHR dopamine concentrations have been reported to be similar to WKY, dopamine turnover appeared to be lower and the dopamine metabolite, homovanillic acid, and the homovanillic acid/dopamine ratio were found to be much lower in several brain areas of SHRs compared to WKYs, including the ventral tegmental area, substantia nigra, striatum, and frontal cortex *(31,32)*. These results suggested that dopamine uptake, storage, and/or metabolism was disturbed in SHRs. Recent evidence suggests that ADHD patients may also have disturbances in dopamine uptake, storage, and/or metabolism *(33,34)*. Using positron emission tomography, Ernst et al. *(34)* showed that [^{18}F] 3,4-dihydroxy-phenylalanine (DOPA) accumulation was increased in midbrain dopamine neurons of ADHD children. However, adults with ADHD were found to have abnormally low [^{18}F](DOPA accumulation in the prefrontal cortex, where DOPA decarboxylase occurs predominantly in noradrenergic terminals *(33)*, possibly suggesting developmental changes or, alternatively, opposite changes in dopaminergic and noradrenergic systems.

4. NORADRENERGIC SYSTEMS

Stimulus-evoked (electrically stimulated or K^+ evoked) release of norepinephrine from prefrontal cortex slices of SHR was similar to that of WKY *(35)*. However, autoreceptor-mediated inhibition of norepinephrine release was less efficient in SHR than in WKY prefrontal cortex and medulla oblongata *(35,36)*. α2-adrenoceptors appear to have been downregulated in SHRs. α2A-adrenoceptor mRNA levels were lower in the central nervous system of SHRs compared to WKYs *(37)*. α2A-adrenoceptor mRNA levels were negatively correlated with systolic blood pressure, whereas mRNA levels of the α1A-adrenoceptor and noradrenaline transporter were positively correlated with systolic blood pressure, suggesting that increased activity of the sympathetic nervous system may contribute to the elevated blood pressure of SHRs *(37)*. Consistent with increased synthesis of norepinephrine, tyrosine hydroxylase gene expression was higher in the ventrolateral medulla oblongata of SHRs than that of WKYs *(38)*. The concentration of norepinephrine was elevated in several brain areas of SHRs compared with WKYs, including locus ceruleus, substantia nigra, and prefrontal cortex *(31)*, suggesting that the disturbance in noradrenergic function is widespread and not restricted to a particular part of the nervous system. Increased norepinephrine is consistent with downregulation of β-adrenoceptors in the frontal cortex of SHRs *(39)*. Increased uptake by synaptosomal preparations of cerebral cortex of SHRs may represent compensatory upregulation of the norepinephrine transporter in an attempt to decrease the extracellular concentration of norepinephrine *(39)*. An increase in norepinephrine transporters would increase uptake of dopamine into noradrenergic terminals and varicosities, which could deplete extracellular dopamine in the prefrontal cortex *(40,41)*. The results suggest that there is an imbalance between dopaminergic and noradrenergic neurotransmission in the prefrontal cortex of SHR *(42)*. Whereas dopamine release is decreased in the SHR prefrontal cortex, norepinephrine concentrations are elevated, and the noradrenergic system appears to be hyperactive *(42)*.

5. GLUTAMATERGIC SYSTEMS

In addition to decreased autoreceptor-mediated inhibition of norepinephrine release from SHR prefrontal cortex slices, glutamate activation of α-amino-3-hydroxy-5-methyl-4-isoxazole propionate (AMPA) receptors caused greater release of norepinephrine from SHR prefrontal cortex slices than WKY *(43,44)*. Neural circuits that use glutamate as a neurotransmitter were suggested to exert greater stimulatory control of norepinephrine function in the prefrontal cortex of SHR *(43,44)*. It is possible that, like dopamine, impulse-stimulated release of norepinephrine is decreased in SHR, but this is compensated by reduced α2-adrenoceptor-mediated feedback inhibition of norepinephrine release and increased glutamate-mediated stimulation of release *(43–45)*. This may increase the spatial and temporal availability of released norepinephrine at postsynaptic and extrasynaptic receptors and thereby return noradrenergic function to normal, but the same does not seem to apply to dopamine *(43–45)*.

The tonic dopamine concentration in the extracellular fluid appears to be regulated by glutamate, which is present in micromolar concentrations in the extracellular space outside the synaptic cleft *(46–50)*. Glutamate inhibits dopamine release by activation of group II metabotropic receptors (mGluR2/3) and stimulates dopamine release by activation of group I receptors (mGluR5) on dopamine terminals in rat striatum *(46,51)*. Dopamine release is also increased by activation of AMPA receptors in rat striatum and stimulation of ventral tegmental dopamine neurons *(52–56)*. As suggested by Seeman and Madras *(57)*, the common defect in ADHD could be decreased extracellular dopamine levels. This deficiency could result from increased expression of DAT, impaired dopamine synthesis or release, or any other cause, including the possibility that regulation of extracellular dopamine by glutamate afferents from the prefrontal cortex, hippocampus, or amygdala is impaired. In vitro activation of AMPA receptors caused similar release of dopamine from SHR and WKY nucleus accumbens core *(54)*. However, glutamate-stimulated release of dopamine from the shell subdivision of SHR nucleus accumbens was significantly lower than from the core subdivision of SHR *(54)*. It is possible that, in addition to reduced stimulus-evoked release of dopamine, low extracellular dopamine concentrations observed in SHR striatum *(16)* may result from reduced glutamate-stimulated release of dopamine in the shell subdivision of the nucleus accumbens.

6. SECOND MESSENGER SYSTEMS

The disturbances in SHR do not appear to be restricted to a single neurotransmitter system. Differences between SHR and WKY suggest that the fundamental defect in SHR affects several, functionally distinct, neurotransmitter pathways. The disturbances of SHR can possibly be attributed to defects in two major second messenger systems, namely, impaired cyclic adenosine monophosphate (cAMP) formation *(8)* and impaired calcium influx into cells *(58)*.

Horn et al. *(59)* showed that synaptic plasma membranes prepared from SHR cerebrum have lower Ca^{2+} adenosine triphosphatase activity than WKY. This implies that Ca^{2+} is removed at a slower rate from SHR cytoplasm than WKY; hence the concentration gradient that drives Ca^{2+} into the cell is not as steep in SHR as in WKY. A lower Ca^{2+} concentration gradient may account for the decreased Ca^{2+} uptake observed in cerebral cortex slices of SHR compared to WKY *(58)*. Decreased Ca^{2+} influx could impair *N*-methyl-D-aspaitate receptor function *(58)*. Because neurotransmitter release is dependent on the influx of Ca^{2+} into presynaptic terminals and varicosities, an underlying disturbance in calcium metabolism could cause compensatory alterations in the regulation of neurotransmitter release.

The hyperactivity observed in ADHD children has been suggested to be because of increased cAMP levels in the prefrontal cortex and striatum *(60)*. Increased expression of *Gi*α genes has been demonstrated in very young SHRs at 2 wk of age *(8)*. Inactivation of Giα proteins by intraperitoneal injection of pertussis toxin into 2-wk-old SHRs delayed the development of hypertension *(61)*. These results suggest that the increased expression of genes for Gi proteins, with a consequent decrease in cAMP levels and impaired regulation of cellular function, precedes the elevation of blood pressure and may contribute to the development of hypertension and ADHD symptoms in SHRs. If striatal Giα proteins are also increased, then activation of D2 receptors may give rise to enhanced D2 receptor-mediated inhibition of dopamine release from SHR nucleus accumbens and caudate-putamen slices *(20–22)*.

Downregulation of α2-adrenoceptors observed in the SHR central nervous system may have been a compensatory response to increased Giα-mediated inhibition of adenylyl cyclase in an attempt to increase stimulus-evoked release of norepinephrine *(37)*.

7. NUCLEUS ACCUMBENS SHELL

In support of a deficit in the nucleus accumbens shell, giving rise to ADHD behavior in SHRs, Papa et al. *(26,27)* found decreased calcium/calmodulin-dependent protein kinase II and reduced c-Fos expression only in the nucleus accumbens shell of SHRs and not the core subdivision when compared to WKYs. The mesolimbic dopamine projection to the shell subdivision of the nucleus accumbens is responsible for motivation; it determines the amount of effort an animal is prepared to exert in order to achieve a reward. Hypofunction of the mesolimbic dopamine system will impair the function of the mesocortical and nigrostriatal dopamine systems, by influencing dopamine release and the cortico-striato-thalamo-cortical circuits that dopamine modulates. This could impair learning and expression of goal-directed behavior, thereby contributing to the ADHD symptoms displayed by SHRs.

A deficiency in the mesolimbic dopamine projection to the nucleus accumbens shell will impair dopamine release in the shell and thereby impair dopamine release in the nucleus accumbens core and dorsal striatum, as these areas are controlled by an ascending spiral that connects the striatum to the midbrain dopamine neurons *(62)*. The ascending spiral circuit regulates dopamine release and integrates information across functionally different parallel cortico-striato-thalamo-cortical circuits *(62)*. The nucleus accumbens is the interface between the limbic system and the motor system *(62,63)*. Limbic structures, such as the orbital and medial prefrontal cortex, hippocampus, amygdala, entorhinal, perirhinal, and anterior cingulate cortex, project to the nucleus accumbens and rostral medial caudate nucleus *(62,64,65)*. The nucleus accumbens projects via the ventral pallidum and substantia nigra to the dorsomedial thalamus, which projects to the dorsolateral prefrontal cortex in an ascending spiral *(62,64)*. The dorsolateral prefrontal cortex, together with the posterior parietal cortex, projects to the head of the caudate nucleus and rostral putamen, which, in turn, project via the globus pallidus/substantia nigra to the ventral anterior nucleus of the thalamus and from there to the supplementary motor, premotor, and motor cortex *(62,64)*. The latter, together with the somatosensory cortex, project to the rostral dorsolateral striatum and putamen, which project via the globus pallidus/substantia nigra to the ventrolateral nucleus of the thalamus and back to the supplementary motor cortex, completing the ascending spiral through which the nucleus accumbens shell influences behavioral expression *(62,64)*.

8. VENTRAL TEGMENTAL AREA DOPAMINE NEURONS

Glutamate plays an important role in stimulating catecholamine release at the somatic level. Disturbances at the level of the dopamine cell body may occur at a very early stage of development, giving rise to subsequent impaired dopamine neuron function in terminal areas such as the nucleus accumbens. The development of ADHD symptoms could be analogous to the process of drug addiction. Children who have been exposed prenatally to drugs of abuse exhibit ADHD-like behavior *(66)*. Exposure to drugs of abuse increases the extracellular dopamine concentration, which activates D1- and D2-like receptors in the ventral tegmental area of the midbrain, which in turn increases glutamate-driven activity in dopamine-containing neurons *(67)*. The mechanism is suggested to involve increased AMPA receptor-mediated excitatory transmission in ventral tegmental area dopamine neurons *(67,68)*. Increased activation by glutamate initially causes sensitization of ventral tegmental dopamine neurons with subsequent adaptations in the nucleus accumbens *(68)*. The increased glutamate drive is suggested ultimately to lead to pathophysiological conditions associated with high intracellular concentrations of Ca^{2+}, which gives rise to impaired function of ventral tegmental dopamine neurons consistent with adaptation *(68)*. Similarly, ADHD symptoms may result from adaptation to initially increased extracellular dopamine in the ventral tegmental area of the midbrain at a very early stage of development, giving rise to increased glutamate drive and subsequent loss of function of dopamine neurons.

Inappropriate activation of ventral tegmental dopamine neurons by glutamate afferents from the prefrontal cortex or other excitatory inputs could have increased dopamine release from ventral tegmental dopamine neurons at an early stage of development, giving rise to sensitization and subsequent impairment of ventral tegmental dopamine neuron function.

Table 1
Summary of Major Differences Between SHR and WKY

Authors names	Date	SHR age	Test used	Differences between SHR and WKY
Knardahl S, Sagvolden T	1979	6 wk	Open-field exploration	SHRs gradually became more active than controls
Myers MM, Whittemore SR, Hendley ED	1981	6 and 10 wk	Norepinephrine uptake and receptor binding studies	SHRs have greater rates of norepinephrine uptake and decreased β-adrenergic receptor density in the frontal cortex
Linthorst ACE, Van Den Buuse M, De Jong W, et al.	1990	4, 8, and 12 wk	In vitro superfusion	Decreased electrically stimulated release of [^{3}H]dopamine from SHR caudate slices. Nomifensine did not influence the difference in release between SHR and WKY
Tsuda K, Tsuda S, Masuyama Y, et al.	1990	adult	In vitro superfusion	Inhibitory effect of α2-adrenoceptor agonist on [^{3}H]norepinephrine release from the medulla oblongata slices of SHR significantly less than WKY
Linthorst ACE, De Lang H, De Jong W, et al.	1991	7–9 wk	Trans-striatal brain dialysis	Extracellular striatal dopamine concentration was lower in SHR. D2 receptor inhibition of dopamine release was greater in SHR
Sagvolden T, Hendley ED, Knardahl S	1992	6–7 wk, adults	Free- and forced-exploration in open-field, plus multiple fixed-interval schedules of reinforcement/extinction	SHRs were more active than controls in the open field. SHRs emitted more lever presses during the extinction component of the schedule than controls. SHRs became more active toward the end of the session
Wultz B, Sagvolden T	1992	adult	Differentially reinforced immobility requiring the rat to remain immobile at a particular place in an operant chamber in order to obtain a reinforcer	SHRs received more reinforcers than controls as long as the schedule did not require long periods of immobility. The total number of movements on target of SHRs increased as the schedule requirements increased.

(Continued)

Table 1
(Continued)

Authors names	Date	SHR age	Test used	Differences between SHR and WKY
Sagvolden T, Metzger MA, Schiørbeck HK, et al.	1992	adult	Multiple fixed-interval extinction schedules of reinforcement	Psychomotor stimulants weakened control by immediate reinforcers and strengthened control by delayed reinforcers
Mook DM, Jeffrey J, Neuringer A	1993	adult	Rewarded 12-arm radial maze	SHRs varied their choices more, making fewer repetition errors than WKYs. When rewards depended on variable sequences of responses on two levers in an operant chamber, SHRs' sequences were more variable than those of WKYs. WKYs learned to repeat more readily than the SHRs
Sagvolden T, Pettersen MB, Larsen MC	1993	adult	Free- and forced-exploration plus two-component multiple schedules of reinforcement with a fixed interval 2 min signaled by houselight on and a 5-min extinction signaled by houselight off.	SHRs were more active than WKYs in free exploration and forced exploration open field tests. SHRs were not overactive initially but activity increased toward the end of the extinction period
Kirouac G, Ganguly P	1993	5 and 15 wk	D1 and D2 receptor autoradiography	Increased D1 receptor density at 5 and 15 wk of age, increased D2 receptor density at 5 wk of age
Linthorst AC, van Giersbergen PL, Gras M, et al.	1994	10 wk	High-performance liquid chromatography (HPLC)	Homovanillic acid (HVA) and the ratios DOPAC/dopamine and HVA/dopamine were lower in sham-treated SHR than in sham-treated WKY
De Jong W, Linthorst AC, Versteeg HG	1995	4, 8, and 12 wk	In vitro and in vivo release of dopamine	No difference in blood pressure at 4 wk of age. Decreased release of [^{3}H]dopamine from SHR caudate slices of 4-wk-old SHRs. Decreased extracellular concentration of dopamine in caudate of 8-wk-old SHRs

(Continued)

Table 1
(Continued)

Authors names	Date	SHR age	Test used	Differences between SHR and WKY
Russell VA, de Villiers A, Sagvolden T, et al.	1995	12–14 wk	In vitro superfusion	Electrically stimulated [^{3}H]dopamine release was lower in caudate-putamen and prefrontal cortex slices of SHR. D2 receptor agonist caused greater inhibition of [^{3}H]dopamine release from SHR caudate-putamen slices. D2 antagonist caused greater increase in [^{3}H]dopamine release from SHR nucleus accumbens slices
De Villiers A, Russell VA, Sagvolden T, et al.	1995	12–14 wk	HPLC	Decreased homovanillic acid, decreased homovanillic acid/ dopamine ratio, and increased norepinephrine in brain of SHR
Horn JL, Janicki PK, Franks JJ	1995	adult	$^{45}Ca^{2+}$ uptake into synaptic plasma membrane vesicles	Diminished $^{45}Ca^{2+}$ uptake into synaptic plasma membrane vesicles prepared from cerebrum of SHR
Papa M, Sagvolden T, Sergeant JA, et al.,	1996	6 wk	Immunocytochemistry	Reduced Ca^{2+}/calmodulin-dependent protein kinase II (CaMKII) in nucleus accumbens shell of SHR
Watanabe Y, Fujita M, Ito Y, et al.	1997	2 and 15 wk	Dopamine transporter, D1 and D2 autoradiography	Increased dopamine transporter at 2 and 15 wk, increased D1 receptors at 15 wk in SHR caudate-putamen
Marcil J, Thibault C, Anand Srivastava MB	1997	3–5 d, 2 wk, 4 wk, and 8 wk	Expression of Giα	Increased expression of Gi-protein in SHR heart at 2 wk and older
Papa M, Sergeant JA, Sadile AG	1997	6 wk	Immunohistochemistry	Decreased *c-fos* and *zif/268* in nucleus accumbens core and shell of SHR
Papa M, Sergeant JA, Sadile AG	1998	6 wk	Immunohistochemistry	Reduced Ca^{2+}/ CaMKII in nucleus accumbens shell of SHR.Decreased *c-fos* and *zif/268* in nucleus accumbens core and shell of SHR

(Continued)

Table 1
(Continued)

Authors names	Date	SHR age	Test used	Differences between SHR and WKY
Russell VA, de Villiers AS, Sagvolden T	1998	12–14 wk	In vitro superfusion	Methylphenidate released less [^{3}H]dopamine from nucleus accumbens slices of SHR. D-Amphetamine released more [^{3}H]dopamine from caudate-putamen, nucleus accumbens, and prefrontal cortex slices of SHR. At low concentration, in vitro methylphenidate increase in electrically stimulated release of [^{3}H]dopamine from caudate-putamen, nucleus accumbens and prefrontal cortex, similar for SHR and WKY
Berger DF, Sagvolden T	1998	8–9 wk	Operant discrimination task—two-component multiple schedule reinforcement with 2-min fixed interval 5-min extinction schedule of water reinforcement	Hyperactive and behavioral extinction deficit toward the end of the extinction component
Carey MP, Diewald LM, Esposito FJ, et al.	1998	4 wk	D1 and D2 receptor autoradiography	SHRs have higher density of D1 receptors in caudate-putamen, nucleus accumbens, and olfactory tubercle which was reversed by methylphenidate treatment (3 mg/kg i.p., for 2 wk). Methylphenidate treatment also downregulated D2 receptors in these areas
Russell VA, Allie S, Wiggins T	2000	4–6 wk	In vitro superfusion	Depolarization-evoked release (resulting from electrical stimulation or exposure to high concentration of K^+) of [^{3}H]norepinephrine from SHR prefrontal cortex was similar to WKY. α2-Adrenoceptor mediated inhibition of [^{3}H]norepinephrine release is decreased in SHR prefrontal cortex

(Continued)

Table 1
(Continued)

Authors names	Date	SHR age	Test used	Differences between SHR and WKY
Russell VA	2000	4–6 wk	In vitro superfusion	Increased glutamate-stimulated release of $[^3H]$norepinephrine from SHR prefrontal cortex slices
Russell VA, de Villiers AS, Sagvolden T	2000	12–14 wk	In vitro superfusion	Methylphenidate (3 mg/kg for 2 wk) did not normalise the decreased electrically stimulated release of $[^3H]$dopamine from SHR caudate-putamen slices. Methylphenidate increased endogenous dopamine activation of D2 receptors in WKY striatum but did not alter D2 receptor function in SHR
Sagvolden T	2000	Review	Reanalysis of data	Overactivity, motor impulsiveness, and deficient sustained attention in SHR
Russell VA	2001	4–6 wk	In vitro superfusion	Increased glutamate-stimulated release of $[^3H]$norepinephrine from SHR prefrontal cortex slices is antagonized by CNQX, an AMPA receptor antagonist
Lehohla M, Russell V, Kellaway L	2001	4–6 wk	NMDA-stimulated uptake of $^{45}Ca^{2+}$ into brain slices in vitro	Decreased $^{45}Ca^{2+}$ uptake into barrel cortex slices of SHR
Christiansen RE, Roald AB, et al.	2002	2, 4, 6, 8 and 10 wk	Blood pressure measurement	SHR and WKY have similar body weight. Mean arterial blood pressure was not different at the age of 2 wk but increased from 4 to 10 wk of age
Ueno KI, Togashi H, Mori K	2002	6 wk, stroke-prone SHR	Open-field exploration	Methylphenidate (0.01–1 mg/kg, i.p.) significantly attenuated locomotor hyperactivity at low doses
Reja V, Goodchild AK, Pilowsky PM	2002	adult	Total RNA was reverse-transcribed into cDNA followed by quantitative fluorescence	Amount of α2A-R mRNA in central nervous system lower in SHR and negatively correlated with systolic blood pressure.

(Continued)

Table 1
(Continued)

Authors names	Date	SHR age	Test used	Differences between SHR and WKY
			detection polymerase chain reaction for cDNA.	Phenylethanolamine-*N*-methyltransferase, noradrenaline transporter, and α1A-R mRNA levels positively correlated with systolic blood pressure in all central tissue investigated
Reja V, Goodchild AK, Phillips JK	2002	adult	Total RNA reverse-transcribed into cDNA followed by quantitative fluorescence detection polymerase chain reaction for cDNA	Increased tyrosine hydroxylase gene expression in the rostral and caudal ventrolateral medulla oblongata of the brainstem of SHR. There was a positive relationship between systolic blood pressure and tyrosine hydroxylase gene expression
Li Y, Anand-Srivastava MB	2002	2 wk	Blood pressure measurement	Inactivation of enhanced expression of G(i) proteins by pertussis toxin attenuates the development of high blood pressure in SHR
Russell VA	2003	4–6 wk	In vitro superfusion	Glutamate-stimulated release of [^{3}H]dopamine from SHR nucleus accumbens core is similar to WKY core while release from SHR shell is lower than SHR core
Yang PB, Amini B, Swann AC	2003	8 wk	Automated activity monitoring system recorded horizontal activity, total distance traveled, rearing, stereotypic movements, and number of discrete movements	Repeated administration of 2.5 mg/kg methylphenidate elicited locomotor sensitization in Sprague-Dawley and WKY rats but not in SHR. Repeated administration of 10 mg/kg methylphenidate induced locomotor tolerance in Sprague-Dawley and WKY rats but variable response in SHR

SHR, spontaneously hypertensive rat; WKY, Wistar–Kyoto rat; DOPAC, 3,4-dihydroxy-phenylacetic acid; i. p., intraperitoneally; AMPA, α–amino-3-hydroxy-5-methyl-4-isoxazole propionate.

In support of this hypothesis, SHRs appear to have a disturbance in the regulation of midbrain dopamine neurons. The effect of psychomotor stimulant drugs was less pronounced in SHRs than in WKYs, whereas psychostimulants strengthened control by delayed reinforcers to a greater extent in WKYs in fixed-interval schedules of reinforcement of bar-presses by water *(4)*. Furthermore, repeated administration of a dopamine uptake blocker, methylphenidate (2.5 mg/kg), elicited locomotor sensitization in Sprague-Dawley and WKY rats, whereas SHRs were not affected by the drug *(69)*. Similarly, a higher dose of methylphenidate (10 mg/kg) produced locomotor tolerance in Sprague-Dawley and WKY rats but not in SHRs *(69)*. This is consistent with in vitro findings where methylphenidate released significantly less dopamine from SHR nucleus accumbens slices than WKY *(22)*. Chronic methylphenidate treatment (3 mg/kg for 2 wk) increased endogenous dopamine activation of D2 receptors in WKY striatum but did not alter D2 receptor function in SHRs probably because regulation of the dopamine pathway was already disturbed and D2 receptors were already upregulated *(70)*. These results suggest that the pathway that is affected by drugs of abuse is also the pathway that is disturbed in SHR.

9. CONCLUSION

In conclusion, SHR provide a good model for ADHD symptoms. Disturbances that have been identified in the central nervous system of SHR have provided insight into the possible neurogenesis of the behavioral disturbances of ADHD. Evidence suggests that the most frequently prescribed psychostimulants, D-amphetamine and methylphenidate, alleviate ADHD symptoms by blocking dopamine reuptake, which increases dopamine availability at postsynaptic and extrasynaptic receptors not only following impulse-triggered release of dopamine from mesolimbic, mesocortical, and nigrostriatal dopamine nerve terminals, but also following glutamate-stimulated release of dopamine from mesolimbic terminals in the nucleus accumbens shell. The nucleus accumbens shell plays an important role in the integration of afferent signals from limbic areas of the brain, particularly the amygdala, hippocampal formation, prefrontal cortex, and cingulate cortex. Transmission of these signals to motor areas of the brain is modulated by mesolimbic dopamine input, which gives rise to reinforcement of appropriate behavior *(71)*. The evidence is consistent with a deficiency in the dopaminergic sytem contributing to the behavioral disturbances of SHR.

ACKNOWLEDGMENTS

The author wishes to thank the University of Cape Town and South African Medical Research Council for financial support.

REFERENCES

1. Kirley A, Hawi Z, Daly G, et al. Dopaminergic system genes in ADHD: toward a biological hypothesis. Neuropsychopharmacology 2002;27:607–619.
2. Sagvolden T. Behavioral validation of the spontaneously hypertensive rat (SHR) as an animal model of attention-deficit/hyperactivity disorder (AD/HD). Neurosci and Biobehav Rev 2000;24:31–39.
3. Berger DF, Sagvolden T. Sex differences in operant discrimination behavior in an animal model of attention-deficit hyperactivity disorder. Behav Brain Res 1998;94:73–82.
4. Sagvolden T, Metzger MA, Schiørbeck HK, Rugland A-L, Spinnangr I, Sagvolden G. The spontaneously hypertensive rat (SHR) as an animal model of childhood hyperactivity (ADHD): changed reactivity to reinforcers and to psychomotor stimulants. Behav Neural Biol 1992;58:103–112.
5. Sagvolden T, Pettersen MB, Larsen MC. Spontaneously hypertensive rats (SHR) as a putative animal model of childhood hyperkinesis: SHR behavior compared to four other rat strains. Physiol Behav 1993;54:1047–1055.

6. Christiansen RE, Roald AB, Tenstad O, Iversen B. Renal hemodynamics during development of hypertension in young spontaneously hypertensive rats. Kidney Blood Press Res 2002;25:322–328.
7. Okamoto K, Aoki K. Development of a strain of spontaneously hypertensive rats. Jpn Circulation J 1963;27:282–293.
8. Marcil J, Thibault C, Anand-Srivastava MB. Enhanced expression of Gi-protein precedes the development of blood pressure in spontaneously hypertensive rats. J Mol Cell Cardiol 1997; 29:1009–1022.
9. Knardahl S, Sagvolden T. Open-field behavior of spontaneously hypertensive rats. Behav Neural Biol 1979;27:187–200.
10. Sagvolden T, Hendley ED, Knardahl S. Behavior of hypertensive and hyperactive rat strains: Hyperactivity is not unitarily determined. Physiol Behav 1992;52:49–57.
11. Wultz B, Sagvolden T. The hyperactive spontaneously hypertensive rat learns to sit still, but not to stop bursts of responses with short interresponse times. Behav Genet 1992;22:415–433.
12. Mook DM, Jeffrey J, Neuringer A. Spontaneously hypertensive rats (SHR) easily learn to vary but not repeat instrumental responses. Behav Neural Biol 1993;59:126–135.
13. Sagvolden T, Sergeant JA. Attention deficit/hyperactivity disorder—from brain dysfunctions to behavior. Behav Brain Res 1998;94:1–10.
14. Myers MM, Musty RE, Hendley ED. Attenuation of hyperactivity in the spontaneously hypertensive rat by amphetamine. Behav Neural Biol 1982;34:42–54.
15. Ueno KI, Togashi H, Mori K, et al. Behavioral and pharmacological relevance of stroke-prone spontaneously hypertensive rats as an animal model of a developmental disorder. Behav Pharmacol 2002;13:1–13.
16. De Jong W, Linthorst AC, Versteeg HG. The nigrostriatal dopamine system and the development of hypertension in the spontaneously hypertensive rat. Arch Mal Coeur Vaiss 1995;88:1193–1196.
17. Linthorst ACE, De Lang H, De Jong W, Versteeg DH. Effect of the dopamine D2 receptor agonist quinpirole on the in vivo release of dopamine in the caudate nucleus of hypertensive rats. Eur J Pharmacol 1991;201:125–133.
18. Linthorst ACE, Van Den Buuse M, De Jong W, Versteeg DHG. Electrically stimulated [3H]dopamine and [14C]acetylcholine release from nucleus caudatus slices: differences between spontaneously hypertensive rats and Wistar-Kyoto rats. Brain Res 1990;509:266–272.
19. Russell VA. The nucleus accumbens motor-limbic interface of the spontaneously hypertensive rat as studied in vitro by the superfusion slice technique. Neurosci Biobehav Rev 2000;24:133–136.
20. Russell VA, de Villiers A, Sagvolden T, Lamm M, Taljaard J. Altered dopaminergic function in the prefrontal cortex, nucleus accumbens and caudate-putamen of an animal model of attention-deficit hyperactivity disorder—the spontaneously hypertensive rat. Brain Res 1995;676:343–351.
21. Russell VA, de Villiers AS, Sagvolden T, Lamm MCL, Taljaard JJF. Impaired vesicular storage of dopamine in an animal model for attention-deficit hyperactivity disorder—the spontaneously hypertensive rat. Soc Neurosci Abstr 1996;22:2082.
22. Russell VA, de Villiers A, Sagvolden T, Lamm M, Taljaard J. Differences between electrically-, ritalin- and d-amphetamine-stimulated release of [^{3}H]dopamine from brain slices suggest impaired vesicular storage of dopamine in an animal model for attention-deficit hyperactivity disorder. Behav Brain Res 1998;94:163–171.
23. Carey MP, Diewald LM, Esposito FJ, et al. Differential distribution, affinity and plasticity of dopamine D-1 and D-2 receptors in the target sites of the mesolimbic system in an animal model of ADHD. Behav Brain Res 1998;94:173–185.
24. Kirouac G, Ganguly P. Up-regulation of dopamine receptors in the brain of the spontaneously hypertensive rat: an autoradiographic analysis. Neurosci 1993;52:135–141.
25. Watanabe Y, Fujita M, Ito Y, Okada T, Kusuoka H, Nishimura T. Brain dopamine transporter in spontaneously hypertensive rats. J Nucl Med 1997;38:470–474.
26. Papa M, Sagvolden T, Sergeant JA, Sadile AG. Reduced CaMKII-positive neurones in the accumbens shell of an animal model of attention-deficit hyperactivity disorder. Neurorep 1996;7:3017–3020.

27. Papa M, Sergeant JA, Sadile AG. Differential expression of transcription factors in the accumbens of an animal model of ADHD. Neurorep 1997;8:1607–1612.
28. Papa M, Sergeant JA, Sadile AG. Reduced transduction mechanisms in the anterior accumbal interface of an animal model of attention-deficit hyperactivity disorder. Behav Brain Res 1998;94:187–195.
29. Jones SR, Gainetdinov RR, Wightman RM, Caron MG. Mechanisms of amphetamine action revealed in mice lacking the dopamine transporter. J Neurosci 1998;18:1979–1986.
30. Moore KE. Amphetamines: biochemical and behavioral actions in animals. In: Iversen LL, Iversen SD, Snyder S, eds. Handbook of psychopharmacology. New York: Plenum Press, 1978; 41–98.
31. De Villiers A, Russell VA, Sagvolden T, Searson A, Jaffer A, Taljaard J. α2-adrenoceptor mediated inhibition of [3H]dopamine release from nucleus accumbens slices and monoamine levels in a rat model for attention-deficit hyperactivity disorder. Neurochem Res 1995;20:427–433.
32. Linthorst AC, van Giersbergen PL, Gras M, Versteeg DH, de Jong W. The nigrostriatal dopamine system: role in the development of hypertension in spontaneously hypertensive rats. Brain Res 1994;639:261–268.
33. Ernst M, Zametkin AJ, Matochik JA, Jons PH, Cohen RM. DOPA decarboxylase activity in attention deficit hyperactivity disorder adults. A [fluorine-18]fluorodopa positron emission tomographic study. J Neurosci 1998;18:5901–5907.
34. Ernst M, Zametkin A, Matochik J, Pascualvaca D, Jons P, Cohen R. High midbrain [^{18}F]DOPA accumulation in children with attention deficit hyperactivity disorder. Am J Psychiatry 1999;156:1209–1215.
35. Russell VA, Allie S, Wiggins T. Increased noradrenergic activity in prefrontal cortex slices of an animal model for attention-deficit hyperactivity disorder—the spontaneously hypertensive rat. Behav Brain Res 2000;117:69–74.
36. Tsuda K, Tsuda S, Masuyama Y, Goldstein M. Norepinephrine release and neuropeptide Y in medulla oblongata of spontaneously hypertensive rats. Hypertension 1990;15:784–790.
37. Reja V, Goodchild AK, Pilowsky PM. Catecholamine-related gene expression correlates with blood pressures in SHR. Hypertension 2002;40:342–347.
38. Reja V, Goodchild AK, Phillips JK, Pilowsky PM. Tyrosine hydroxylase gene expression in ventrolateral medulla oblongata of WKY and SHR: a quantitative real-time polymerase chain reaction study. Auton Neurosci 2002;98:79–84.
39. Myers MM, Whittemore SR, Hendley ED. Changes in catecholamine neuronal uptake and receptor binding in the brains of spontaneously hypertensive rats (SHR). Brain Res 1981;220:325–338.
40. Mazei MS, Pluto CP, Kirkbride B, Pehek EA. Effects of catecholamine uptake blockers in the caudate-putamen and subregions of the medial prefrontal cortex of the rat. Brain Res 2002;936:58–67.
41. Moron JA, Brockington A, Wise RA, Rocha BA, Hope BT. Dopamine uptake through the norepinephrine transporter in brain regions with low levels of the dopamine transporter: evidence from knock-out mouse lines. J Neurosci 2002;22:389–395.
42. Russell VA. Hypodopaminergic and hypernoradrenergic activity in prefrontal cortex slices of an animal model for attention-deficit hyperactivity disorder—the spontaneously hypertensive rat. Behav Brain Res 2002;130:191–196.
43. Russell VA. Increased AMPA receptor function in slices containing the prefrontal cortex of spontaneously hypertensive rats. Metab Brain Dis 2001;16:143–149.
44. Russell VA, Wiggins T. Increased glutamate-stimulated norepinephrine release from prefrontal cortex slices of spontaneously hypertensive rats. Metab Brain Dis 2000;15:297–304.
45. Russell VA, Allie S, Wiggins T. Increased noradrenergic activity in prefrontal cortex slices of an animal model for attention-deficit hyperactivity disorder—the spontaneously hypertensive rat. Behav Brain Res 2000;117:69–74.
46. Baker DA, Xi ZX, Shen H, Swanson CJ, Kalivas PW. The origin and neuronal function of in vivo nonsynaptic glutamate. J Neurosci 2002;22:9134–9141.

47. Glowinski J, Cheramy A, Romo R, Barbeito L. Presynaptic regulation of dopaminergic transmission in the striatum. Cell Mol Neurobiol 1988;8:7–17.
48. Grace AA. Phasic versus tonic dopamine release and the modulation of dopamine system responsivity: a hypothesis for the etiology of schizophrenia. Neuroscience 1991;41:1–24.
49. Howland JG, Taepavarapruk P, Phillips AG. Glutamate receptor-dependent modulation of dopamine efflux in the nucleus accumbens by basolateral, but not central, nucleus of the amygdala in rats. J. Neurosci. 2002;22:1137–1145.
50. Kulagina NV, Zigmond MJ, Michael AC. Glutamate regulates the spontaneous and evoked release of dopamine in the rat striatum. Neurosci 2001;102:121–128.
51 Golembiowska K, Konieczny J, Ossowska K, Wolfarth S. The role of striatal metabotropic glutamate receptors in degeneration of dopamine neurons: Review article. Amino Acids 2002;23:199–205.
52. Legault M, Wise RA. Injections of *N*-methyl-D-aspartate into the ventral hippocampus increase extracellular dopamine in the ventral tegmental area and nucleus accumbens. Synapse 1999;31:241–249.
53. Maione S, Biggs CS, Rossi F, Fowler LJ, Whitton PS. Alpha-amino-3-hydroxy-5-methyl-4-isoxazolepropionate receptors modulate dopamine release in rat hippocampus and striatum. Neurosci Lett 1995;193:181–184.
54. Russell VA. In vitro glutamate-stimulated release of dopamine from nucleus accumbens core and shell of spontaneously hypertensive rats. Metab Brain Dis 2003; 18:161–168.
55. Vorel SR, Campos A, Gardner EL. Prolonged electrical stimulation of the medial forebrain bundle elicits cocaine-seeking behavior. Program No. 876.8. 2002 Abstract Viewer/Itinerary Planner. Washington, DC: Society for Neuroscience, 2002.
56. Vorel SR, Liu X, Hayes RJ, Spector JA, Gardner EL. Relapse to cocaine-seeking after hippocampal theta burst stimulation. Science 2001;292:1175–1178.
57. Seeman P, Madras B. Methylphenidate elevates resting dopamine which lowers the impulse-triggered release of dopamine: a hypothesis. Behav Brain Res 2002;130:79–83.
58. Lehohla M, Russell V, Kellaway L. NMDA-stimulated Ca^{2+} uptake into barrel cortex slices of spontaneously hypertensive rats. Metab Brain Res 2001;16:165–174.
59. Horn JL, Janicki PK, Franks JJ. Diminished brain synaptic plasma membrane Ca^{2+}-ATPase activity in spontaneously hypertensive rats: association with reduced anesthetic requirements. Life Sci 1995;56:427–432.
60 Andersen SL. Changes in the second messenger cyclic AMP during development may underlie motoric symptonms in attention deficit/hyperactivity disorder (ADHD). Behav Brain Res 2002;130:197–201.
61. Li Y, Anand-Srivastava MB. Inactivation of enhanced expression of G(i) proteins by pertussis toxin attenuates the development of high blood pressure in spontaneously hypertensive rats. Circ Res 2002;91:247–254.
62. Haber SN, Fudge JL, McFarland NR. Striatonigral pathways in primates form an ascending spiral from the shell to the dorsal striatum. J Neurosci 2000;20:2369–2382.
63. Morgenson GJ, Douglas LJ, Yim CY. From motivation to action: functional interface between the limbic system and the motor system, Prog Neurobiol 1980;14:69–97.
64. Alexander GE, De Long MR, Strick PL. Parallel organization of functionally segregated circuits linking basal ganglia and cortex. Ann Rev Neurosci 1986;9:357–381.
65. Parkinson JA, Willoughby PJ, Robbins TW, Everitt BJ. Disconnection of the anterior cingulate cortex and nucleus accumbens core impairs Pavlovian approach behavior: further evidence for limbic cortical-ventral striatopallidal systems. Behav Neurosci 2000;114:42–63.
66. Mick E, Biederman J, Faraone SV, Sayer J, Kleinman S. Case-control study of attention-deficit hyperactivity disorder and maternal smoking, alcohol use, and drug use during pregnancy. J Am Acad Child Adolesc Psychiatry 2002;41:378–385.
67. Bonci A, Bernardi G, Grillner P, Mercuri NB. The dopamine-containing neuron: maestro or simple musician in the orchestra of addiction? TIPS 2003;24:172–177.

68. Carlezon WA, Nestler EJ. Elevated levels of GluR1 in the midbrain: a trigger for sensitization to drugs of abuse? TINS 2002;25:610–615.
69. Yang PB, Amini B, Swann AC, Dafny N. Strain differences in the behavioral responses of male rats to chronically administered methylphenidate. Brain Res 2003;971:139–152.
70. Russell VA, de Villiers AS, Sagvolden T, Lamm MCL, Taljaard JJF. Methylphenidate affects striatal dopamine differently in an animal model for attention-deficit/hyperactivity disorder—the spontaneously hypertensive rat. Brain Res Bull 2000;53:187–192.
71. Everitt BJ, Parkinson JA, Olmstead MC, Arroyo M, Robledo P, Robbins TW. Associative processes in addiction and reward. The role of amygdala-ventral striatal subsystems. Ann NY Acad Sci 1999; 877:412–438.

5

The Roles of Norepinephrine and Serotonin in Attention Deficit Hyperactivity Disorder

Robert D. Oades

1. INTRODUCTION

Norepinephrine (NE) belongs to the chemical group of the catecholamines and is also known outside the Americas as noradrenaline. Serotonin, an indoleamine, is better described chemically as 5-hydroxytryptamine (5-HT). Together with the catecholamines dopamine (DA) and epinephrine (adrenaline), they are known as the "monoamines." These monoamines have an agent role in transmission between neurons—often in the synapse between neurons and their elements in apposition, sometimes between release and receptor sites that are further apart. Then the role is more reminiscent of hormonal communication. Both roles are subsumed as neurotransmission. These transmitters are located in well-characterized, similar neural pathways throughout the vertebrates.

This chapter is essentially concerned with the roles of NE and 5-HT in the central nervous system (CNS) and how characteristics of 5-HT and NE transmission could contribute to the principal features of attention deficit hyperactivity disorder (ADHD). This review starts with the basic aspects of monoamine biochemistry and neurochemical anatomy and proceeds over mechanisms of function (animal research) to investigations of their role in the neuropsychology and nosology thought to underlie ADHD. However, throughout these considerations it should not be overlooked that both 5-HT and NE pathways are widely distributed peripherally with functions additional to those considered here.* It is also important to bear in mind in the ensuing discussion of NE and 5-HT function that many of the effects simply attributed to the activity of one or the other monoamine are, through multiple interactions, additionally dependent on another monoamine.

2. BIOCHEMISTRY

5-HT and NE synthesis depends on the availability of the amino acids tryptophan and phenylalanine, respectively. Tryptophan is hydroxylated in the rate-limiting step by tryptophan hydroxylase to the precursor 5-hydroxytryptophan (5-HTP) prior to conversion to 5-HT by decarboxylation.

*For example, 5-HT has a prominent role in pulmonary and renal blood flow, as well as the enteric autonomic system (smooth muscle contraction): NE, released from postganglionic sympathetic neurons, also actively modulates vasoconstriction/dilation, especially heart and smooth muscle function (also the uterus, intestine, bronchi, and iris). In addition NE modulates insulin secretion and several metabolic activities (note also that NE is the precursor to epinephrine synthesis in the adrenal medulla).

From: *Attention Deficit Hyperactivity Disorder: From Genes to Patients*
Edited by: D. Gozal and D. L. Molfese © Humana Press Inc., Totowa, NJ

For NE synthesis, phenylalanine is hydroxylated to tyrosine prior to the rate-limiting hydroxylation to L-3, 4-dehydroxy-phenylalanine (Fig. 1). Decarboxylation then produces DA, which can be dehydroxylated to NE. Many studies examining the effects of enhancing or depleting NE make use of the crucial role of tyrosine hydroxylase (TOH) and dopamine β-hydroxylase (DBH). Studies of 5-HT depletion often use diets free of tryptophan for examining the effect of reducing 5-HT activity. Thus it is not surprising that dietary effects on the availablity of factors needed for transmitter synthesis have been part of the agenda in some ADHD studies.

Breakdown (catabolism) occurs following postsynaptic uptake of the neurotransmitter, when the transmitter remains unused in the synapse, or after presynaptic reuptake when not stored in vesicles. In detail the NE and 5-HT catabolic pathways can differ. Several enzymes are involved in both. But primary is the oxidation process (monoamine oxidase [MAO]). For 5-HT this leads to 5-hydroxy-indoleacetic acid (5-HIAA; Fig. 2); for NE there are many intermediates resulting from the activities of several enzymes.

Three trends emerge from metabolic studies that help the interpretation of clinical results. First, the primary products of stimulated central NE synthesis are mostly 3-methoxy- and dihydroxy-phenyl-glycol (MHPG, DHPG), whereas extraneuronal products also include metanephrine (MN) and normetanephrine (NMN) *(1)*. As these latter metabolites, along with vanillomandelic acid (VMA), do not cross the blood-brain barrier, peripheral measures of these metabolites likely reflect peripheral sources. Second, these metabolites (e.g., NMN, VMA), often measured peripherally, can be excreted partially, after further metabolism, as homovanillic acid (HVA). This leads to some confusion over identifying the relative roles of NE and DA activity. Third, NE and 5-HT are the preferred substrates for MAO type A, whereas tyramine, tryptamine, and DA are the preferred substrates of MAO type B; however, the separation of function between these two isoenzymes is not tight (e.g., selective inhibitors of both MAO-A [clorgyline] and MAO-B [selegiline] can reduce 5-HT catabolism).

3. CNS PATHWAYS

3.1. *Norepinephrine*

In the 1950s, pioneer work demonstrated NE to be a chemical transmitter that has its cells of origin in the brain stem *(2,3)*. The locus ceruleus (LC; A6) is located in the dorsolateral pontine tegmentum just lateral to the fourth ventricle *(4,5*; Fig. 3). It and the nearby A5, A7 nuclei (subceruleus) give rise to NE fibers innervating the forebrain (dorsal noradrenergic bundle), diencephalon, cerebellum, and local brainstem nuclei. Some fibers also descend in the spinal cord *(6)*. A more ventral bundle with fibers from the nucleus tractus solitarius (A2) also innervates the diencephalon and a number of subcortical limbic regions *(7)*. The LC in humans is about 15 mm long and in adults including some 40,000–60,000 NE-containing cells. Of interest for animal models, there is much similarity between the LC in humans and that of the rat—even if the latter contains only 3% of the number of neurons in the human LC. Other transmitting agents, such as neuropeptide Y, galanin, and γ-aminobutyric acid (GABA) may also be colocalized in these neurons.

To understand the function of the NE system it is important to appreciate that there is much dendrite branching locally within the LC and axonal branching between widely separate areas innervated by the same neuron *(8)*. If one considers the vast areas of cortex innervated it may be that as few as 5% of transmitter-containing varicosities are located in

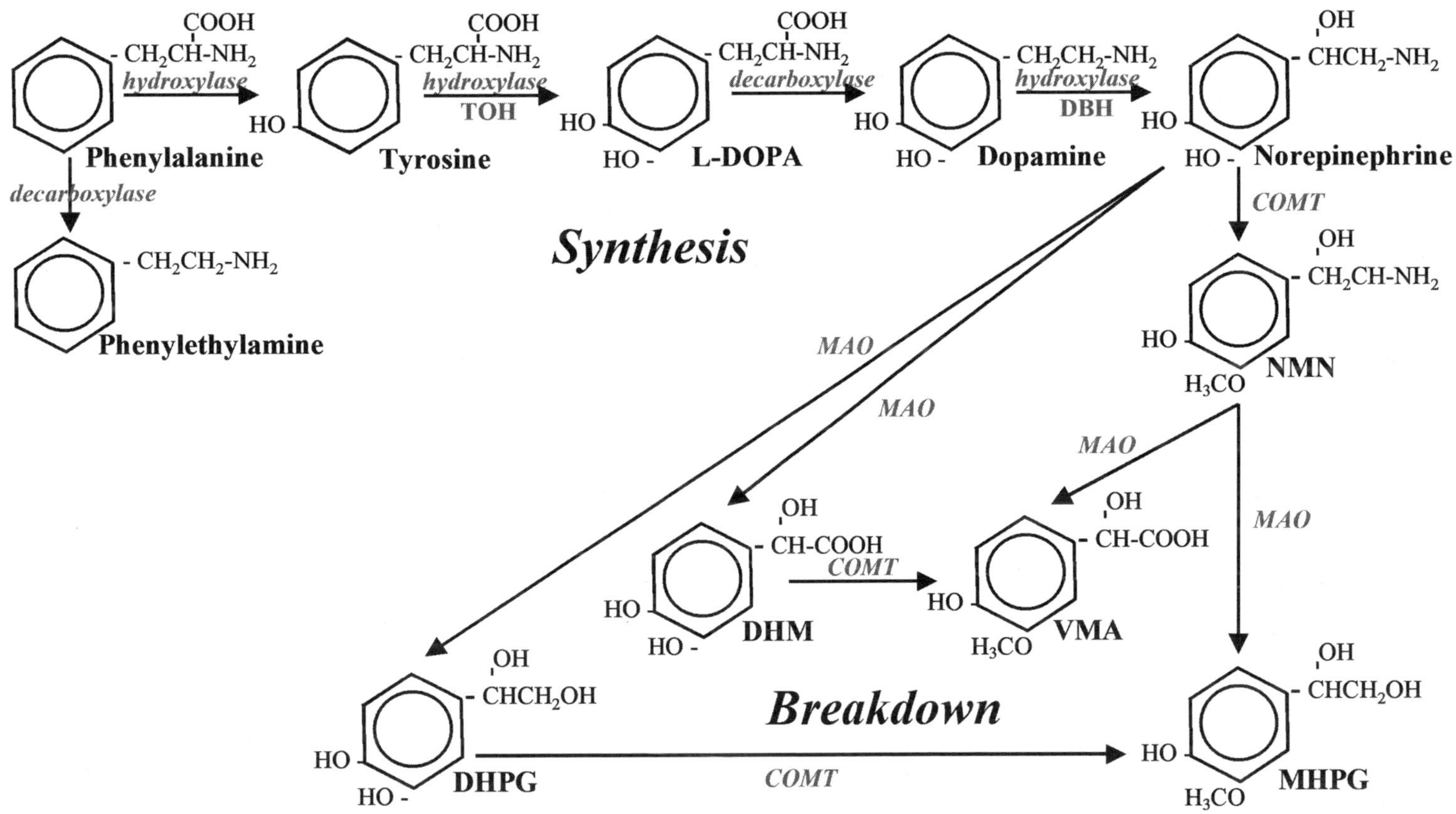

Fig. 1. Norepinephrine (NE) metabolism: Biochemical pathways showing the synthesis and breakdown of NE. COMT, Catechol-*O*-methyltransferase; DHM, 3,4-dihydroxymandelic acid; DHPG, 3,4-dihydroxyphenylethylglycol; l-DOPA, *laevo*-dihydroxyphenylalanine; MAO, monoamine oxidase; MHPG, 3-4-hydroxyphenylethylglycol; NMN, normetanephrine; VMA, vanillomandelic acid.

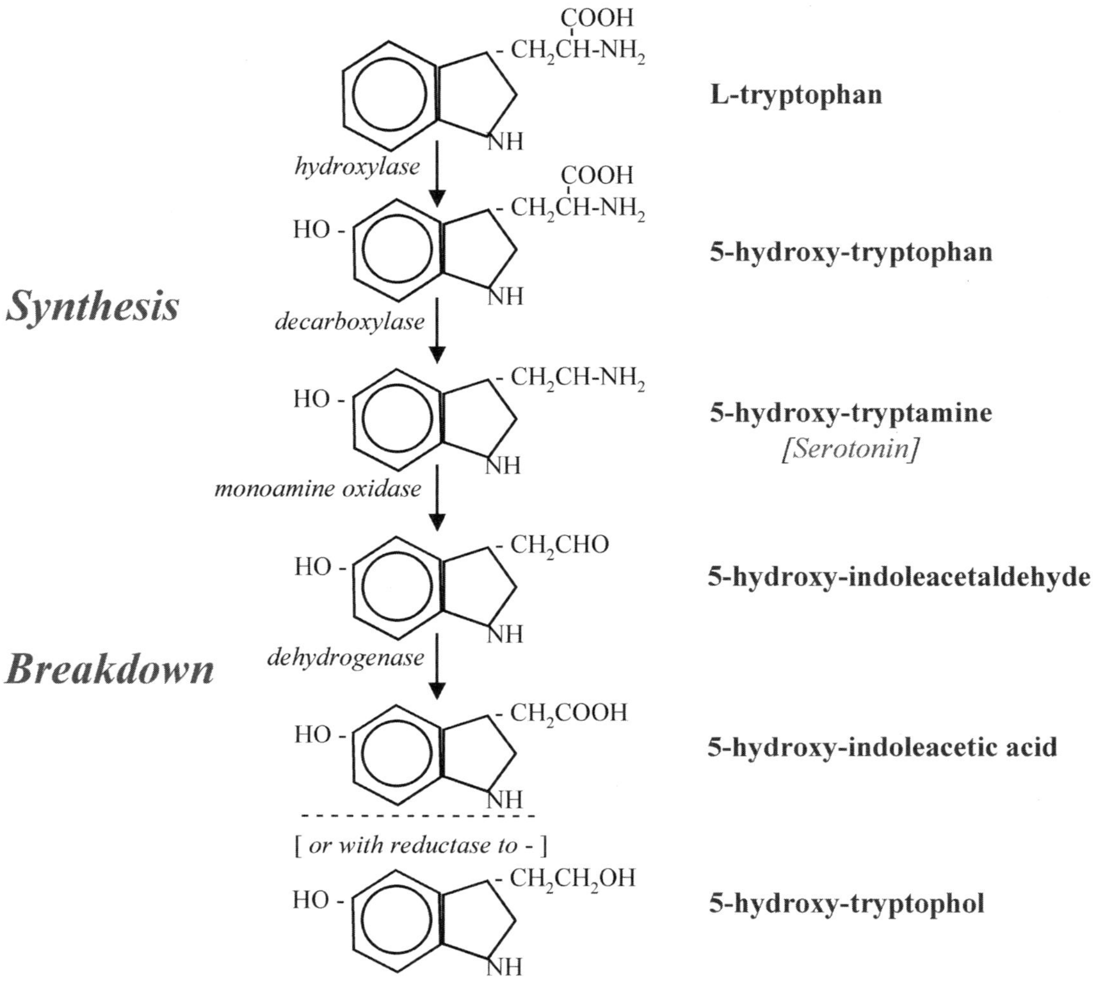

Fig. 2. Serotonin (5-HT) metabolism: Biochemical pathways showing the synthesis and breakdown of 5-HT.

conventional synapses *(9)*. Most of the transmitter released has its effect at a distance from the end of the axon. The densest input is to the laminae III and IV *(10)*. α-1 and α-2 receptor types that can be pre- or postsynaptically located are distributed more across the superficial laminae, whereas β sites may be found in most cortical laminae (α2a have a primarily frontal, α2b a more thalamic, and α2c a brainstem distribution).

3.2. 5-HT

5-HT was first demonstrated in the CNS of cats and dogs about 50 yr ago *(11,12)*. The development of fluorescence histochemistry 10 yr later led to the description of the basic components of the 5-HT projection system *(13)*. In succeding decades the development of antibodies and of immunohistochemical *(13)* and immunocytochemical methods led to the current understanding of the cell body origins and their heterogeneous termination patterns *(14)*. For 5-HT there are nine cell groups (B1–B9). B1–B5 are small cell groups located in the midline from the mid-pons to the caudal medulla (Fig. 4). They project locally and down the dorsal and ventral horns of

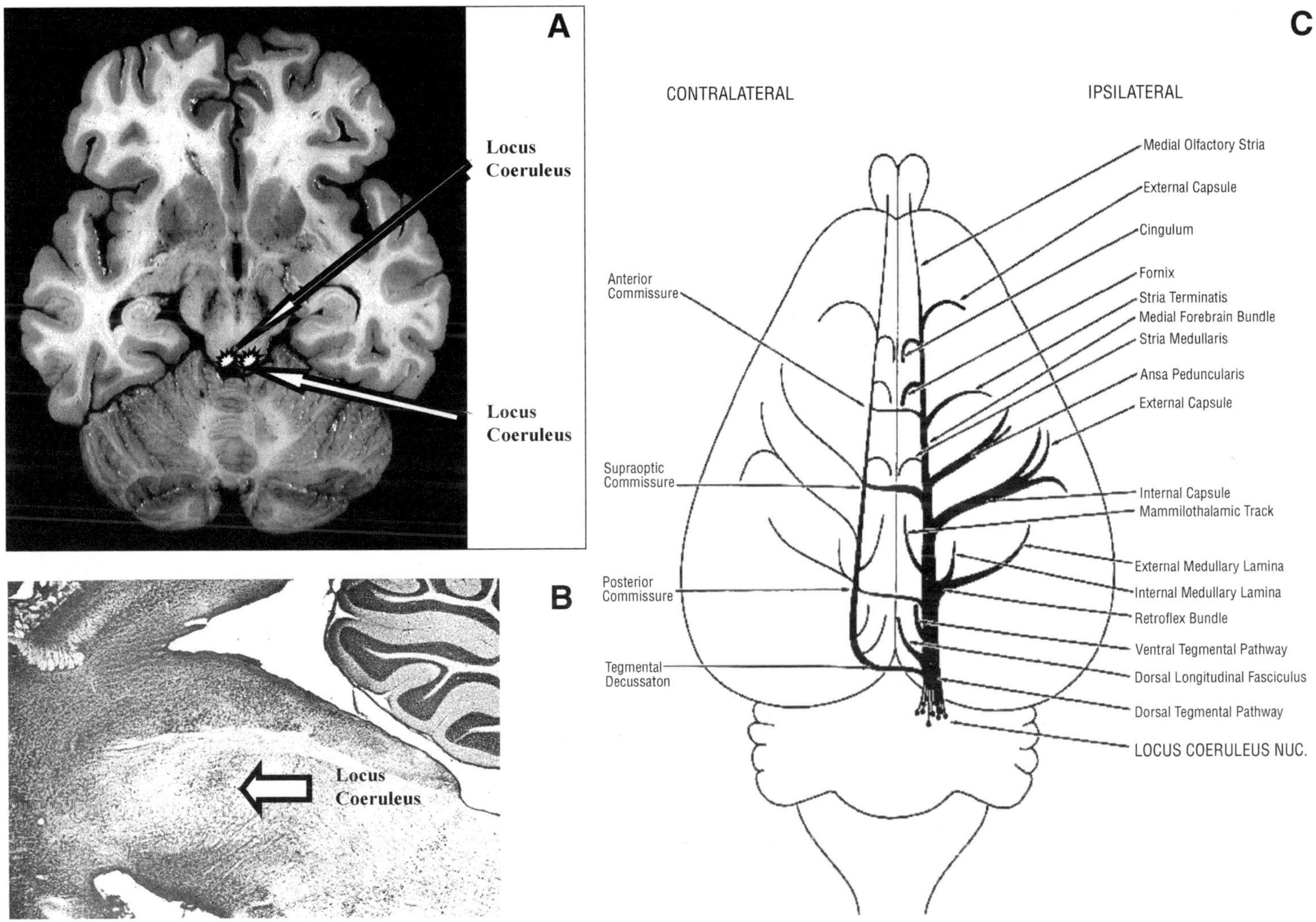
A
Locus Coeruleus
Locus Coeruleus
B
Locus Coeruleus
C
CONTRALATERAL
IPSILATERAL
Anterior Commissure
Supraoptic Commissure
Posterior Commissure
Tegmental Decussaton
Medial Olfactory Stria
External Capsule
Cingulum
Fornix
Stria Terminatis
Medial Forebrain Bundle
Stria Medullaris
Ansa Peduncularis
External Capsule
Internal Capsule
Mammilothalamic Track
External Medullary Lamina
Internal Medullary Lamina
Retroflex Bundle
Ventral Tegmental Pathway
Dorsal Longitudinal Fasciculus
Dorsal Tegmental Pathway
LOCUS COERULEUS NUC.

Fig. 3.

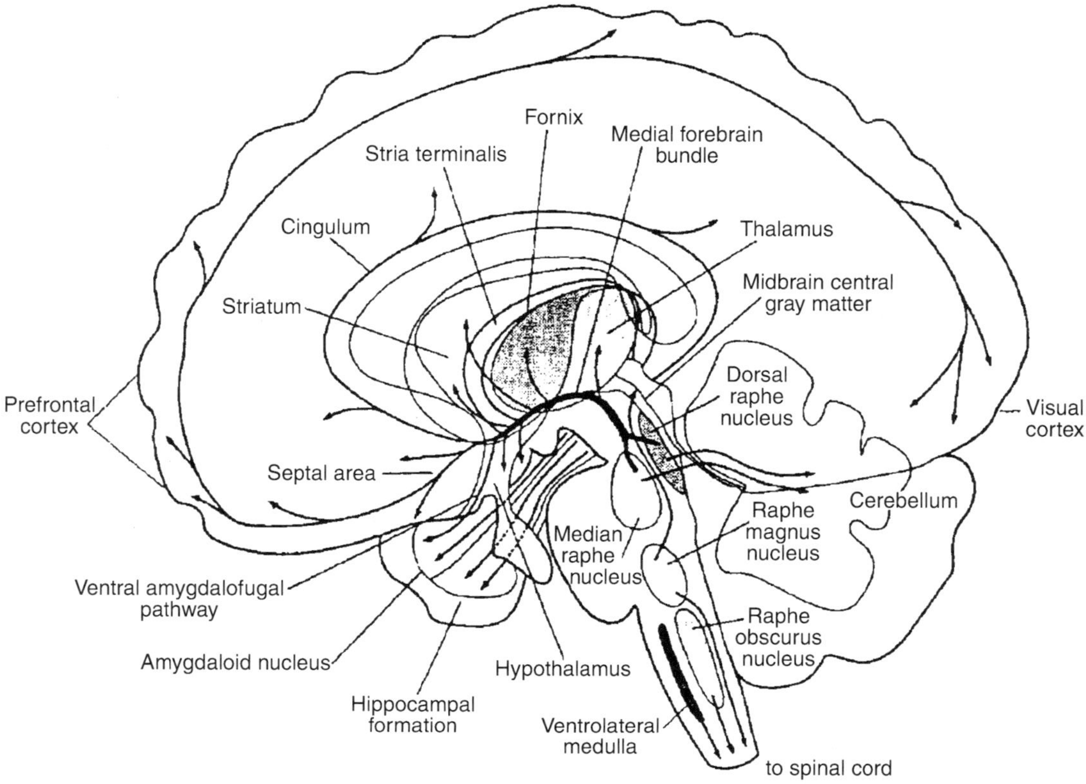

Fig. 4. Representation of the serotonin (5-HT) projections ascending in the medial forebrain bundle from the dorsal and median raphe nuclei in the brain stem. Branching occurs above the thalamus to the limbic system, basal ganglia and cerebral cortices. 5-HT projections descend to the spinal cord from the raphe magnus and obscurus in the ventrolateral medulla. (Taken from ref. *15* with permission of the NY Academy of Sciences.)

the spinal cord. More significant for the current discussion are B6 and B7 (the dorsal raphe nuclei) that lie along the floor of the fourth ventricle near the LC, and ventrally the B8 group (the median raphe) on the borders of the pons and midbrain. The dorsal raphe is the larger group but along with the median raphe, both contain neurons using other transmitters (e.g., DA; *15*).

There is a fairly broad overlap for the forebrain innervation from these two nuclei. The emphasis is on the neostriatum and frontal lobe for the dorsal raphe (with a decreasing gradient over the more caudal cortical regions), whereas the median raphe projects more to diencephalic and limbic structures. Output from the median raphe relays not just to the hippocampus, but extends to the cingulate and fairly evenly through the parietal and neighboring cortices. The sensory and motor cortices show a mixed pattern, some with much 5-HT

Fig. 3. Anatomical location of the locus ceruleus (LC) and the ascending pathways: **(A)** bilateral brain stem locations of the LC in a horizontal section of the human brain (with the cerebellum just behind); **(B)** sagittal view from the side through a rat brain with arrow pointing to the norepinephrine path deriving from the LC above; **(C)** diagram of the ascending and commissural pathways arising from the LC in the rat brain. Innervation of the hippocampus proceeds via the fornix, whereas that of the medial and dorsal cortex passes through the cingulum with anterior cortex innervated by the rostral extension of the medial forebrain bundle. Adapted from refs. *4,5* with permission from Elsevier.

innervation (e.g., auditory and somatosensory cortex) and some with less (e.g., motor cortex). Some areas receive high and low patches of input (visual cortex). There are morphologically two quite different forms of innervation, although their functional relevance remains obscure. The one with fine axons and small varicosities (inclusions) is found throughout cortical terminal regions, and is largely of dorsal raphe origin. The other is coarser with a large beaded form, is more sparsely distributed (mostly frontoparietal and hippocampal regions) and mostly of median raphe origin *(15–17)*. 5-HT1a binding sites are found as autoreceptors, as well as postsynaptically on cholinergic neurons, and those using amino acid transmission. It is noteworthy that 5-HT2a sites are frequently found on DA and NE neurons (*see* refs. *18* and *19*).

4. INTERACTIONS BETWEEN MONOAMINES

4.1. 5-HT–NE Interactions

Many central effects of monoamines are modified by activity in pathways releasing other monoamines. Indeed, some of the autonomic effects of 5-HT of central origin are exerted via 5-HT2a receptors on processes of the NE networks arising in the N. tractus solitarius *(20)*. Interactions between the brainstem nuclei work both ways. NE can facilitate 5-HT release (e.g., via α-1 binding sites; *21,22*), although 5-HT can reduce NE activity *(23,24)*. This latter effect can occur in the brainstem via 5-HT1a sites potentiating local NE inhibitory feedback *(25)*. However, in the cortices, NE usually inhibits 5-HT release (via α-2 receptors; *26*), whereas 5-HT can facilitate or reduce NE release (5-HT2a [heteroceptor] or 5-HT2c binding sites [autoreceptors] depending on their pre-/postsynaptic loci; *27,28*).

4.2. 5-HT–DA Interactions

Many of the central effects of 5-HT arise via modulation of activity in DA paths. Often the levels of DA and 5-HT metabolites in samples of cerebrospinal fluid (CSF) drawn from healthy subjects are highly intercorrelated *(29)*. Indeed, in ADHD children high levels of 5-HIAA and HVA decreased together in those reponding to psychostimulant treatment *(30)*. Thus it is not surprising to learn that increases of amphetamine-induced locomotion *(31)* and the associated induced release of DA *(32)* are modulated by 5-HT at 5-HT2a receptors: both effects are suppressed by 5-HT2a antagonists. Other ADHD-like features modeled in animals show DA/5-HT interactions. Shifts of attention and stimulus-reward learning, facilitated by methylphenidate, are impaired by reduced 5-HT synthesis *(33)*. A separate psychostimulant action on reinforcement—the amphetamine-induced enhancement of response for conditioned reward—is suppressed by 5-HT stimulation (at mesolimbic 5-HT1b sites; *34*).

Reverse influences of DA on 5-HT activity should not be overlooked. Neonatal damage to DA systems leads to large increases of 5-HT in the basal ganglia and cerebellum, though not in the cortex *(35)*. There are potential consequences of such interactions in terms of treatment. Impulsivity in ADHD has a basis in the reponsiveness of 5-HT neurons (*36*; Subheading 8.1.) and the stimulation by 5-HT2 agonists of premature responses in rats performing a choice task can be brought under control with DA antagonists *(37)*.

A number of receptor sites underlie these mechanisms. Currently the 5-HT2a/2c sites are among those that are better understood. 5-HT2a sites are often located on neurons with projections ascending from the ventral tegmental area *(38)* and modulate active DA transmission, whereas 5-HT2c sites affect tonic DA outflow *(39)*. Agonism at these two sites suppresses, whereas antagonism stimulates DA outflow. This action is better documented for mesocortical sites with 5-HT2a, and for mesolimbic sites with 5-HT2c sites *(40–42)*. Effects of the 5-HT1 receptor classes on DA release are less well-understood *(26,43)*.*

4.3. NE–DA Interactions

NE activity modulates the stimulation by amphetamine of DA release *(46)*. But the mechanisms seem to differ between subcortical and cortical areas. In mesolimbic regions NE α-1 sites are needed for amphetamine to raise DA levels and elicit locomotion (e.g., 1b-knockout mice; *47*). α-2 agonists decrease mesolimbic DA levels, whereas α-2 antagonists are without effect *(48)*. Mesolimbic DA release is also influenced by NE at β-sites *(49)*. But, in cortical regions α-1 sites can interfere with DA D1 function *(50)* and blocking α-2 sites can raise DA levels like DA D2 antagonists (*51*; *see* Subheading 9.2.).

In cortical regions the interactions are complicated by an extra mechanism that has consequences for understanding ADHD treatment. Considerable extrasynaptic levels of DA are likely to interact with the numerous extrasynaptic DA receptors. But, this DA can also be taken up and cleared by NE transporters *(52)*. So it is not surprising that chronic imipramine blockade of these sites leads to a downregulation of D1 sites *(53)*. Clearance of DA by both DA and NE transporters has been confirmed *(54)*. But, further, a comparison of NE-innervated cortices with those receiving more or less DA innervation has shown that in both cases NE and DA levels can be reduced by α-2 agonists (e.g., clonidine) and increased by α-2 antagonists (e.g., idazoxan; *55*). This demonstrates the corelease of DA from NE transporters. Thus, uptake and release of DA was recorded at NE uptake sites in the cortices (but not the basal ganglia). Inhibition of NE transporters influences both mesocortical NE- and DA-dependent functions.

5. DEVELOPMENT

5.1. Norepinephrine

Catecholamine synthesis in the brainstem is in place in the middle of the second month of gestation. This matures up to around 13 wk in parallel with the development of the ascending pathways (medial forebrain bundle) that penetrate the cortical plate at this time *(56)*. Animal studies suggest that development lags behind that for DA at first, but overtakes it later *(57)*.

Rodent and primate studies suggest that basal and stress-induced NE activity soars prepubertally, but falls back in adolescence, whereby changes in those reared away from their mother are less marked *(58–60)*. Cortical α-2 receptors are evident before α-1 sites, but the latter expand postnatally while the α-2 concentration levels off. In puberty α-1 levels fall more than α-2 concentrations *(61)*. Efficient control of NE function is mirrored by transporter mechanisms that also decline through puberty but rise again somewhat on attaining adulthood *(62,63)*. These developmental changes are reflected in 24-h urine collections in human subjects *(64)*. Compared with 8- to 12-yr-old children, in groups of younger and older teenagers NE levels fell by approx 40% and its metabolite (MHPG) by two-thirds (implying a halving of turnover activity). Yet by 20 yr of age levels of both substances had again increased by a third.

It is not clear whether there are gender differences in the development of the NE system. In contrast in the DA system a more marked overproduction of D2- and D1-like receptors

*Differences between reports likely reflect separate site-specific presynaptic roles on newly synthesized vs basal DA levels, which in turn may vary between brain regions. For example, 5-HT1a sites are mostly presynaptic in the brainstem, but postsynaptic in many projection areas. Thus, the presence of 5-HT1a sites on dendrites in the VTA suggests a disinhibitory role *(44)*, whereas 5-HT1b mesolimbic sites facilitate DA release *(45)*.

between birth and puberty is reported for males. Indeed, in rodents mesolimbic D1 binding appears to remain elevated in males *(65)*.*

5.2. 5-HT

Reports on the 5-HT system in animals show that the fine-axon system develops steadily from birth, with the fibers gradually concentrating in the first three layers of the cortex. The larger, more beaded neurons develop later, but they also innervate the first three cortical layers and are forming pericellular innervation arrays by adolescence *(66)*. 5-HT turnover remains relatively steady early in development although DA activity is rapidly increasing. However 5-HT activity, sensitive to stressors, may be depressed, for example, by rearing in isolation *(67,68)*. CSF measures taken from premature neonates to 6-mo-old infants broadly confirm a large increase of DA metabolism although 5-HT turnover remains steady *(69)*. Across this age range the HVA/5-HIAA ratio doubled. This should not disguise, of course, that there is a large continuing prepubertal development of the 5-HT innervation of limbic and cortical areas in terms of binding sites and activity. However, the pace is moderate by comparison with the DA system *(60,70)*.

Human studies (platelet binding, postmortem reports) suggest that from the age of 10 yr, and certainly from adolescence, 5-HT turnover and binding for 5-HT2a and transporter sites decrease markedly *(71–73)*. Indeed, an associated downregulation of 5-HT2a sites has been monitored electrophysiologically *(74)*. Concordant with this a drop of 50% or more was noted for 5-HT and its metabolite in urinary measures between 8- and 12- and 14- and 17-yr-olds *(64)*. This resulted in a halving of turnover rates, which only partially recovered in young adults. In summary, the cortical innervation by 5-HT neurons is basically in place by birth, hyperinnervation is evident during childhood, and this is cut back over puberty and adolescence. Details of the timing and localization of spurts and pauses are notable for numerous examples that are not in phase with DA developments. This provides many sensitve moments when environmental influences could disturb the balance of DA/5-HT interactions with largely unknown consequences.

6. EVIDENCE FOR MONOAMINERGIC CONTRIBUTION TO ADHD—GENETIC STUDIES

6.1. Norepinephrine

Ten years after Hechtman's review *(76)*, studies are only starting to get under way to test her argument that genetic influences on NE will inform on ADHD. Genetic studies of features important to NE transmission and relevant to the ADHD condition have been few. They have concentrated on the α-2a site for which NE has high affinity (where increased binding has been related to stress and frontal lobe cognition *[77,78]*) and the reuptake site, which if blocked (like the α-2a site) will lead to a decrease of neuronal firing *(79)*. Metabolic enzymes (DBH, Catechol-*O*-methyl transferase [COMT], and MAO; Fig. 1) have also received some attention. MAO activity, relevant for the breakdown of all the monoamines, has been inversely related to the expression of personality features thought to be relevant for groups or subgroups of ADHD subjects (e.g., impulsiveness, aggression, and sensation-seeking; *see* discussion in *80*).

*This difference may be further exaggerated by a leftward bias in males compared to a rightward bias of D1 binding in females. However, with maturation there is a decrease in the asymmetry in terms of DA and its metabolism (75).

A study using a so-called "line-item" approach to the α-2a receptor (approximately the inverse of more conventional studies with single base-pair polymorphisms) found an allele associated with clusters of symptoms relevant to ADHD along with oppositional and conduct disorders *(81)*. In contrast to this, another allele the study examined related to anxiety and schizoid features. Studies focusing on this receptor seem promising. In contrast to the situation with DA, first reports on several polymorphisms relating to the NE transporter (NET1) have drawn a blank *(82,83)*. There is no evidence as yet that the NET is relevant to the heritability of the ADHD phenotype.

COMT activity is relevant to both DA and NE metabolism (Fig. 1). There is a low activity allele with methionine substitutions that is reported to be preferentialy transferred in male Han Chinese with ADHD, whereas the high-activity form with valine substitutions was more common in the females *(84)*. Although there is support for the transmission of the valine form in Israeli triads *(85)*, in view of negative results from three other countries, the situation remains controversial.

Several polymorphisms have figured in studies of the genetic transmission of DBH (also for TOH), but there is little evidence for preferential transmission in ADHD (*see* ref. *86*) and none for linkage *(87)*. Consideration of MAO heritability also seems irrelevant to questions concerning the roles of NE and 5-HT in ADHD. Associations were reported from a case-control study of ADHD with comorbid externalizing problems *(88)* but earlier reports of relationships to novelty-seeking have not been replicated *(89)*.

6.2. 5-HT

Little is known in relation to mental health about the genetic bases of the 22 or so subtypes of 5-HT binding sites currently known. Most studies have concentrated on the following:

1. Variants of the 5-HT1 class of receptors (especially 5-HT1b).
2. The 5-HT2 class (because of an association with DA release and motor activity *[45]*, and an association of 5-HT2a blockade with reduced impulsivity in animals *[90]* and "harm avoidance"* in healthy adults *[91]*).
3. The transporter (5-HTT). For 5-HTT there are some features (alleles) that are transmitted and associated with a risk for ADHD *(92,93)*. Compared with a long form of the allele there is a short form with less efficient transcription efficency and diminished 5-HT uptake.

Temperament contributes strongly to the normal response to novelty. The challenge of novel stimuli, as in the form of a stranger, naturally can lead to anxiety in the very young. This is important as temperamental or internalizing coping responses characterize ADHD children with very different comorbid problems. It is therefore of some interest that more anxiety was recorded to strangers in infants homozygous for the short form of the 5-HTT-linked promoter region (LPR) length polymorphism, but less anxiety was observed in those with genotypes including one or more copies of the long form *(94)*. Auerbach et al. *(95)* also reported that infants homozygous for the short form were less easily distressed and tended to be more withdrawn, needing a longer latency to smile. Yet it may emerge that the absence of the short form characterizes vulnerability for a heritable form of ADHD *(96)*, for if it is associated with higher thresholds for provoking anxiety, it may coincide with the ease of risk-taking evident in many ADHD subjects. One awaits the results from prospective infant studies with interest.

---

*Harm avoidance is one of three personality dimensions on the Cloninger scales. The other two dimensions, novelty-seeking and reward-dependence, were not related to 5-HT2a binding in this study.

With respect to 5-HT1b receptors, a recent report on 115 ADHD families using the transmission disequilibrium test for a particular polymorphism (G861C) showed a tendency for parental transmission of this allele, and in particular for paternal transmission to the child that was affected *(97,98)*. Quist et al. *(99)* had already pointed out a linkage disequilibrium of the 5-HT2a receptor (polymorphism His 452Tyr allele) with ADHD in these families, indicating a preferential transmission of the 452Tyr allele to the affected offspring. Although this was not confirmed by Hawi et al. *(97)*, data from a symptomatic adult group also suggest that the gene for 5-HT2a sites played a role in the ADHD pathology recorded *(100)*. Clearly one is still too close to the onset of such studies to be able to draw firm conclusions.

7. METHODS

Invasive methods for measuring transmitter activity in the CNS in vivo are available in animals (e.g., dialysis probes, electrochemistry) and adult humans (e.g., position emission tomography studies of ligand binding) but are not justified from an ethical standpoint in children. Measures must be conducted peripherally. There are three possible points of access along the route of elimination of excess monoamines and their metabolic products. These are the CSF, blood (including plasma and platelets), and urine. Opinions differ widely on the extent to which these peripheral measures can reflect CNS function. Somatic sources of 5-HT are particularly high. As there is no reason to suspect that in otherwise somatically healthy ADHD children central systems are differentially impaired with respect to peripheral systems, crude indicators may be sought in the comparison of baseline measures between groups. The effects of challenges with monoaminergic drugs or environmental conditions on biochemical measures represent a good method for testing the functionality of NE and 5-HT pathways.

The extracerebral release of transmitters does not interfere with CNS transmission, as there is a blood–brain barrier with a powerful pump that transports them from brain to blood. What can cross the blood–brain barrier out of the brain and influence concentrations measured peripherally? Basically all the monoamines can pass with varying degrees of ease passively or actively out of CNS tissue (review, ref. *101*), although as acid metabolites do not equilibrate across the blood–brain membranes, they are sensitive to active transport mechanisms *(101)*. These mechanisms of active clearance may contribute to differences reported between blood or plasma and CSF measures. (Regions where the blood–brain barrier does not so function include the circumventricular and subfornical organs, the choroid plexus, and the area postrema of the medulla.) However, measures derived from venous blood and urine often reflect challenges to the system, at least at a qualitative level. Peripheral and central monoamine activities are often correlated: if the correlations are not good, they are still strong enough to be relevant to the study of behavior *(103)*.

Some limits and influences on the study of monoamine activity from peripheral sources should also be recognized. In most cases changes in a peripheral catchment cannot not be attributed to over-or underactivity in any particular part of the CNS.* Further, it should not be overlooked that just as the processes of synthesis, release, and uptake of transmitters change with age, so do the characteristics of the blood–brain barrier *(104)*. These are poorly

*Usually blood samples for plasma or platelet analyses are collected from the arm. However, a series of studies compared venoarterial gradients form the left/right jugular, hepatosplanchnic, forearm, and cardiac vessels and showed that it is possible to separate the contributions from various somatic organs, as well as cortical vs subcortical contributions (e.g., *101,107–109*).

documented. The integrity of the blood–brain membranes may receive insult from illness and their properties may be influenced by drug treatment. For example, it has been suggested that neuroleptic treatment can increase permeability *(105)*.

An alternative approach is with the use of models that represent the specific feature of interest rather than the whole system. Relevant choices here include selection of the platelet fraction from blood to examine receptor function: thus, the binding characteristics of platelet 5-HT transporters model precisely those of the central transporter *(106)*. A rather different type of model involves study of a particular breed of animal whose CNS responsivity resembles in certain ways that of children with ADHD.

8. ANIMAL MODELS

8.1. *Rodent*

Two widely cited models come to mind. One proposes to "model" hyperactivity with chemical lesion of DA pathways with 6-hydroxydopamine (usually using desipramine to protect NE terminals). The other compares some symptom dimensions shown by spontaneous hypertensive rats (SHR) in comparison to their genetic controls, the Wistar–Kyoto strain (WKY). In this second example, although largely peripheral NE systems contribute to the dominant feature of hypertension, the changes do not leave central NE systems unaffected. Further, 5-HT systems are also partly involved in the control of blood pressure.*

The strength of the lesion model lies in the reliable stimulation of increased locomotion. However there is an overriding weakness. Although the lesion renders the system hypofunctional in one sense, DA receptors become supersensitive to DA stimulation to produce the activity. This form of DA hyperactivity is not the basis for motor hyperactivity in ADHD subjects where there is much evidence for a (relatively) hypo-DA function. Nonetheless, as both psychostimulants and agents acting on other monoaminergic systems can calm ADHD patients (*see* Section 10), it is important that not only methylphenidate antagonizes hyperlocomotion in lesioned rats, but antagonists of 5-HT and NETs also reduce the locomotion elicited from lesioned rats *(110)*. Indeed, the 5-HT modulation is not limited to the transporter and DA D2 mechanisms. 5-HT2 antagonists (e.g., ritanserin) also prevent D1 stimulation of hyperlocomotion arising from a lesion-induced supersensitive neostriatum *(111)*. Clearly this most dopaminergic of symptoms, motor activity, can also be modulated by activity of the other monoamines, one way in psychopathology and in another way perhaps with succesful treatment.

What features pertinent to ADHD does the SHR model, which may also be influenced by NE and 5-HT? The SHR explores more *(112)*, though activity can be context-dependent *(113)*, reminiscent of situational rather than pervasive hyperkinetic children. SHRs may learn Hebb-mazes, active-avoidance tasks, and multiple reversals faster than controls *(114,115)*, yet this sometimes reflects poor WKY performance *(113)*. Sometimes the SHR has difficulty with passive avoidance, water-maze extinctions, longer-term working memory, and delayed response learning (e.g., temporarily withholding response for gratification; *116,117*). To a degree these difficulties, especially the last one, do mirror some of the features of ADHD.

Unfortunately neither quantitative relationships of NE and 5-HT activity to SHR behavioral function nor their responses to pharmacological challenge have been much studied. A

*Regulation of blood pressure by the nucleus of the tractus solitarius is upregulated by increased 5-HT turnover in SHR *(118)*; hypertension may reflect an increase of sensitivity to stimulation of 5-HT2 receptors *(119,120)*.

few reports suggest that NE and 5-HT systems function differently, but even here the locus of control is poorly understood. Basal release of NE in slices of prefrontal cortex does not differ between SHR and WKY rats *(121)*. The vesicular stores are not depleted. But brainstem, cortical *(122)*, and even CSF levels *(123)* of NE are higher than normal. These levels are managed better after treatment with α-2 agonists that specifically reduce NE release (*121*; *see* Subheading 9.1.). Thus, autoreceptor-mediated control of NE release seems to be poorly regulated in the prefrontal cortex of SHRs *(124)* even though synaptosomal NE uptake is also reported to be higher in SHRs vs WKY controls *(125)*.

What about the 5-HT system? An analysis of amines and metabolites in the prefrontal cortex and parts of the brainstem containing the LC and raphe *(122)* showed a significant decrease of 5-HT turnover in the brainstem (and a nonsignificantly lower turnover in the cortex). Although this may simply reflect the bases for hypertension, one should recognize the influence this could have on mesocortical NE and DA activity (*see* Section 4). Further, considering the difficulty that SHRs (and ADHD children) have in witholding response on interval schedules, data consistent with the SHR neurochemistry just described comes from a study of blockade of NE and 5-HT uptake on differential responding at low rates of response (a 72-s schedule; *126*). This study reported that a range of NE uptake inhibitors enhanced, whereas a range of 5-HT uptake inhibitors impaired, the efficiency of witholding responses appropriate to the delays of the schedule. One may conclude that the rodent model provides evidence for the "potential" for NE and 5-HT control of higher (dys)functions relevant to ADHD.

In looking to the future, it is appropriate to introduce a potentially useful model based on a new genetic variant of mouse, the Coloboma strain. Hyperactivity in this animal appears to result from a reduction of SNAP-25, a protein that regulates presynaptic exocytotic catecholamine release *(127)*. Unexpectedly, whereas DA utilization is low, calcium-dependent NE concentrations are high. Also unexpected is that use of a neurotoxin specific to NE terminals (DSP-4) reduces not only NE but also hyperactivity. This suggests a link between NE transmission and motor activity, and prompts the search for other potentially relevant mouse models that are suitable to study with genetic knockout techniques. One concerns neurexin proteins involved in exocytotic mechanisms and in the binding to postynaptic neuroligins *(128)*. This promotes the coupling of impulse-related transmitter release to efficient postsynaptic docking. Arguably this mechanism in its (in)efficiency could make an important contribution to aspects of the ADHD condition.

Last, in the absence of an established model of developmental processes leading to ADHD, a brief mention is made of the potential for further study of the role of perinatal anoxia/hypoxia. The model involves placing rat pups in a nitrogen atmosphere for about 25 min. After 3–9 wk DA and 5-HT metabolism is unusually high in the hippocampus and neostriatum *(129)*, a feature that leads animals to make many errors on tests of sustained attention *(130)*. The stages of a rat's development are difficult to equate with those of a child, but considering that major (differential) changes of 5-HT activity were noted during development (*See* Section 5), closer study could prove valuable. Another effect of anoxia is to alter CNS and peripheral levels of neuropeptide Y (NPY) *(131)*. NPY is commonly localized in NE neurons; raised NPY levels have been reported in many ADHD children *(132)*, as would be expected from raised NE levels. Work with the SHR shows increased NPY binding, that NPY enhances the effects of α-2 receptor agonism (e.g., vasoconstriction) and that whereas NPY administration decreases motor activity in normotensive animals, it increases it in the SHR *(133,134)*. Clearly there are several leads in the developmental hypoxia model and the SHR that should be followed up.

8.2. Primate

Recent reviews on the contribution of transmitter systems to ADHD give prominence to NE alongside DA, to the neglect of 5-HT and other candidates *(135)*. These views are predicated on the undisputed role of impaired frontal activity in ADHD performance where delayed reinforcement *(136)*, response inhibition, and error- *(137)* and change-detection were studied *(138)*. But the weight of the argument lies on a series of studies demonstrating that stimulation of NE activity in monkeys, when catecholamines are depleted, enhances working memory (WM) task performance: too little transmitter impairs, facilitated by α-2 stimulation; too much transmitter impairs, reflecting α-1 stimulation (where the low affinity of α-1 sites for NE means that they are active at high NE concentrations; *77,139*). Yet the evidence for WM dysfunction rather than impairments of other executive functions in ADHD remains equivocal. A few studies have reported impairments of digit/arithmetic *(140,141)* and visuospatial span *(142–144)*. But the impairments are often small (~1 standard deviation; *145*), more of a problem for those with comorbid reading/learning difficulties *(146)* or are found only where the task loads on attentional capacity *(147)*. Indeed, many of the differences disappear after covarying for IQ *(148)* and with increasing age *(149–151)*. It is doubtful if impaired WM performance is a salient part of the neuropsychological profile of ADHD *(152)* or contributes significantly to other executive functions, such as planning *(153,154)*.

It is therefore important to define the role of NE in tasks pertinent to ADHD. NE activity relates to vigilance, signal-detection abilities, and attention-related processes. NE activity can alter (tune) the signal to noise ratio improving attention to relevant stimulation (For review, *see* refs. *10,155*). A series of studies has shown that fluctuations of neuronal discharge in the LC of monkeys correlate with performance on a continuous performance test (CPT) of sustained attention *(156)*. These authors have shown that while phasic LC firing is associated with good performance, elevated tonic discharge rates are associated with errors of commission, decreased sensitivity (d′), and increased criterion levels for stimulus identification (β decreased). The latter situation was improved by clonidine. Although clonidine does not seem to help ADHD children on the CPT (the sedative action seems to dominate), guanfacine can improve performance *(157)*. Nonetheless, although the monkey model provides some insight as to what could be happening in ADHD, it is not surprising that this complex relationship is not mirrored in a simple relationship between MHPG and CPT performance. Neither urinary nor plasma nor CSF levels of MHPG were related to CPT errors of omission or commission *(158–160)*. However, the latter study *(160)* did mention a trend for a negative relationship between the HVA/MHPG ratio with d′. This suggests there is a potentially important imbalance between the two main catecholamine actors in ADHD in the determination of “currently” relevant stimulation. The question remains open whether action at the α-2 receptor is the best way to “tune” the NE role in tuning in ADHD cognition.

9. EVIDENCE FOR MONOAMINE CONTRIBUTIONS TO ADHD—NE AND 5-HT ACTIVITY

9.1. Evidence From Group Comparisons

Does the metabolism of NE and 5-HT differ between children with ADHD and those without a psychiatric or medical diagnosis? The question is based on the following assumptions:

1. Pathological–developmental factors affecting transmitters in the body will affect peripheral and central metabolism similarly.
2. Transmitter metabolism underlies the expression of the behavioral and cognitive measures typical of ADHD.

To a degree both assumptions are equivocal. The main limit to interpretation of the answer (apart from the caveat over the sample's source) lies with the knowledge that there are many other factors involved in the efficient coupling of nervous activity to the appropriate postsynaptic response that have not been studied, and may not necessarily influence the metabolic parameters as currently measured.

Analyses of CSF, blood compartments, and urine (Table 1) indicate that in the ADHD condition MHPG levels (NE metabolite) are usually lower than normal; less clearly, NE levels may be increased. Overall this suggests a decreased turnover. There is a hint that other catabolic pathways may be differentially affected (NMN levels). The severity of the core symptoms do not influence the results *(161,162)*. But, over the 4–5 yr from pre- to post-puberty when a number of symptoms regress, MHPG levels have been noted to increase or normalize *(163)*. Further, some studies that deliberately contrasted subgroups find that several comorbidities (independent of their nature) appear to counteract the metabolic decrease: e.g., in those with a reading disorder *(159)*, and in 15 subjects with high levels of anxiety (not in table; *103*).

The results for the 5-HT system are more limited, reflecting in part the methodological issues (*see* Section 7). However, if one brings the separate findings together, there is an indication of an increase of 5-HT turnover, largely reflecting decreases in 5-HT levels (Table 1). Nonetheless, as with NE, it must be recognized that there will be subgroups, however defined, for which the effects associated with the core symptoms will be masked by other features. One such example is shown by the contrast between ADHD boys brought up in families with or without alcoholic fathers *(164)*. Those with this experience showed a larger cortisol response to a challenge dose of fenfluramine than those without an alcoholic father. This was interpreted as reflecting increased 5-HT receptor sensitivity.

Another example of the influences of comorbidity on 5-HT activity concerns impulsivity. Impulsive aggression (oppositional behaviors; *30,165*) has been associated with low plasma and CSF 5-HIAA and synaptic availability of 5-HT. This contrasts with the generalization noted in the preceding paragraph. Intriguingly, Oades et al. *(36)* compared the binding characteristics of the platelet 5-HT T with clinical ratings (impulsivity/distractibility, externalizing/ aggression) and the (in)ability to withhold responses on the stop–signal task (cognitive impulsivity). Decreased affinity correlated with poor response inhibition (cognitive impulsiveness) but not clinical ratings, even though the cognitive and clinical indices of impulsivity were related. In contrast, aggressive behavior related to increased 5-HT T affinity (*see* Subheading 6.2.: genetic control of 5-HT availability by the transporter [HTTLPR]).*

Cognitive impulsivity might be expected to reveal itself on the CPT test of sustained attention in the form of an increased rate of false alarms. However, as yet, both high (blood; *166*) and low levels of 5-HT (tryptophan depletion; *167*) have been related to more errors of commission. But d′ reflecting target sensitivity, was reported to decrease as the excretion of the 5-HT metabolite increased *(160)*, which supports interpretations of the aforementioned platelet study.

---

*Reductions of binding site affinity should normally be offset by increased receptor capacity. If this does not occur then more 5-HT remains available in the synapse.

Table 1
Comparisons of Components of NE and 5-HT Metabolism in Urine, Blood, and CSF Samples From ADHD and Controls.

Source	Hyperactives	Controls	Metabolite	Monoamine	Change vs controls	Reference
Urine	9	6	MHPG		none	*232*
Urine	7	12	MHPG & *NMN*		decrease & increase	*233*
Urine	13	14	MHPG	NE	none & increase	*234*
Urine	15	13	MHPG		decrease	*235*
Urine	10	10	MHPG		increase	*236*
Urine	9	9	MHPG		decrease	*237*
Urine	73	51	MHPG		decrease	*238*
Urine	28	23	MHPG		decrease	*239*
Urine (2 h)	20	22	MHPG NMN, MN, VMA, NMN/NE	NE	none & none all increase	*103*
Urine (1 h)	15	16	DOPEG	NE	decrease & none	*240*
Urine	13	13	MHPG/NE, MHPG, HVA/MHPG	NE	decrease none & none trend increase	*241*
Urine	14	9	MHPG/NE, MHPG,	NE	trend decrease none & increase	*132*
Urine	15(37)	21	MHPG		none	*180*
Urine	31	26	MN, NMN & NMN/NE		none	*186*
Urine	x (severe)	y (mild)	VMA	NE	none & none	*162*
Serum	35	19		NE	none	*242*
Serum	49	11		NE	none	*243*
Plasma	12	11		NE	trend increase	*244*
Plasma	8 (+RD)	14 (RD)	MHPG		decrease (if no RD)	*159*
Plasma	14	9	*NE*		trend increase	*132*
Plasma	35 (many vs few symptoms)		*NE*		none	*161*
CSF	29 (vs 20 conduct disorder)		MHPG		trend increase	*158*
Urine	13	13	5-HIAA/5-HT, 5-HIAA, HVA/5-HIAA	5-HT	none, increase, & decrease decrease	*241*
Urine	14	9	5-HIAA/5-HT, 5-HIAA,	5-HT	trend increase, increase, & decrease	*132*

(Continued)

Table 1
(Continued)

Source	Hyperactives	Controls	Metabolite	Monoamine	Change vs controls	Reference
Urine	15(37)	21	5-HIAA		none	*180*
Blood	25	vs norm		5-HT	decrease	*245*
Blood	49	11		5-HT	none	*243*
Blood	70	vs norm		5-HT	decrease	*246*
Serum	11	11		5-HT	decrease	*246*
Platelet	17	75	5-HIAA		none	*241*
Platelet	55	38		5-HT	none	*247*
Plasma	35 (many vs few symptoms)			5-HT	decrease	*161*
CSF	24	6	5-HIAA		none	*248*
CSF	6	16	5-HIAA		none	*249*
CSF	29 (vs 20 conduct disorder)		5-HIAA		none	*158*

Finally, another indication that there may be 2 ADHD subgroups differing in the sensitivity of the 5-HT system comes from neurophysiological study of the augmenting-reducing response using event-related potentials. The N1/P2 component may increase (augment) or decrease (reduce) in response to increases of salience (loudness of sounds). An augmenting response is a feature of sensation-seeking *(168)*, and ADHD subjects who respond to amphetamine *(169)*. Increasing stimulus intensity-dependence relates to decreasing 5-HT activity (and vice versa; cf. effects of alcohol and lithium; *170*). Among ADHD subjects who do not respond to amphetamine, a reducing response to auditory stimuli is typical *(169)*. It remains unclear how closely coupled 5-HT activity is with the augmenting-reducing phenomenon. But, it would be worthwhile combining biochemical measures in ADHD subjects with/without the conduct problems that are influenced by 5-HT activity with this paradigm.

9.2. Evidence From Pharmacological Treatments

The question addressed here is whether there is evidence that treatments that exert a good effect on the ADHD condition also exert a minor or major effect by way of the NE or 5-HT systems. "As noted 20 yr ago, the large number of efficacious drugs do not support any single neurotransmitter defect hypothesis" *(171)*. Here, we ask if there is convincing evidence that NE and 5-HT should be ruled in, rather than out of any potentially explanatory model for ADHD. Let us first consider the agents that have proved most efficacious in the treatment of ADHD, the psychostimulants methylphenidate and amphetamine (and pemoline; Fig. 5). Below, evidence from other agents with significant effects on the NE and 5-HT systems that result in more modest but significant clinical effects in patients with ADHD are considered.

The dominant effect of *methylphenidate* is to block reuptake of impulse-released DA at the DA transporter, resulting in increased extracellular availability of DA (the oral dose to block 50% of sites is about 0.25 mg/kg: *172*). But it also binds to the NE transporter strongly and the 5-HT T very weakly. *Amphetamine* binds with each monoamine transporter and can raise extracellular levels by stimulating the release of extravesicular newly

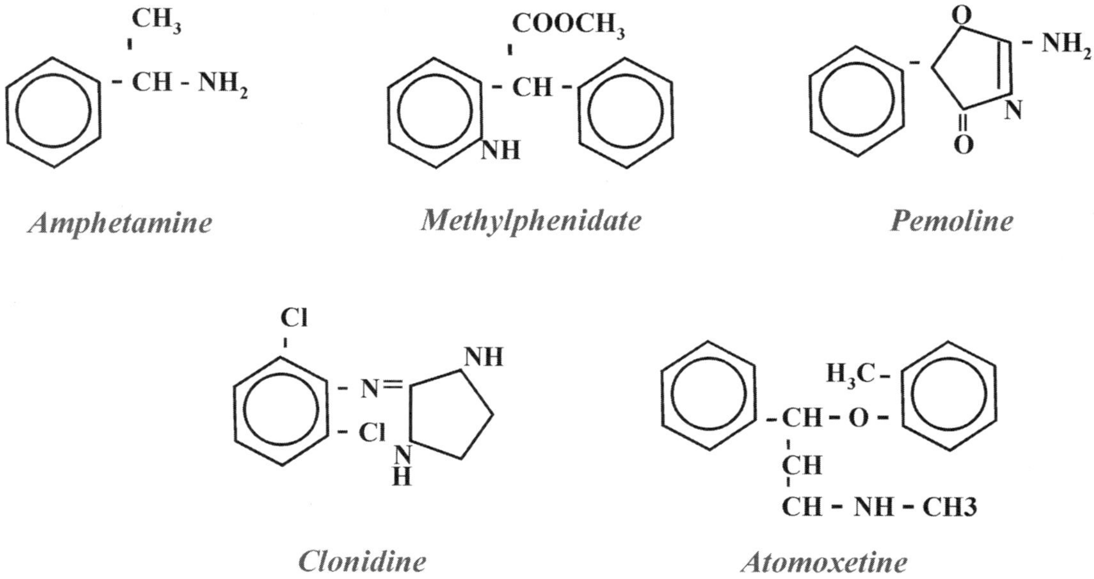

Fig. 5. The biochemical structure of five agents with therapeutic effects on attention deficit hyperactivity disorder. Amphetamine, methylphenidate, and pemoline are psychostimulants that block the presynaptic reuptake of monoamines, clonidine is an α-2 agonist at norepinephrine (NE) binding sites (including somatic autoreceptors), atomoxetine relatively specifically blocks NE reuptake.

synthesized transmitter and blocking reuptake. The former mechanism is usually emphasized, as treatments that block catecholamine synthesis inhibit the effects of amphetamine more than methylphenidate. (Caveat: the mechanism of stimulating the transporter to release transmitter or block the reuptake varies with dose, and specific data vary with measures made in vitro or in vivo; *173*.) A modest degree of MAO inhibition has also been reported. Pemoline (caveat: liver toxicity) will not be further discussed; its effects are specific to the release and uptake of DA *(174)*.

In preclinical studies in rodents, methylphenidate (0.75–3.0 mg/kg, intravenous) does not increase motor activity or mesolimbic levels of DA, but it does increase extracellular levels of NE (e.g., in the limbic system; *175*). Similar doses of amphetamine (subcutaneous) increase limbic and frontal levels of NE to a greater extent (and release DA; *173*). Although higher doses (e.g., 20 mg/kg) of methylphenidate still release NE they do not increase levels of 5-HT. Nonetheless, such pharmacological doses have been reported to enhance 5-HT metabolite levels in frontostriatal regions *(176)*. In contrast, 2.5–3.0 mg/kg amphetamine can raise 5-HT levels threefold and increase its metabolism (e.g., neostriatum; *177*). Subchronic amphetamine treatment has been reported to sensitize brainstem 5-HT1a, but not 5-HT2a sites *(178)*.

Do the biochemical responses to the psychostimulants reflect expectations from the preclinical results? First, care must be taken with the interpretation of results as the variability between reports, whether from different or the same authors, can be marked for measures taken from the CSF, plasma, or urine. Second, HVA levels, as noted above, can reflect peripheral NE metabolism,* and also tend to decrease/normalize after methylphenidate treatment, whether or not the patients responded clinically (urine, *180*; CSF, *30*). Both studies noted that although 5-HT metabolism was not necessarily high, levels tended to decrease with treatment following corrections of high levels of DA metabolism and symptom improvement.

The only clear result for NE, 5-HT, and their metabolites is that urinary MHPG levels decrease after amphetamine (seven of seven studies) but not after methylphenidate treatment (three of three studies; Table 14.1 in *181*). VMA levels were also reduced after amphetamine in three of three studies. For other metabolites, increases and decreases have been reported and no clear pattern emerges. It is surprising that unequivocal changes of NE levels are not usually recorded after methylphenidate treatment. At first sight it is enigmatic that the frequently reported low turnover for NE in ADHD patients should be further lowered in those who respond to psychostimulant treatment *(182)*. A possible explanation derives from electrophysiological recordings in primates *(183)*. A parallel is drawn between an overly tonic firing mode for the LC during poor CPT performance and the sustained attention problems in ADHD. Low activity facilitates interactions with many stimuli rather than focused attention. Stimulants decrease the tonic activity and facilitate a transition to a phasic firing mode. This counteracts the 'hypoarousal' in the system. The coupling of information transfer is improved, even though the overall NE turnover rate decreases further.

Raising the issue of arousal encourages mention of the biochemical support for the concept of hypoarousal in ADHD from measures of adrenaline and phenylethylamine (PEA). Adrenaline levels tend to be low in urine samples from ADHD children and the adrenergic (and cortisol) response to stress is reduced *(184–186)*.† Adrenaline levels rise with methylphenidate or amphetamine treatment *(187–189)*. This is consistent with the simple concept of low levels of arousal becoming partially normalized by stimulant treatment. PEA is a naturally occurring amphetamine-like derivative that results from decarboxlation of phenylalanine, a precursor to normal catecholamine synthesis (Fig. 1). Levels are frequently found to be raised in a range of psychiatric, excited conditions (e.g., acute schizophrenia, bipolar disorder, some obsessive-compulsive and psychopathic conditions) but reduced in depression *(190–193)*. They are lower in ADHD, even if PEA levels are not significantly correlated with symptom severity itself *(180,194)*. Psychostimulant treatments raise PEA levels *(195,196)*. PEA levels may reflect endogenous homeostatic mechanisms for promoting catecholamine activity (e.g., like amphetamine, PEA increases CSF levels of NE and DA in nonhuman primates *[197]*). In summary, although both psychostimulants lead to an increase of extracellular catecholamines, they differ in the following:

1. On the mechanism at the transporter.
2. On its relation to impulse flow.
3. At clinically relevant doses, only amphetamine significantly influences 5-HT activity; yet it is clear that specific effects of methylphenidate (and atomoxetine) at the NE T can bring about significant changes in the activity of both catecholamines, especially in mesocortical regions.

---

*Peripheral NA metabolites were reported to be high in the ADHD urinary samples *(179)*.

†However, in highly anxious children, usually with internalizing problems, urinary adrenalin levels can indeed be high with respect to patients without prominent anxiety *(180)*. Slightly higher levels of plasma adrenaline reported in ADHD children *(132)* may likewise have reflected the cognitive testing that occurred around the same time.

The relatively recent introduction of *atomoxetine*, a selective NE T inhibitor, as an efficacious form of ADHD treatment merits attention; however, independent studies of the nature of the improvement and biochemical effects remain sparse. In rodents it raises mesocortical NE and DA levels threefold. Like methylphenidate it is without influence on the 5-HT system, but in contrast it is without effect on nigrostriatal or mesolimbic catecholamines *(198)*. (Note that methylphenidate also raises mesocortical NE and DA levels to a similar degree.) The focus of attention on the mechanisms underlying its efficacy return to the role of cortical NE transporters on the availability of both catecholamines (*see* Subheading 4.3.). Atomoxetine improves each of the diagnostically important symptom clusters (inattention, impulsivity, and activity; *199*), but results of more specific tests of attentional abilities or of cognitive impulsivity remain unclear.

A range of well-known antidepressants can also positively influence ADHD symptoms (e.g., MAO inhibitors, desipramine; for review, *see* ref. *200*). In seven trials *desipramine* (DMI), known for its blockade of NE uptake, is reported to modestly improve hyperactivity, impulsivity, distractibility, and some limited aspects of learning (paired associates) and recall (match to familiar figures; *201,202*). Yet it has no apparent effect on the CPT measure of sustained attention *(202,203)*. Cardiac side effects discourage the use of DMI, but, as with other "helpful" treatments, DMI can decrease NE excretion, along with its central and peripheral metabolites *(204)*. DMI may not so much alter basal levels of NE but increase those arising from stimulus-coupled release of NE, a parallel to methylphenidate's action *(10)*. Unfortunately there is little information on dose-dependent biochemical effects or correlations with the reported behavioral improvements.

Less well-documented are effects of DMI on the 5-HT system. This is surprising, as tertiary antidepressants like imipramine, with an effect on the 5-HT transporter, exert modest improvements like the secondary antidepressants (e.g., DMI; *205*). Recently Overtoom and colleagues *(206)* reported on a left-right discrimination test in ADHD children treated with either DMI, methylphenidate, levo-3,4,-dihydroxy-phenylalanine (L-DOPA), or placebo. The discrimination became a stop-signal test with a no-go tone rapidly following some of the discriminanda. Methylphenidate treatment speeded reaction times and decreased omissions and discrimination errors. That L-DOPA (promoting postsynaptic DA levels) had no effect does not show that DA had no effect, as the synaptic mechanisms differ from the other agents investigated. But it promotes speculation that methylphenidate was at least in part influencing the NE system. More intriguing still is that inhibition on the stop-task improved only after DMI treatment. Fortunately the authors recorded prolactin responses to treatment. These decreased as expected after the two "DA" treatments, but increased after DMI. The supposition that this was a 5-HT effect was confirmed by their finding that serum 5-HIAA levels decreased. This seems to confirm the proposition (*see* Subheading 9.1.) that changes in the 5-HT system may relate to cognitive impulsivity, whereas other attentional effects may reflect NE/catecholaminergic activity.

Clonidine is not a treatment of first choice. This reflects its side effects (high blood pressure, sedation, dizziness) and that its efficacy is largely restricted to oppositional problems (e.g., aggression,* frustration tolerance, cooperation; *207*). However, some improvements in hyperactivity and impulsivity have been reported (meta-analysis, *208*), especially when coadministered with methylphenidate *(209,210)*. Further, performance on some specific tests

*Relevant to the study of NE's role in comorbid aspects of ADHD is that β-NE blockers also yield positive results in treating problems related to aggression, despite potential cardiac problems with this form of treatment *(215)*.

of frontal executive functions can be enhanced *(211)*, and response speed and errors on tests of sustained attention improved with clonidine treatment *(212)*. Two reports *(213,214)* confirmed the inhibitory effects of clonidine expected from preclinical studies by showing that MHPG levels decreased in ADHD children and young adults. (The literature on hypertension also shows falling NE concentrations.) It is therefore of interest to look at clonidine's agonist activity at α-2 NE receptors.

A direct action at α sites was assumed to underlie the enhanced growth hormone response to a pharmacological challenge with clonidine *(214)*. Although an increased receptor sensitivity may be consistent with simple interpretations of clonidine's inhibitory influence, and perhaps that of guanfacine, the implication from platelet α-2 receptor binding is different *(216)*. This group used the platelet model of binding to predict stimulant response. They found a generally low level of binding: ADHD children with relatively normal binding responded to treatment, and those with low levels were nonresponders. However, other interpretations of clonidine's action are possible, and some expectations can be generated from animal studies. Using systemic doses in the range of 0.1–1 mg/kg (and local treatments), clonidine not only reduces NE release (in the brainstem and cortices) but reduces brainstem and cortical 5-HT release *(21,217)*. These studies show that α-1 and α-2 sites exert opposite facilitatory and inhibitory influences on 5-HT release. Further, of interest for the interpretation of the roles of mesocortical DA and NE (*see* Subheading 4.3.), the stimulation of increases of cortical DA and NE (e.g., by clozapine treatment) can be prevented by quite moderate doses of clonidine (0.015 mg/kg; *218*).

In summary, clinical and preclinical work with clonidine show the following:

1. Limited but significant improvements in some areas of function relevant to ADHD.
2. Reduced 5-HT release could underlie the modulation by clonidine of aggressive and impulsive behavior *(15)*.
3. A mechanism for reduced NE release incurs reduced DA release, which could have both helpful effects (e.g., on hyperactivity) and less helpful ones (e.g., on the appreciation of reinforcement).

In a similar vein, lowering NE release may enhance sustained attention performance *(212)*, and it may raise the degree to which α-2 rather than α-1 receptors (with a lower NE affinity) might assist cortical function (e.g., working memory and related executive functions; *219*). Nonetheless, hard evidence for binding differences in ADHD children is lacking, and treatments aimed at the α-2 receptor could be counter productive in the appropriate control of responses to stress.

Two of three open trials of *guanfacine*, an agonist at α-2 NE sites, found a modest improvement of ratings of attention and impulsivity, with one demonstrating fewer errors on the CPT *(157,220,221)*. Controlled trials (vs amphetamine) in adult ADHD patients showed comparable reductions of symptoms and even an improvement of the Stroop color-word naming, so often impaired in childhood ADHD *(222)*. In children with ADHD and comorbid tics teacher ratings improved in half the patients, who also performed a CPT more accurately *(223)*. Thus, a modest degree of success for Arnsten's α-2 NE hypothesis *(139)* appears to be realized, although with a certain risk of lethargy, bradycardia, and hypotension the agent should perhaps be held in reserve for psychostimulant nonresponders.

Despite indications that some treatments may achieve therapeutic effects (e.g., impulsivity) by an action on 5-HT systems, direct attempts using agents with unequivocal effects on 5-HT metabolism have been largely without success (e.g., the precursor amino acid tryptophan *[224]*, fenfluramine that facilitates 5-HT release *[187]*; an agonist at 5-HT1a sites, buspirone [review: ref. *225*]). It is sobering and important to note that although a particular agent may reduce symptoms and alter monoaminergic metabolism, it is not known that the metabolic changes are related to the psychopathological changes. The report of Donnelly and colleagues *(187)* is salutary. Fenfluramine treatment (0.6–2 mg/d) had no significant therapeutic effect on ADHD boys aged 6–12 yr. However, urinary NE, MHPG, VMA, and epinephrine all decreased significantly, as did plasma MHPG and platelet 5-HT levels. Yet for those with impulsive aggression and delinquency there is a clear relationship with low 5-HT activity, be it expressed as reduced platelet binding of imipramine (e.g., *226*), plasma 5-HIAA *(165)*, or prolactin response to fenfluramine challenge *(227)*.

10. GENERAL ISSUES

Early proposals that NE could have a causal role in ADHD, and hyperkinetic behavior in particular *(228)*, were based on the effect of amphetamine to reduce NE activity during arousal. Now there is a widespread belief that children with ADHD are under- rather than overaroused, yet there is an increasing consensus that NE function has something to do with the symptoms *(205)*. Evidence in this chapter shows that NE activity undoubtedly modulates attentional mechanisms both directly (tuning signal-to-noise ratios) and indirectly (via the control of mesocorticolimbic DA release). NE may influence other relevant behaviors depending on their dependence on cognitive mechanisms (e.g., environmental stimulation facilitating hyperkinesis) and the nature of the mechanisms underlying comorbid conditions. Crucial mechanisms include the control of catecholamine availability in the cortex (via the transporter) and phasic firing modes in the LC. Both of these should be targets for treatment.

Common to a consideration of the relative role of NE and 5-HT in ADHD is the increasing appreciation of a crucial role for the transporter in determining the availability of monoamines. Thus, cortical NE Ts can release DA *(55)*, the DA transporter is regulated by a variety of substrates including 5-HT *(229)* and the NE T (compare knockout mice) modulates the perception of reinforcement *(230)*. This latter finding has implications for understanding the aversion to accepting delays between response and reward, and the reinforcement gradients associated with the SHR and with ADHD subjects *(231)*.

5-HT mechanisms are also relevant to the expression of features of ADHD by direct (transporter-mediated reuptake mechanisms) and indirect mechanisms (modulation of DA activity, especially in the initiation of behavioral responses). These have been underresearched in view of more clearly established relations of 5-HT activity to the expression of externalizing responses more frequent in comorbid conditions. Now it is appreciated that 5-HT activity has a role in information processing (modulating gain) and cognitive impulsivity. The appreciation of these roles and the *interactions* of the three monoamines should make it easier to tailor treatment to the particular individual (im)balance of the pattern of cognitive, motivational, and motor bases to be found in a given patient.

REFERENCES

1. Moleman P, Tulen JHM, Blankestijn PJ, Man in t'Veld A, Boomsma F. Urinary excretion of catecholamines and their metabolites in relation to circulating catecholamines: siz-hour infusion of epinephrine and norepinephrine in healthy volunteers. Arch Gen Psychiat 1992;49:568–572.
2. Carlsson A, Falck B, Hillarp NA. Cellular localization of brain monoamines. Acta Physiol Scand 1962;56(Suppl 1):1–28.

3. Vogt M. The concentration of sympathin in different parts of the central nervous system under normal conditions and after administration of drugs. J Physiol (London) 1954;123:451–481.
4. Anderson CD, Pasquier DA, Forbes WB, Morgane PJ. Locus coeruleus-to-dorsal raphe input examined by electrophysiological and morphological methods. Brain Res Bull 1977;2:209–221.
5. Jones BE, Moore RY. Ascending projections of the locus coeruleus in the rat. II. Autoradiographic study. Brain Res 1977;127:23–53.
6. Loughlin SE, Foote SL, Bloom FE. Efferent projections of nucleus locus coeruleus: topographic organization of cells of origin demonstrated by three-dimensional reconstruction. Neurosci 1986; 18:291–306.
7. Delfs JM, Zhu JP, Druhan JP, Aston-Jones GS. Origin of noradrenergic afferents to the shell subregion of the nucleus accumbens: anterograde and retrograde tract-tracing studies in the rat. Brain Res 1998;806:127–140.
8. Chan-Palay V, Asan E. Quantitation of catecholamine neurons in the locus coeruleus in human brains of normal young and older adults and in depression. J Comp Neurol 1989;287: 357–372.
9. Descarries L, Watkins KC, Lapierre Y. Noradrenergic axon terminals in the cerebral cortex of rat.III. Topometric ultrastructural analysis. Brain Res 1977;133:197–222.
10. Berridge CW, Waterhouse BD. The locus coeruleus–noradrenergic system: modulation of behavioral state and state-dependent cognitive processes. Brain Res Rev 2003;42:33–84.
11. Amin AH, Crawford TBB, Gaddum JH. The distribution of substance P and 5-hydroxytryptamine in the central nervous system of the dog. J Physiol 1954;126:596–618.
12. Twarog BM, Page ICH. Serotonin content of some mammalian tissues and urine and method for its determination. Am J Physiol 1953;175:479–485.
13. Dahlström A, Fuxe K. Evidence for the existence of monoamine containing neurons in the central nervous system. I. Demonstration of monoamines in cell bodies of brain neurons. Acta Physiol Scand 1964;62(Suppl 232):1–55.
13. Steinbusch HWM. Distribution of serotonin-immunoreactivity in the central nervous system of the rat: cell bodies and terminals. Neurosci 1981;6:557–618.
14. Kosofsky BE, Molliver ME. The serotonergic innervation of the cerebral cortex: different classes of axon terminals arise from the dorsal and median raphe nuclei. Synapse 1987;1:153–168.
15. Törk I. Anatomy of the serotonergic system. Ann NY Acad Sci 1990;600:9–34.
16. Hornung J-P, Fritschy J-M, Törk I. Distribution of subsets of serotoninergic axons in the cerebral cortex of the marmoset. J Comp Neurol 1990;297:165–181.
17. Molliver ME. Serotonergic neuronal systems: what their anatomic organization tells us about function. J Clin Psychopharmacol 1987;7:3S–23S.
18. De Haes JI, Bosker FJ, Van Waarde A, et al. 5-HT1A receptor imaging in the human brain: effect of tryptophan depletion and infusion on [18F]MPPF binding. Synapse 2002;46:108–115.
19. Wright DE, Seroogy KB, Lundgren KH, Davis BM, Jennes L. Comparative localization of serotonin$_{1A,1C}$ and $_2$ receptor subtype mRNAs in rat brain. J Comp Neurol 1995;351:357–373.
20. Nosjean A, Hamon M, Darmon M. 5-HT2A receptors are expressed by catecholaminergic neurons in the rat nucleus tractus solitarii. NeuroReport 2003;13:2365–2369.
21. Bortolozzi A, Artigas F. Control of 5-hydroxytryptamine release in the dorsal raphe nucleus by the noradrenergic system in rat brain. Role of alpha-adrenoceptors. Neuropsychopharmacol 2003;28:421–434.
22. Pudovkina OL, Cremers TI, Westerink BHC. The interaction between the locus coeruleus and dorsal raphe nucleus studied with dual-probe microdialysis. Eur J Pharmacol 2002;445:37–42.
23. Birthelmer A, Ehret A, Amtage F, et al. Neurotransmitter release and its presynaptic modulation in the rat hippocampus after selective damage to cholinergic or/and serotonergic afferents. Brain Res Bull 2002;59:371–381.
24. Szabo ST, Blier P. Effects of serotonin (5-hydroxytryptamine, 5-HT) reuptake inhibition plus 5-HT(2A) receptor antagonism on the firing activity of norepinephrine neurons. J Pharmacol Exp Ther 2002;302:983–991.

25. Ruiz-Ortega JA, Ugedo L. Activation of 5-HT1A receptors potentiates the clonidine inhibitory effect in the locus coeruleus. Eur J Pharmacol 1997;333:159–162.
26. Gobert A, Rivet J-M, Audinot V, Newman-Tancredi A, Cistarelli L, Millan MJ. Simultaneous quantification of serotonin, dopamine and noradrenaline levels in single frontal cortex dialysates of freely-moving rats reveals a complex pattern of reciprocal auto- and heteroceptor-mediated control of release. Neurosci 1998;84:413–429.
27. Gobert A, Millan MJ. Serotonin 5-HT 2a receptor activation enhances dialysate levels of dopamine and noradrenaline, but not 5-HT, in the frontal cortex of freely-moving rats. Neuropharmacol 1999;38:315–318.
28. Millan MJ, Dekeyne A, Gobert A. Serotonin (5HT2c) receptors tonically inhibit dopamine (DA) and noradrenaline (NA), but not 5-HT, release in the frontal cortex in vivo. Neuropharmacol 1998;37:953–955.
29. Geracioti TD, Keck PE, Ekhator NN, et al. Continuous covariability of dopamine and serotonin metabolites in human cerebrospinal fluid. Biol Psychiat 1998;44:228–233.
30. Castellanos FX, Elia J, Kruesi MJP, et al. Cerebrospinal fluid homovanillic acid predicts behavioral response to stimulants in 45 boys with attention deficit/hyperactivity disorder. Neuropsychopharmacol 1996;14:125–137.
31. O'Neill MF, Heron-Maxwell CL, Shaw G. 5-HT2 receptor antagonism reduces hyperactivity induced by amphetamine, cocaine and MK-801 but not D-1 agonist c-APB. Pharmacol Biochem Behav 1999;63:237–244.
32. Porras G, Di Matteo V, Fracasso C, et al. 5-HT(2A) and 5-HT(2C/2B) receptor subtypes modulate dopamine release induced in vivo by amphetamine and morphine in both the rat nucleus accumbens and striatum. Neuropsychopharmacol 2002;26:311–324.
33. Rogers RD, Blackshaw AJ, Middleton HC, et al. Tryptophan depletion impairs stimulus reward learning while methylphenidate disrupts attentional control in healthy young adults: implications for the monoaminergic basis of impulsive behaviour. Psychopharmacol 1999; 146:482–491.
34. Fletcher PJ, Korth KM. Activation of 5-HT1B in the nucleus accumbens reduces amphetamine induced enhancement of responding for conditioned reward. Psychopharmacol 1999;142: 165–174.
35. Luthman J, Fredeiksson A, Sundström E, Jonsson G, Archer T. Selective lesion of central dopamine or noradrenaline neuron systems in the neonatal rat: motor behavior and monoamine alterations at adult stage. Behav Brain Res 1989;33:267–277.
36. Oades RD, Slusarek M, Velling S, Bondy B. Serotonin platelet-transporter measures in childhood attention-deficit/hyperactivity disorder (ADHD): clinical versus experimental measures of impulsivity. World J Biol Psychiat 2002;3:96–100.
37. Koskinen T, Sirviö J. Studies on the involvement of the dopaminergic system in the 5-HT2 agonist DOI-induced premature responding in a five-choice serial reaction time task. Brain Res Bull 2001;54:65–75.
38. Nocjar C, Roth BL, Pehek EA Localization of 5-HT(2A) receptors on dopamine cells in subnuclei of the midbrain A10 cell group. Neuroscience 2002;111:163–176.
39. Lucas G, Spampinato U. Role of striatal serotonin$_{2A}$ and serotonin$_{2C}$ receptor subtypes in the control of the in vivo dopamine outfow in the rat striatum. J Neurochem 2000;74:693–701.
40. Di Giovanni G, Di Matteo V, Di Mascio M, Esposito E. Preferential modulation of mesolimbic vs. nigrostriatal dopaminergic function by serotonin$_{2c/2b}$ receptor agonists: a combined in vivo electrophysiological and microdialysis study. Synapse 2000;35:53–61.
41. Di Matteo V, Cacchio M, Di Giulio C, Esposito E. Role of serotonin (2C) receptors in the control of brain dopaminergic function. Pharmacol Biochem Behav 2002;71:727–734.
42. Hutson PH, Barton CL, Jay M, et al. Activation of mesolimbic dopamine function by phencyclidine is enhanced by 5-HT2C/2B receptor antagonists: neurochemical and behavioural studies. Neuropharmacol 2000;39:2318–2328.
43. Kuroki T, Dai J, Meltzer HY, Ichikawa J. *R*(+)-8-OH-DPAT, a selective 5-HT1A receptor agonist, attenuated amphetamine-induced dopamine synthesis in rat striatum, but not nucleus accumbens or medial prefrontal cortex. Brain Res 2000;872:204–207.

44. Doherty MD, Pickel VM. Targeting of serotonin 1a receptors to dopaminergic neurons within the parabrachial subdivision of the ventral tegmental area in rat brain. J Comp Neurol 2001;433: 490–500.
45. Yan QS, Yan SE. Activation of 5.HT1B/(1D) receptors in the mesolimbic dopamine system: increases dopamine release from the nucleus acumbens. Eur J Pharmacol 2001;418:55–64.
46. Pan WHT, Sung JC, Fuh SMR. Locally application of amphetamine into the ventral tegmental area enhances dopamine release in the nucleus accumbens and the medial prefrontal cortex through noradrenergic neurotransmission. J Pharmacol Exp Ther 1996;278:725–731.
47. Auclair A, Cotecchia S, Glowinski J, Tassin J-P. D-amphetamine fails to increase extracellular dopamine levels in mice lacking alpha 1b-adrenergic receptors: relationship between functional and nonfunctional dopamine release. J Neurosci 2002;22:9150–9154.
48. Yavich L, Lappalainen R, Sirviö J, Haapalinna A, MacDonald E. α_2-Adrenergic control of dopamine overflow and metabolism in mouse striatum. Eur J Pharmacol 1997;339:113–119.
49. Tuinstra T, Cools AR. High and low responders to novelty: effects of adrenergic agents on the regulation of accumbal dopamine under challenged and non-challenged conditions. Neurosci 2000;99:55–64.
50. Gioanni Y, Thierry A-M, Glowinski J, Tassin J-P. α_1-Adrenergic, D1 and D2 receptors interactions in the prefrontal cortex: implications for the modality of action of different types of neuroleptics. Synapse 1998;30:362–370.
51. Hertel P, Fagerquist MV, Svensson TH. Enhanced cortical dopamine output and antipsychotic-like effects of raclopride by α_2 adrenoceptor blockade. Science 1999;286:105–107.
52. Carboni E, Tanda GL, Frau R, Di Chiara G. Blockade of the noradrenaline carrier increases extracellular dopamine concentrations in the prefrontal cortex: evidence that dopamine is taken up in vivo by noradrenergic terminals. J Neurochem 1990;55:1067–1070.
53. De Montis G, Devoto P, Gessa GL, et al. Central dopaminergic transmission is selectively increased in the limbic system of rats chronically exposed to antidepressants. Eur J Pharmacol 1990;180:31–35.
54. Wayment HK, Schenk JO, Sorg BA. Characterization of extracellular dopamine clearance in the medial prefrontal cortex: role of monoamine uptake and monoamine oxidase inhibition. J Neurosci 2001;21:35–44.
55. Devoto P, Flore G, Pani L, Gessa GL. Evidence for co-release of noradrenaline and dopamine from noradrenergic neurons in the cerebral cortex. Mol Psychiatr 2001;6:657–664.
56. Zevcevic N, Verney C. Development of the catecholamine neurons in human embryos and fetuses, with special emphasis on the innervation of the cerebral cortex. J Comp Neurol 1995;351:509–535.
57. Tomasini R, Kema IP, Muskiet FAJ, Neiborg G, Staal MJ, Go KG. Catecholaminergic development of fetal ventral mesencephalon: characterization by high performance liquid chrmatography with electrochemical detection and immunohistochemistry. Exp Neurol 1997;145:434–441.
58. Choi S-J, Kellogg CK. Adolescent development influences functional responsiveness of noradrenergic projections to the hypothalamus in male rats. Dev Brain Res 1996;94:144–151.
59. Clarke AS, Hedeker DR, Ebert MH, Schmidt DE, McKinney WT, Kraemer GW. Rearing experience and biogenic amine activity in infant rhesus monkeys. Biol Psychiat 1996;40:338–352.
60. Miguez JM, Aldegrunde M, Paz-Valinas L, Recio J, Sanchez-Barcelo E. Selective changes in the contents of noradrenaline, dopamine and serotonin in rat brain areas during aging. J Neur Transm 2000;106:1089–1098.
61. Hartley EJ, Seeman P. Development of receptors for dopamine and noradrenaline in rat brain. Eur J Pharmacol 1983;91:391–397.
62. Moll GH, Mehnert C, Wicker M, et al. Age-associated changes in the densities of the presynaptic monoamine transporters in different regions of the rat brain from early juvenile life to late adulthood. Dev Brain Res 2000;119:251–257.
63. Roux JC, Mamet J, Perrin J, et al. Neurochemical development of the brainstem catecholaminergic cell groups in rat. J Neur Transm 2003;110:51–65.

64. Oades RD, Roepcke B, Schepker R. A test of conditioned blocking and its development in childhood and adolescence: relationship to personality and monoamine metabolism. Dev Neuropsychol 1996;12:207–230.
65. Andersen SL, Teicher MH. Sex differences in dopamine receptors and their relevance to ADHD. Neurosci Biobehav Rev 2000;24:137–141.
66. Vu DH, Törk I. Differential development of the dual serotonergic fiber system in the cerebral cortex of the cat. J Comp Neurol 1992;317:156–174.
67. Jones GH, Hernandez TD, Kendall DA, Marsden CA, Robbins TW. Dopaminergic and serotonergic function following isolation rearing in rats: study of behavioural responses and postmortem and in vivo neurochemistry. Pharmacol Biochem Behav 1992;43:17–35.
68. Santana C, Rodriguez M, Alfonso D, Arevalo R. Dopaminergic neuron development in rats: biochemical study from prenatal life to adulthood. Brain Res Bull 1992;29:7–13.
69. Silverstein FS, Donn S, Buchanan K, Johnston MV. Concentrations of homovanillic acid and 5-hydroxyindoleacetic acid in cerebrospinal fluid from human infnats in the perinatal period. J Neurochem 1984;43:1769–1772.
70. Murrin LC, Gibbens DL, Ferrer JR. Ontogeny of dopamine, serotonin and spirodecanone receptors in rat forebrain—an autoradiographic study. Develop Brain Res 1985;23:91–109.
71. Konradi C, Kornhuber J, Sofic E, Heckers S, Riederer P, Beckmann H. Variations of monoamines and their metabolites in the human brain putamen. Brain Res 1992;579:285–290.
72. Retz W, Kornhuber J, Riederer P. Neurotransmission and the ontogeny of human brain. J Neur Transm 1996;103:403–419.
73. Sigurdh J, Spigset O, Allard P, Mjörndahl T, Hägglof B. Binding of [^{3}H]lysergic acid diethylamide to serotonin 5-HT$_{2A}$ receptors and of [^{3}H]paroxetine to serotonin uptake sites in platelets from healthy children, adolescents and adults. Neuropsychobiol 1999;40:183–187.
74. Zhang ZW. Serotonin induces tonic firing in layer V pyramidal neurons of rat prefrontal cortex during postnatal development. J Neurosci 2003;23:3373–3384.
75. Rodriguez M, Martin L, Santana C. Ontogenic development of brain asymmatry in dopaminergic neurons. Brain Res Bull 1994;33:163–171.
76. Hechtman L. Genetic and neurobiological aspects of attention deficit hyperactive disorder: a review. J Psychiatr Neurosci 1994;19:193–201.
77. Arnsten AFT. Catecholamine regulation of the prefrontal cortex. J Psychopharmacol 1997;1: 151–162.
78. Flugge G, van Kampen M, Meyer H, Fuchs E, Alpha2A and alpha2C-adrenoceptor regulation in the brain: alpha2A changes persist after chronic stress. Eur J Neurosci 2003;17:917–928.
79. Linner L, Arborelius L, Nomikos GG, Bertilsson L, Svensson TH. Locus coeruleus neuronal activity and noradrenaline availability in the frontal cortex of rats chronically treated with imipramine: effect of α2-adrenoceptor blockade. Biol Psychiat 1999;46:776–774.
80. Fahlke C, Garpenstrand H, Oreland L, Suomi SJ, Higley JD. Platelet monoamine oxidase activity in nonhuman primate model of type 2 excessive alcoholconsumption. Am J Psychiat 2002;159: 2107–2109.
81. Comings DE, Gonzalez NS, Cheng LS-C, MacMurray J. A "line-item" approach to the identification of genes involved in polygenic behavioral disorders: the adrenergic α_{2A} (ADRA2A) gene. Am J Med Genet 2003;118B:110–114.
82. Barr CL, Kroft J, Feng Y, et al. The norepinephrine transporter gene and attention deficit hyperactivity disorder. Am J Genet 2002;114:255–259.
83. McEvoy B, Hawi Z, Fitzgerald M, Gill M. No evidence of linkage or association between norepinephrine transporter (NET) gene polymorphisms and ADHD in the Irish population. Am J Med Genet 2002;114:656–666.
84. Qian Q, Wang Y, Zhou R, et al. Family based and case control association studies of catechol-*O*-methyltransferase in attention deficit hyperactivity disorder suggest genetic sexual dimorphism. Am J Med Genet 2003;118B:103–109.

85. Eisenberg J, Mei-Tal G, Steinberg A, et al. Haplotype relative risk study of catechol-*O*-methyltransferase (COMT) and attention deficit hyperactivity disorder (ADHD): association of the high-enzyme activity Val allele with ADHD impulsive-hyperactive phenotype. Am J Med Genet 1999;88:497–502.
86. Kirley A, Hawi Z, Daly G, et al. Dopaminergic system genes in ADHD: toward a biological hypothesis. Neuropsychopharmacol 2002;27:607–619.
87. Wigg K, Zai G, Schachar R, Tannock R, et al. Attention defict hyperactivity disorder and the gene for dopamine beta hydroxylase. Am J Psychiat 2002;159:1046–1048.
88. Lawson DC, Turie D, Langley K, et al. Association analysis of monoamine oxidase A and attention deficit hyperactivity disorder. J Med Genet 2003;116B:84–89.
89. Garpenstrand H, Ekblom J, Hallman J, Oreland L. Platelet monoamine oxidase activity in relation to alleles of dopamine D4 and tyrosine hydroxylase genes. Acta Psychiat Scand 1997;96:295–300.
90. Dalley JW, Theobald DE, Eagle DM, Passetti F, Robbins TW. Deficits in impulse control associated with tonically-elevated serotonergic function in rat prefrontal cortex. Neuropsychopharmacol 2002;26:716–728.
91. Moresco FM, Dieci M, Vita A. In vivo serotonin 5HT(2A) receptor binding and personality traits in healthy subjects: a positron emission tomography study. NeuroImage 2002;17:1470–1478.
92. Kent L, Doerry U, Hary E, et al. Evidence that variation at the serotonin transporter gene influences susceptibility to attention deficit hyperactivity disorder (ADHD): analysis and pooled analysis. Mol Psychiat 2002;7:908–912.
93. Smeraldi E, Zanardi R, Benedetti F, Di Bella D, Perez J, Catalano M. Polymorphism within the promoter of the serotonin transporter gene and antidepressant efficacy of fluvoxamine. Mol Psychiat 1998;3:508–511.
94. Lakatos K, Nemoda Z, Birkas E, et al. Association of D4 dopamine receptors gene and serotonin transporter promoter polymorphisms with infants'response to novelty. Mol Psychiat 2003;8: 90–97.
95. Auerbach JG, Faroy M, Ebstein R. The association of the dopamine D4 receptor gene /DRD4) and the serotonin transporter promoter gene (5-HTTLPR) with temperament in 12-month-old infants. J Child Psychol Psychiat 2001;42:777–783.
96. Zoroglu SS, Erdal ME, Alasehirli B, et al. Significance of the serotonin transporter gene 5-HTTLPR and variable number tandem repeat polymorphism in attention deficit hyperactivity disorder. Neuropsychobiology 2002;45:176–181.
97. Hawi Z, Dring M, Kirley A, et al. Serotonergic system and attention deficit hyperactivity disorder (ADHD): a potential suscepptibility locus at the 5-HT1B receptor gene in 273 nuclear families from a multicentre sample. Mol Psychiat 2002;7:718–725.
98. Quist JF, Barr CL, Schachar R, et al. The serotonin 5-HT1B receptor gene and attention deficit hyperactivity disorder. Mol Psychiat 2003;8:98–102.
99. Quist JF, Barr CL, Schachar R, et al. Evidence for the serotonin HTR2A receptor gene as a susceptibility factor in attention deficit hyperactivity disorder (ADHD). Mol Psychiat 2000;5:537–541.
100. Levitan RD, Masellis M, Basile VS, et al. Polymorphism of the serotonin-2A receptor gene (HTR2A) associated with childhood attention deficit hyperactivity sidorder (ADHD) in adult women with seasonal affective disorder. J Affect Disord 2002;71:229–233.
101. Lambert GW, Horne M, Kalff V, et al. Central nervous noradrenergic and dopaminergic turnover in response to acute neuroleptic challenge. Life Sci 1995;56:1545–1555.
102. Potter WZ, Manji HK. Are monoamine metabolites in cerebrospinal fluid worth measuring? Arch Gen Psychiat 1993;50:653–656.
103. Plizka SR, Maas JW, Javors MA, Rogeness GA, Baker J. Urinary catecholamines in attention-deficit hyperactivity disorder with and without comorbid anxiety. J Am Acad Child Adolesc Psychiat 1994;33:1165–1173.
104. Tohgi H, Takahashi S, Abe T. The effect of age on concentrations of monoamines, amino acids and their related substances in the cerebrospinal fluid. J Neur Transm (PD section) 1993;5:215–226.

105. Müller N, Empl M, Riedel M, Schwarz M, Ackenheil M. Neuroleptic treatment increases soluble IL-2 receptors and decreases soluble IL-6 receptors. Eur Arch Psychiat Clin Neurosci 1997;247:308–313.
106. Cheetham SC, Viggers JA, Slater NA, Heal DJ, Buckett WR. [^{3}H] Paroxetine binding in rat frontal cortex strongly correlates with [^{3}H] 5HT uptake: effect of administration of various antidepressant treatments. Neuropharmacol 1993;32:737–743.
107. Lambert GW, Cox HS, Horne M, et al. Direct determination of homovanilic acid release from the human brain, an indicator of central dopaminergic activity. Life Sci 1991;49:1061–1072.
108. Lambert GW, Eisenhofer G, Jennings GL, Esler MD. Regional homovanillic acid production in humans. Life Sci 1993;53:63–75.
109. Lambert GW, Ferrier C, Kaye DM, et al. Monoaminergic neuronal activoity in subcortical brain regions in essential hypertension. Blood Press 1994;3:55–66.
110. Davids E, Zhang K, Kula NS, Tarazi FI, Baldessarini RJ. Effects of norepinephrine and seotonin transporter inhibitors on hyperactivity induced by neonatal 6-hydroxydopamine lesioning in the rat. J Exp Pharmacol Ther 2002;301:1097–1102.
111. Bishop C, Kamdar DP, Walker PD. Intrastriatal serotonin 5-HT2 receptors mediate dopamine D1-inducd hyperlocomotion in 6-hydrosxydopamine-lesioned rats. Synapse 2003;50:164–170.
112. Sagvolden T, Metzger MA, Schiorbeck HK, Rugland A-L, Spinnangr I, Sagvolden G. The spontaneously hypertensive rat (SHR) as an animal model of childhood hyperactivity (ADHD): changed reactivity to reinforcers and to psychomotor stimulants. Behav Neur Biol 1992;58: 103–112.
113. Rogers LJ, Sink MS, Hambley JW. Exploration, fear and maze learning in spontaneously hypertensive and normotensive rats. Behav Neur Biol 1988;49:222–233.
114. Lukaszewska I, Niewiadomska G. The difference in learning abilities between hypertensive (SHR) and Wistar normotensive rats are cue dependent. Neurobiol Learn Memory 1995;63: 43–53.
115. Nakamura-Palacios EM, Caldas CK, Fiorini A, Chaga KN, Vasquez EC. Deficits of spatial learning and working memory in spontaneously hypertensive rats. Behav Brain Res 1996;74: 217–221.
116. Gattu M, Pauly JR, Boss KL, Summers JB, Buccafusco JJ. Cognitive impairment in spontaneously hypertensive rats: role of central nicotinic receptors. Part I Brain Res 1997;771:89–103.
117. Sagvolden T, Pettersen MB, Larsen MC. Spontaneously hypertensive rats (SHR) as a putative animal model of childhood hyperkinesis. Physiol Behav 1993;54:1047–1055.
118. Dev BR, Philip L. Extracellular catechol and indole turnover in the nucleus of the solitary tract of spontaneously hypertensive and Wistar–Kyoto normotensive rats in response to drug-induced changes in arterial blood pressure. Brain Res Bull 1996;40:111–116.
119. Bagdy G, Szemeredi K, Listwak SJ, Keiser HR, Goldstein DS. Plasma catecholamine, renin activity and ACTH responses to the serotonin agonist DOI in juvenile spontaneously hypertensive rats. Life Sci 1993;53:1573–1582.
120. Tsukamoto K, Sved AF, Ito S, Komatsu K, Kanmatsuse K. Enhanced serotonin-mediated responses in the nucleus tractus solitarius of spontaneously hypertensive rats. Brain Res 2000; 863:1–8.
121. Russell V, Allie S, Wiggins T. Increased noradrenergic activity in prefrontal cortex slices of an animal model for attention-deficit hyperactivity disorder—the spontaneously hypertensive rat. Behav Brain Res 2001;117:69–74.
122. De Villiers AS, Russell VA, Sagvolden T, Searson A, Jaffer A, Taljaard JF. α2-adrenoceptor mediated inhibition of [^{3}H]dopamine release from nucleus accumbens slices and monoamine levels in a rat model for attention-deficit hyperactivity disorder. Neurochem Res 1995;20:427–433.
123. Togashi H, Matsumoto M, Yoshioka M, Hirokami M, Minami M, Saito H. Neurochemical profiles in cerebrospinal fluid of stroke-prone spontaneously hypertensive rats. Neurosci Lett 1994;166:117–120.

124. Russell V. Hypodopaminergic and hypernoradrenergic activity in prefrontal cortex slices of an animal model for attention-deficit hyperactivity disorder—the spontaneously hypertensive rat. Behav Brain Res 2002;130:191–196.
125. Davids E, Zhang K, Tarazi FI, Baldessarini RJ. Animal models of attention-deficit hyperactivity disorder. Brain Res Rev 2003;42:1–21.
126. Dekeyne A, Gobert A, Auclair A, Girardon S, Millan MJ. Differential modulation of efficiency in a food-rewarded a differential reinforcement of low rate 72-s schedule in rats by norepinephrine and serotonin reptake inhibitors. Psychopharmacol 2002;162:156–167.
127. Jones MD, Hess EJ. Norepinephrine regulates locomotor hyperactivity in the mouse mutant coloboma. Pharmacol Biochem Behav 2003;75:209–216.
128. Missler M, Zhang W, Rohlmann A, et al. α-Neurexins couple Ca^{2+} channels to synaptic vesicle exocytosis. Nature 2003;423:939–948.
129. Dell'Anna ME, Luthman J, Lindqvust E, Olson L. Development of monoamine systems after neonatal anoxia in rats. Brain Res Bull 1993;32:159–170.
130. Puumala T, Ruotsalainen S, Jakala P, Koivisto E, Riekkinen P, Sirviö J. Behavioral and pharmacological studies on the validation of a new animal model of attention deficit hyperactivity disorder. Neurobiol Learn Memory 1996;66:198–211.
131. Poncet L, Denoroy L, Dalmaz Y, Pèquignot JM, Jouvet M. Alteration in central and peripheral substance P and neuropetide Y like immunoreactivity after chronic hypoxia in the rat. Brain Res 1996;733:64–72.
132. Oades RD, Daniels R, Rascher W. Plasma neuropeptide Y levels, monoamine metabolism, electrolyte excretion and drinking behavior in children with attention deficit hyperactivity disorder (ADHD). Psychiat Res 1998;80;177–186.
133. Dumont Y, Martel JC, Fournier A, St-Pierre S, Quirion R. Neuropeptide Y and neuropeptide Y receptor subtypes in brain and peripheral tissue. Prog Neurobiol 1992;38:125–167.
134. Lehmann J. Neuropetide Y: an overview. Drug Dev Res 1990;19:329–351.
135. Castellanos FX. The psychobiology of attention-deficit/hyperactivity disorder. In: Quay HC, Cohen TP, eds. Handbook of sisruptive behavior disorders. New York: Kluwer Academic/Plenum Publishers, 1999:179–198.
136. Ernst M, Kimes AS, London ED, et al. Neural substrates of decision making in adults with attention deficit hyperactivity disorder. Am J Psychiat 2003;160:1061–1070.
137. Rubia K, Smith AB, Brammer MJ, Taylor E. Right inferior prefrontal cortex mediates response inhibition while mesial prefrontal cortex is responsible for error detection. NeuroImage 2003; 20:351–358.
138. Oades RD, Dittmann-Balcar A, Schepker R, Eggers C. Auditory event-related potentials and mismatch negativity in healthy children and those with attention-deficit- or Tourette-like symptoms. Biol Psychol 1996;43:163–185.
139. Arnsten AFT. Dopaminergic and noradrenergic influences on cognitive functons mediated by prefrontal cortex. In: Solanto MV, Arsten AFT, Castellanos FY, eds. Stimulant drugs and ADHD: basic and clinical neuroscience. Oxford: Oxford University Press, 2001:185–208.
140. Kalff AC, Hendriksen JGM, Kroes M, et al. Neurocognitive performance of 5- and 6-yr old children who met criteria for attention deficit/hyperactivity disorder at 18 months follow-up: results from a prospective population study. J Abnorm Child Psychol 2002;30:589–598.
141. Stevens J, Quittner AL, Zuckerman JB, Moore S. Behavioral inhibition, self-regulation of motivation, and working memory in children with attention deficit hyperactivity disorder. Dev Neuropsychol 2002;21:117–139.
142. Barnett R, Maruff P, Vance A, et al. Abnormal executive function in attention deficit hyperactivity disorder: the effect of stimulant medication and age on spatial working memory. Psychol Med 2001;31:1107–1115.
143. Karetekin C, Asarnow RF. Working memory in childhood-onset schizophrenia and attention-deficit/hyperactivity disorder. Psychiatr Res 1998;80:165–176.

144. Tripp G, Ryan J, Peace K. Neuropsychological functioning in children with DSM-IV combined type attention deficit hyperactivity disorder. Aust NZ J Psychiatr 2003;36:771–779.
145. Muir-Broaddus J, Rosenstein LD, Medina DE, Soderberg C. Neuropsychological test performance of children with ADHD relative to test norms and parent behavioral ratings. Arch Clin Neuropsychol 2002;17:671–689.
146. Roodenrys S, Koloski N, Grainger J. Working memory function in attention deficit hyperactivity disordered and reading disabled children. Br J Dev Psychol 2001;19:325–337.
147. Oie M, Sundet K, Rund BR. Contrasts in memory functions between adolescents with schizophrenia or ADHD. Neuropsychologia 1999;37:1351–1358.
148. Kuntsi J, Oosterlaan J, Stevenson J. Psychological mechanisms in hyperactivity; I. Response inhibition deficit, working memory impairment, delay aversion, or something else? J Child Psychol Psychiat 2001;42:199–210.
149. Barkley RA, Edwards G, Laneri M, Fletcher K. Executive functioning, temporal discounting and sense of time in adolescents with attention deficit hyperactivity disorder (ADHD) and oppositional defiance disorder (ODD). J Abnorm Child Psychol 2001;29:541–556.
150. Shallice T, Marzocchi GM, Coser S, Del Salvio M, Meuter RF, Rumiati RI. Executive function profile of children with attention deficit hyperactivity disorder. Dev Neuropsychol 2002; 21:43–71.
151. Siegel LS, Ryan EB. The development of working memory in normally achieving and subtypes of learning disabled children. Child Dev 1989;60:973–980.
152. Sergeant JA, Geurts H, Oosterlaan J. How specific is a deficit of executive function for attention-deficit/hyperactivity disorder? Behav Brain Res 2002;130:3–28.
153. Sonuga-Barke EJS, Dalen L, Daley D, Remington B. Are planning, working memory, and inhibition associated with individual differences in preschool ADHD symptoms? Dev Neuropsychol 2002;21:255–272.
154. Welsh MC, Satterlee-Cartnell T, Stine M. Towers of Hanoi and London: contribution of working memory and inhibition to performance Brain Cogn 1999;41:231–242.
155. Oades RD. The role of noradrenaline in tuning and dopamine in switching between signals in the CNS. Neurosci Biobehav Rev 1985;9:261–283.
156. Usher M, Cohen JD, Servan-Schreiber D, Rajkowski J, Aston-Jones GS. The role of the locus coeruleus in the regulation of cognitive performance. Science 1999;283:549–554.
157. Chappell PB, Riddle MA, Scahill L, et al. Guanfacine treatment of comorbid attention-deficit hyperactivity disorder and Tourette's syndrome: preliminary clinical experience. J Am Acad Child Adolesc Psychiatry 1995;34:1140–1146.
158. Castellanos FX, Elia J, Kruesi MJP, et al. Cerebrospinal fluid monoamine metabolites in boys with attention-deficit hyperactivity disorder. Psychiatr Res 1994;52:305–316.
159. Halperin JM, Newcorn JH, Koda VH, Pick L, McKay K.E, Knott P. Noradrenergic mechanisms in ADHD children with and without reading disabilities: a replication and extension. J Am Acad Child Adolesc Psychiatry 1997;36:1688–1697.
160. Oades RD. Differential measures of 'sustained attention' in children with attention-deficit/hyperactivity or tic disorders: relations to monoamine metabolism. Psychiatr Res 2000;93: 165–178.
161. Spivak B, Vered Y, Yoran-Hegesh R, Averbuch E, Mester R, Graf E. Circulatory levels of catecholamines, serotonin and lipids in attention deficit hyperactivity disorder. Acta Psychiatr Scand 1999;99:300–304.
162. Uzbekov MG, Misionzhnik EY. Changes in urinary monoamine excretion in hyperkinetic children. Hum Psychopharmacol 2003;18:493–497.
163. Pick LH, Halperin JM, Schwartz ST, Newcorn JH. A longitudinal study of neurobiological mechanisms in boys with attention-deficit hyperactivity disorder: preliminary findings. Biol Psychiatry 1999;45:371–373.
164. Schulz KP, McKay KE, Newcorn JH, Sharma V, Gabriel S, Halperin JM. Serotonin function and risk for alcoholism in boys with attention-deficit hyperactivity disorder. Neuropsychopharmacol 1998;18:10–17.

165. van Goozen SHM, Matthys W, Cohen-Kettenis PT, Westenberg H, van Engeland H. Plasma monoamine metabolites and aggression: two studies of normal and oppositional defiant disorder children. Eur Neuropsychopharmacol 1999;9:141–147.
166. Cook EH, Stein MA, Ellison T, Unis AS, Leventhal BL. Attention deficit hyperactivity disorder and whole blood serotonin levels: effects of comorbidity. Psychiatr Res 1995;57:13–20.
167. Walderhaug E, Lunde H, Nordvik JE, Landro NI, Refsum H, Magnusson A. Lowering of serotonin by rapid tryptophan depletion increases impulsiveness in normal individuals. Psychopharmacol 2002;164:385–391.
168. Juckel G, Schmidt LG, Rommelspacher H, Hegerl U. The tridimensional personality questionnaire and the intensity dependence of auditory evoked dipole source activity. Biol Psychiatry 1995;37:311–317.
169. Buchsbaum MS, Wender PH. Averaged evoked responses in normal and minimally brain dysfunctioned children treated with amphetamine. A preliminary report. Arch Gen Psychiatry 1973; 29:764–770.
170. Hegerl U, Juckel G. Auditory evoked dipole source activity: indicator of central serotonergic dysfunction in psychiatric patients? Pharmacopsychiatry 1994;27:75–78.
171. Zametkin AJ, Rapoport JL. Neurobiology of attention deficit disorder with hyperactivity: where have we come in 50 years? J Am Acad Child Adolesc Psychiatry 1987;26:676–686.
172. Swanson J, Volkow ND. Pharmokokinetic and pharmacodynamic properties of methylphenidate in humans. In: Solanto MV, Arsten AFT, Castellanos FY, eds. Stimulant drugs and ADHD: basic and clinical neuroscience. Oxford: Oxford University Press, 2001:259–282.
173. Kuczenski R, Segal D. Regional norepinephrine response to amphetamine using dialysis: comparison with caudate dopamine. Synapse 1992;11:164–169.
174. Patrick KS, Markowitz JS. Pharmacology of methylphenidate, amphetamine enantiomers and pemoline in attention deficit hyperactivity disorder. Hum Psychopharmacol 1997;12:527–546.
175. Kuczenski R, Segal D. Exposure of adolescent rats to oral methylphenidate: preferential effects on extracellular norepinephrine and absence of sensitization and cross-sensitization to methamphetamine. J Neurosci 2002;22:7264–7271.
176. Kuczenski R, Segal DS, Leith NJ, Applegate CD. Effects of amphetamine, methylphenidate and apomorphine on regional brain serotonin and 5-hydroxyindole acetic acid. Psychopharmacol 1987;93:329–335.
177. Kuczenski R, Segal D. Effects of methylphenidate on extracellular dopamine, serotonin and norepinephrine: comparison with amphetamine. J Neurochem 1997;68:2032–2037.
178. Bonhomme N, Cador M, Stinus L, Le Moal M, Spampinato U. Short and long-term changes in dopamine and serotonin receptor binding sites in amphetamine-sensitized rats: a quantitative autoradiographic study. Brain Res 1995;675:215–223.
179. Plizka SR, McCracken JT, Maas JW. Catecholamines in attention-deficit hyperactivity disorder: current perspectives. J Am Acad Child Adolesc Psychiatry 1996;35:264–272.
180. Kusaga A, Yamashita Y, Koeda T, et al. Increased urine phenylethylamine after methylphenidate treatment in children with ADHD. Ann Neurol 2002;52:371–374.
181. Plizka SR. Comparing the effects of stimulant and non-stimulant agents on catecholamine function: implications for theories of ADHD. In: Solanto MV, Arnsten AFM, Castellanos FX, ed. Stimulant drugs and ADHD: basic and clinical neuroscience. Oxford: Oxford University Press, 2001:332–352.
182. Oades RD. Attention deficit disorder and hyperkinetic syndrome: biological perspectives. In: Sagvolden T, Archer T, eds. Attention Deficit Disorder: Clinical and Basic Research, Hillsdale, NJ: Lawrence Erlbaum, 1989:353–368.
183. Aston-Jones G, Rajkowski J, Cohen J. Role of locus coeruleus in attention and behavioral flexibility. Biol Psychiatry 1999;46:1309–1320.
184. Hanna GL, Ornitz EM, Hariharan M. Urinary epinephrine excretion during intelligence testing in attention-deficit hyperactivity disorder and normal boys. Biol Psychiatry 1996a;40:553–555.
185. King JA, Barkley RA, Barrett S. Attention-deficit hyperactivity disorder and the stress response. Biol Psychiatry 1998;44:72–74.

186. Konrad K, Gauggel S, Schurek J. Catecholamine functioning in children with traumatic brain injuries and children with attention-deficit/hyperactivity disorder. Cogn Brain Res 2003;16:425–433.
187. Donnelly M, Zametkin AJ, Rapoport JL, et al. Treatment of childhood hyperactivity with desipramine: plasma drug concentration, cardiovascular effects, plasma and urinary catecholamine levels, and clinical response. Clin Pharmacol Ther 1986;39:72–81.
188. Elia J, Borcherding BG, Potter WZ, Mefford IN, Rapoport JL, Keysor CS. Stimulant drug treatment of hyperactivity: biochemical correlates. Clin Pharmacol Ther 1990;48:57–66.
189. McCracken JT, Hinshaw SP, Henker B, Whalen CK, Zupran B. Urinary catecholamine differences in ADHD versus normal children and effects of methylphenidate. Society for Research in Child and Adolescent Psychopathology, Los Angeles, 1990 (cit. Plizka 2001).
190. Boulton AA. Phenylethylaminergic modulation of catcholaminergic neurotransmission. Prog Neuropsychopharmacol Biol Psychiatry 1991;15:139–156.
191. De Groot CM, Bornstein RA, Baker GB. Obsessive-compulsive symptom clusters and urinary amine correlates in Tourette syndrome. J Nerv Ment Dis 1995;183:224–230.
192. Karoum F, Linnoila M, Potter WZ, Chuang LW, Goodwin FK, Wyatt RJ. Fluctuating high urinary phenylethylamine excretion rates in some bipolar affective disorder patients. Psychiatry Res 1982;6:215–222.
193. O'Reilly R, Davis BA, Durden DA, Thorpe L, Machnee H, Boulton AA. Plasma phenylethylamine in schizophrenic patients. Biol Psychiatry 1991;30:145–150.
194. Baker GB, Bornstein RA, Rouget AC, Ashton AC, Van Muyden JC, Coutts RT. Phenylethylaminergic mechanisms in attention deficit disorder. Biol Psychiatry 1991;29:15–22.
195. Chuang LW, Karoum F, Wyatt RJ. Different effects of behaviorally equipotent doses of amphetamine and methamphetamine on brain biogenic amines: specific increase of phenylethylamine by amphetamine. Eur J Pharmacol 1982;81:385–392.
196. Zametkin AJ, Karoum F, Linnoila M, et al. Stimulants, urinary catecholamines and indoleamines in hyperactivity: a comparison of methylphenidate and amphetamine. Arch Gen Psychiatry 1985;42:251–255.
197. Perlow MJ, Chieuh CC, Lake CR, Wyatt RJ. Increased dopamine and norepinephrine concentrations in primate CSF following amphetamine and phenylethylamine administration. Brain Res 1980;186: 469–473.
198. Bymaster FP, Katner JS, Nelson DL, et al. Atomoxetine increases extracellular levels of norpeinephrine and dopamine in prefrontal cortex of the rat: a potential mechanism for efficacy in attention deficit/hyperactivity disorder. Neuropsychopharmacol 2002;27:699–711.
199. Michelson D, Adler L, Spencer T, et al. Atomoxetine in adults with ADHD: two randomized placebo-controlled studies. Biol Psychiatry 2003;53:211–220.
200. Spencer T, Biederman J, Wilens TE, Harding M, ,Donnell D, Griffin S. Pharmacotherapy of attention-deficit hyperactivity disorder across the life cycle. J Am Acad Child Adolesc Psychiatry 1996;35:409–432.
201. Garfinkel BD, Wender PH, Sloman L, O'Neill I. Tricyclic antidepressant and methylphenidate treatment of attention deficit disorder in children. J Am Acad Child Adolesc Psychiatry 1983;22:343–348.
202. Rapport MD, Carlson GA, Kelly KL, Pataki C. Methylphenidate and desipramine in hospitalized children: I. Separate and combined effects on cognitive function. J Am Acad Child Adolesc Psychiatry 1993;32:333–342.
203. Gualtieri CT, Keenan PA, Chandler M. Clinical and neuropsychological effects of desipramine in children with attention deficit disorder. J Clin Psychopharmacol 1991;11:155–159.
204. Donnelly M, Rapoport JL, Potter WZ, et al. Fenfluramine and dextroamphetamine treatment of childhood hyperactivity. Clinical and biochemical findings. Arch Gen Psychiatry 1989;46:205–212.
205. Biederman J, Spencer T. Attention-deficit/hyperactivity disorder (ADHD) as a noradrenergic disorder. Biol Psychiatry 1999;46:1234–1242.
206. Overtoom CCE, Verbaten MN, Kemner C, et al. Effects of methylphenidate, desipramine and L-dopa on attention and inhibition in children with attention deficit hyperactivity disorder. Behav Brain Res 2003;145:7–15.

207. Simeon JV, Wiggins DM. Pharmacotherapy of attention-deficit-hyperactivity disorder. Canad J Psychiatry 1993;38:443–448.
208. Connor DF, Fletcher KE, Swanson JM. A meta-analysis of clonidine for symptoms of attention-deficit disorder. J AM Acad Child Adolesc Psychiatry 1999;38:1551–1559.
209. Connor DF, Barkley RA, Davis HT. A pilot study of methylphenidate, clonidine, or a combination in ADHD comorbid with aggressive oppositional defiant or conduct disorder. Clin Pediatr 2000;39;15–25.
210. Hazell PL, Stuart JE. A randomized control trial of clonidine added to psychostimulant medication for hyperactive and aggressive children. J Am Acad Child Adolesc Psychiatry 2003;42:886–894.
211. Berridge CW, Arnsten AFT, Foote SL. Noradrenergic modulation of cognitive function: clinical implications of anatomical, electrophysiological and behavioural studies in animal models. Psychol Med 1993;23:557–564.
212. Van der Meere J, Gunning B, Stemerdink N, The effect of methylphenidate and clonidine on response inhibition and state regulation in children with ADHD. J Child Psychol Psychiatry 1999;40:291–298.
213. Halliday RA, Callaway E, Lannon R. The effects of clonidine and yohimbine on human information processing. Psychopharmacol 1989;99:563–566.
214. Hunt RD, Cohen DJ, Anderson G, Clark L. Possible change in noradrenergic receptor sensitivity following methylphenidate treatment: growth hormone and MHPG response to clonidine challenge in children with attention deficit disorder and hyperactivity. Life Sci 1984;35:885–897.
215. Campbell M, Cueva JE. Psychopharmacology in child and adolescent psychiatry: a review of the past seven years. Part 1. J Am Acad Child Adolesc Psychiatry 1995;34:1124–1132.
216. Shekim WO, Bylund DB, Hodges K, Glaser R, Ray-Prenger C, Oetting G. Platelet alpha 2-adrenergic receptor binding and the effects of d-amphetamine in boys with attention deficit hyperactivity disorder. Neuropsychobiol 1994;29:120–124.
217. Pudovkina OL, Cremers TI, Westerink BHC. Regulation of the release of serotonin in the dorsal raphe nucleus by alpha1 and alpha2 adrenoceptors. Synapse 2003;50:77–82.
218. Devoto P, Flore G, Vacca G, et al. Co-release of noradrenaline and dopamine from noradreneergic neurons in the cerebral cortex induced by clozapine, the prototype atypical antipsychotic. Psychopharmacol 2003;167:78–84.
219. Franowicz JS, Arnsten AFT. Actions of alpha-2 noradrenergic agonists on spatial working memory and blood pressure in rhesus monkeys appear to be mediated by the same receptor subtype. Psychopharmacol 2002;162:304–312.
220. Horrigan JP, Barnhill LJ. Guanfacine for the treatment of attention deficit hyperactivity disorder in boys. J Child Adolesc Psychopharmacol 1995;5:215–223.
221. Hunt RD, Arnsten AFT, Asbell MD. An open trial of guanfacine in the treatment of attention deficit hyperactivity disorder. J Am Acad Child Adolesc Psychiatry 1995;34:50–54.
222. Taylor FB, Russo J. Comparing guanfacine and dextroamphetamine for the treatment of adult attention-deficit/hyperactivity disorder. J Clin Psychopharmacol 2001;21:223–228.
223. Scahill L, Chappell PB, Kim YS, et al. A placebo-controlled study of guanfacine in the treatment of children with tic disorders and attention deficit hyperactivity disorder. Am J Psychiatry 2001;158:1067–1074.
224. Nemzer ED, Arnold LE, Vololato NA, McConnell H. Amino acid supplementation as therapy for attention deficit disorder. J Am Acad Child Adolesc Psychiatry 1986;25:509–513.
225. Popper CW. Pharmacologic alternatives to psychostimulants for the treatment of attention-deficit/ hyperactivity disorder. Child Adolesc Psychiatr Clin N Am 2000;9:605–646.
226. Birmaher B, Stanley M, Greenhill L, Twomey J, Gavrilescu A, Rabinovich H. Platelet imipramine binding in children and adolescents with impulsive behavior. J Am Acad Child Adolesc Psychiatry 1990:29:914–918.
227. Halperin JM, Schulz, KP, McKay KE, Sharma V, Newcorn JH. Familial correlates of central serotonergic function in children with disruptive behavior disorders. Psychiatr Res 2003;119: 205–216.
228. Kornetsky C. Psychoactive drugs in the immature organism. Psychopharmacol 1970;17:105–136.

229. Gulley JM, Zahniser NR. Rapid regulation of dopamine transporter function by substrates, blockers and presynaptic ligands. Eur J Pharmacol 2003;479:139–152.
230. Rocha B. Stimulant and reinforcement effects of cocaine in monoamine transporter knockout mice. Eur J Pharmacol 2003;479:107–115.
231. Sagvolden T, Johansen EB, Aase H, Russell VA. A dynamic developmental theory of attention-deficit/hyperactivity disorder (ADHD) predominantly hyperactive/impulsive and combined subtypes. Behav Brain Sci 2005, in press.
232. Wender PH, Epstein RS, Kopin IJ, Gordon EK. Urinary monoamine metabolites in children with minimal brain dysfunction. Am J Psychiatry 1971;127:1411–1415.
233. Shekim WO, Dekirmenjian H, Chapel JL. Urinary catecholamine metabolites in hyperactive boys treated with D-amphetamine. Am J Psychiatry 1977;134:1276–1279.
234. Rapoport JL, Mikkelsen EJ, Ebert MH, Brown GL, Weise VL, Kopin IJ. Urinary catecholamine and amphetamine excretion in hyperactive and normal boys. J Nerv Ment Dis 1978;66:731–737.
235. Shekim WO, Dekirmenjian H, Chapel JL. Urinary MHPG in minimal brain dysfunction and its modification by D-amphetamine. Am J Psychiatry 1979;136:667–671.
236. Khan AU, Dekirmenjian H. Urinary excretion of catecholamine metabolites in hyperkinetic child syndrome. Am J Psychiatry 1981;138:108–112.
237. Shekim WO, Javaid J, Dans JM, Bylund DBN. Urinary MHPG and HVA excretion in bos with attention deficit disorder and hyperactivity treated with D-amphetamine. Biol Psychiatry 1983;18:707–714.
238. Shen Y-C, Wang Y-F. The effect of methylphenidate on urinary catecholamine excretion in hyperactivity: a partial replication. Biol Psychiatry 1988;350–356.
239. Shekim WO Sinclair E, Glaser RD, Horwitz E, Javaid J, Bylund DB. Norepinephrine and dopamine metabolites and educational variables in boys with attention deficit disorder and hyperactivity. J Child Neurol 1987;2:50–56.
240. Hanna GL, Ornitz EM, Hariharan M. Urinary catecholamine excretion and behavioral differences in ADHD and normal boys. J Child Adolesc Psychopharmacol 1996b;6:63–73.
241. Oades RD, Müller BW. The development of conditioned blocking and monoamine metabolism in children with attention-deficit-hyperactivity disorder or complex tics and healthy controls: an exploratory analysis. Behav Brain Res 1997;88:95–102.
242. Rapoport JL, Quinn PO, Scribanic N, Murphy DL. Platelet serotonin of hyperactive school age boys. Br J Psychiat 1974;125:138–140.
243. Ferguson HB, Pappas BA, Trites RL, Peters DA, Taub H. Plasma free and total tryptophan, blood serotonin, and the hyperactivity syndrome: no evidence for the serotonin deficiency hypothesis. Biol Psychiat 1981;16:231–238.
244. Ionescu G, Kiehl R, Eckert S, Zimmerman T. Abnormal plasma catecholamines in hyperkinetic children. Biol Psychiat 1990;28;547–551.
245. Coleman M. Serotonin concentrations in whole blood of hyperactive children. J Pediatr 1971;78:985–990.
246. Saul RC, Ashby CD. Measurement of whole blood serotonin as a guide in prescribing psychostimulant medication for children with attentional deficits. Clin Neuropharmacol 1986;9:189–195.
247. Bhagnan HN, Coleman M, Coursina DB. The effect of pyridoxine hydrochloride on blood serotonin and pyridoxal phopsphate contents in hyperactive children. Pediatrics 1975;55:437–441.
248. Irwin M, Belendink K, McCloskay K, Freedman DX. Trypotophan metabolism in children with attention deficit disorder. Am J Psychiatry 1981;138:1082–1085.
249. Shetty T, Chase TN. Central monoamines and hyperkinesis of childhood. Neurol 1976;26;1000–1002.
250. Shaywitz BA, Cohen DJ, Bowers MB. CSF amine metabolites in children with minimal brain dysfunction: evidence for alteration of brain dopamine—a preliminary report. J Pediatr 1977;90: 67–71.

6

Intermittent Hypoxia During Sleep as a Model of Environmental (Nongenetic) Contributions to Attention Deficit Hyperactivity Disorder

Barry W. Row and David Gozal

1. INTRODUCTION

Attention deficit hyperactivity disorder (ADHD) is a clinically heterogenous neuropsychiatric syndrome of persistent and developmentally inappropriate levels of hyperactivity, inattention, and impulsivity, typically of juvenile onset. Research on this disease has been complicated by the fact that the specific features and presentations of ADHD show substantial variability between individuals, and that no single pathophysiological profile of ADHD has been identified *(1,2)*. Although the exact cause of ADHD is still unknown, both genetic and environmental factors are now recognized to play a role in the development of the disease *(3–5)*. Children who suffer from sleep-disordered breathing (SDB) have been reported to experience learning disabilities, hyperactivity, and impaired attention in much the same manner as children with ADHD, suggesting that SDB and some forms of ADHD may share common pathophysiological mechanisms (*see* Chapter 19). These findings in clinical populations with sleep disorders have led to the hypothesis that exposure to intermittent hypoxia, such as that encountered in SDB, during critical developmental periods is an important environmental contributor to the development of ADHD-like behavioral problems, and may be particularly important in individuals with a genetic predisposition to develop ADHD. In support of this hypothesis, data from animal experiments has shown that exposure to intermittent hypoxia, the primary hallmark of SDB, replicates many of the behavioral features of ADHD and may provide insight into the neurobiological mechanisms underlying some nongenetic forms of ADHD-like pathology.

2. PATHOPHYSIOLOGY OF ADHD

The most generally accepted hypothesis of ADHD is that the behavioral manifestations of the disease represent a dysfunction of frontosubcortical systems involved in attention and motor behavior, particularly the dorsal prefrontal cortex *(1,6,7)*. Evidence supporting a role of the prefrontal cortex in ADHD has originated from findings indicating that ADHD patients have similar behavioral symptoms as those with injuries or diseases of the prefrontal cortex (PFC) *(1,8–10)*. Additionally, animal studies have shown that lesions of the PFC lead to ADHD-like hyperactivity and cognitive deficits *(11,12)*. However, because of the complexity

From: *Attention Deficit Hyperactivity Disorder: From Genes to Patients*
Edited by: D. Gozal and D. L. Molfese © Humana Press Inc., Totowa, NJ

of the frontal cortical circuitry, it is unclear whether ADHD represents dysfunction at the level of the frontal cortex or in brain areas with frontal cortical projections. Functional and structural neuroimaging studies have revealed abnormalities in both the frontal cortex and striatum of ADHD patients, although there is some disagreement between studies on the specific locus of the abnormalities, presumably because no one region will be abnormal in all patients *(13)*. Prefrontal cortical influences on planning, motivation, and cognition are largely dependent on dopaminergic projections arising from the ventral tegmental area (VTA), although noradrenergic systems arising from the locus ceruleus (LC) also play a role *(14–17)*. The dopaminergic neurons arising from the VTA are organized into two major systems, the mesolimbic and mesocortical systems. The cells of the mesolimbic system project primarily to the ventral striatum (nucleus accumbens [NA] and olfactory tubercule), the nuclei of the stria terminalis, the amygdala, the hippocampus, the lateral septal nuclei, and the frontal, anterior cingulate, and entorhinal cortices. The projections from the NA to the PFC are thought to be particularly important in ADHD, as this nucleus receives convergent input from the amygdala, hippocampus, entorhinal area, anterior cingulate, and parts of the temporal lobe and is thought to act as a gating mechanism for information from these regions *(18,19)*. Dopaminergic neurons in the mesocortical system originate in the VTA and project to the neocortex, with the densest projection to the PFC *(20,21)*.

Given the clinical complexity of ADHD, it is unlikely that a single mechanism underlies ADHD in all patients, especially given that reviews of the neurobiology of ADHD have concluded that no single pathophysiological profile exists *(1,4)*. The majority of drugs that provide effective medication of ADHD, such as psychostimulants, tricyclic antidepressants, α2 adrenoceptor agonists, and dopamine transporter (DAT) blockers, act on catecholaminergic systems *(1)*. However, as many as 30% of children with ADHD do not respond favorably to psychostimulant medications, raising the possibility that multiple biological factors underlie ADHD *(22)*. Although there is generalized agreement that ADHD is associated with dysfunction of frontosubcortical pathways controlling attention and motor behavior, a number of different hypotheses of ADHD, such as dysregulation of subcortical dopaminergic and noradrenergic systems, disruption of the neuronal circuitry underlying executive functions, behavioral inhibition, and/or reward processes, as well as generalized dysfunction of the prefrontal cortex and/or regions sending afferent projections to the PFC, such as the hippocampus and NA, have all been proposed *(2,6,23–27)*. None of the existing neurobiological hypotheses of ADHD should be considered mutually exclusive, as the existence of direct connections between the PFC, NA, and the hippocampus, as well as the existence of reciprocal connections involving the nucleus accumbens and the PFC, suggest that these structures operate as an integrated unit *(28)*. Evidence from human studies and animal models indicates that functional disruption of the components of this circuitry elicits ADHD-like symptoms, and may underlie the clinical heterogeneity of the disease. Therefore, a unitary causal model of ADHD may be insufficient to account for the clinical complexity of the disease, and both genetic and nongenetic factors may underlie different subtypes of this disorder.

3. ANIMAL MODELS OF ADHD

Animal models have been widely used to investigate the pathophysiology of ADHD, primarily because of the fact that they allow experimental control of factors that may be involved in/contribute to this condition. In addition, animal models permit avoidance of the effects of existing comorbidities, previous drug exposure, family interactions, and other social and environmental factors encountered in human ADHD patients *(29)*. Animal models have typically attempted to replicate the primary behavioral symptoms of ADHD, such as hyperactivity, learning deficits, and attentional disorders/impulsivity, although no single animal model has been able to reliably replicate all aspects of the disease *(29)*. The discrepancies between the animal model and the human condition likely reflect the heterogeneity of the latter, and therefore data from animal models should be interpreted with caution and used primarily to investigate specific components of the disease.

The majority of animal models of ADHD have focused on naturally occurring or artificially engineered genetic mutations that lead to abnormalities in catecholaminergic transmission and/or regulation. Examples of such animal models include the spontaneously hypertensive rat (SHR), the Naples High-Excitability rat (NHE), the dopamine transporter knockout mouse (DAT-KO), and the coloboma mutant mouse, and have been the subject of extensive reviews *(29,30)*. Although these models have clearly implicated catecholaminergic systems in ADHD, the central questions of exactly how these systems are dysregulated still remains unresolved. Locomotor hyperactivity has been associated with hypodopaminergic and hyperdopaminergic animal models, indicating that imbalances in dopamine (DA) systems rather than the actual level of DA can produce behavioral and cognitive dysregulation *(31–35)*. The complex regulation of DA release may account for at least some of the observations of both increased and decreased DA activity in models of ADHD. DA release in striatal regions occurs via two different mechanisms: a phasic DA release dependent on excitation of DA cell firing, and a basal tonic DA release regulated by glutaminergic inputs to this region *(36)*. Grace *(36)* has proposed a model whereby the glutamatergic projections of the PFC and the hippocampus affect the activity of subcortical DA systems. Decreased glutaminergic input to the NA, because of either prefrontal or hippocampal disturbances, may eventually result in reduced tonic DA release and decreased activation of DA autoreceptors that regulate the phasic release of DA. This results in decreased basal extracellular DA, and ultimately a lower level of inhibition of DA release by presynaptic autoreceptors. The absence of these local autoregulatory suppressive mechanisms will result in increased phasic release of DA when bursts of action potentials reach the DA terminals. Thus, a reduced tonic DA activity may coexist with an increased spike-dependent DA release *(37,38)*. Alternatively, increased tonic extrasynaptic dopamine is also required to regulate dopamine release by activating D4 heteroreceptors that inhibit glutamate release from cortical afferents in the striatum *(30,39)*. Additionally, it should also be noted that the influences of other neurotransmitters on ADHD need to be considered, as both epinephrine and norepinehrine are potent agonists of the D4 receptor *(40,41)*, and that serotoninergic influences have been also been implicated *(29)*. Taken together, the findings illustrate that the behavioral symptoms of ADHD likely are owing to disruption of multiple neurotransmitter systems.

Damage to the neuroanatomical systems involved in locomotor activity, learning, and attention produce replicates many of the behavioral symptoms of ADHD. For example, selective removal of forebrain DA projections in the neonatal rat, neonatal anoxia, hippocampal X-irradiation, as well as exposure to environmental toxins have all been shown to induce ADHD-like enhancement of locomotor activity coupled with learning impairments and/or deficits in attention (reviewed in ref. *29*). These findings clearly indicate that exposure to environmental factors that disrupt the neuroanatomical circuity of brain regions implicated in ADHD, such as the PFC and NA, as well as brain regions that exert modulatory effects on these structures, such as the hippocampus, may underlie some forms of ADHD-like behavioral pathology, especially if these exposures occur during critical developmental periods.

4. INTERMITTENT HYPOXIA AS A MODEL OF ADHD

The repeated episodes of upper airway obstruction during sleep and the resultant episodic or intermittent hypoxia (IH) associated with forms of SDB, such as obstructive sleep apnea (OSA), are thought to contribute to the cognitive deficits seen in these patients (*see* Chapter 19). Children who suffer from SDB and children with ADHD present similar behavioral profiles, suggesting that disruption of similar neuronal networks may underlie the functional sequelae in both groups, at least in some cases. Hypoxia is a major pathological factor inducing neuronal cell injury, neurodegeneration, and cell death that is frequent encountered in neonatal and pediatric pathology *(42)*. The brain is particularly vulnerable to hypoxia during periods of maturation and development. Hypoxic episodes occurring during these critical periods have a serious impact on brain maturation with anatomical consequences ranging from cell death to hampered differentiation of dendrites and axons, and to compromised outgrowth and synapse formation *(42–44)*. These anatomical abnormalities may underlie the behavioral and psychological dysfunctions commonly observed after hypoxia. Although severe perinatal and postnatal forms of hypoxia hypoxia/ischemia or prolonged anoxia are associated with cognitive and motor impairments and, in some cases, death *(45–47)*, epidemiological studies indicate that milder forms of perinatal and postnatal hypoxias are associated with increased risk for disorders, such as ADHD *(48–50)*.

Disruption of the neuroanatomical integrity is a possible consequence of SDB. Neuroimaging studies have reported that adult patients who suffer form OSA, the most common form of SDB, display gray-matter loss and alterations in markers of neuronal integrity *(51–53)*. The effects of IH on neural function can not be assessed in humans for obvious ethical reasons. However, we have recently developed a rodent model of SDB that mimics the oscillations in oxygenation during the sleep cycle usually seen in SDB patients. In this model, adult male rats undergo exposure to an intermittent hypoxia profile consisting of alternating 90-s epochs of hypoxia (10% O_2) and room air for 14 d during habitual sleep times. Such exposure is associated with increased apoptosis and cytoarchitectural disorganization in the hippocampal CA1 region and the frontoparietal cortex, which peak after 1 and 2 d of IH, and decrease thereafter *(54)*. Moreover, although apoptosis was extensively present in the CA1 region, the CA3 region and dorsocaudal brainstem were virtually unaffected. Behaviorally, adult male rats exposed to IH display cognitive deficits consistent with impaired functioning of the hippocampus and/or PFC *(54–58)*. These findings were not unexpected considering the effects of episodic/sustained hypoxia on brain function. For example, experimental rats were exposed for 8 h daily to varying fractional concentrations of inspired oxygen (FiO_2) and carbon dioxide ($FiCO_2$) for 35 d. These exposures consisted of brief (3–6 s) episodic (twice every min), eucapnic (3.5% FiO_2 and 10% $FiCO_2$, $n = 6$), or hypocapnic (3.5% FiO_2 and 0% $FiCO_2$, $n = 14$) challenges with hypoxia or room air (21% FiO_2 and 0.03% $FiCO_2$, $n = 15$). Norepinephrine, DA, serotonin, and their metabolites in the hypothalamus, hippocampus, and adrenal glands were measured by high-performance liquid chromatography (HPLC). Spontaneous behavioral activity was assessed for 30 min by automated activity monitors. Episodic hypocapnic hypoxia produced a decrease in DA turnover and eucapnic hypoxia increased norepinephrine levels in the hypothalamus. Animals exposed to hypocapnic hypoxia also exhibited a consistent increase in horizontal (walking) and vertical (rearing) activity, as well as in total activity time. From these results, it would seem that episodic eucapnic and hypocapnic hypoxia may affect metabolism of different neurotransmitters in the CNS *(59)*.

There also appears to be a unique developmental window of neuronal vulnerability to IH in the rat. Rat pups exposed to IH at 10–25 d of postnatal age display marked increases in hippocampal and cortical apoptosis in comparison to both neonatal and adult rats *(60)*. This is consistent with previous findings that the juvenile rat is more susceptible to the effects of hypoxia–ischemia *(61,62)*. Exposure to IH during this unique period of susceptibility is also associated with learning impairments and a gender-dependent behavioral hyperactivity in male, but not in female, rats, displaying increased locomotor activity in the open field when tested at 30 d of age *(56)*. Locomotor hyperactivity was also observed in rat pups exposed to intermittent hypoxia at 7–11 d of postnatal age and tested at 35 d of age, although no effect of gender was observed in this study *(58,63)*. The discrepancies in locomotor activity between these two studies likely reflect differences in the degree and duration of the intermittent hypoxia used in each study, as well as the age at which the animals were tested. The enhanced locomotor activity observed in juvenile rats is in marked contrast to the absence of altered locomotor activity the adult rat under similar exposures (Row and Gozal 2003, unpublished observations).

Exposure to IH has long-term consequences as well. Adult males exposed to IH show only partial recovery of learning after 2 wk of recovery *(54)*. Juvenile rats exposed to IH from postnatal day 7–11 display working memory impairments when tested at 65 d of age as well as enhanced expression of vesicular monamone transporter (VMAT) and D1 DA receptors in the striatum at 80 d of age *(58)*. Although these findings clearly indicate that IH has long-term consequences in the rat, it is unclear whether these changes are directly owing to the IH, or represent compensatory changes brought about by damage to other neural sites *(64)*.

The selective disruption of hippocampal and cortical neurons observed after exposure to IH, particularly in the developing animal, has important implications for the development of ADHD-like pathology. Because of their anatomical relationships and their established role during working memory tasks, the PFC and hippocampal formation are functionally associated *(28)*. The PFC is involved in higher order functions, such as working memory, attentional and executive processes, and the organization and planning of responses *(31,65)*. The hippocampus plays a role in some forms of selective attention, learning and memory, and locomotor activity, and is also thought to play a major role in neurodevelopmental disorders involving dysregulation of dopaminergic systems, such as schizophrenia *(66–71)*. Both the PFC and the hippocampus innervate the NA, which plays an essential role in integrating information from the limbic and cortical regions into goal-directed behavior *(28)*. The PFC, the hippocampus, and the NA all receive dopaminergic afferents from the ventral mesencephalon (the VTA and the substantia nigra pars compacta [SNC]), which plays a crucial role in the function of these structures *(31)*. In turn, these structures all send direct or indirect projections back to the VTA and SNC, where the dopaminergic cell bodies are located.

The ventral and dorsal parts of the vertebrate hippocampus are connected with different sets of extrahippocampal structures. The ventral hippocampus primarily projects to the amygdala, NA (predominately the shell), and the PFC, whereas the dorsal hippocampus projects primarily to the core of the NA *(72)*. This suggests that the functions of the ventral and dorsal hippocampus, as well as the effects of ventral and dorsal hippocampal manipulations, may differ, although the difference in projections may be partially offset because of strong intrahippocampal projections. Hippocampal-dependent learning has been shown to be more vulnerable to dorsal hippocampal lesions, although the anatomical data suggest that locomotor activity may depend more on the ventral than on the dorsal hippocampus *(68,73–77)*. However, consistent differences between the effects of ventral and dorsal hippocampal lesions have not been demonstrated. Complete or partial hippocampal lesions produce hyperactivity in rats *(68,78–81)*, as well as rendering them more susceptible to the locomotor-stimulating effects of dopamine agonists. Pharmacological manipulation of both the dorsal and ventral hippocampus have been shown to modulate locomotor activity in the rat; however, the effects are more pronounced in the ventral hippocampus *(82)*. Ventral hippocampal activity appears to be linearly related to locomotor activity, primarily resulting from the effects of the substantial projection of the ventral hippocampus to the VTA *(68)*. In contrast, both pharmacological deactivation and stimulation of the dorsal hippocampus have been found to increase locomotor activity. The hyperactivity following ventral and dorsal hippocampal lesions illustrate that hippocampal activity is important to inhibiting locomotor activity, and that both the ventral and dorsal hippocampus are involved. However, studies suggest that locomotion is primarily driven by ventral hippocampal activity, and that the dorsal hippocampus plays a modulatory role (reviewed in ref. *68*).

Regulation of DA in the NA by the direct hippocampal–NA projections has been proposed as one of the mechanisms by which the hippocampus modulates locomotor activity in the rat *(83,84)*, although the hippocampal projections to the PFC and the VTA are also involved *(28,72,85,86)*. Traditionally, the ventral hippocampus has been presumed to have a greater influence on midbrain dopaminergic neurons; however, the strong dorsal and ventral intrahippocampal connections make this distinction gradual rather than absolute. Nevertheless, the strong projections of the dorsal hippocampus to the core of the NA indicate that behaviors mediated by this structure, such as delay aversion, may be especially sensitive to dorsal hippocampal disruption *(32)*. Hippocampal lesions remove the prominent hippocampal projections to the NA *(83,84)*. Hippocampal lesions reduce dopaminergic innervation of forebrain sites, including the NA *(87)*. These alterations in locomotor activity observed after hippocampal damage are consistent with the idea that the hippocampus in involved in inhibitory control of physiological and behavioral processes, such as the dopaminergic tonus of the NA *(79)*.

One of the potential mechanisms of neuronal damage in IH involves the neurotransmitter glutamate. During transient ischemia or hypoxia, increased glutamate release occurs in the synaptic cleft and can lead to overstimulation of glutamate receptors. These receptors, and more specifically *N*-methyl-D-aspartate (NMDA) receptors, have been extensively implicated in neuronal excitotoxicity *(88,89)*. Rats exposed to chemical hypoxia with carbon monoxide displayed an immediate and significant increase in glutamate release, followed days later by neuronal damage in the frontal cortex *(90)*. Additionally, significant reductions in NMDA receptor immunoreactivity are observed within the cortex and CA1 region following IH *(54)*. This is consistent with the hypothesis that a chronic, slowly evolving glutamate excitotoxicity is one of the factors that underlie the structural and behavioral consequences of intermittent hypoxia. Glutamate excitotoxicity has been implicated in hypoxia/ischemia-induced neuronal damage, as both hypoxia and ischemia will induce increased release of excitatory amino acids, such as glutamate, that can potentially lead to excessive activation of ionotropic NMDA receptors, eventually resulting in programmed cell death *(91–96)*. Coupled with previous findings that alterations in NMDA NR2 receptor subunit expression, as well as reductions in NMDA glutamate receptor binding sites, were observed in the hippocampus following hypobaric hypoxia and that NMDA receptor antagonists exert a neuroprotective effect in hypoxia/ischemia-induced neuronal damage and oxidant tissue injury *(97–100)*, it is suggested that NMDA glutamate receptor expressing cells within the hippocampus appear to be especially vulnerable to IH. The structural and neurobehavioral consequences of IH exposure in the adult rat involve a number of interrelated pathways, namely glutamate excitoxicity, oxidative stress, mitochondrial dysfunction, upregulation of proinflammatory mediators, and altered regulation of pro- and antiapoptotic gene cascades *(54,55,57,101–104)*.

The increased release of glutamate during hypoxic conditions and the parallel increases in oxidative stress may have important implications for cell survival. For example, the lipid peroxidation product 4-hydroxy-2,3,-nonenal (4HN) has been shown to directly modulate NMDA channel activity, causing increases in NMDA-induced intracellular Ca^{2+} levels, as well as being associated with increased phosphorylation of the NR1 receptor subunit, suggesting that such compounds may play a role in the pathological responses of neurons to oxidative stress by directly acting on glutamate receptors *(105)*. This is consistent with the hypothesis of a vicious cycle in which NMDA receptor activation by glutamate leads to generation of reactive oxygen species, which, in turn, will enhance the release of glutamate, as well as inhibit its reuptake and inactivation, ultimately leading to cellular death *(106–108)*. Murata and colleagues *(109)* have recently demonstrated that administration of the NMDA receptor antagonist MK-801 in conjunction with a free-radical scavenger attenuated the neurotoxicity associated with hypoxia/reoxygenation even when treatment was administered during reoxygenation, suggesting that the combination of increased glutamate release and free-radical production that occurs with reoxygenation may be responsible for the observed neuronal damage. This is consistent with observations that even when the magnitude of the hypoxic exposure is insufficient to induce marked increases in neuronal apoptosis when administered as a sustained paradigm, substantial increases in programmed cell death and gliosis develop when the hypoxic exposure is administered in a cyclical fashion *(54)*. Thus, it seems that the intermittent nature of the hypoxic stimulus, rather than the level of hypoxia *per se*, may trigger a differential array of tissue responses that underlie the observed cellular damage and subsequent behavioral impairments. The cellular damage that occurs in response to IH likely involves a number of interrelated pathways that include mitochondrial dysfunction, excitoxicity, oxidative stress, and altered regulation of pro- and antiapoptotic gene cascades. The repeated reoxygenations that occur in IH may serve to deplete or compromise the innate defense mechanisms of the cell although failing to appropriately recruit inducible defense processes, ultimately resulting in increased vulnerability and apoptosis within sensitive brain regions. This may be especially important in the juvenile animal, as age-dependent changes in the balance of between proapoptotic and antiapoptotic members of the Bcl and caspase 2 gene families, as well as increased expression of NMDA receptors during development have been observed *(88,110)*.

In conclusion, our working hypothesis suggests that exposure to IH is detrimental to the functioning of hippocampus, PFC, and related subcortical structures. Additionally, the existence of a unique period of susceptibility in the developing animal indicates that exposure to intermittent hypoxia insults may have important consequences in the development of ADHD-like pathology, and that IH paradigms may be useful in the elucidation of specific mechanisms underlying particular aspects of ADHD-associated manifestations.

REFERENCES

1. Faraone SV, Biederman J. Neurobiology of attention-deficit hyperactivity disorder. Biol Psychiatry 1998;44:951–958.
2. Solanto MV. Dopamine dysfunction in AD/HD: integrating clinical and basic neuroscience research. Behav Brain Res 2002;130:65–71.
3. Palomo T, Beninger RJ, Kostrzewa RM, Archer T. Brain sites of movement disorder: genetic and environmental agents in neurodevelopmental perturbations. Neurotox Res 2003;5:1–26.
4. Biederman J, Faraone SV. Current concepts on the neurobiology of attention-deficit/hyperactivity disorder. J Atten Disord 2002;6 Suppl 1:S7–S16.
5. Biederman J, Faraone SV, Monuteaux MC. Differential effect of environmental adversity by gender: Rutter's index of adversity in a group of boys and girls with and without ADHD. Am J Psychiatry 2002;159:1556–1562.
6. Barkley RA. Behavioral inhibition, sustained attention, and executive functions: constructing a unifying theory of ADHD. Psychol Bull 1997;121:65–94.
7. Durston S. A review of the biological bases of ADHD: what have we learned from imaging studies? Ment Retard Dev Disabil Res Rev 2003;9:184–195.
8. Benson DF. The role of frontal dysfunction in attention deficit hyperactivity disorder. J Child Neurol 1991;6 Suppl:S9–S12.
9. Niedermeyer E, Naidu SB. Attention-deficit hyperactivity disorder (ADHD) and frontal-motor cortex disconnection. Clin Electroencephalogr 1997;28:130–136.
10. Itami S, Uno H. Orbitofrontal cortex dysfunction in attention-deficit hyperactivity disorder revealed by reversal and extinction tasks. Neuroreport 2002;13:2453–2457.
11. de Bruin JP, van Oyen HG, Van de Poll N. Behavioural changes following lesions of the orbital prefrontal cortex in male rats. Behav Brain Res 1983;10:209–232.
12. Yee BK. Cytotoxic lesion of the medial prefrontal cortex abolishes the partial reinforcement extinction effect, attenuates prepulse inhibition of the acoustic startle reflex and induces transient hyperlocomotion, while sparing spontaneous object recognition memory in the rat. Neuroscience 2000;95:675–689.
13. Biederman J, Spencer T. Attention-deficit/hyperactivity disorder (ADHD) as a noradrenergic disorder. Biol Psychiatry 1999;46:1234–1242.
14. Papp M, Bal A. Separation of the motivational and motor consequences of 6-hydroxydopamine lesions of the mesolimbic or nigrostriatal system in rats. Behav Brain Res 1987;23:221–229.
15. Mogenson GJ, Yang CR. The contribution of basal forebrain to limbic-motor integration and the mediation of motivation to action. Adv Exp Med Biol 1991;295:267–290.
16. Hollerman JR, Tremblay L, Schultz W. Involvement of basal ganglia and orbitofrontal cortex in goal-directed behavior. Prog Brain Res 2000;126:193–215.
17. Sesack SR, Carr DB. Selective prefrontal cortex inputs to dopamine cells: implications for schizophrenia. Physiol Behav 2002;77:513–517.
18. O'Donnell P, Grace AA. Synaptic interactions among excitatory afferents to nucleus accumbens neurons: hippocampal gating of prefrontal cortical input. J Neurosci 1995;15:3622–3639.
19. Grace AA. Gating of information flow within the limbic system and the pathophysiology of schizophrenia. Brain Res Rev 2000;31:330–341.
20. Albanese A, Minciacchi D. Organization of the ascending projections from the ventral tegmental area: a multiple fluorescent retrograde tracer study in the rat. J Comp Neurol 1983;216:406–420.
21. Williams SM, Goldman-Rakic PS. Widespread origin of the primate mesofrontal dopamine system. Cereb Cortex 1998;8:321–345.
22. Madras BK, Miller GM, Fischman AJ. The dopamine transporter: relevance to attention deficit hyperactivity disorder (ADHD). Behav Brain Res 2002;130:57–63.

23. Altman J. Morphological and behavioral markers of environmentally induced retardation of brain development: an animal model. Environ Health Perspect 1987;74:153–168.
24. Castellanos FX, Tannock R. Neuroscience of attention-deficit/hyperactivity disorder: the search for endophenotypes. Nat Rev Neurosci 2002;3:617–628.
25. Castellanos FX. Neural substrates of attention-deficit hyperactivity disorder. Adv Neurol 2001;85:197–206.
26. Russell VA. Hypodopaminergic and hypernoradrenergic activity in prefrontal cortex slices of an animal model for attention-deficit hyperactivity disorder—the spontaneously hypertensive rat. Behav Brain Res 2002;130:191–196.
27. Solanto MV, Abikoff H, Sonuga-Barke E, et al. The ecological validity of delay aversion and response inhibition as measures of impulsivity in AD/HD: a supplement to the NIMH multimodal treatment study of AD/HD. J Abnorm Child Psychol 2001;29:215–228.
28. Thierry AM, Gioanni Y, Degenetais E, Glowinsky J. Hippocampo-prefrontal cortex pathway: anatomical and electrophysiological characteristics. Hippocampus 2000;10:411–419.
29. Davids E, Zhang K, Tarazi FI, Baldessarini RJ. Animal models of attention-deficit hyperactivity disorder. Brain Res Brain Res Rev 2003;42:1–21.
30. Russell VA. Dopamine hypofunction possibly results from a defect in glutamate-stimulated release of dopamine in the nucleus accumbens shell of a rat model for attention deficit hyperactivity disorder—the spontaneously hypertensive rat. Neurosci Biobehav Rev 2003;27:671–682.
31. Arnsten AF. Catecholamine regulation of the prefrontal cortex. J Psychopharmacol 1997;11:151–162.
32. Cardinal RN, Pennicott DR, Sugathapala CL, Robbins TW, Everitt BJ. Impulsive choice induced in rats by lesions of the nucleus accumbens core. Science 2001;292:2499–2501.
33. Giros B, Jaber M, Jones SR, Wightman RM, Caron MG. Hyperlocomotion and indifference to cocaine and amphetamine in mice lacking the dopamine transporter. Nature 1996;379:606–612.
34. Shaywitz BA, Yager RD, Klopper JH. Selective brain dopamine depletion in developing rats: an experimental model of minimal brain dysfunction. Science 1976;191:305–308.
35. Viggiano D, Grammatikopoulos G, Sadile AG. A morphometric evidence for a hyperfunctioning mesolimbic system in an animal model of ADHD. Behav Brain Res 2002;130:181–189.
36. Grace AA. Phasic versus tonic dopamine release and the modulation of dopamine system responsivity: a hypothesis for the etiology of schizophrenia. Neuroscience 1991;41:1–24.
37. Floresco SB, West AR, Ash B, Moore H, Grace AA. Afferent modulation of dopamine neuron firing differentially regulates tonic and phasic dopamine transmission. Nat Neurosci 2003;6:968–973.
38. Grace AA, Moore H, O'Donnell P. The modulation of corticoaccumbens transmission by limbic afferents and dopamine: a model for the pathophysiology of schizophrenia. Adv Pharmacol 1998;42:721–724.
39. Russell VA. In vitro glutamate-stimulated release of dopamine from nucleus accumbens core and shell of spontaneously hypertensive rats. Metab Brain Dis 2003;18:161–168.
40. Lanau F, Zenner MT, Civelli O, Hartman DS. Epinephrine and norepinephrine act as potent agonists at the recombinant human dopamine D4 receptor. J Neurochem 1997;68:804–812.
41. Newman-Tancredi A, Audinot-Bouchez V, Gobert A, Millan MJ. Noradrenaline and adrenaline are high affinity agonists at dopamine D4 receptors. Eur J Pharmacol 1997;319:379–383.
42. Nyakas C, Buwalda B, Luiten PG. Hypoxia and brain development. Prog Neurobiol 1996;49:1–51.
43. Nyakas C, Markel E, Schuurman T, Luiten PG. Impaired learning and abnormal open-field behaviours of rats after early postnatal anoxia and the beneficial effect of the calcium antagonist nimodipine. Eur J Neurosci 1991;3:168–174.
44. Nyakas C, Buwalda B, Kramers RJ, Traber J, Luiten PG. Postnatal development of hippocampal and neocortical cholinergic and serotonergic innervation in rat: effects of nitrite-induced prenatal hypoxia and nimodipine treatment. Neuroscience 1994;59:541–559.
45. Gray PH, Tudehope DI, Masel JP, et al. Perinatal hypoxic-ischaemic brain injury: prediction of outcome. Dev Med Child Neurol 1993;35:965–973.

46. Tuor UI, Del Bigio MR, Chumas PD. Brain damage due to cerebral hypoxia/ischemia in the neonate: pathology and pharmacological modification. Cerebrovasc Brain Metab Rev 1996;8: 159–193.
47. du Plessis AJ, Johnston MV. Hypoxic-ischemic brain injury in the newborn. Cellular mechanisms and potential strategies for neuroprotection. Clin Perinatol 1997;24:627–654.
48. Krageloh-Mann I, Toft P, Lunding J, Andresen J, Pryds O, Lou HC. Brain lesions in preterms: origin, consequences and compensation. Acta Paediatr 1999;88:897–908.
49. Zappitelli M, Pinto T, Grizenko N. Pre-, peri-, and postnatal trauma in subjects with attention-deficit hyperactivity disorder. Can J Psychiatry 2001;46:542–548.
50. Lou HC. Etiology and pathogenesis of attention-deficit hyperactivity disorder (ADHD): significance of prematurity and perinatal hypoxic-haemodynamic encephalopathy. Acta Paediatr 1996;85:1266–1271.
51. Kamba M, Suto Y, Ohta Y, Inoue Y, Matsuda E. Cerebral metabolism in sleep apnea. Evaluation by magnetic resonance spectroscopy. Am J Respir Crit Care Med 1997;156:296–298.
52. Kamba M, Inoue Y, Higami S, Ogawa T, Chen W. Cerebral metabolic impairment in patients with obstructive sleep apnoea: an independent association of obstructive sleep apnoea with white matter change. J Neurol Neurosurg Psychiatry 2001;71:334–339.
53. Macey PM, Henderson LA, Macey KE, et al. Brain morphology associated with obstructive sleep apnea. Am J Respir Crit Care Med 2002;166:1382–1387.
54. Gozal D, Daniel JM, Dohanich GP. Behavioral and anatomical correlates of chronic episodic hypoxia during sleep in the rat. J Neurosci 2001;21:2442–2450.
55. Gozal D, Row BW, Gozal E, et al. Temporal aspects of spatial task performance during intermittent hypoxia in the rat: evidence for neurogenesis. Eur J Neurosci 2003;18:2335–2342.
56. Row BW, Kheirandish L, Neville JJ, Gozal D. Impaired spatial learning and hyperactivity in developing rats exposed to intermittent hypoxia. Pediatr Res 2002;52:449–453.
57. Row BW, Lui R, Xu W, Kheirandish L, Gozal D. Intermittent hypoxia is associated with oxidative stress and spatial learning deficits in the rat. Am J Respir Crit Care Med 2003;167:1548–1553.
58. Decker MJ. Hue GE, Caudle WM, et al. Episodic neonatal hypoxia evokes executive dysfunction and regionally specific alterations in markers of dopamine signaling. Neuroscience 2003;117:417–425.
59. Li R, Bao G, el-Mallakh RS, Fletcher EC. Effects of chronic episodic hypoxia on monoamine metabolism and motor activity. Physiol Behav 1996;60:1071–1076.
60. Gozal E, Row BW Shurr A, Gozal D. Developmental differences in cortical and hippocampal vulnerability to intermittent hypoxia in the rat. Neurosci Lett 2001;305:197–201.
61. Towfighi J, Mauger D, Vannucci RC, Vannucci SJ. Influence of age on the cerebral lesions in an immature rat model of cerebral hypoxia-ischemia: a light microscopic study. Brain Res Dev 1997;100:149–160.
62. Vannucci RC, Rossini A, Towfighi J, Vannucci SJ. Measuring the accentuation of the brain damage that arises from perinatal cerebral hypoxia-ischemia. Biol Neonate 1997;72:187–191.
63. Decker MJ, Rye DB. Neonatal intermittent hypoxia impairs dopamine signaling and executive functioning. Sleep Breath 2002;6:205–210.
64. Robinson TE, Castaneda E, Whishaw IQ. Compensatory changes in striatal dopamine neurons following recovery from injury induced by 6-OHDA or methamphetamine: a review of evidence from microdialysis studies. Can J Psychol 1990;44:253–275.
65. Levy R, Goldman-Rakic PS. Segregation of working memory functions within the dorsolateral prefrontal cortex. Exp Brain Res 2000;133:23–32.
66. Altman J, Brunner RL, Bayer SA. The hippocampus and behavioral maturation. Behav Biol 1973;8:557–596.
67. Csernansky JG, Bardgett ME. Limbic-cortical neuronal damage and the pathophysiology of schizophrenia. Schizophr Bull 1998;24:231–248.
68. Bast T, Feldon J. Hippocampal modulation of sensorimotor processes. Prog Neurobiol 2003;70: 319–345.
69. O'Donnell P, Grace AA. Dysfunctions in multiple interrelated systems as the neurobiological bases of schizophrenic symptom clusters. Schizophr Bull 1998;24:267–283.

70. Olton DS, Papas BC. Spatial memory and hippocampal function. Neuropsychologia 1979;17: 669–682.
71. Vinogradova OS. Hippocampus as comparator: role of the two input and two output systems of the hippocampus in selection and registration of information. Hippocampus 2001;11:578–598.
72. Amaral DG, Witter MP. Hippocampal formation. In: the rat nervous system. Paxinos G, ed. San Diego: Academic Press 1995;443–494.
73. Amaral DG, Witter MP. The three-dimensional organization of the hippocampal formation: a review of anatomical data. Neuroscience 1989. 31:571–591.
74. Bannerman DM, Yee BK Good MA, Heupel MJ, Iversen SD, Rawlins JN. Double dissociation of function within the hippocampus: a comparison of dorsal, ventral, and complete hippocampal cytotoxic lesions. Behav Neurosci 1999;113:1170–1188.
75. Caine SB, Humby T, Robbins TW, Everitt BJ. Behavioral effects of psychomotor stimulants in rats with dorsal or ventral subiculum lesions: locomotion, cocaine self-administration, and prepulse inhibition of startle. Behav Neurosci 2001;115:880–894.
76. Hock BJ, Jr. Bunsey MD. Differential effects of dorsal and ventral hippocampal lesicns. J Neurosci 1998;18:7027–7032.
77. Sinnamon HM, Freniere S, Kootz J. Rat hippocampus and memory for places of changing significance. J Comp Physiol Psychol 1978;92:142–155.
78. Cassel JC, Cassel S, Galani R, Kelche C, Will B, Jarrard L. Fimbria-fornix vs selective hippocampal lesions in rats: effects on locomotor activity and spatial learning and memory. Neurobiol Learn Mem 1998;69:22–45.
79. Coutureau E, Galani R, Jarrard LE, Cassel JC. Selective lesions of the entorhinal cortex, the hippocampus, or the fimbria-fornix in rats: a comparison of effects on spontaneous and amphetamine-induced locomotion. Exp Brain Res 2000;131:381–392.
80. Gray JA, McNaughton N. Comparison between the behavioural effects of septal and hippocampal lesions: a review. Neurosci Biobehav Rev 1983;7:119–188.
81. Lipska BK, Jaskiw GE, Karoum F, Phillips I, Kleinman JE, Weinberger DR. Dorsal hippocampal lesion does not affect dopaminergic indices in the basal ganglia. Pharmacol Biochem Behav 1991;40:181–184.
82. Zhang WN, Bast T, Feldon J. The ventral hippocampus and fear conditioning in rats: different anterograde amnesias of fear after infusion of N-methyl-D-aspartate or its noncompetitive antagonist MK-801 into the ventral hippocampus. Behav Brain Res 2001;126:159–174.
83. Kelley AE, Domesick VB. The distribution of the projection from the hippocampal formation to the nucleus accumbens in the rat: an anterograde- and retrograde-horseradish peroxidase study. Neuroscience 1982;7:2321–2335.
84. Groenewegen HJ, Vermeulen-Van der Zee E, te Kortschot A, Witter MP. Organization of the projections from the subiculum to the ventral striatum in the rat. A study using anterograde transport of Phaseolus vulgaris leucoagglutinin. Neuroscience 1987;23:103–120.
85. Takahata R, Moghaddam B. Glutamatergic regulation of basal and stimulus-activated dopamine release in the prefrontal cortex. J Neurochem 1998;71:1443–1449.
86. Moghaddam B. Stress preferentially increases extraneuronal levels of excitatory amino acids in the prefrontal cortex: comparison to hippocampus and basal ganglia. J Neurochem 1993;60:1650–1657.
87. Swerdlow NR, Braff DL, Geyer MA. Animal models of deficient sensorimotor gating: what we know, what we think we know, and what we hope to know soon. Behav Pharmacol 2000;11: 185–204.
88. Mishra OP, Fritz KI, Delivoria-Papadopoulos M. NMDA receptor and neonatal hypoxic brain injury. Ment Retard Dev Disabil Res Rev 2001;7:249–253.
89. Sattler R, Tymianski M. Molecular mechanisms of glutamate receptor-mediated excitotoxic neuronal cell death. Mol Neurobiol 2001;24:107–129.
90. Piantadosi CA, Zhang J, Levin ED, Folz RJ, Schmechel DE. Apoptosis and delayed neuronal damage after carbon monoxide poisoning in the rat. Exp Neurol 1997;147:103–114.
91. Albin RL, Greenamyre JT. Alternative excitotoxic hypotheses. Neurology 1992;42:733–738.

92. Choi DW. Ischemia-induced neuronal apoptosis. Curr Opini Neurobiol 1996;6:667–672.
93. Nicholls D, Attwell D. The release and uptake of excitatory amino acids. Trends Pharmacol Sci 1990;11:462–468.
94. Rothman SM, Olney JW. Glutamate and the pathophysiology of hypoxic-ischemic brain damage. Ann Neurol 1986;19:105–111.
95. Sattler R, Tymianski M. Molecular mechanisms of calcium-dependent excitotoxicity. J Mol Med 2000;78:3–13.
96. Schurr A, Payne RS, Heine MF, Rigor BM. Hypoxia, excitotoxicity, and neuroprotection in the hippocampal slice preparation. J Neurosci Methods 1995;59:129–138.
97. Gozal E, Rowell PP. Differential NMDA glutamate receptor changes following sustained or intermittent hypoxia in the rat brain. Sleep 2002;25:A333.
98. Pichiule P, Chavez JC, Boero J, Arregui A. Chronic hypoxia induces modification of the N-methyl-D-aspartate receptor in rat brain. Neurosci Lett 1996;218:83–86.
99. Said SI, Pakbaz H, Berisha HI, Raza S. NMDA receptor activation: critical role in oxidant tissue injury. Free Radic Biol Med 2000;28:1300–1302.
100. Michaelis EK. Molecular biology of glutamate receptors in the central nervous system and their role in excitotoxicity, oxidative stress and aging. Prog Neurobiol 1998;54:369–415.
101. Goldbart A, Row BW, Kheirandish L, et al. Intermittent hypoxic exposure during light phase induces changes in cAMP response element binding protein activity in the rat CA1 hippocampal region: water maze performance correlates. Neuroscience 2003;122:585–590.
102. Gozal D, Row BW, Kheirandish L, et al. Increased susceptibility to intermittent hypoxia in aging rats: changes in proteasomal activity, neuronal apoptosis and spatial function. J Neurochem 2003;86:1545–1552.
103. Li RC, Row BW, Gozal E, et al. Cyclooxygenase 2 and intermittent hypoxia-induced spatial deficits in the rat. Am J Respir Crit Care Med 2003;168:469–475.
104. Row BW, Goldbart A, Gozal E, Gozal D. et al. Spatial pre-training attenuates hippocampal impairments in rats exposed to intermittent hypoxia. Neurosci Lett 2003;339:67–71.
105. Lu C, Chan SL, Haughey N, Lee WT, Mattson P. et al. Selective and biphasic effect of the membrane lipid peroxidation product 4-hydroxy-2,3-nonenal on N-methyl-D-aspartate channels. J Neurochem 2001;78:577–589.
106. Palmer LJ, Buxbaum SG, Larkin E, et al. A whole-genome scan for obstructive sleep apnea and obesity. Am J Hum Genet 2003;72:340–350.
107. Pellegrini-Giampietro DE, Pulsinelli WA, Zukin RS. NMDA and non-NMDA receptor gene expression following global brain ischemia in rats: effect of NMDA and non-NMDA receptor antagonists. J Neurochem 1994;62:1067–1073.
108. Barth A, Barth L, Newell DW. Combination therapy with MK-801 and alpha-phenyl-tert-butyl-nitrone enhances protection against ischemic neuronal damage in organotypic hippocampal slice cultures. Exp Neurol 1996;141:330–336.
109. Murata T, Omata N, Fujibayashi Y, et al. Posthypoxic reoxygenation-induced neurotoxicity prevented by free radical scavenger and NMDA/non-NMDA antagonist in tandem as revealed by dynamic changes in glucose metabolism with positron autoradiography. Exp Neurol 2000;164:269–279.
110. Mooney SM, Miller MW. Expression of bcl-2, bax, and caspase-3 in the brain of the developing rat. Brain Res Dev 2000;123:103–117.

7

The Psychological Evaluation of Attention Deficit Hyperactivity Disorder in School-Aged Children

A Clinical Approach Based on Recent Practice Guidelines

Dean W. Beebe

1. INTRODUCTION

Through the early 1990s, the evaluation and treatment of attention deficit hyperactivity disorder (ADHD) was often directed by the theoretical orientation and professional experience of each clinician. Though important empirically driven clinical guides were published (e.g., ref. *1*), their impact was diluted by the sheer volume of clinical approaches that largely ignored the growing research literature. Thankfully, recent years have witnessed the development and dissemination of well-articulated practice parameters that are guided by research and the consensus of recognized experts. These include guidelines for the assessment of individuals with ADHD published by the American Academy of Child and Adolescent Psychiatry in 1997*(2)*, the National Institutes of Health in 1998 *(3)*, the American Academy of Pediatrics (AAP) in 2000 *(4)*, and the Institute for Clinical Systems Improvement in 2003 *(5)*.

The goal of this chapter is to translate these practice parameters into a practical approach for the everyday clinical work of psychologists, psychiatrists, social workers, and other mental health professionals who work with school-age children. To allow for a focused discussion of issues related to ADHD, the chapter assumes that the reader has a reasonable foundation in child clinical assessment. Readers who are interested in broad discussions of child clinical assessment are referred to excellent texts by Sattler *(6)* and Merrell *(7)*. Although data-driven, this chapter will not represent a comprehensive review of the research literature; for this, the reader is referred to the wealth of information found in the balance of this volume, as well as other comprehensive texts (e.g., *8*). The reader is also directed to other chapters in this volume for research on treatment approaches; this chapter will focus on assessment. Finally, for brevity purposes, emphasis will be placed on work with school-age children, who represent the largest group seen for ADHD assessment *(8)*. Readers who are interested in adult ADHD are referred to recent books by Resnick *(9)* and Goldstein and Ellison *(10)*. Those who work extensively with preschool children are referred to work by Connor *(11)*, Shepard et al. *(12)*, and McGoey et al. *(13)*.

This chapter follows a proposed sequence of assessment steps, summarized in Fig. 1 and illustrated further in tables and brief case vignettes throughout the chapter. The assessment steps are presented for heuristic value and, though following a logical progression, should

From: *Attention Deficit Hyperactivity Disorder: From Genes to Patients*
Edited by: D. Gozal and D. L. Molfese © Humana Press Inc., Totowa, NJ

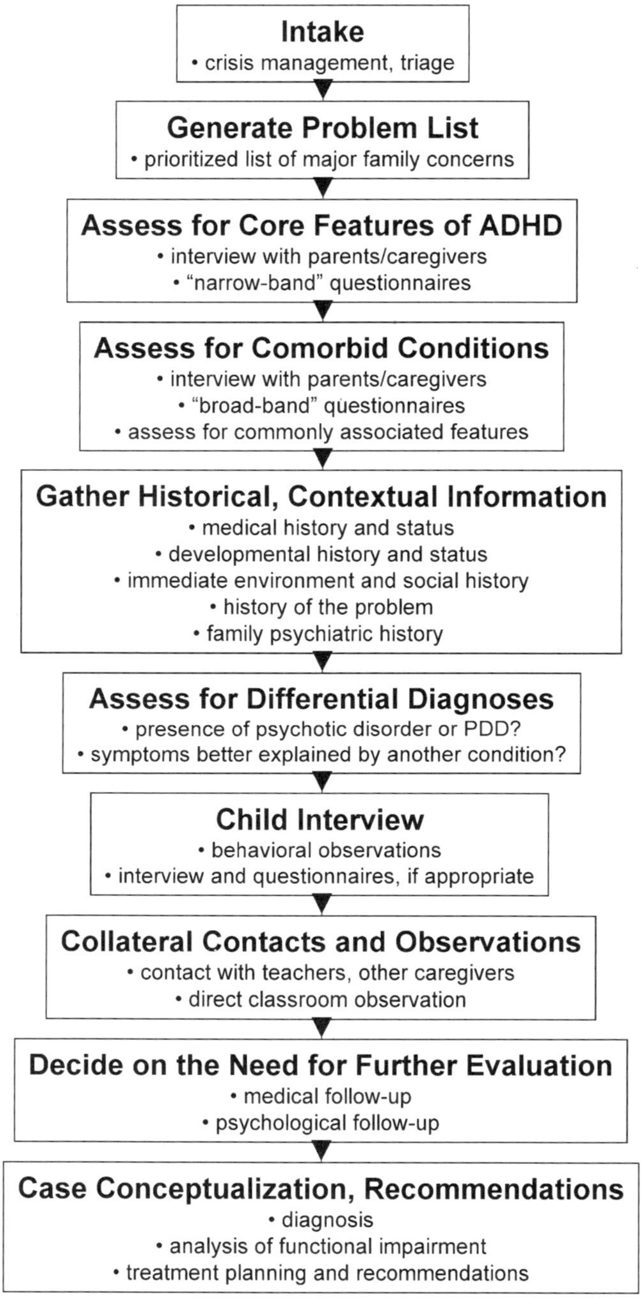

Fig. 1. Overview of a procedural heuristic for the assessment of suspected ADHD.

not be viewed as immutable. Clinicians are welcomed to change the order of the steps as they adapt the recommendations presented here to their own practices.

2. STEP 1: INTAKE

An often overlooked step in the assessment process occurs at the time of initial telephone contact with the family. This step is sometimes undertaken by the assessing clinician, but central intake workers often fill this role in larger group- and clinic-based practices. Key decisions made at this step include the appropriateness of the referral, the "fit" with services and talents available within the practice, and the procedural route the referral will follow. Presenting concerns of parents* of children with ADHD include not only inattention, impulsivity, or hyperactivity, but also anger management difficulties, disrespect, aggression, poor conduct, disorganization, oppositionality, "laziness," "immaturity," poor school performance (often in contrast to what is perceived to be a bright child), and frequent teacher complaints. As with any mental health referral, an important consideration is whether the child or family is in acute crisis, as in cases of potential imminent harm to the child or another person, or in the immediate threat of life-altering events (e.g., school expulsion, legal action). In these cases, the "routine" handling of the chronic disorder, such as ADHD, must be set aside in favor of immediate crisis intervention *(5)*.

3. STEP 2: GENERATE THE PROBLEM LIST

Although surprises abound in mental health assessment, in cases where ADHD is present, a solid intake process will have raised relevant concerns prior to the first clinic visit. Even in these cases, however, it is prudent to ask for a broad overview of the presenting concerns, often in list form. Overlooking this step places the clinician at risk for missing areas of concern that are important for diagnosis and treatment, prematurely biases the clinician toward a diagnosis that may be inappropriate or insufficient, makes the erroneous assumption that the clinician knows more about the situation than does the family, and misses a valuable opportunity to develop rapport early in the process. Asking the family to rank or prioritize their concerns can further provide structure and direction for the subsequent clinical interview in a way that resonates with the family's perspective.

> *Case 1*: Johnny, age 7, has such significant impulsivity and other behavior problems that his mother fears that even if he does not hurt himself (he has impulsively run through glass panes and fallen off of a high deck), she may resort to abuse in an effort to gain control of the home. The intake worker sets up an "emergency appointment" with a clinician, and provides guidance on acute support services, including a 24-h hotline and emergency admission procedures. Thorough assessment of Johnny's possible ADHD can wait until the crisis is managed.
>
> *Case 2*: In reviewing the intake materials for a new client, a young clinician notes that the parent has expressed concerns about a child's ability to pay attention. Fresh out of a seminar on diagnosing ADHD, he begins the clinical interview with direct questions about ADHD. The family, a bit taken aback but eager to obtain help, goes along. It is not until the last 5 min of the session that the clinician learns that the family is actually more concerned about the possibility of a learning disability, and that the child's behavior problems seem to be most evident during arithmetic lessons and homework. Valuable time and opportunities have been squandered by an errant, if well-intentioned, clinical approach.

* It is acknowledged that family structures differ tremendously. The general term "parent" is used here for ease of presentation, but refers more broadly to primary caregivers and guardians.

4. STEP 3: ASSESS FOR CORE FEATURES OF ADHD

For the purpose of this chapter, it is assumed that concerns about attention, impulse control, or activity level figure prominently in the problem list. In this case, the clinician should inquire further regarding these core features of ADHD, avoiding a simple recitation of Diagnostic and Statistical Manual for Mental Disorders (DSM-IV) criteria at first to obtain a more complete picture of the nature, frequency, severity, pervasiveness, and duration of symptoms. The prevailing diagnostic criteria according to the DSM-IV *(14)* are reviewed elsewhere in this volume. In short, DSM-IV requires the "childhood onset of adaptive impairment due to significant inattention, impulsivity, or hyperactivity that persists at least six months. These symptoms must be present across multiple situations and must not be better accounted for by another mental disorder."

Table 1 provides broad questions that can be stated in a conversational tone to elicit information relevant to DSM-IV criteria. Following these are more specific questions that can be used to further "flesh out" a diagnosis, especially when the clinician is having difficulty eliciting useful information with broad questions. Although a conversational tone is important to build and maintain rapport, in the end it is important to ask enough specific questions to be able to address the diagnostic criteria *(8)*. Sattler *(6)* recommends a progression from open-ended questions to close-ended questions over the course of the interview; the more open-ended questions allow the parents the most freedom to express their concerns and perspective, whereas close-ended questions may be necessary to understand whether specific diagnostic criteria have been met. Readers who prefer a more structured interview format, as well as students who are just learning how to interview with DSM-IV in mind, are directed to Rogers' extensive review of empirically established structured child clinical interviews *(15)*.

Several parent- and teacher-report questionnaires have been developed that directly inquire about the key features of ADHD. "Narrow-band" ADHD forms that focus primarily on ADHD symptoms are more effective in assisting diagnostic decisions than are "broad-band" indexes that cover a wide array of symptoms *(4)*. Comprehensive reviews of narrow-band questionnaires are presented elsewhere *(8,16–18)*, but the most common will be listed here. Several authors have provided simple translations of ADHD items into questionnaire formats, such as Barkley's Disruptive Behavior Disorders Rating Scale *(16)* and DuPaul and colleagues' ADHD Rating Scale *(19)*. Others have developed more comprehensive behavior questionnaires, from which relevant narrow-band subscale scores can be derived. These include the attention and hyperactivity subscales from the Behavior Assessment System for Children *(20)*, the attention subscale from Achenbach's Child Behavior Checklist and Teacher Report Form *(21)*, and the ADHD Index and Hyperactivity subscale from the Conners Parent Rating Scales and Teacher Rating Scales *(22)*. Each of these questionnaires has strong psychometric qualities and offers both parent and teacher report forms.

Standardized narrow-band questionnaires and questionnaire subscales have several selling points. In contrast to clinician-constructed questionnaires or nonstandardized interviews, standardized questionnaires have established psychometric properties. Well-characterized normative data can help address exactly how unusual a child's behaviors are for his or her age (or gender). This is especially important in differentiating the extreme and impairing behaviors that characterize ADHD from more common developmental variations, such as

Table 1
Sample Questions for Core Features of ADHD

Broad, conversational questions

- You mentioned that he/she has problems with [inattention/being overactive/acting without thinking...]. Can you tell me more about what you see?
- Can you provide examples?
- Has this gotten him/her into trouble? In what situations?
- What happens because he/she (fill in behavior)? What is the impact?
- Are there times when this isn't a problem? Tell me more about those times.
- How long has this been a problem? When did you first notice it?
- What do members of your family (his/her teacher, etc.) think about this behavior?

Follow-up/specific questions

- Does he/she have problems paying attention to certain things? What things?
- Is he/she easily distracted?
- Does he/she make careless mistakes at school, at home, or in other situations?
- Is it hard for him/her to remember what you or his/her teachers say?
- Does it seem like he/she does not listen to you or his teachers? When *does* he/she listen?
- Does he/she have problems following instructions?
- Does he/she have problems following through on things?
- How organized is he/she? Is his/her locker, desk, bookbag, bedroom, or playroom a mess?
- Does he/she avoid tasks that require him/her to pay close attention?
- Does he/she lose things a lot? Are worksheets, assignments, books, or coats unintentionally left behind?
- Does he/she get into trouble for fidgeting, squirming, or having problems sitting still?
- Does he/she get into trouble for running around or climbing on things when he/she shouldn't?
- Is he/she able to stay in his/her seat at school, home, restaurants, church, or other places?
- Does it seem like he/she just can't slow down or stay in one place?
- Can he/she play quietly? Doing what?
- Can he/she stick with an activity without switching quickly? Which activities seem to be hard to stick with?
- Does he/she interrupt, talk out of turn, or blurt out answers at school?
- Does it seem like he/she never stops talking?
- How does he/she do with waiting his/her turn in games or lines?
- Does he/she butt into games or conversations?
- Does he/she usually think before acting, or act before thinking?
- Does he/she end up doing dangerous things without thinking, like jumping from heights or running into the street without looking? Is he/she thrill-seeking or just not thinking?

the high activity level and short attention span that occurs in very young children (*see also* ref. *4*). Such questionnaires are also readily understood by a wide variety of parents and teachers. Finally, they can be completed outside the testing office, and are especially useful for obtaining the perspectives of caregivers and teachers whom the clinician may not otherwise contact.

Nevertheless, *diagnostic decisions cannot be made based on questionnaires alone (5)*. Questionnaires, no matter how well-developed, are prone to rater/observer biases, idiosyncratic item interpretation, rater-specific tolerance levels for certain behaviors, and the degree to which the rater actually knows the child. Like all clinical assessments, the diagnostic evaluation of a child with suspected ADHD involves integrating information from multiple sources, assessing the reliability and validity of these sources, and drawing conclusions based on the weight of the evidence.

One key limitation of the behavioral questionnaires is that they rarely address the environmental contingencies that surround problem behaviors. Using the ABC (antecedents-behaviors-consequences) model of describing environmental contingencies, the clinician should conduct an analysis of the circumstances and consequences surrounding problem behaviors. A related limitation of band-questionnaires is that, by design, most focus on *symptoms* of ADHD, not the functional *impairment* caused by these symptoms. Signs of impairment, not symptoms, are the primary cause of most referrals and mediate the long-term adverse effects of ADHD *(23)*. As such, while inquiring about the specific symptoms of ADHD, it is equally, if not more, important to determine the environmental contingencies and functional impact of these symptoms.

It can be informative to ask about the situations in which the child does *not* seem impaired. This reframing of the ABC model may provide insight into potential environmental interventions, or alternative hypotheses for the meaning of problem behaviors (e.g., impulsivity that is present only in anxiety-provoking or highly stimulating situations). In other cases, it can initiate an educational process for the parents. Some parents assume, for example, that a child who can watch television or play video games for hours cannot have ADHD. In fact, the attention span required for such activities is often quite brief, and the reinforcement the child experiences while doing so is immediate and powerful *(4)*. Television and video game programmers earn their living by maintaining people's attention; in some ways, they may be better at behavior modification than many psychologists!

It is important to inquire about the child's behaviors across multiple contexts *(2)*. Not only is this required to make a formal diagnosis, but it can provide additional insight into the environmental contingencies that prompt, perpetuate, or suppress problem behaviors. The diagnosis of ADHD does not require impairment across all situations—in fact, the degree and nature of impairment often vary across settings—but impairment must be present in multiple settings. Typically, but not always, the greatest impairment arises in situations that place high expectations on the child to regulate his or her attention and behavior, but which are characterized by a low degree of external structure and support in doing so. Because of this, it is especially important to ask about behaviors and performance at school, where the greatest concerns are often seen.

Case 3: The parents of Mark, age 8, come to the office at odds. His mother is frustrated with frequent teacher complaints of off-task behaviors, as well as her own experience of his grabbing at objects while shopping and his apparent inability to complete homework at an age-appropriate level. However, when she forces him to sit with her and go through each homework item one by one, he learns well. Mark's father, who works second shift and sees him mostly during the weekend, observes that he has boundless energy, but that this doesn't get him into trouble around the house. He questions the motives and competence of the teacher and has difficulty supporting his wife when he has not seen the same problems.

The clinician is cautioned to take into consideration ethnic and cultural issues at this and other steps in the assessment process. ADHD assessment is not unique in this respect, and the reader is referred to Suzuki et al. *(24)*, Sattler *(6)*, and Merrell *(7)* for guidelines for culturally sensitive assessment. Reid *(25)* has provided one of the few comprehensive reviews of the use of ADHD behavior rating scales across cultural groups. Although the data have been "weak and inconsistent" on whether the disruptive behavior disorders, including ADHD, vary in true prevalence across racial or ethnic lines within the United States *(26)*, certain subpopulations do tend to score higher on ADHD questionnaires than others *(19,25,27,28)*. Also, it is clear that, across countries, the apparent prevalence of ADHD varies dramatically *(29)*. One key concern with all disruptive behavior disorders is the degree to which a behavior is socially accepted. Barkley *(16)* recommends that if a parent from a minority group endorses a specific symptom, the clinician should follow up with: "Do you consider this to be a problem for your child compared to other children of the same ethnic or minority group?" Although helpful, such add-on questions do not fully address the issue of cross-cultural awareness. When working with families who differ from the dominant European-American culture (on which both DSM-IV and most standardized questionnaires and interviews were based), the clinician is cautioned that the language used to describe behaviors, and the significance and meaning attributed to a given behavior, are at least partially culturally determined *(25)*.

5. STEP 4: ASSESS FOR COMORBID CONDITIONS

It is estimated that as many as 70% of children with ADHD may also be diagnosed with one or more comorbid psychiatric conditions *(2,30)*. As summarized in Table 2, children with ADHD show much higher rates of a variety of other conditions than is present in the general pediatric population.

The problem list generated above provides a good launching point for inquiring about comorbid conditions. Each problem on the list should be explored, with an eye toward means by which core features of ADHD might influence the presence or manifestation of the other reported problems (and the converse situation). Thorough discussion of the assessment of each potential comorbid condition extends beyond the bounds of this chapter. For initial guidance, however, Table 2 provides sample screening questions to be used when the clinician suspects the presence of several of the more common comorbid conditions. Obviously, the clinician is not limited to these questions, and should consider the full range of potentially comorbid disorders when reviewing the presenting problem list.

Broad-band questionnaires can be an important adjunct to interviews in assessing for the presence, nature, and severity of comorbid pathology, and have been endorsed for such use in multiple practice parameters *(2–5)*. Commonly used broad-band questionnaires, such as the Child Behavior Checklist/Teacher Report Form, Conners Parent and Teacher Rating Scales, and Behavior Assessment System for Children can alert the clinician to areas outside the core symptoms to focus on further. As with their narrow-band counterparts, their strengths include strong psychometric support and convenience, but they also share the potential biases inherent in any questionnaires.

In clinical practice, when the question of ADHD arises, I typically request that at least one parent and at least one teacher who know the child well complete both a broad band questionnaire and narrow-band ADHD instrument. When possible, forms are mailed out and received prior to the first interview. The combined information can provide a powerful launching point for dialogue, even during the initial session, and can prompt discussion of areas that might

Table 2
Population and Comorbidity Rates for Common Comorbid Conditions and Sample Screening Questions

Condition	Pop. rate	Rate in ADHD	Sample screening questions
Oppositional–defiant disorder	2–16%	35–50%	• Does he/she openly defy you or a teacher, actually saying "no" or ignoring you? • Does he/she seem annoyed easily? What sorts of things bother him/her? • Does he/she seem to annoy other people on purpose? Who? Where? • Does he/she seem angry, "hot-tempered," resentful, or full of spite?
Conduct disorder	2–3%	14–50%	• Does he/she lie a lot? About what? • Does he/she get into physical fights? Has he/she used a weapon? • Has he/she hurt or tried to intimidate people or animals? • Has he/she ever stolen or damaged other people's things? Tell me more about what happened.
Anxiety disorders	9%	20–34%	• Does he/she seem nervous or anxious? How can you tell? • Are there times when he/she seems panic-stricken or "frozen" by anxiety? • Are there certain things or situations that he/she is very afraid or nervous around, or tries to avoid? • Is he/she very shy, more than other children the same age? • Does he/she repeat certain actions over and over, like a ritual?
Depression/dysthymia	2–8%	15–20%	• Does he/she seem to feel sad, blue, or down? How can you tell? • Is he/she irritable, cranky, or moody? • What does he/she do for fun? Are there things he/she used to enjoy but doesn't anymore? • Does he/she talk about hurting him/herself? Has he/she actually tried to do so?
Bipolar disorder	1%	Unclear	• Are there times when he/she seems to think he/she can do anything or be anything? • Are there times when he/she is unusually energetic, almost "high," but without drugs? • Are there times when he/she hardly sleeps but seems not to be affected by it the next day? • Does he/she seem to have thoughts that come so fast he or she could not keep up with them?
Learning disability, cognitive delay	2–10%	10–25%	• Even when he/she is paying attention, is it hard for him/her to learn? • Are there certain subjects that he/she just doesn't seem to get?

(Continued)

Table 2
(*Continued*)

Condition	Pop. rate	Rate in ADHD	Sample screening questions
			• How does he/she do with (reading/writing/arithmetic)? How about (fill in another academic subject)? • Has he/she ever been classified as having a learning disability or educational handicap? Tell me more.
Tourette's/ tic disorder	<1%	11%	• Does he/she have certain movements that happen often but are not intentional? For example, blinking, making an odd face, shrugging, or moving an arm the same way a lot? • Does he/she make noises without meaning to, like grunting, sniffing, or saying certain words?
Substance abuse	Varies by age	Varies by age	• Do you suspect that he/she smokes, uses drugs, or drinks alcohol? What makes you suspect this? How much do you think he/she does this?

From refs. *2,14,30,44,52–55*.

have been overlooked in the initial problem list. They can also form the foundation for discussion of concerns raised by one party (e.g., a parent) but not another (e.g., a teacher).

Although not in themselves diagnostic, associated features of ADHD should also be assessed. These include poor social skills, motor coordination problems, low sense of self-esteem or self-efficacy (particularly around schoolwork), and poor "executive functioning" (e.g., difficulty dealing with changes in routine, poor emotion regulation, poor planning, disorganization, poor self-monitoring) *(8)*. To supplement the clinical interview, the Behavior Rating Inventory of Executive Functioning (BRIEF) *(31)* has parent and teacher-report questionnaire forms that provide information on multiple aspects of executive functioning in daily life, and can be a useful complement to narrow-band ADHD scales and broad-band psychopathology screeners. Similarly, Barkley *(1,8,16)* has advocated the use of questionnaire screeners for social skills deficits (e.g., the Social Skills Rating System *[32]*) and the pervasiveness of behavior problems (Home and School Situation Questionnaires *[1,8,16]*). Although beyond the scope of this review, even more comprehensive questionnaire batteries can be constructed, if needed, to examine issues of parental psychological functioning, marital adjustment, parenting stress and social support, parenting practices, and dyadic and family interactions *(33)*.

6. STEP 5: GATHER HISTORICAL AND CONTEXTUAL INFORMATION

As with all psychiatric assessment, the assessment of children with suspected ADHD requires eliciting information regarding the child's history. Though it is nearly impossible to psychometrically validate such instruments, general background questionnaires, such as those published by Sattler *(6)* and Barkley *(16)*, can help structure the assessment process, ensuring that important historical and contextual information is addressed. When these are gathered ahead of time, such forms also provide a frame of reference for the clinician prior to the clinical interview. Table 3 lists the historical and contextual domains that should be addressed in the assessment of a child with suspected ADHD.

Table 3
Important Historical and Contextual Information

Medical history and status

- Prenatal history, including maternal substance use, toxin exposure, length of gestation, and pregnancy complications
- Perinatal history, including complications during labor and delivery, health at time of delivery
- History of significant neurological injuries (e.g., traumatic brain injury) or neurodevelopmental conditions (e.g., genetic disorder, thyroid condition)
- Potential exposure to neurotoxins, including lead
- General health history of the child, including chronic illnesses, the frequency and recency of medical attention, vision and hearing screening results, and current and past medications
- Sleep functioning of the child

Developmental history and status

- Attainment of language and motor milestones
- Development of adaptive and self-help skills
- History of protracted stalling or regression in developmental and adaptive milestones
- Presence and persistence of difficulties with language or motor functioning
- Current academic and adaptive status

Immediate environment and social history

- Nature of housing, neighborhood (e.g., public housing)
- Members of immediate household
- Stability of household (e.g., frequent moves, entries into and departures from the household)
- Description of the school environment currently and over the years
- Parenting and disciplinary style
- Other sources of environmental support (e.g., church, supportive relatives)
- History of abuse or neglect (both personal and witnessed)
- Family stresses (e.g., job loss, divorce, deaths in families)
- Cultural affiliation of family and degree of identification with local cultural mainstream

History of the problem

- Presence of symptoms prior to age 7
- When symptoms first drew the attention of parents/teachers/professionals
- First symptoms in hindsight
- Changes in symptoms and development of comorbidities over time
- Prior psychological, psychiatric, and academic evaluations
- Prior attempts at intervention, including discipline at home and school intervention plans (Individualized education plans, "504 plans")

Family psychiatric history

- Family history of learning, scholastic, attention, or behavior problems
- Family history of neurological disorders
- Family history of psychiatric disorders, including disruptive behavior disorders and chemical dependency

Though most mental health workers are not physicians, it is important to obtain a basic understanding of the medical factors most likely to affect the cognitive and behavioral functioning of a child. This typically involves asking questions regarding pre- and perinatal medical histories, as well as any history of neurological injuries (e.g., head injury with signs of concussion) or neurodevelopmental conditions (e.g., chromosomal abnormality, familial or idiopathic epilepsy). Each of these factors may cause or contribute to behavioral disruption, and may warrant additional evaluation by relevant specialists and consideration in case conceptualization and recommendations. If there is any suspicion of neurotoxin exposure, such as lead exposure if the child has lived in pre-1970s-built housing with cracked or flaking paint, the child should undergo formal screening by medical professionals.

The general health history of the child should also be understood, not only because of the potential direct effect of medical problems on functioning (e.g., effect of frequent ear infections on hearing and subsequent speech development) but also because significant medical events often alter the parent-child relationship, with secondary effects on child behavior. A history of frequent physical injuries should prompt further inquiry, as these may relate to impulsivity or inattention, motor coordination problems, environmental circumstances, or even physical abuse. Finally, as is covered in greater detail in Chapter 19, the clinician should inquire about the child's sleep functioning. Although the nature of the relationship between sleep problems and ADHD remains hotly debated, there is little question that a very high proportion of children with ADHD are reported by their parents to have sleep problems *(34–36)*. Given that pediatric sleep disorders are often quite treatable, interventions in this area have the potential to dramatically improve quality of life.

The developmental history and status of the child places his or her behavioral difficulties in a larger developmental context. The diagnosis of ADHD requires that the observed or reported symptoms are substantially out of step with a child's developmental level. When there is a suspicion of significant developmental delays, the child's attention and behavior regulation must be determined to be proportionately poorer still. The clinician should inquire regarding the attainment and progression of language, motor, adaptive, and self-help skills. Any protracted stalling or regression of developmental or adaptive milestones should be explored thoroughly, as these often signal the presence of a significant medical or environmental stressor. The clinician should also attempt to understand the child's current academic and adaptive status, both under "typical" circumstances and when the child is in an optimized environment (e.g., how well does the child learn with one-on-one instruction and behavioral cues?).

As outlined in Chapter 2 of this volume, ADHD has a significant genetic component. As such, it is important to solicit information regarding the psychiatric, scholastic, and neurological histories of immediate family members. From a practical perspective, knowledge of first- and second-degree relatives generally suffices. Even given substantial heritability to ADHD, however, its behavioral phenotype is substantially affected by environmental and social factors. The clinician should solicit information regarding the multiple spheres of environmental influence, including the school, immediate family, neighborhood, and other domains (e.g., church). Changes in these spheres and major family stresses should be noted, with particular attention to the relationship between these events and changes in the child's behaviors.

If they were not already assessed when discussing the parents' primary concerns, the symptom history should be traced. This is especially important when children present for treatment during middle or late childhood, as the current criteria for ADHD require the presence of symptoms prior to age 7*. This is not to say that the problems must have been noted prospectively by age 7; in some cases, behaviors can be overlooked (e.g., with primarily inattentive children who are not behaviorally disruptive in the class), normalized or dismissed as a transient "phase," or

* Barkley *(8,29)* has questioned the validity of the "under 7 cutoff," but still emphasizes the importance of establishing childhood onset.

minimized by environmental accommodations (e.g., small classroom size, considerable one-on-one support). Indeed, the impact of inattention and the related symptoms of poor planning and disorganization may increase across childhood, with the progressive increase in expectations for independent work. However, the presence of significant symptoms during early childhood, even in hindsight, is required for the diagnosis. The temporal relationship of symptom development, especially with respect to environmental changes and the development of comorbid conditions, can suggest points of potential causality and intervention.

Some children will have undergone prior evaluation by another clinician or the school; records from these evaluations help to track symptoms and impairment, and can either suggest or obviate the need for some follow-up assessments *(see* Section 10*)*. Even less structured assessment documents, such as report cards, provide a valuable record of the functional impact of a child's symptoms. Finally, understanding the interventions that have already been tried can provide insights into the coping resources and behavior management approaches of the family and school, as well as tips on intervention paths that are likely to meet with the greatest success and least systemic resistance.

Although obtaining historical information is essential to the assessment process, the clinician should also recognize that retrospective reports can be inaccurate and inadvertently biased toward the reporter's explicit or implicit hypotheses about the child's behaviors. This emphasizes the need to maintain clinical objectivity during the assessment process, and to gather prospectively generated information (e.g., school records, medical chart information) whenever possible.

7. STEP 6: ASSESS FOR DIFFERENTIAL DIAGNOSES

The DSM-IV diagnosis of ADHD requires that "the symptoms do not occur exclusively during the course of a Pervasive Developmental Disorder, Schizophrenia, or other Psychotic Disorder and are not better accounted for by another mental disorder (e.g., Mood Disorder, Anxiety Disorder, Dissociative Disorder, or a Personality Disorder)." Typically, most of the needed information is solicited in the problem list and assessment of comorbid conditions. If there is any concern regarding hallucinations or delusions, this should be followed on in a frank and detailed manner, as the diagnosis and treatment for childhood-onset psychotic disorders are much different from those for ADHD.

Although DSM-IV does not allow for the concurrent diagnosis of ADHD and pervasive developmental disorder (PDD; e.g., autism, Asperger's disorder, PDD not otherwise specified), research data call this prohibition into question *(37)*. Even so, clinicians are cautioned against overdiagnosing ADHD in the context of PDD. If a child displays qualitative impairments in social interaction, coupled with restricted repetitive and stereotyped patterns of behavior, interests, and activities *(14)*, the clinician should conduct careful follow-up. By virtue of their normal intellectual skills, many children with "high functioning" autism or Asperger's disorder are not identified until middle or late childhood, after having endured numerous misdiagnoses and the failure of relevant interventions *(38)*. Often, one of these misdiagnoses is ADHD. In children of apparently normal intellectual ability, the clinician should move beyond the stereotype of the disengaged "autistic" child who is engaged in isolated repetitive behaviors. Rather, the assessor should inquire more carefully regarding the reciprocity of social interactions (even if the child is socially interested) and the presence of narrow and intense interests (e.g., amassing a huge knowledge base of baseball statistics) that interfere with daily functioning *(39)*. In these cases, although treatments for inattention, hyperactivity, or impulsivity may be useful, the overall case conceptualization and treatment plan must be framed around the PDD diagnosis to be most effective (*see also* refs. *38,39*).

The issue of whether symptoms are better explained by another mental disorder can be tricky, and is not unique to ADHD; nearly all DSM-IV diagnoses have a similar "rule out" criterion. Important considerations to take into account when making such decisions include the relative severity of symptoms, the contexts in which symptoms are most obvious, family/genetic influences, and the relative timing of onset and exacerbation of symptoms of each disorder. A careful functional behavioral analysis, including delineation of antecedents and consequences related to each problem behavior, can further allow for better diagnostic accuracy *(40)*. The determination of which diagnoses or conditions are primary is not academic; diagnoses carry specific connotations and expectations, and can dictate which treatments are attempted.

8. STEP 7: CHILD INTERVIEW

The timing of the child interview in the diagnostic process is rather arbitrary, though it is often ideal to have spoken at length with the parents first to have a better idea of what to expect when the child comes in, as well as key issues to explore further with him or her. As with the parent interview, the reader is directed to more comprehensive child assessment texts (e.g., refs. *6,7*) for an overview of key issues in child clinical interviews. This chapter will focus on issues that are relatively specific to ADHD.

When working with a child with suspected ADHD, it is essential to understand that he or she may not show inattention, hyperactivity, or impulsivity in the office. After all, the office setting is typically novel, one-on-one, stimulating and—depending on the assessor's talents—fun. Thus, although the presence of symptoms is noteworthy, the absence of symptoms is not particularly informative *(23)*. Also, because of the novelty of the situation and the child's unique perspective and attempts at image-setting, his or her report during a clinical interview may be quite discrepant from that obtained from parents and teachers. An important challenge for the clinician is to integrate this information.

Despite the challenges inherent in effective child interviewing, when ADHD is suspected, the child interview is an essential part of the diagnostic process for several reasons. First, the child's view of the situation can give important clues as to how he or she will respond to

Case 4: The mother of 6-yr-old Miguel expresses frustration with her son's lack of response to stimulant medications prescribed by his pediatrician. One of the most distressing behaviors is his lack of attention to her directives. He is not reported to be markedly inattentive or have a behavior problem at school or with his grandparents. Further inquiry reveals that, even when his attention is gathered by his mother, he often reacts angrily or refuses to do as she asks. Many times, after a protracted battle, his mother decides it is easier to give up than to force the issue. A thorough evaluation reveals long-standing difficulty with parent limit-setting across multiple situations. In the absence of additional evidence of ADHD, oppositional defiant disorder is considered the primary diagnosis. Behavioral therapy focused on parent training is undertaken, and displays success even after the pediatrician discontinues the stimulants.

potential interventions. Second, parents and teachers may be unaware of certain child behaviors, moods, and cognitions that turn out to be key to the overall case conceptualization. Third, the child may reveal historical information that was not revealed by the parent, such as abuse or neglect. Fourth, especially for older children, a firsthand account of his or her symptoms and their functional impact can be quite cogent.

The nature of the interview will vary. With young children, it is often helpful to conduct the child assessment while playing a game. The emphasis should *not* be on "play therapy" or "play assessment," both of which emphasize the symbolic content of play, but rather on providing a context for behavioral observation and, as important, a tool for increasing the child's comfort with the examiner during the interview. With older children and adolescents, the give-and-take of an interview may be more comfortable.

Notwithstanding the limitations of behavioral observation in the office setting, how the child behaves during the session can be important. If present, signs of impulsivity, fidgeting, hyperactivity, distractibility, disorganization, and difficulty with dual-tasking (e.g., talking and playing at the same time) are often significant. Receptive and expressive communication skills, social skills, motor coordination or stereotypies, thought processes, and apparent mood and affective state and stability should all be noted.

Insofar as a clinical interview is possible, it is important to obtain a sense of the child's experience of the home, school, and other environments, and their ability to meet others' expectations in those settings. In the context of a more free-flowing discussion, specific questions, aimed at the developmental level of the child, should address the core symptoms of ADHD and common comorbid conditions. The functional impact of these symptoms can sometimes be strikingly described by the child, although on many occasions he or she will tend to downplay any impact or focus on others' actions *(16)*. The more developmentally advanced and forthcoming the child, the more closely the interview may parallel the parent interview. When working with a developmentally able child, it can also be helpful for him or her to complete questionnaires for which child report forms have been developed (e.g., refs. *20,21*). However, perhaps even more than with adult-report questionnaires, the findings from child-report questionnaires must consider the source of information, and carefully weigh the resulting information with the balance of the other available information *(18)*.

Case 5: The parents of 15-yr-old Susan bring her in for evaluation because of declining school grades and apparent inattention at school. She was reported to have been "spacey" as a young child, but this was dismissed as "just Susan." Based on the parent report alone, the clinician suspected that she had lived with undiagnosed inattentive-type ADHD for some time, the functional impact of which was growing because of increased demands for independent work. After a rapport-building period during the child interview, Susan tearfully admitted to "being under a lot of stress." On further inquiry, she revealed that she had taken to "partying" with her friends without her parents' knowledge, including escalating drug use. She also tearfully reported a history of "date rape" by an older acquaintance. Although the possibility of long-standing ADHD was still a consideration, the situation was obviously more complex.

9. STEP 8: COLLATERAL CONTACTS AND OBSERVATIONS

It is critical to gather information from multiple sources. At a minimum, this typically requires the use of parent- and teacher-report questionnaires. On many occasions, it can also be helpful to talk directly with teachers and additional caregivers (e.g., after-school care or daycare providers, relatives). By necessity, these conversations are often brief and target the specific presenting concerns. Again following the ABC model, the antecedents and consequences of behaviors are important facets of the assessment. As part of the antecedent assessment, the clinician should inquire about the general classroom setting (e.g., number of children and adults in class, size of room, degree of structure, seating arrangement, typical teaching methods). The clinician should also attempt to understand how long the reporter has known the child and under what circumstances. Prior attempts at intervention beyond those reported by the parents should also be solicited. Finally, although not part of the diagnostic process itself, it can be of further assistance to ask the reporter what he or she thinks the child needs, and what untapped support options might be available for the child.

In some cases, direct classroom observation is possible or has been conducted by others (e.g., as part of a comprehensive school evaluation). The advantages of direct observation include the opportunity to see the child's "typical" environment, his or her behaviors in that environment, and the functional effects of these behaviors. Several formal behavior observations techniques have been developed (e.g., refs. *7,20,21*) that provide a structured means for recording behaviors and comparing them against a frame of reference (e.g., norms, a matched "control" child in the class). Disadvantages of behavior observation include the reactance of the child (or of others around him or her) to the presence of the observer, difficulties with logistics (e.g., scheduling, billing), and the possibility that the brief behavioral "snapshot" does not capture the child's typical behaviors. Analog assessments, in which child behavior is observed in an office-based *simulated* classroom (or other) environment, have been developed in an attempt to overcome some of these limitations (e.g., ref. *41*). Although viewed as promising, to date these analog approaches have been inadequately studied to support their clinical use *(42)*.

10. STEP 9: DECIDE ON NEED FOR FURTHER EVALUATION

In the majority of cases, the above steps are sufficient to make an accurate diagnosis and to formulate a case conceptualization and recommendations. From a medical perspective, the AAP has found that blood work, structural or functional neuroimaging, and standard or quantitative electroencephalography are *not* clinically indicated in the routine evaluation of children with suspected ADHD *(4)*. However, there are instances in which further medical consultation is needed. If a medical condition, such as toxin exposure, epilepsy, or a history of significant head trauma, is suspected, the clinician should refer the child for appropriate specialist evaluation. Similarly, if a psychiatric condition that is outside the clinician's area of expertise is suspected (e.g., substance abuse, PDD), the clinician is ethically obliged to consult with a specialist on that condition *(43)*. If a receptive or expressive speech/language delay is suspected, the child should be referred for formal evaluation of these skills, though clinical experience suggests some caution. Just as psychiatric assessment has a bias toward understanding aberrant behaviors (not language functioning), speech and language assessments are poor substitutes for a psychiatric assessment. I have worked with children who had previously undergone a speech and language evaluation and were diagnosed with "central auditory processing disorder" because audition/language was the only modality assessed, then they were inadequately treated because the broader impact of ADHD was overlooked.

The astute reader will have noticed that this chapter has not yet addressed formal one-on-one cognitive or personality tests of the child. This is because, in many cases, such testing is not needed. Multiple reviewers, based on comprehensive evaluations of a broad research literature, have come to the conclusion that the *routine use of formal cognitive and personality tests of the child with suspected ADHD is unwarranted (4,5)*. This includes the routine use of one-on-one continuous performance tests (CPTs) which, although in widespread use by mental health practitioners and pediatricians, do not provide adequate sensitivity and specificity to guide diagnosis, case conceptualization, or treatment planning *(2,4,44)*. Other psychological tools, such as empirically derived factors from intelligence tests, have even less research support as diagnostic tools, and should not be used to rule ADHD in or out *(45)*.

Nevertheless, when comorbid learning problems are suspected or there are concerns about cognitive delay, follow-up cognitive or educational testing is appropriate *(2)*. Many schools are well prepared to address this issue, although some parents are understandably concerned that the school may not handle a given child well. Private psychologists who specialize in work with children with ADHD or learning disabilities (those who specialize in one almost invariably are experienced with the other) are also well-qualified to conduct such evaluations, although obtaining third-party (e.g., insurance) reimbursement can be difficult. In rare cases when a frank neurological disorder is suspected (e.g., epilepsy, brain injury), a neuropsychological assessment, administered by a psychologist with the appropriate pre- and postdoctoral specialty training, can be a helpful adjunct to a medical workup, providing a more comprehensive determination of the impact of the medical condition and recommendations for intervention.

Follow-up psychological evaluation may be warranted in cases where there is suspicion of significant abnormalities of cognitive contents or processes (unusual or bizarre thoughts, schematic/interpretive biases) or mood disorders. Again, psychologists with specialization in the specific concerns surrounding a child should be consulted; the use of psychological tests by non psychologists or psychologists without adequate training and experience is unethical and, in many cases, illegal.

Psychologists are cautioned to take into account the potential impact of ADHD symptoms on the testing process and outcome. Generally speaking, unless the specific symptoms of ADHD are being assessed, it is ideal to minimize the impact of these symptoms in the testing room. This may include holding off on assessment until medications are initiated and appropriately titrated. At a minimum, the testing environment should be artificially structured: decreasing visual and auditory distractions, having a clean testing space, setting clear behavioral expectations, using frequent cues and immediate reinforcement for on-task behaviors, encouraging the child to take his or her time (if appropriate to the task), refocusing the child prior to instructions and item administration (e.g., "Ready?"), keeping a brisk testing pace for impulsive patients (e.g., avoiding excessive test setup and cleanup time), physically structuring the space to limit impulsive movement, and taking frequent breaks to allow for movement and discussion of distractions at appropriate times. The goal is to obtain the most clear and accurate assessment by reducing the "noise" generated by ADHD symptoms. Of course, in doing so, the testing situation becomes quite different from the child's typical setting (e.g., the classroom). The challenge for the clinician, then, is to estimate the relative and cumulative impact of ADHD symptoms and non-ADHD psychological test findings on daily functioning in order to plan the most effective interventions.

In sum, as a behavioral diagnosis, ADHD does not call for the routine clinical use of medical or psychological assessment tools that extend beyond the assessment of primary symptoms of ADHD, screening for comorbid conditions, or determination of functional impairment. In a majority of cases, more elaborate assessments result in a waste of precious family resources, a delay in effective treatment, and the loss of availability of clinical resources to others who need them. Nevertheless, more intensive assessments are most certainly warranted in specific cases, and they have an important place in research as well. The clinician who sees children with suspected ADHD is well advised to develop a network of potential referral and follow-up assessment options to access when needed.

11. STEP 10: DEVELOP CASE CONCEPTUALIZATION AND RECOMMENDATIONS FOR TREATMENT

The assessment process has multiple goals. On one level, the assessment is intended to result in accurate diagnosis. DSM-IV recognizes three subtypes of ADHD, based on whether at least six of nine inattentive or hyperactive/impulsive symptoms are observed. The *primarily inattentive type* occurs when this threshold is reached for only inattentive items. The *primarily hyperactive/impulsive type* occurs when this threshold is reached for items only in the hyperactivity and impulsivity list. The *combined type* is diagnosed when the "six of nine" threshold is reached for both sets of items. For adolescents and adults who previously displayed full ADHD symptoms but no longer do so, an "*in partial remission*" code may be used. A final code provided in DSM-IV, "ADHD Not Otherwise Specified," is *not* recommended for routine use, because little supportive information is provided in DSM-IV and very little research has been devoted to this code.

The present diagnostic nomenclature, though empirically guided, has limitations. There is some question whether the DSM-IV symptom list, which was based on the behavioral presentation of grade-school children with ADHD, applies well to other age groups (preschool-age, adolescents, and adults) or across gender and ethnic groups *(4,8)*. Moreover, categorical assessments of psychopathology, such as DSM-IV, are vulnerable to criticisms that human behavior shows little sign of such naturally occurring categories, but instead is best viewed in terms of continua *(46)*. Given these limitations, clinical judgment is called on when making diagnoses. Nevertheless, the clinician is cautioned against

> *Case 6*: Eight-year-old Tamicka had a history of poor academic performance, although her parents were fairly certain she was a bright girl. She often stared out the window or fidgeted with objects on her desk during class, and never seemed to be able to complete assignments and homework as quickly as other children. She had begun to dislike school and was labeled by teachers as "lazy" and "unmotivated." After she was appropriately diagnosed with ADHD (inattentive type), she was placed on a stimulant medication and received classroom accommodations, such as preferential seating and extended testing time. The overall goal was to improve her classroom performance, not just her attention. The difference was dramatic. The intellect that her parents had long suspected began to show in strong school grades. In addition to being more attentive, she seemed happier and more confident.

using idiosyncratic standards or criteria that stray from the prevailing nomenclature; doing so hampers communication, may result in frank misdiagnosis, contributes to the community perception of mental health as subjective and biased, and risks misapplication of the results of extensive treatment research.

Accurate diagnosis is often critical to obtaining needed services. Both Section 504 of the Vocational Rehabilitation Act of 1973 (sometimes simplified to "Section 504") and the Individuals with Disabilities Education Act of 1997 contain language that calls for public school accommodations or services for individuals with diagnosed disabilities, and have been widely applied to ADHD when it has been appropriately diagnosed. Accurate diagnosis also facilitates communication among professionals and, at least in theory, provides guidance on the most effective treatments *(40)*.

Nevertheless, the assessment process should not stop with diagnosis. The presenting concerns are often about *functional impairment* and there is increasing recognition that the ultimate goal of treatment is reduction or elimination of functional impairment *(23)*. As such, a key goal of the assessment process is to formulate and summarize impressions on the relationship between primary ADHD symptoms, associated and comorbid conditions, and other medical, environmental, and historical factors in determining current impairment. Assume multiple directions of causality. In even the most "hard-wired genetic case," there will be environmental contingencies that affect the behavioral presentation and degree of impairment. Conversely, one must be careful not to overestimate the effect of the environment on the child; the environment is typically structured to some degree as a response to the child's behaviors.

At this point in the development of the field, the formulation and presentation of a functional assessment of the child's behaviors is a uniquely clinical step in the assessment process, and cannot be guided by actuarial rules or tables. Nevertheless, it is not trivial, as such a formulation can allow for a fundamental reframing of the child's behaviors, with attribution of the impairment shifted away from an unproductive blaming stance to a more useful identification of targets for direct intervention.

The case formulation should be constructed to suggest key points of potential intervention. Although ADHD treatment is often considered synonymous with psychopharmacological treatment, intervention is best viewed as a multifaceted enterprise. In many cases, residual impairment remains even with aggressive medication management *(8)*. This should not be surprising in light of the high degree of comorbidity of ADHD with other syndromes, as well as its associated features (e.g., falling behind in school, poor social skills). As such, treatment should address needs in multiple domains: symptoms at home and at school, comorbid conditions, mood, cognitive and educational skills, adaptive and self-help skills, social skills, family relations, and relations with teachers and other important figures *(47)*.

Chapters 21 and 22 in this volume provide up-to-date information on medication interventions, and many subsequent chapters provide pearls of wisdom on other management strategies. In addition, a number of excellent, empirically driven references are available from leaders in the field, such as Barkley *(8,48)*, DuPaul and Stover *(49)*, and Pelham et al. *(50)* and well-formulated practice parameters have been published by the AAP *(51)*, American Academy of Child and Adolescent Psychiatry *(2)*, Institute for Clinical Systems Improvement *(5)*, and the Natural Institute of Health *(3)*. These publications converge to suggest that certain interventions have demonstrated effectiveness (medications, behavior therapy), whereas others have been discredited or have undergone inadequate research to document effectiveness (e.g., cognitive therapy, play therapy, dietary modifications, chiropractics, biofeedback, sensory integration therapy). A knowledge of the treatment options available, and the research evidence on each, is essential for those who assess children with ADHD. A detailed discussion of interventions for ADHD would extend well beyond the boundaries of this chapter, however, so the reader is referred to the earlier references for further information.

12. CONCLUDING COMMENTS

There is little doubt that, in recent years, ADHD has received more attention in the popular media than has any other mental disorder that affects children. Lay and professional opinions abound and threaten to drown out the well-constructed research that has led to significant advances in the identification, management, and quality of life for the many children who have experienced significant adaptive impairment because of ADHD. Thankfully, recent consensus statements and empirical summaries provide concise, research-grounded recommendations and guidelines. The goal of this chapter was to present one model for the psychological assessment of children with suspected ADHD that is consistent with these consensus statements and summaries. It was intended to provide an overall guide for such assessment, to be used flexibly in a child- and family-friendly manner. Readers are encouraged to adapt the recommendations presented here, as well as assessment models presented by leaders in the field (e.g., refs. *6,8*), with the goal of providing the best care for each child and family who presents in their office.

REFERENCES

1. Barkley RA. Attention deficit hyperactivity disorder. New York: Guilford Press, 1990.
2. American Academy of Child and Adolescent Psychiatry. Practice parameters for the assessment and treatment of children, adolescents, and adults with attention-deficit/hyperactivity disorder. J Am Acad Child Adolesc Psychiatry 1997;36:85S–121S.
3. National Institutes of Health. Diagnosis and treatment of attention deficit hyperactivity disorder (ADHD). NIH Consensus Statement 1998;16:1–37.
4. American Academy of Pediatrics. Clinical practice guideline: diagnosis and evaluation of the child with attention-deficit/hyperactivity disorder. Pediatrics 2000;105:1158–1170.
5. Institute for Clinical Systems Improvement. Health care guideline: diagnosis and management of attention deficit hyperactivity disorder in primary care for school age children and adolescents. Institute for Clinical Systems Improvement, 2003.
6. Sattler JM. Assessment of children: Behavioral and clinical applications (4th ed.). La Mesa, CA: Author published, 2002.
7. Merrell KW. Behavioral, social, and emotional assessment of children and adolescents. Mahwah, NJ: Lawrence Erlbaum Associates, 2003.
8. Barkley RA. Attention-deficit hyperactivity disorder: A handbook for diagnosis and treatment. New York: Guilford Press, 1998.
9. Resnick RJ. The hidden disorder: a clinician's guide to attention deficit hyperactivity disorder in adults. Washington, DC: American Psychological Association, 2000.
10. Goldstein S, Ellison AT. Clinician's guide to adult ADHD. San Diego, CA: Academic Press, 2002.
11. Connor DF. Preschool attention deficit hyperactivity disorder: A review of prevalence, diagnosis, neurobiology, and stimulant treatment. J Dev Behav Pediatrics 2002;23:S1–S9.
12. Shepard BA, Carter AS, Cohen JE. Attention-deficit/hyperactivity disorder and the preschool child. In: Brown T, ed. Attention-deficit disorders and comorbidities in children, adolescents, and adults. Washington, DC: American Psychiatric Publishing, 2000:407–436.
13. McGoey KE, Eckert TL, DuPaul GJ. Early intervention for preschool-age children with ADHD: A literature review. J Emotional Behav Disord 2002;10:14–28.

14. American Psychiatric Association. Diagnostic and statistical manual of mental disorders (4th ed). Washington, DC: American Psychiatric Association, 1994.
15. Rogers R. Handbook of diagnostic and structured interviewing. New York: Guilford Press, 2001.
16. Barkley RA. Defiant children: a clinician's manual for assessment and parent training. New York: Guilford, 1997.
17. Volpe RJ, DuPaul GJ. Assessment with brief behavior rating scales. In: Andrews JJW, Saklofske DH, Janzen HL, eds. Handbook of psychoeducational assessment: ability, achievement, and behavior in children. San Diego, CA: Academic Press, 2001:357–387.
18. Reitman D, Hummel R, Franz DZ, Gross AM. A review of methods and instruments for assessing externalizing disorders: theoretical and practical considerations in rendering a diagnosis. Clin Psychol Rev 1998;18:555–584.
19. DuPaul GJ, Power TJ, Anastopoulos AD, Reid R. ADHD rating scale—IV: checklists, norms, and clinical interpretation. New York: Guilford, 1998.
20. Reynolds CR, Kamphaus RW. BASC—behavioral assessment system for children manual. Circle Pines, MN: American Guidance Service, 1992.
21. Achenbach TM. Integrative Guide for the 1991 CBCL/4–18, YSR, and TRF profiles. Burlington, VT: University of Vermont Department of Psychiatry, 1991.
22. Conners C. Conners' rating scales revised. North Tonawanda, NY: Multi-Health Systems, 1997.
23. Pelham W. Attention deficit hyperactivity disorder: diagnosis, assessment, nature, etiology, and treatment: Unpublished manuscript, 2002.
24. Suzuki LA, Ponterotto JG, Meller PJ. Handbook of multicultural assessment: clinical, psychological, and educational applications. San Francisco, CA: Jossey-Bass/Wiley, 2001.
25. Reid R. Assessment of ADHD with culturally different groups: The use of behavioral rating scales. Sch Psychol Revi 1995;24:537–560.
26. Lahey BB, Miller TL, Gordon RA, Riley AQ. Developmental epidemiology of the disruptive behavior disorders. In: Quay HC, Hogan AE, eds. Handbook of disruptive behavior disorders. New York: Klewer Academic/Plenum Publishers, 1999:23–48.
27. Reid R, Casat CD, Norton HJ, Anastopoulos AD, Temple EP. Using behavior rating scales for ADHD across ethnic groups: The IOWA Conners. J Emotional Behav Disord 2001;9:210–218.
28. Reid R, DuPaul GJ, Power TJ, et al. Assessing culturally different students for attention deficit hyperactivity disorder using behavior rating scales. J Abnorm Child Psychol 1998; 26:187–198.
29. Barkley RA. Attention-deficit hyperactivity disorder. In: Mash EJ, Barkley RA, eds. Child psychopathology. New York: Guilford Press, 2003:75–143.
30. MTA Cooperative Group. A 14-month randomized clinical trial of treatment strategies for attention-deficit/hyperactivity disorder. Archi Gen Psychiatry 1999;56:1073–1086.
31. Gioia GA, Isquith PK, Guy SC, Kenworthy L. BRIEF—Behavior rating inventory of executive function. Odessa, FL: Psychological Assessment Resources, 2000.
32. Gresham F, Elliott S. Social skills rating system. Circle Pines, MN: American Guidance Systems, 1990.
33. Frauenglass S, Routh DK. Assessment of the disruptive behavior disorders: Dimensional and categorical approaches. In: Quay HC, Hogan AE, eds. Handbook of disruptive behavior disorders. New York: Kluwer Academic/Plenum Publishers, 1999:49–71.
34. O'Brien LM, Ivanenko A, Crabtree VM, et al. Sleep Disturbances in children with attention deficit hyperactivity disorder. Pediatr Res 2003;54:237–243.
35. O'Brien LM, Holbrook CR, Mervis CB, et al. Sleep and neurobehavioral characteristics of 5- to 7-year-old children with parentally reported symptoms of attention-deficit/hyperactivity disorder. Pediatrics 2003;111:554–563.
36. Corkum P, Tannock R, Moldofsky H. Sleep disturbances in children with attention-deficit/hyperactivity disorder. J Am Acad Child Adolesc Psychiatry 1998;37:637–646.
37. Frazier JA, Biederman J, Bellordre CA, et al. Should the diagnosis of attention-deficit/hyperactivity disorder be considered in children with pervasive developmental disorder? J Attention Disord 2001;4:203–211.

38. Klin A, Volkmar FR, Sparrow SS. Asperger syndrome. New York: Guilford Press, 2000.
39. Beebe D, Risi S. Treatment of adolescents and young adults with high-functioning autism and Asperger syndrome. In: Reinecke MA, Dattilio FM, Freeman A, eds. Cognitive therapy with children and adolescents: a casebook for clinical practice. New York: Guilford Press, 2003: 369–401.
40. Scotti JR, Morris TL. Diagnosis and classification. In: Hersen M, Ammerman RT, eds. Advanced abnormal child psychology (2nd ed). Mahwah, NJ: Lawrence Erlbaum Associates, 2000:15–32.
41. Barkley RA, DuPaul GJ, McMurray MB. Comprehensive evaluation of attention deficit disorder with and without hyperactivity as defined by research criteria. J Consult Clini Psychol 1990; 58:775–789.
42. Mori LT, Armendariz GM. Analogue assessment of child behavior problems. Psychol Assess 2001;13:36–45.
43. American Psychological Association. Ethical principles of psychologists and code of conduct. Am Psychologist 2002;57:1060–1073.
44. Agency for Health Care Policy and Research. Diagnosis of attention deficit/hyperactivity disorder: technical review 3. Rockville, MD: U.S. Department of Health and Human Services, Agency for Health Care Policy and Research, 1999.
45. Reinecke MA, Beebe DW, Stein MA. The third factor of the WISC-III: it's (probably) not freedom from distractibility. J Am Acad Child Adolesc Psychiatry 1999;38:322–328.
46. Achenbach TM. Assessment of psychopathology. In: Sameroff AJ, Lewis M, Miller SM, eds. Handbook of developmental psychopathology (2nd ed.). New York: Kluwer Academic/Plenum Publishing, 2000:41–56.
47. Casat CD, Pearson DA, Casat JP. Attention-deficit/hyperactivity disorder. In: Vance HB, Pumariega A, eds. Clincial assessment of child and adolescent behavior. New York: John Wiley and Sons, 2001:263–306.
48. Barkley RA. Taking charge of ADHD, revised edition: the complete, authoritative guide for parents. New York: Guilford Press, 2000.
49. DuPaul GJ, Stoner G. ADHD in the schools: assessment and intervention strategies. New York: Guilford Press, 2003.
50. Pelham W, Wheeler T, Chronis A. Empirically supported psychosocial treatments for ADHD. J Child Clin Psychol 1998;27:190–205.
51. American Academy of Pediatrics. Clinical practice guideline: treatment of the school-aged child with attention-deficit/hyperactivity disorder. Pediatrics 2001;108:1033–1044.
52. American Academy of Child and Adolescent Psychiatry. Practice parameters for the assessment and treatment of children and adolescents with bipolar disorder. J Am Acad Child Adolesc Psychiatry 1997;36:157S–76S.
53. American Academy of Child and Adolescent Psychiatry. Practice parameters for the assessment and treatment of children and adolescents with anxiety disorders. J Am Acad Child Adolesc Psychiatry 1997;36:69S–84S.
54. American Academy of Child and Adolescent Psychiatry. Practice parameters for the assessment and treatment of children and adolescents with substance use disorders. J Am Acad Child Adolesc Psychiatry 1997;36:140S–56S.
55. American Academy of Child and Adolescent Psychiatry. Practice parameters for the assessment and treatment of children and adolescents with conduct disorder. J Am Acad Child Adolesc Psychiatry 1997;36:1225–1395.

8
Executive Function

Martha Bridge Denckla

1. INTRODUCTION: SCOPE AND AIMS

It is not the purpose of this chapter to instruct the reader on the topic of attention deficit hyperactivity disorder (ADHD) in general behavioral terms, to review evidence for the neurobiological nature thereof, or to analyze ADHD in terms of models of cognitive neuropsychology; these matters may be reviewed by the reader in this volume, as well as some recent publications *(1–3)*. Resolutely atheoretical, this chapter aims to set forth many questions (but few answers) on the limited (yet multifaceted) issues, important both for research studies and clinical evaluations, connecting the domain of executive function (EF) and/or certain deficits thereof, executive dysfunction (EDF), with the diagnosis of any subtype of ADHD.

At once the reader must want to know why this is important for research, for clinical evaluation, or for both. It is because the implication of EDF with the diagnostic entities subsumed under the term ADHD (a term already superbly critiqued by Russell Barkley in many publications) *(4,5)* provides at least three directions toward clinical and scientific understanding of ADHD and, reciprocally, at least one useful dimension (the fourth dimension—time—as in development) that clarifies the nonunitary nature of EF. The three directions in which EDF clarifies ADHD are:

1. EDF provides information about issues of subtypes, gender, and adult "false negatives" or misunderstandings generated by the historical interview or "ratings" approaches to diagnosis.
2. EDF goes far to explain ADHD as comorbid with learning disorders (LD), both as a complicating/exacerbating factor, as well as "on its own" an increasing-over-time reason for academic underachievement, vocation failure/fading, and social maladjustment that increases with life's demands for self-control/independence.
3. EDF anchors ADHD in the brain, and not exclusively in the frontal lobes (in contradistinction to Sergeant et al. *[6]*, thanks to two decades of literature expanding the EF domain to more than one regional partner in a frontal-subcortical circuit *[7]* and to a decade of neuroimaging research revealing cerebellar and striatal structural deficits in children with ADHD *[8,9]*).

What is the reciprocal of the elucidation of EF/EDF through studying the domain/deficit in association with ADHD? The advantage of experience with this association is that afforded by observations and measurements of a fairly common developmental disorder, by no means neurologically homogeneous, elucidating in developmental progression those components of EF that emerge in early childhood, late childhood, adolescence, and young adulthood. Such a perspective is not only empirical but also brain-driven, sensitive to the developmental

From: *Attention Deficit Hyperactivity Disorder: From Genes to Patients*
Edited by: D. Gozal and D. L. Molfese © Humana Press Inc., Totowa, NJ

unfolding of brain–environment/nature–nurture mutuality and interdependency. The neurodevelopmental perspective helps to throw off the tyranny of theory-derived terms such as the "central executive" while substituting for such a "mystery cloaked in an enigma" a dynamic definition in which complexity arises from connecting, integrating, and reinforcing earlier-established components rather than a static reductionism to theoretically proposed diagrams.

The developmental perspective also puts into the spotlight, via a neurological "systems/circuits" analysis, the close scrutiny of motor control (MC). Unlike Barkley *(2)*, who subsumes MC under "cognitive" aspects of ADHD, and unlike the many clinicians who set aside MC as another comorbidity (the Diagnostic and Statistical Manual of Mental Disorders, 4th ed. [DSM-IV]), developmental motor coordination disorder (DMCD) is curiously frequent, on the order of LD; the neurologist who is also a developmental neuropsychologist has historically appreciated the parallel developmental status of MC and cognitive control, even in the 1970s diagnostic "dark ages" when hyperactivity or hyperkinesis rather than attention deficit demarcated disorders involving self-control *(10,11)*. An entity called minimal brain dysfunction (MBD) at that time (mid-1960s to 1980) encompassed what we now refer to as ADHD, LD, and DMCD (and more); recent reincarnation as the Swedish category titled developmental attention, motor, and perception disorder (or DAMP *[12]*, which may be thought of as overlapping with a Canadian "cousin" called nonverbal learning disabilities, NLD *[13]*). Because the terminology of the DSM-IV *(14)* in general and of ADHD in particular did not enter usage until or after 1980, it may be useful to review how the characteristics of hyperactivity (subsumed under MBD) *(10)* came to have relevance to cognitive issues then thought to underlie learning disabilities, such as dyslexia, then also thought to overlap with MBD (except for the rarer purely genetic or familial developmental dyslexia). The basic assumption of the MBD label was that for educational purposes, once one's IQ was deemed adequate, one needed to dichotomize "organic" (i.e., brain-based) from "emotional" (i.e., psychodynamic) reasons for academic failure. In at least one state—New Jersey—there were special classes for the neurologically impaired, distinct from classes for the mentally retarded; because MBD (with at least average intelligence documented) provided the eligibility for such classes, neurologists became involved in making the diagnosis for admission to such classes even prior to Law 94–142 *(15)*, which broadened special education. Because the examination of basic movement capabilities, disappearance of primitive reflexes, and appearance of age-appropriate motor coordination attainments was (and remains) the core of developmental neurology, the diagnosis of MBD leaned heavily on such indicators of "organicity" or (more colloquially) "brain maturity at risk here" and is not limited to "brain damage." Little by little, pediatricians and neurologists joined forces to create standard, structured, and/or semiquantitative motor evaluations; out of these grew a distinction between abnormalities of MC (strength, tone, reflexes, and certain qualitative types of incoordination or involuntary movements) and developmental "delays," or immaturities *(16–19)*. It remains unknown to this day whether the developmental delays, either all of them or some of them, eventually disappear with maturation; alternatively, as is known with mental retardation, what looks like delay in childhood might hit a plateau that, while subtle, represents a lifelong deficiency. The subtle nature of all the motor signs, both classic and developmental, used in the diagnosis of MBD meant that in reality daily life was not prominently impaired (nothing as severe as a direct consequence of cerebral palsy was the impact) but eligibility for special classes was conferred by means of the implications of the motor signs with respect to "brain factors at risk here." (There were direct consequences—often poor handwriting, sometimes poor athletic skills—but these were viewed as peripheral issues complicating but not interacting with the brain-based cognitive deficits indirectly "certified" by the motor signs.) Thus there was a clinical pragmatic rationale of close scrutiny of the motor system in children referred to pediatricians (some of whom began to specialize as developmental pediatricians) and child neurologists, motivated by services directed at educational (and presumably cognitive) impairment (Table 1). This clinical–pragmatic situation inspired some academic neurologists to design and study, as researchers, relatively brief and portable quantified motor coordination examinations such as that which evolved into the Physical and Neurological Examination for Subtle Signs (PANESS) *(19–21)*. Such examination data began to find its way into research, because educationally oriented studies of cognitive factors underlying reading failure began to demand more precise delineation of the subject characteristics of the populations of "poor" vs "adequate" readers. It was then, long before EF or even "frontal lobe functions" had become the focus of concern for developmental neuropsychology, that the MC status of some "poor readers" began to suggest to neurologically trained researchers (PhD as well as MD in their credentials) that here there was a marker for cognitive control circuit. Some motor signs suggested subcortical anomalies of development (basal ganglia or cerebellum), whereas other signs suggested frontal inadequacies *(10)*. Progressing from "smoke" to "fire," neurologically oriented researchers inferred from signs of impaired MC that adjacent cognitive control circuits might be powerfully interactive with more conventionally emphasized cognitive systems, such as language, perception, and widely distributed attentional components *(22)*.

All of the "smoke to fire" train of thought converged with the flowering of interest in frontal-lobe functions inspired after the official adoption of ADHD as a diagnosis *(14)* that placed cognition in the spotlight and all but buried MBD. Although some child psychiatrists continue to talk about (and treat for) hyperactivity as a "behavioral" issue completely separated from cognition or educational disability and some researchers focused on LD continue (largely through misunderstanding of the ADHD syndrome) to deny that ADHD implies any cognitive component relevant to education, for the most part there has been an appreciation of the complexity of the "frontal" system with respect to behavioral self-control, cognitive control, and (overlapping at the edges) MC. Thus, although given its own diagnostic code number and named DMCD, MC remains a clinical and conceptually useful neighbor to ADHD. (Barkley, in his influential and conceptually profound 1997 book *ADHD and the Nature of Self-Control [4]*, cites research on motor control as among the strongest influences on his formulation of the EFs developing out of the basic inhibitory control function.) When this chapter turns to a review of functional magnetic resonance imaging as a source of clarification of the association of EDF with ADHD, the MC component will gain renaissance status.

2. CLINICAL APPROACHES AND USES OF EF IN THE DIAGNOSIS AND TREATMENT OF PATIENTS WITH ADHD

Since the 1980s, clinicians desiring to add direct testing for ADHD to the established diagnostic methods of history-taking, structured interview, and questionnaires/rating scales (increasingly computer-scored) have followed one or both of the following two paths:

1. Attempts to operationalize the leading word "attention" in a variety of continuous performance tests and related attentional challenges.
2. Attempts to transfer from adult neuropsychology tests/tasks reputed to probe the integrity of "frontal" systems.

Table 1
Motor System Signs as Parallels to Executive Function and/or ADHD, From MBD to DAMP

First author	Reference in this chapter	Age range in years	Signs	Statistics
Touwen, 1977	*16*	4–14	Many	No
Camp, 1978	*18*	6–12	Many	Yes
Denckla, 1978	*10*	6–12	Many	No
Denckla, 1978	*11*	6–11	Overflow	Yes
Nichols, 1981	*22*	1–7	Hop, line walk	Yes
Wolff, 1985	*17*	6–12	Choreiform movements	Yes
Rasmussen, 2000	*12*	4–22	Many	Yes

When dealing with children, of course, developmental concerns were bound to arise, so customized "child-friendly" and child-normed versions began in research and gradually (usually despite contradictions between research findings) were picked up and used in clinical settings. Broadly speaking, the continuous performance tests (CPTs) have not provided the direct evidence, the desired confirmation, or probabilistic exclusion of the diagnosis of ADHD that had been hoped would emerge *(5,6)*. The best of the CPTs have provided limited evidence, but only with certain designs, for inhibitory "no-go" deficits *(23)* or for slow and variable reaction times *(24,25)*. Rather than confirming deficits of attention, most CPTs appeared to redirect clinicians' and researchers' attention to output-linked issues of response inhibition and response preparation.

Beyond generating a pragmatic reason for examining cognition and motor function, clinical experiences have been great hypothesis generators for research. The surprising inadequacy of measures purporting to assess diagnostically relevant attention in ADHD candidates and the unanticipated reliability of measures of response preparation/response inhibition strengthened the conviction of clinicians that the interface between cognition and action, the executive control system, must be assessed. Not until recently, however, owing to the work of the Delis–Kaplan team, has there been available to clinicians the widely normed, psychometrically sound EF measures applicable to children; the California Verbal Learning Test—Children's Version® (CVLT-C) *(26)*, as well as the Delis–Kaplan Executive Function System™ (D-KEFS) *(27)* should be included in this category.

Meanwhile, the clinician attempting to assess perceptual and memory functions stumbled repeatedly and was taken by surprise when executive task demands of presumably otherwise-constructed tasks interfered with taking these at face value. First to fall under the suspicion of susceptibility to EF "masking" was the Benton Visual Retention Test, Multiple Choice Form BVRT-mc *(28)*. As perfectly summarized by Frank Woods, the BVRT-mc requires "careful looking and reflective responding" (personal communication with Frank Wood, 2003). Longitudinal clinical experience furthermore revealed that children who performed miserably on their first or even second encounter with the BVRT-mc would usually perform quite well or even leap forward into superiority at a later "double digit" age (10 or more years old). The "lag-and-leap" group often did well at all ages, whether contemporaneously with failure or success on BVRT-mc, on the Wechsler Intelligence Scale for Children (WISC) Block Design, and in "real-world" visuospatial/visuomnemonic attainments. The clinician began to notice, on the other hand, that the observable failure of "careful looking and reflective responding" *(28)* on the BVRT-mc occurred in children referred to clinic for probable ADHD; this began the private suspicion that for clinical purposes BVRT-mc might well be renamed the "Benton Visual Attention Test."

Next on the "entry requirement for EF" reanalysis list was another Benton laboratory test, the Judgment of Line Orientation Test (JLO) *(29)*. If asked quickly in the corridor of a professional meeting what/where the JLO assesses, most neuropsychologists say almost reflexively "visuospatial ability/right parietal lobe." The exceptions to this reflex answer prove extraordinarily helpful to the developmental neuropsychologist; namely, those who study patients with Parkinson's disease will tell the inquirer that because of "task demands," not visuospatial deficit, their adult patients deal poorly with JLO. This minority report on the construct validity of JLO was very helpful to developmental clinicians who found, as with the BVRT-mc, that some patients whose WISC Block Design (and, by history, puzzle and block-building prowess) seemed to indicate robust visuospatial capacities, were falling down on JLO performance. The analogy to a "subcortically dysexecutive" group's troubles coping with JLO powerfully motivated a reanalysis of task demands on JLO, taking note along the way of its peculiar format (not at all similar to the multiple choice format experienced by school children); researchers were suddenly struck by the leading word, "judgment," in the name of the test. As in the case of the BVRT-mc, longitudinal clinical experience (of a duration rarely afforded by research studies) elucidated a kind of "task demand threshold effect," i.e., the developmental attainment of a certain level of EF sufficient to allow visuospatial perception to emerge as that which JLO then in fact measured. It could then be inferred that a critical threshold for necessary and sufficient "judgment" must be reached developmentally in order for the task to permit "line orientation" as a spatial–cognitive factor to be revealed. (As an important fringe benefit of this clinical experience with ADHD-bearing-EDF impact on JLO, research focused on NLD *[13]* has been facilitated, because JLO is so often a research task thought to probe visuospatial perception as a domain of central importance to NLD). From a strictly clinical, differential diagnostic point of view, affording what researchers call "specificity," only those learning-disabled children under the age of 10 who did beautifully on BVRT-mc and JLO were entirely free of signs or symptoms of ADHD.

Another clinically derived set of observations helpful in the emerging awareness of EDF came from inspection of many WISC profile discrepancies between scaled scores on Block Design (model provided) and Object Assembly (internal model and/or label required). This pattern had long been taken into account when educational psychologists' reports commented on the examinee's "organization." A little more probing is needed in order to derive from Digit Span the age-related "pass/fail" relationship between digits forward and digits backward. Pennington and Ozonoff were among the first to use digits backward as an exemplar of working memory, if considered in relation to the limit set by digits forward *(30)*. (There is an ancient set of papers affiliating digits forward with left- and digits backward with right-hemisphere integrity; a right frontal affiliation for digits backward would be interesting in association with recent similar structural imaging findings in children with ADHD.)

The concept of discrepancies between pairs of tests or scores on the same test (such as the Stroop Color–Word Interference Test attempts) turns out to be clinically useful. In the clinic, a child with ADHD often shows an EDF profile like the following:

1. A normal Beery-Buktenica Visual-Motor Integration Test *(28)* score is coupled with a discrepantly poor-for-age copy of the Rey-Osterreith Complex Figure *(31)*.
2. Semantic category Word Fluency is easily performed at a securely normal acceptable level, whereas Controlled Word Association, its more rule-governed (and filtering-requiring) partner, is poorly performed and, at most, barely within normal limits *(32)*.

It is thus viewed within each pair of tests that the one requiring more EF (working memory, inhibition, planning, organization) reveals the difficulties of the child with ADHD.

More surprising still is the clinical finding that, within a test composed of a set of developmentally graded subtests, restoration to the testing of the kindergarten subtest increases the difficulty for the child with ADHD. This was observed within the several pages of a Cancellation test *(33)*; the child with ADHD, now at least 7 yr old, failed miserably *not* on the pages of "search and circle" involving a numerical or alphabetical target, but rather on the kindergarten page of shapes (with a target diamond). Repeatedly, the child who has formed and used the habit of scanning and marking alphanumeric symbols in school but has left shapes far in the past fails to mount a search strategy when confronted with stimuli that are no longer habitually encountered. Tannock *(34)* found a similar phenomenon with the color-naming component of the Rapid Automatized Naming Test (RAN); children with ADHD but good at reading named alphanumeric symbols at age-expected speeds, confirming the RAN relationship with fluent reading *(35)*, but failed to come up to speed on the kindergarten reading-prediction subtest of color-naming. As with the cancellation task profile, on the RAN it is "remotely used, non-habitual, re-experienced-as-novel" stimuli that successfully demonstrate the very basic EF deficit of response preparation in children with ADHD.

In recent years, the availability of the CVLT-C *(26)* has added to the clinician's repertoire a psychometrically sound instrument within which can be probed the discrepancy between "what" is the status of memory functions and "how" memorization as a process unmasks EDF. Particularly when children with ADHD are verbally gifted, their Level of Recall scores may be superior but their Semantic Cluster Ratio scores may be far inferior to the mean for peers. Less obvious but also clinically useful (again, particularly when verbal abilities are otherwise unimpeachable) is the repetitiousness (erroneously labeled "perseverations") within each recall trial; it is probably an indication of verbal working memory in the "central executive" sense, although an alternative interpretation would be that faulty self-monitoring could cause excessive self-repetition. In either interpretation, the *z*-scores for this kind of error document one aspect of EDF in association with ADHD.

Filling in the gap between traditionally "mental-health-derived" questionnaire ratings and direct (but of necessity limited-sample) examinations of EF is the Behavioral Ratings Inventory of Executive Functions (BRIEF) *(36)*. Similar in computer-scored graphic display, also in the parent and teacher forms, to the Conners traditional type *(40)*, the BRIEF surveys age-related, real-life self-control in daily activities. For a review of the BRIEF, the reader is referred to ref. *37*.

Before leaving the section of this chapter devoted to clinical evaluation of executive function, the following two important topics remain:

1. The "inhibitory insufficiency" summary score.
2. The very common confounding factor of language disorder, language-based LD, or more circumscribed still, dyslexia (as currently understood).

As exemplified by Barkley, *(2,4)* contemporary understanding of ADHD and the pharmacological stimulant treatment thereof leans heavily on the concept of inhibitory insufficiency as either *a* or *the* fundamental neurological deficit of ADHD. It is therefore of great importance to take note and list during clinical evaluation those occurrences or errors indicative of deficient inhibition. For school-aged children between 6 and 14 yr of age, there are, conveniently, observable "milestones" of the disappearance of movement spreading beyond the neuromuscular target of intended movement; these are "overflow movements," occurring cortically either adjacent to or contralateral to primary movements (contralateral overflow is called "mirror movement"). Normal up to a certain age within a certain topography, adjacent spread (e.g., feet to hands) cortically disappearing before contralateral spread (mirroring of finger sequences) does, cortical overflow is not consciously experienced or dysfunctional. (Most observers of young children are familiar with the "workings" of a protruding tongue accompanying the laborious procedural learning of pencil control for letter formation; this is an example within left motor association cortex of adjacent spread from graphomotor to tongue region.) Knowledge of "inhibitory milestones" observable at 6, 10, and 14 yr of age gives the evaluator power to observe an EF component without necessitating conscious/engaged cooperation of the examinee. Clinical experience shows that such observable inhibitory insufficiency is more reliable than commission errors on CPTs (and more "consumer-friendly" in children's views) as documentation of this clinical EDF in ADHD. Other signs of deficient inhibition are there for the observant evaluator, ready for noting. On any multiple-choice format task, "leap before you look" at all choices is a common-sense instantiation of cognitive impulsivity. Already mentioned above is the particularly useful BVRT-mc, wherein the sample is in working memory and the match to sample therefore stresses "reflective responding." The Boston Naming Test *(28)* tempts the verbally gifted but ADHD examinee to give many "*x*, no *y*" impulsive responses. By giving a "first correct answer (*x*)" divided by the ultimate self-generated correct answer (*y*) score, the evaluator can document inhibitory insufficiency (also interpretable as "thinking out loud" or failing to "put brain in gear before moving mouth"). On two other verbal measures, Controlled Word Association Test of Fluency and CVLT-C, there are off-task words to be noted—"rule-breaks" and "intrusions." On the word fluency task, proper nouns or multiple grammatical transforms of the same root word constitute "rule-breaks," and whereas low productivity *per se* may be the milder version of an ADHD EDF sign, in many younger (or severe) cases of ADHD deviations from the rules are overtly spoken. CVLT-C intrusions, especially when occurring on uncued trials (*see* following paragraph for *caveat* about cued trials) indicate names of items "retrieved" from sources other than the list to be learned and thus resemble "*x*, no *y*" responses on the Boston Naming Test.

The previous sections have frequently mentioned "verbally adequate" or "verbally gifted" persons with ADHD; it cannot have escaped the notice of the reader that much of the clinical evaluation targeting EDF involves verbal tasks. The developmental clinician, however, is often seriously challenged by the need to find evidence of ADHD/EDF in children with some cognitive limitation in that spectrum of "language-based learning disabilities" that encompasses at its severe end mixed spoken language disorder ("mixed" referring to receptive and expressive) all the way over to the subtle end represented by "pure" dyslexia, conceived of as a phonological-level disorder (yet still involving some nonreading expressive spoken issues). The comorbidity of ADHD and some language impairment is considered to anywhere from 20 to 35% *(38)*, but in clinical practice it probably runs higher (because all clinics see more comorbidity than is epidemiologically documented). Under circumstances of linguistic inadequacy, even of the subtle "phonological" type, there is the possibility that discrepancies cannot be interpreted with confidence as evidence of EDF. Digits backward depend on capacity for digits forward *(30)*, so lack of discrepancy makes EDF a moot point. Repetitiousness (so-called "perseverations") on the CVLT-C may reflect the "phonological loop" (a "slave system" to the "central executive" within that model of working memory) *(39)*. Cued intrusions on CVLT-C can mean the same EDF-inhibitory deficit as do free-recall intrusions but, when solo, suggest the overly categorical paraphasia-in-kind characteristic of word-retrieval (classically "dysnomic") deficiency. Cluster ratios become deceptive when there is a low denominator, thus failing to distinguish the high-categorical/low specific recall of the language impaired from normal EF (strategy). When there is true comorbidity, it is to the developmental motor evaluation and to the multiple-choice perceptual or perceptual-memory observations that we must turn for the EDF falling outside the verbally-mediated subdomain of presumptive EF tasks. Sometimes the absence of nonverbal EDF helps to clarify not comorbidity but pseudo-ADHD, especially of the "predominantly inattentive type." (Even the mental health-derived Conners Scales *(40)* include an ambiguous amalgamated dimensional T-score for "Cognitive Problems/Inattention," and one extreme school of thought considers the Inattentive type of ADHD likely to be some totally alien processing disorder, presumably more akin to an LD *(2)*. In short, the comorbid presence of language deficits, even subtle ones limited to "phonology," and ADHD can reduce the number of interpretable discrepancy-derived inferences as to EDF; but the absence of motor- or multiple choice–nonverbal issues in a case that by history seems typical of "inattentive type" ADHD can suggest that ADHD is not truly an issue in the case. (Whether or not stimulant pharmacotherapy helps is not at all diagnostic of the presence/absence of ADHD.)

Some nuances help to clarify the LLD/ADHD confound, especially with respect to those developmentally sensitive task sets, Cancellation *(33)* and RAN *(35)*. The pseudo-ADHD/LLD cases perform developmentally, not (as noted for ADHD) stressed by "ancient, no longer habitual" subtest but dealing expeditiously with target-search for shapes and naming colors quickly enough while slowing down for number-search/number-naming and slower still in responses to alphabet letters. Habit and practice do not facilitate fluent automaticity in those whose language circuitry for "see it/say it" is presumably biologically weak.

An interesting reverse diagnostic issue is seen when young fluent readers with ADHD who show mastery of both use-of-phonics in their decoding and sight words "fail" for age/grade on tests of phonological awareness. This paradox is again easily understood by referring back to the Cancellation and RAN profiles. (Kindergarten is long past.) Even more important is to extract the principle that executive demands loom large in any task named "awareness" or "judgment" (as in JLO, *see* earlier discussion).

3. MORE USEFUL EXTENSIONS OF CLINICAL EDF EVALUATIONS

The issue (reciprocal in some overlaps) of pseudo-ADHD manifested with language deficits (and the source of ambiguity owing to comorbidity, or ADHD/LLD moot points) enhances the value of careful clinical documentation of EDF in cases of suspected ADHD. In very bright children, older adolescents or young adults, and in girls or women at most ages, revelations of underlying neurobiology clarifying the meaning of ADHD as a brain-based developmental disorder are forthcoming. Authorities on ADHD recognize the shortcomings of the historical approach, skillfully multifaceted and compounded as it is of structured interview, questionnaires, ratings, and so forth *(2,41,42)*. Research has not yet caught up with the richness of clinical EDF data (*see* later discussion), so the clinician must be humble and tentative while conveying the impressions of decades. Longitudinal clinical follow-up is very illuminating when bright youngsters with suspected ADHD return every year or two and repeatedly copy the Rey–Osterreith Complex Figure in the same hodgepodge disorganized fashion; because feedback/correction is never given, the "natural" state of EDF continues unaltered. The same child who passes the more structured in-a-box Beery Buktenica Visual Motor Integration test at ages below "teens" where the designs are predominantly familiar practiced shapes, returns as a young teenager to fail at the plan-requiring and more stop–restart-requiring items toward the 13-yr, 8-mo "ceiling" level of the test.

Table 2
Specificity to ADHD of Executive Dysfunction

First author	Year	Reference this chapter	Contrasting disorders	Which EF task(s) show ADHD specificity?
Pennington	1993	*38*	Reading disability	TOH
Pennington	1996	*30*	Autism, Tourette's syndrome[a]	Stroop
Schuerholz	1996	*54*	Tourette's syndrome ± ADHD	Go/no-go
Ozonoff	1999	*55*	Autism, Tourette's syndrome[a]	Stroop
Tannock	2000	*34*	Reading disability	Color Rapid Naming[b]
Sergeant	2002	*6*	Review, all of above plus oppositional defiant and conduct disorders	Not consistent across studies: best SSRT

[a]No subdivision by ± ADHD, unlike Schuerholz et al., 1996.
[b]Tannock may explain and reduce significance of Stroop.
TOH, Tower of Hanoi, SSRT, stop-signal reaction time.

The youngster whose raw power of verbal memory saw him through earlier encounters with the CVLT-C (albeit with diagnostically dysexecutive low semantic closer ratios) becomes a teenager who no longer can equal his peers even in level of recall because peers (but not our person with ADHD) strategically enhance their memorization to recall far more items. The examination for EF reveals over time the developmental lag (in some cases, the plateau) associated with ADHD, such that although mental health-generated severity ratings may appear to moderate toward normal, especially with respect to hyperactivity, the cognitive correlate of ADHD, the EDF, appears increasingly prominent. In other words, as the normal developmental progress toward independent life leaps forward, the dysexecutive person with ADHD seems more clearly left behind. The nature of the disorder is clarified and the importance of making or retaining the diagnosis is demonstrated; otherwise the person is liable to be the recipient of teachers' (or parents') epithets, such as "irresponsible," "lazy," and "unmotivated" (*see* Table 2).

Girls and women with ADHD are even more likely to be misunderstood and to develop secondary reactive emotional problems than those of the male gender *(42)*. There is no folk saying equivalent to "boys will be boys" and, although the considerable feminine sensitivity to social rewards tends to modulate all but the most severely affected girls toward social acceptability (so that they are less often seen as young children to be significantly hyperactive or outwardly impulsive), by mid-childhood, around late third grade, girls may slide both academically and socially. Removal of structure and feedback at short intervals reveals such girls to have problems with the "how" and "when" essential elements of EF; yet even when meeting criteria for "inattentive type," some impulsive elements are present in the profiles of girls with ADHD (such as interrupting social conversations and blurting out answers without raising a hand to be called on in school). The impulsivity items do not often rise to the number or severity necessary to reach the threshold for a full-syndrome diagnosis, yet the impact of ADHD is insidiously undermining these girls' adaptive adjustment.

Women with ADHD often present themselves on referral from mental health facilities, where the comorbidities of anxiety or depression have been under treatment and necessarily preempt the focus of concern. Often the underlying and still-symptomatic ADHD is masked and all-but-impossible to differentiate from the comorbidities unless detailed neuropsychological assessment probes for LD and EDF. (Clinical experience highlights the executive demands of running a household, as well as the unabated societal expectation that women manage and organize family life; as with girls, women with ADHD of mild-to-moderate severity meet with far less tolerance or sympathy than do men with a similar condition *(41,42)*. The direct clinical evaluation of EF is more helpful with girls than with women, because of the unfortunate confound represented by the cognitive impact of the comorbid anxiety or depression. This cognitive impact is often substantial with the EF domain. (A major gap in the clinician's fund of knowledge is the specificity factor; it is unknown whether the profile of EDF is differentially structured by ADHD, anxiety, and/or by depression.)

4. HOW USEFUL ARE PUBLISHED PSYCHOMETRIC "BATTERIES" OF EF? (*SEE* TABLE 3)

The Neuropsychological Examination for Young Children (NEPSY™) *(32)* is a battery for children (ages 4–12 yr) within which the Attention/EF Domain consists of tasks whose selection was guided by published literature, some clinical and some with research designs, supporting discriminative power with respect to certain syndromes (ADHD foremost among these) and localized injuries (frontal lobe) *(43)*. Although the NEPSY also encompasses a domain called Sensorimotor Functions, there is little evidence that the relationships between this domain and that of Attention/EFs have been overtly utilized in the interpretation chapter of the manual; rather, as in the days of MBD, the Sensorimotor domain is justified on the basis of its subtests serving as "markers of normal development or as indicators of atypical development." (NEPSY Manual) The validity chapter of the NEPSY does indeed indicate that children with ADHD are significantly handicapped on most of the Attention/EF subtests but no more so than on the Language Domain subtests, and only marginally more so than on the Sensorimotor Domain subtests, especially "tactile localization." This profile resembles what has already earlier been emphasized, namely, EF enters into many test scores not directly aimed at probing EF. From a clinical perspective, however, the manual (p. 218) points out that "impaired performance in individual children was relatively low," so that group data was not mirrored by clinical diagnostic data. A "profile analysis approach," recommended at the conclusion of the chapter on validity, is not implemented with a diagnostic orientation, as explicitly voiced (p. 237) in the chapter on interpretation.

With respect to fulfilling diagnostic criteria, ADHD is not addressed by the NEPSY *per se*. A critique of the interpretation offered for the Attention/EFs Domain is that the manual does not offer guidance with respect to contrasts or covariates of the executive demands, except for a hierarchical approach to the "more basic" (presumed to be attentional) and successively "more advanced" (plan, organize, use strategy) elements. There is no appreciation of the reciprocal dilemma of interpretation of EF entering into tasks otherwise named/intended and of the cognitive specifics of tasks, especially when abundantly endowed, obviating the EF demands at younger ages; the NEPSY as a clinical instrument offers almost no guidance as to how to operationalize the within-individual discrepancies that permit clinical inferences about EDF.

The D-KEFS™ *(27)* is a recent addition to the clinical (and possible research) capabilities of the neuropsychologist wishing to address EF/EDF. Entirely on topic, it is applicable to

Table 3
Recent Batteries Inclusive of Executive Function

Test battery	Reference this chapter	Non-EF domains	Age range	Psychometric properties
NEPSY	*32*	Several	4–12	Modest
D-KEFS	*27*	No	8–80	Robust
CANTAB	*47*	Minimal	4–12	Preliminary

only half—the older half—of the NEPSY age range, but it is a welcome addition to the assessment of teenagers and young adults (especially the middle-schoolers often previously omitted from any neuropsychological instrument). The EF probes of D-KEFS are all toward the advanced end of the developmental range of the domain. The clinician using the D-KEFS will be at an advantage if separate probes of the motor domain (NEPSY sensorimotor and/or PANESS) are added onto the D-KEFS and if response preparation, response inhibition, and speed items (which can be extracted from the Process/Efficiency scores) are particularly emphasized. Response Initiation Measures can also be teased out of D-KEFS. The manual (p. 53) provides sophisticated "caveats" about correlations that "can dissociate in the damaged brain … in particular clinical populations."

Pilot studies with children, including the clinical population of some with fetal alcohol syndrome, clarified diagnostic dissociation between baseline conditions (like naming colors and reading words) and EF-increased-demand condition (color-word interference inhibition and inhibition/switching conditions) as critical for EDF interpretation. The D-KEFS is constructed with built-in baseline tasks and "value-added" EF-demand tasks that are content-controlled. Although clinical experience with this system is still in its early days, the prognosis looks bright/good with respect to the D-KEFS for older children and, especially for teenage adolescents.

5. TESTS FROM CLINICAL RESEARCH STUDIES OF ADHD's EDF

Most studies designed to address the sensitivity of EDF as a discriminator of ADHD from normal status have assembled tests/tasks from clinical experience, initially following the "frontal lobe battery" approach derived from literature concerning adults with acquired brain lesions or degenerative diseases *(43)*. Several recent publications have reviewed much of the data on children and young adolescents. To a minor and tentative extent, some of these reviews have raised the issue of specificity-within-developmental disorders; others confine themselves to sensitivity with respect to normal developmental status.

This chapter will continue its anamnestic approach to reviewing the topic under its mandate by going into detail about a decade of research heavily invested in discovering the role of EDF as the central mediating cognitive domain underlying aspects of both LD and ADHD. An unintended byproduct of this decade of research was that of casting doubt on the meaningfulness of one subdomain of LD, that initially called NLD and extensively conceptualized by Rourke and colleagues for more than a quarter of a century *(13,44)*. In addition, because brain imaging was concurrently undertaken with all neurological/neuropsychological research observations, findings about the brain—when localization suggested the involvement of certain areas within EF-related circuits—provided feedback to improve the design to probe populations for the diagnosis of ADHD. A review of this decade's work leads to the conclusion that brain-based hypotheses are more likely to be confirmed by data than are those based on theory or model of cognition. Perhaps this is because when studying developing brains, the researchers cannot at any given moment in the age range reliably operationalize the elements of the theory or the model of cognition in their chosen tasks. Thus, task analysis (as in the clinical review earlier in this chapter) may reveal cognitive elements at one stage in development overshadowing what, in stable later stages of life, is the intended cognitive probe; in addition, knowledge of LD implies awareness that at any stage/age processing capabilities/talents vary widely. At any given age or stage, there exists among research subjects a range of capabilities in the specific ingredient of cognition intended to be manipulated as a probe of EF or its opposite, EDF.

A prime example of the problem is the Stroop Color-Word Interference Test *(45)*. An EF task variously described as one of selective attention, inhibition, or interference control, the Stroop is not intended for the illiterate; yet although the Stroop bases its rationale on the "well-established habit" of reading printed words rather than naming the color of the ink in which such words are printed, most studies (Cox *[45]* being an exception recently influencing some studies) ignore the variation in automaticity/fluency that characterizes the habit of reading in most population samples. The Cox effect *(45)* points out that the Stroop Interference Score varies as a function of reading skill rather than being a valid reflection of interference control in all persons who are technically considered "literate." A second factor gnawing away, as it were, at the construct validity of the Stroop's final score is that of slow response preparation exemplified by the color subtest of RAN *(35)* and indeed reported (without appropriate discussion) in recent articles concerning Stroop scores within an EF battery purporting to differentiate the EDF of ADHD *(46)*.

The Wisconsin Card Sort Test (WCST), an early candidate for sensitivity to the EDF of ADHD in children, has proven disappointing, all the more so in its computerized form *(24,25)*. Particularly inconsistent has been the sought-after perseverations score *(6)*, whereas errors of set maintenance, not popularly emphasized, have modest claims to ADHD/EDF sensitivity *(6,24,25)*. Another computerized executive battery with developmental aspirations, the Cambridge Neuropsychological Test Automated Battery *(47)*, has so far proven disappointing in terms of sensitivity to the EDF of ADHD; of all its subtests, only the most difficult (lengthiest) level of spatial working memory has been inordinately difficult for children with ADHD *(48)*.

Experience with tower tasks has been inconsistent, again raising the possibilities that either how gifted in its visuospatial ingredient or how experienced with similar toys are the ADHD and control subjects in the sample might blur any differences contributed by the EDF of ADHD *(49)*.

Several tasks suffer from such variability in terms of wide ranges of normal for children that, methodologically, it would appear unlikely that a relatively subtle childhood developmental disorder like ADHD would result in an obviously significant EDF differential mean score; such tasks include the copying (scored for organization) of the Rey–Osterreith Complex Figure *(31)* and the Contingency Naming Task *(50)*.

Research using a particularly "frontal" CPT called the test of variables of attention (TOVA) has been successful in the conventional sense of yielding discriminative EDF of ADHD *(24,25)*; yet this "go/no-go" challenge did not yield results for ADHD as anticipated (failure to inhibit on infrequent "no-go" trials) but simply indicated slow and excessively variable reaction times on correct "go" trials, plus (less often) elevated anticipatory responses. What really displaced the TOVA from research was its inappropriateness for longitudinal studies; simply put, children refused to experience the TOVA again, thus jeopardizing second and subsequent research study visits. Other, more "consumer-friendly" measures of reaction time came to be substituted both in the clinic and in the research unit.

The most robust survivors in research that made the crossover from the clinic were Verbal Fluency (Controlled Word Association) and CVLT-C *(26)*. As in the clinic, the confound of verbal and linguistic ingredients of cognition had to be taken into account, but in certain well-defined populations wherein EDF of ADHD was suspected but language functions were impeccable, the EF probe stood up well *(51)*. It remains important, however, to use an appropriate covariate (like WISC-derived Vocabulary for the Controlled Oral Word Association Test [COWAT] and Information for the CVLT-C) lest one ignore determinants other than EDF entering into poor scores.

Research lessons learned through studies of "special" neurogenetic groups and imaging loops us back to EF. For a decade, the Learning Disabilities Research Community at Kennedy Krieger Institute/Johns Hopkins University focused on "neurodevelopmental pathways" to LD, whereby "gene to brain to cognition" would hopefully be elucidated. In two of the three populations chosen for study, the linkage of ADHD to parts of the brain established to have EF/EDF implications emerged as more central and major than had been anticipated; to review this decade seems instructive. Tourette's syndrome is well-known to exist in children with a 60% ADHD comorbidity; ADHD not infrequently is the presenting clinical picture, followed by the multiple tics, waxing and waning over time, that are the defining characteristics of Tourette's syndrome. Not withstanding this well-known comorbidity, Tourette's syndrome nonetheless appeared in the neuropsychological literature characterized by several deficits (often labeled "visual-perceptual-motor") in publications remarkably innocent of analyses of the 40% with "pure" noncorbid Tourette's syndrome *(52–54)*. In the research of the Learning Disabilities Research Community, however, both neuropsychology and neuroimaging revealed a marked distinction, in that the ADHD comorbidity carried with it almost all the cognitive disability (including the "visual-perceptual-motor") and an imaging "signature" consistently in the direction of smaller-than-normal anatomic structures (globus pallidus, rostral corpus callosum, left frontal gray matter); in contrast, "pure" Tourette's syndrome was associated with unanticipatedly superior cognitive (and motor) function, except for a still-puzzling finding confined to low output/slow mental search on COWAT *(54,55)*. Imaging aberrations among "pure" Tourette's cases were subtle asymmetry attenuation in basal ganglia plus enlarged white-matter components of the right frontal lobe and rostral corpus callosum *(56–58)*. The import of all this research was to reveal that, stripped of ADHD comorbidity, Tourette's syndrome was a very different cognitive entity and a very circumscribed movement disorder, both observationally and neuroanatomically. (The white-matter enlargement might even fit closely the very recent concept of tics as failures of "bottom-up" afferent gating mechanisms, as clinically suggested by the premonitory sensations of tic sufferers who are more or less successful in suppressing the urge to move in response.)

The similarity of the comorbid-with-Tourette's ADHD to the larger ADHD population, both observationally and neuroanatomically, helps to confirm that which is applicable across heterogeneous causes of ADHD. This is expanded by the next instance. Neurofibromatosis-1 (NF-1), the most common dominant neurogenetic disorder and half the time because of a new mutation, is recognized as a cause of learning disabilities in the context of low-to-normal IQ. Studied relative to siblings and parents who are unaffected, children with NF-1 have lower-than-expected (yet normal) IQs plus school-related underachievements; they are also poorly coordinated.

Initially hypothesized on the basis of published literature *(59,60)* to suffer in school from NLD, children with NF-1 turned out to have major oral (and secondary written) language disorders, DMCD, and a statistically significant within-family excess of ADHD diagnoses *(61,62)*. The ADHD association with NF-1, although no surprise to clinicians, had never been included in the designs of neuropsychological studies and hence had never been raised as an issue with respect to the most frequently emphasized finding, that of low scores on the JLO, which played such a major role in the designation "NLD" as the specific cognitive deficit caused by NF-1. Not only did the DMCD, so highly reliably reported with NF-1 (if looked for) suggest the "smoke" to the "fire" of probable ADHD, but the brain localization of the specific "lesions" of NF-1 strongly suggested that the syndrome of ADHD might be anticipated; these "lesions" are seen first and foremost in the basal ganglia and second most commonly in the cerebellum *(63,64)*. Even more similar to the insights afforded by structural-anatomic imaging in NF-1 is the fact that when ADHD is present in a child with NF-1, the brain volume will move from large to average, whereas, if free of ADHD, the child with NF-1 tends toward showing a larger-than-average brain. Without going into all the complex details of NF-1-related brain imaging, the researcher interested in ADHD can find within-NF-1 evidence that neurobiological factors resulting in the ADHD clinical picture are, whatever the underlying causes, mediated by reduced volume of brain tissue most prominently in the frontal lobes, basal ganglia, and cerebellum *(65,66)*. Thus, regardless of how "special" the sample studied, the pattern of anatomy and its affiliation with EF remain strikingly consistent in their relevance to the developmental disability category called ADHD for clinical diagnostic purposes. In addition, the NF-1 research reveals that ADHD, through factors of EDF impinging on task demands, may permeate volumes between whose covers chapter after chapter on specific neurobiological syndromes concludes that all share the NLD profile. The term "nonverbal" may turn out to be accurate in its diffuseness but less specifically about a set of perceptual (and particularly social) deficits than its usage implies. This is not to say that nobody exists who has a visual–perceptual, visual–spatial, or social–affect processing disorder; but the burden of proof remains on researchers claiming to document such profiles, because the possibility of EDF disrupting the task is rarely part of the study design. Task score validity (i.e., what a poor score really means) is not frequently discussed as a limitation of the results of studies. Even using ADHD as categorical covariate, without controlling for a range of executive abilities introducing variance, may not suffice.

6. WHAT HAS FUNCTIONAL MULTIRESONANCE IMAGING REVEALED ABOUT EF/EDF IN CHILDREN WITH ADHD?

Excitement and high anticipation about functional magnetic resonance imaging (fMRI) providing insights concerning the EDF of children with ADHD has been tempered by the realization that the method itself imposes limitations on designs. First of all, "executive" tasks should involve doing, but activity is severely constrained by the fMRI environment. Active output tasks (other than those involving small muscle movements) cannot be employed; in fact, the baseline requirement for inhibition of most activity means that, particularly for children, there are major executive task demands before any specific task is presented, just to fulfill the condition "lie still."

A second pervasive problem, less limited to children, is that task instructions must be held in working memory, usually of the verbally mediated type. Thus, two important elements within the executive domain—whole-body inhibition and working memory—are lurking in the baseline of most fMRI studies. Any "executive" probe is constrained by these baseline activations, so that even while limited in scope of "execution" the probe must be able to increase over baseline task-specific demands for either stronger or more focal activation. Developmental studies using fMRI have focused primarily on the basic and presumably early-onset EF elements of inhibition and working memory, particularly the former. This is particularly true because of widespread interest in and acceptance of the central role of inhibitory insufficiency at the core of the ADHD syndrome *(68,69)*. When "immature" patterns of widespread distributed fMRI activations are found in normally developing children, relative to adolescents and adults, what is revealed is all too seldom discussed; namely, EDF is precisely what most defines normal childhood immaturity. Thus, the fMRI baseline EF requirements introduce significant confounds into the search for potential signature patterns of EDF associated with ADHD. In fact, the possibility exists that preliminary training (e.g., in a mock scanner) to "lie still" may activate in children with ADHD and/or normal younger children (whom the children with ADHD resemble) precisely those regions of interest, such as frontal lobes, that the researchers wish to attempt to activate by means of "stop" or "go/no-go" tasks.

Some studies have adopted the strategy of studying children with ADHD and controls under stimulant-medicated compared with unmedicated conditions. Vaidya et al. *(69)* reported in such an fMRI design that inhibitory activation when medicated differs only in striatum (increases in ADHD) but not in frontal regions, in which all the children studied increase activation when stimulant-medicated. Indeed when unmedicated, children with ADHD activated striatum "less" than control children even when responses were successfully inhibited. No interpretation was made, however, of the higher-than-control unmedicated frontal activation among the group with ADHD (*see* baseline issue in previous paragraph). Furthermore, "less vs more" activation is difficult to interpret securely, because normative studies have shown not only the more diffuse network activated by inhibitory control but also more activity in some critical regions, e.g., frontal and/or striatal in children, becoming more focal and less extensive locally in adults *(68,70)*. When one then reflects back on the small numbers *(6–10)* and relatively broad age range *(8–13)* of the Vaidya et al. *(69)* study, one is struck by the potential confound introduced by groupwise analysis; even if exquisitely pairwise-matched, the fMRI activation data need scrutiny in terms of the distinction between ADHD as "immature-for-age" and ADHD as "anomalous-for-age" in inhibitory signature. Studies of ADHD populations at adolescent or adult ages and employing other tasks to operationalize inhibitory control as fMRI activator have not as yet shed any new or improved light on the executive system.

In summary, fMRI has thus far done more to raise questions about the development of the executive system and heighten researchers' sensitivity to the pervasive and implicit executive demands of tasks than to clarify what is going on in association with ADHD that is dysexecutive.

7. FUTURE DIRECTIONS IN PURSUIT OF THE ADHD MANIFESTATION OF EDF

Although clinical and research experiences have improved our understanding of EDF, both within and outside ADHD concerns, the definitive way to document EDF, necessitating more of the paired-task approach, has not been fully operationalized over the decade since it was articulated *(76)*. Individual clinical reports can be phrased, "For such a highly verbal child, such a poor showing on word fluency strongly suggests executive dysfunction." When it comes to documentation of the discriminative power of EDF in ADHD groupwise research, however, researchers still encounter not only conflicting results from other centers but also failure to replicate their own local results with subsequent samples. The clinician who is also a researcher suspects that variance in several confounds renders the quest for EDF so elusive; variances in age, gender, and specific ingredients-of-task talents/endowments are among these confounds. What has become clearer, however, is that the more basic EF components with earlier onset and steep developmental trajectory over the prepubertal years are the most substantive for research to focus on (and not only because such elements as "inhibitory control" transfer most smoothly to fMRI) and from which to build complexity in stepwise fashion; cognitive neuroscience can expect to learn more about the structure of the EF domain by observing the developmental progression toward adult architecture. It is also possible that within the heterogeneous category of ADHD there are some persistently "immature" profiles that can reveal over time just what is a necessary and/or sufficient progression of EF elements, or when a "lag" may come to look like a "lesion." Finally, intervention with children with ADHD may be a source of greater understanding of how much EF can be taught and learned, plus how early learned elements may facilitate later EF development.

REFERENCES

1. Tannock R. Attention deficit hyperactivity disorder: Advances in cognitive, neurobiological, and genetic research. J Child Psychol Psychiatry 1998;39:65–99.
2. Barkley RA. Issues in the diagnosis of attention deficit/hyperactivity disorder in children. Brain Dev 2003;25:77–83.
3. Denckla M. ADHD: topic update. Brain Dev 2003;25:383–389.
4. Barkley RA. ADHD and the Nature of Self Control. New York: Guilford Press, 1997.
5. Barkley RA. ADHD part I: The executive functions and ADHD. J Am Acad Child Adolesc Psychiatry 2000;39:1064–1068.
6. Sergeant JA, Geurts H, Oosterlaan J. How specific is a deficit of executive functioning for attention deficit/hyperactivity disorder. Behav Brain Res 2002;130:3–28.
7. Denckla MB, Reiss AL. Prefrontal-subcortical circuits in developmental disorders. In: Krasnegor NA, Lyon GR, Goldman-Rakic PS, eds. Development of the prefrontal cortex: evolution, neurobiology, and behavior. Baltimore, MD: Paul H. Brooks, 1997:283–293.
8. Castellanos FX, Lee PP, Sharp W. Developmental trajectories of brain volume abnormalities in children and adolescents with attention deficit/hyperactivity disorder. JAMA 2002;288:1740–1748.
9. Durston S. A review of the biological bases of ADHD: What have we learned from imaging studies. Ment Retard Dev Disabil Res Rev 2003;9:84–195.
10. Denckla M. Minimal brain dysfunction. In: Chall J, Mirsky A, ReLage K, eds. National Society for the Study of Education: education and the brain. Chicago: University of Chicago Press, 1978:223–268.
11. Denckla M, Rudel R. Anomalies of motor development in hyperactive boys without learning disabilities. Ann Neurol 1978;3:231–233.
12. Rasmussen P, Gillberg C. Natural outcome of ADHD with developmental coordination disorder at age twenty-two years: a controlled longitudinal community-based study. J Am Acad Child Adolesc Psychiatry 2000;39:1424–1431.
13. Rourke BP, Strang JD. Neuropsychological significance of variations in patterns of academic performance: motor, psychomotor, and tactile-perceptual abilities. J Pediatr Psychol 1978;3: 62–66.
14. Diagnostic and Statistical Manual of Mental Disorders, 4th Edition (DSM-IV™). Washington, DC: American Psychiatric Association, 1994.
15. Henderson K. Update 2001: overview of ADA, IDEA, and Section 504. ERIC EC Digest 2001; E606:12–13.
16. Touwen B, Prechtl H. The neurological examination of the child with minor nervous dysfunction. Philadelphia: JB Lippincott, 1977.

17. Wolff PH, Gunnoe CE, Cohen C. Neuromotor maturation and psychological performance: a developmental study. Dev Med Child Neurol 1985;27:344–354.
18. Camp JA, Bialer I, Sverd J, et al. Clinical usefulness of the NIMH physical and neurological examination for soft signs. Am J Psychiatry 1978;135:362–364.
19. Denckla MB. Revised PANESS. Psychopharm Bull 1985;21:773–800.
20. Denckla MB. Development of motor coordination in normal children. Dev Med Child Neurol 1974;16:729–741.
21. Denckla MB. Motor coordination in dyslexic children: theoretical and clinical implications. In: Frank SH, Duffy H, Geschwind N, eds. Dyslexia: a neuroscientific approach to clinical evaluation. Boston: Little, Brown, 1985:187–95.
22. Nichols P, Chen T. Minimal brain dysfunction: a prospective study. Hillsdale, NJ: Erlbaum Associates, 1981:219–241.
23. Conners CK. Conners' Continuous Performance Test Computer Program, Version 3.0. Toronto, Canada: Multi-health Systems, 1994.
24. Reader MJ, Harris EL, Schuerholz LJ, et al. Attention deficit hyperactivity disorder and executive dysfunction. Dev Neuropsychol 1994;10:493–512.
25. Denckla MB. Research on executive function in a neurodevelopmental context: application of clinical measures. Dev Neuropsychol 1996;12:5–15.
26. Fridlund AJ, Delis DC. California Verbal Learning Test-Children's Version®. The Psychological Corporation. San Antonio, TX: Harcourt Brace & Company, 1998.
27. Delis-Kaplan Executive Function System™. San Antonio, TX: The Psychological Corporation, 2001.
28. Spreen O, Straus E. A compendium of neuropsychological tests. New York: Oxford University Press, 1991.
29. Benton AL, Hamsher K, Varney NR, et al. Contributions to neuropsychological assessment: a clinical manual. New York: Oxford University Press, 1983.
30. Pennington BF, Ozonoff S. Executive functions and developmental psychopathologies. J Child Psychol Psychiatr Ann Res Rev 1996;37:51–87.
31. Bernstein JH, Waber DP. Developmental scoring system for the Rey-Osterreith complex figure: professional manual. Odessa, FL: Psychological Assessment Corporation, 1996.
32. Korkman M, Kirk U, Kemp S. Developmental neuropsychological assessment NEPSY™. San Antonio, TX: Psychological Corporation, 1998;64:156–157.
33. Rudel RG, Denckla MB, Broman M. Rapid silent responses to repeated target symbols by dyslexic and nondyslexic children. Brain Lang 1978;6:52–58.
34. Tannock R, Martinussen R, Frijters J. Naming speed performance and stimulant effect indicate effortful semantic processing deficits in attention deficit/hyperactivity disorder. J Abnorm Child Psychol 2000;28:237–252.
35. Denckla MB, Rudel RG. Rapid automatized naming (RAN) dyslexia differentiated from other learning disabilities. Neuropsychologia 1976;14:471–479.
36. Gioia GA, Isquith PK, Guy SC, et al. Behavior rating inventory of executive function. Lutz FL: Psychological Assessment Resources, 2000.
37. Denckla MB. The Behavior Rating Inventory of Executive Function: commentary. Child Neuropsychol 2002;8:304–306.
38. Pennington BF, Groisser D, Welsh MC. Contrasting cognitive deficits in attention deficit hyperactivity disorder versus reading disability. Dev Psychol 1993;299:511–523.
39. Bayliss DM, Roodenrys S. Executive processing and attention deficit hyperactivity disorder: An application of the supervisory attentional system. Dev Neuropsychol 2000;17:161–180
40. Connors K. Conners' Rating Scales. North Tonawanda, NY: Multi-Health Systems, Inc., 1997.
41. Gershon J. A meta-analytic review of gender differences in ADHD. J Atten Disord 2002;5: 143–154.
42. Gaub M, Carlson CL. Gender differences in ADHD: A meta-analysis and critical review. J Am Acad Child Adolesc Psychiatry 1997;36:1036–1045.

43. Grodzinsky GM, Diamond R. Frontal lobe functioning in boys with attention deficit hyperactivity disorder. Dev Neuropsychol 1992;8:427–445.
44. Rourke BP. The syndrome of nonverbal learning disabilities: Developmental manifestations in neurological disease, disorder, and dysfunction. Clin Neuropsychol 1988;2:293–330.
45. Cox CS, Chee E, Chase GA, et al. Reading proficiency affects the construct validity of the Stroop test interference score. Clin Neuropsychol 1997;11:105–110.
46. Seidman LJ, Biederman J, Faraone SV, et al. Toward defining a neuropsychology of attention deficit hyperactivity disorder: performance of children and adolescents from a large clinical sample. J Consult Clin Psychol 1997;65:150–160.
47. Luciana M, Nelson CA. Assessment of neuropsychological function through use of the Cambridge Neuropsychological Testing Automated Battery: performance in 4- to 12-year-old children. Dev Neuropsychol 2002;22:595–624.
48. Goldberg MC, Mostofsky SH, Cutting LE, et al. Subtle executive impairment in children with autism and children with ADHD. Submitted.
49. Klorman R, Hazel-Fernandez LA, Shaywitz SE. Executive functioning deficits in attention-deficit/hyperactivity disorder are independent of oppositional defiant or reading disorder. J Am Acad Child Adolesc Psychiatry 1999;38:1148–1155.
50. Taylor HG. Learning disabilities. In: Mash EJ, ed. Behavioral assessments of childhood disorders (2nd ed.). New York: Guilford Press, 1988:402–405.
51. Romans SM, Roeltgen DP, Kushner H. Executive function in females with Turner syndrome. Dev Neuropsychol 1997;13:23–40.
52. Bornstein RA. Neuropsychological performance in children with Tourette syndrome. Psychiatry Res 1990;33:73–81.
53. Yeates KO, Bornstein RA. Attention deficit disorder and neuropsychological functioning in children with Tourette syndrome. Neuropsychology 1994;8:65–74.
54. Schuerholz LJ, Baumgardner TL, Singer HS, et al. Neuropsychological status of children with Tourette syndrome with and without attention deficit hyperactivity disorder Neurology 1996;46:958–965.
55. Ozonoff S, Jensen J. Brief report specific executive function profiles in three neurodevelopmental disorders. J Autism Dev Disord 1999;29:171–177.
56. Singer HS, Reiss AL, Brown JE, et al. Volumetric MRI changes in basal ganglia of children with Tourette syndrome. Neurology 1993;43:950–956.
57. Baumgardner TL, Singer HS, Denckla MB, et al. Corpus callosum morphology in children with Tourette syndrome and attention deficit hyperactivity disorder. Neurology 1996;4:477–482.
58. Fredericksen KA, Cutting LE, Kates WR, et al. Disproportionate increases of white matter in right frontal lobe in Tourette syndrome. Neurology 2002;58:85–89.
59. Eldridge R, Denckla MB, Bien E, et al. Neurofibromatosis type 1 (Recklinghausen's disease). Am J Dis Child 1989;143:833–837.
60. Cutting LE, Koth CW, Denckla MB. How children with neurofibromatosis type 1 differ from "typical" learning disabled clinic attenders: nonverbal learning disabilities revisited. Dev Neuropsychol 2000;17:29–47.
61. North K, Joy P, Yuille D, et al. Cognitive function and academic performance in children with neurofibromatosis type 1. Dev Med Child Neurol. 1995;37:427–436.
62. Hofman KJ, Harris EL, Bryan RN, et al. Neurofibromatosis type 1: the cognitive phenotype. J Pediatr 1994;124:S1–S8.
63. Itoh T, Magnaldi S, White RM, et al. Neurofibromatosis type 1: the evolution of deep gray and what matter MR abnormalities. Am J Rad 1994;15:1513–1519.
64. Moore BD, Slopis JM, Schomer D, et al. Neuropsychological significance of areas of high signal intensity on brain MRIs of children with neurofibromatosis. Neurology 1996;46:1660–1668.
65. Cutting, LE, Koth, CW, Burdette, C, et al. The relationship of cognitive functioning, whole brain volumes, and T-2 weighted hyperintensities in neurofibromatosis type 1. J Child Neurol 2000;15:157–160.

66. Cutting LE, Cooper KL, Koth CW, Mostofsky SH, et al. Megalencephaly in NF-1: Predominantly white matter contribution and mitigation by ADHD. Neurology 2002;59:1388–1394.
67. Rubia K, Overmeyer S, Taylor E, et al. Hypofrontality in attention deficit hyperactivity disorder during higher-order motor control: a study with functional MRI. AM J Psychiatry 1999;156:891–896.
68. Durston S, Thomas KM, Yang Y, et al. The development of neural systems involved in overriding behavioral responses: an event-related fMRI study. Dev Sci 2002;5:F9–F16.
69. Vaidya CJ, Austin G, Kirkorian G. Selective effects of methylphenidate in attention deficit hyperactivity disorder: a functional magnetic resonance study. Proc Nat Acad Sci 1998;95:14,494–14,499.
70. Luna B, Thulborn KR, Munoz DP, et al. Maturation of widely distributed brain functions subserves cognitive development. Neuroimage 2001;13:786–793.

9

The Neuropsychology of Attention Deficit Hyperactivity Disorder

Validity of the Executive Function Hypothesis

Erik G. Willcutt, Kimberly Brodsky, Nomita Chhabildas, Michelle Shanahan, Benjamin Yerys, Ashley Scott, and Bruce F. Pennington

1. INTRODUCTION

A literature search at the end of 2003 revealed more than 200 published studies that compared groups with and without attention deficit hyperactivity disorder (ADHD) on neuropsychological measures. This rapid accumulation of new knowledge illustrates the potential utility of neuropsychological methods as a tool to refine our understanding of the pathophysiology of ADHD. Yet these studies also underscore the complexity of the neuropsychology of ADHD, and clearly demonstrate how much remains to be learned.

The overarching objective of this chapter is to evaluate the executive function (EF) hypothesis, one of the most prominent neuropsychological models of ADHD *(1,2)*. In the first section of the chapter we provide a brief overview of the syndrome of ADHD and summarize current knowledge regarding the genetic and environmental influences that are associated with ADHD. We then describe the construct of EF and summarize four key criteria that must be met if the EF theory of ADHD is correct. We then present a meta-analytic review of studies of selected EF tasks that have been administered most frequently in previous studies of ADHD, and describe the implications of these results for the EF theory. Finally, we compare the support for the EF model vs other neuropsychological theories of ADHD, and suggest several directions for future research that are needed to develop a comprehensive model of the neuropsychology of ADHD.

2. THE NATURE OF ADHD

Approximately 5% of children meet the diagnostic criteria for ADHD described in the fourth edition of the *Diagnostic and Statistical Manual of Mental Disorders* (*DSM*-IV) *(3)*, making it one of the most common disorders of childhood *(4,5)*. Few disorders have undergone as many changes in name and diagnostic criteria as ADHD, perhaps because few disorders have been the subject of as much taxonomic study. Based on factor analytic studies *(6,7)* and results of the DSM-IV clinical field trials for the disruptive behavior disorders *(8)*, the diagnostic criteria for DSM-IV ADHD incorporate two symptom dimensions. The first includes symptoms that describe maladaptive levels of inattention and disorganization, and the second consists of

From: *Attention Deficit Hyperactivity Disorder: From Genes to Patients*
Edited by: D. Gozal and D. L. Molfese © Humana Press Inc., Totowa, NJ

symptoms of hyperactivity and impulsivity. DSM-IV distinguishes among individuals who exhibit maladaptive levels of both inattention and hyperactivity-impulsivity (combined type), maladaptive levels of inattention only (predominantly inattentive type), and maladaptive levels of hyperactivity-impulsivity alone (predominantly hyperactive-impulsive type).

In this chapter we describe key results from the Colorado Learning Disabilities Research Center (CLDRC) *(9)*, our ongoing study of the etiology of learning difficulties and DSM-IV ADHD. We also emphasize studies of DSM-IV ADHD in the meta-analysis when sufficient data are available. However, because relatively few studies of DSM-IV ADHD have incorporated EF measures, we also review studies that used previous or alternative definitions of ADHD to provide the most complete account of current knowledge regarding the relation between ADHD and EF.

2.1. *Etiology of ADHD*

Recent etiologically informative studies provided important information regarding the genetic and environmental influences that increase susceptibility to ADHD. These methods and results are described in detail in other reviews *(10,11)*. For the purposes of this chapter we provide a streamlined summary of these findings and focus on the implications of these results for neuropsychological theories of ADHD.

2.1.1. *Family and Twin Studies*

Family studies clearly demonstrate that ADHD is familial *(12,13)*, and twin studies suggest that this familiality is the result of genetic influences. Specifically, studies of more than 10,000 twin pairs have found that individual differences in ADHD symptoms are largely attributable to genetic influences, with an average heritability of approx 75% (e.g., *14,15*, reviewed in ref. *11*). These same studies indicate that the remaining phenotypic variance in ADHD symptoms is attributable to nonshared environmental influences; estimates of shared environmental influences were not significant in any previous study.

2.1.2. *Linkage and Candidate Gene Studies*

Once a trait such as ADHD has been shown to be significantly heritable, two main methods can be used to localize the genes that increase risk for ADHD. Family-based linkage analysis can be used to screen the entire genome to identify chromosomal regions that may contain a gene or genes that increase risk for ADHD. In contrast, the candidate gene approach examines specific genes that are targeted because they play a role in a biological system that is associated with the disorder (*see* refs. *16,17* for a more detailed description of candidate gene and linkage studies).

More than 80 published studies have tested for an association between ADHD and 27 different candidate genes *(11)*, and a series of studies by one group has examined more than 20 additional candidate genes in a sample of individuals with ADHD and Tourette's syndrome *(18)*. Most of these studies have focused on genes that influence dopamine (DA), norepinephrine, and serotonin, owing to evidence that these neurotransmitters may play a role in the pathophysiology of ADHD and other psychopathology *(19)*. For 14 of the 27 candidate genes a significant association with ADHD has been reported in at least one study; however, many of these results have been replicated inconsistently or await independent replication. Moreover, each of these genes appears to account for a relatively small proportion of the variance in ADHD symptoms *(10,20)*, suggesting that none is likely to be necessary or sufficient to cause ADHD.

Because the known candidate genes are not sufficient to fully explain the genetic etiology of ADHD, two recent studies used linkage analysis to screen the entire genome for additional genes that influence ADHD *(21,22)*. Each study revealed strong evidence for linkage in two regions (chromosome *16p13* and *17p11* in *22*; *7p13* and *15q15* in *21*) and preliminary evidence for genes with smaller effects elsewhere in the genome. However, only a single region on chromosome 5p13 was significant in both studies, and neither genome scan detected linkage in the regions of most of the known candidate genes for ADHD, underscoring again the variability of results across studies.

In summary, candidate gene and linkage studies clearly indicate that multiple genes are involved in the etiology of ADHD, and suggest that none of these genes is necessary or sufficient to cause ADHD. Although these results have no definitive implications for the neuropsychology of ADHD, the fact that the etiology of ADHD is complex and multifactorial suggests that the neurocognitive correlates of ADHD are likely to be complex and heterogeneous.

3. THE EF HYPOTHESIS

To successfully navigate our ever-changing environmental context, we must continually select from a large set of possible actions. In many cases these actions may be directed toward achieving a positive outcome in a simulated future context, and must therefore compete with alternative actions that might maximize initial benefits but have larger long-term costs *(23)*. EFs are defined as cognitive functions that serve to maintain an appropriate problem-solving set in order to attain a future goal *(24)*. In an oversimplified model of decision-making processes, EFs represent "top-down" cognitive inputs that facilitate decision making by maintaining information about possible choices in working memory and integrating this knowledge with information about the current context to identify the optimal action for the current situation. Although EFs involve several distributed brain networks, the primary neural circuit includes the thalamus, basal ganglia, and prefrontal cortex *(23,25)*.

A large body of research indicates that groups with ADHD differ significantly from groups without ADHD on a variety of neurocognitive measures *(2)*. More specifically, several authors have proposed that ADHD may be attributable to a general EF deficit or a core deficit in one or more EF domains *(1,2,26,27)*. The EF hypothesis is largely based on the observation that prefrontal lesions in experimental animals and human patients sometimes produce behavioral hyperactivity, distractibility, or impulsivity, as well as deficits on EF tasks *(28–30)*.

The neural circuits involved in EF have reciprocal connections with many other brain regions, including the mesolimbic pathway, a neural network comprised of the limbic system, anterior cingulate, and orbital frontal cortex. This substrate is primarily responsible for the adjustment of motivational state in response to reward and punishment cues *(31)*, and Sonuga-Barke *(32)* has hypothesized that dysfunction in this network may lead to the aversion to delay that is well documented in children with ADHD *(33,34)*. Therefore, although we focus primarily on EF in this chapter, it is important to also recognize the importance of these "bottom-up" motivational processes for a comprehensive understanding of the neuropsychology of ADHD. We return to this point at the end of the chapter when we compare the EF model to other models in the literature and describe important directions for future research.

3.1. Structure of EFs

Previous theorists have criticized the construct of EFs as weakly defined and overly broad *(35)*. Theoretical definitions of EF often include a wide range of processes that appear to involve multiple neurocognitive functions. Moreover, because many putative EF tasks are relatively nonspecific, poor performance could be attributable to a weakness in any of several different functions that a given task requires.

Table 1
Exploratory Factor Analysis of Executive Function and Processing Speed Measures

	Factor loadings on the four extracted factors			
Measure	Verbal working memory	Processing speed	Response inhibition/ execution	Set-shifting
Counting span	**0.71**	—	—	—
Sentence span	**0.72**	0.28	—	—
WISC-R digits forward	**0.73**	—	—	—
WISC-R digits backward	**0.76**	—	—	—
Trails part A	—	**0.78**	—	—
Trails part B	—	0.55	—	0.44
WISC-R coding	0.25	**0.68**	0.26	—
WISC-III symbol search	—	**0.55**	0.33	—
CPT commission errors	—	—	**0.83**	0.27
CPT omission errors	—	0.30	**0.71**	—
Stop-signal reaction time	0.26	—	**0.57**	—
CANTAB spatial working memory	0.24	0.34	—	**0.60**
WCST perseverative errors	—	—	—	**0.83**
Eigenvalue	4.28	1.44	1.11	1.01
Percent of variance explained	18.44	15.39	14.75	11.54

— indicates factor loading less than 0.20. Loadings in boldface indicate primary factor loading.
CANTAB, Cambridge Neuropsychological Test Automated Battery.

Factor analyses clearly demonstrate the multifactorial nature of the tasks that are commonly included in the overarching construct of EF *(35–40)*. Despite differences in diagnostic criteria, sampling procedures, and the specific EF measures included in each study, all these analyses revealed that EF tasks comprise more than one latent dimension of neurocognitive functioning. The overall pattern of results across all these studies suggests that EF tasks may consist of at least four factors:

1. Response inhibition.
2. Working memory/updating.
3. Set-shifting/task-switching.
4. Interference control.

In addition, most EF models distinguish between verbal and spatial working memory *(40–42)*, and many include additional domains, such as planning, vigilance, and fluency *(43)*.

To examine the structure of EF in our sample, we conducted an exploratory factor analysis of all putative EF tasks in the CLDRC battery (Table 1). Our EF battery includes measures of response inhibition (stop-signal reaction time [SSRT] and continuous performance test [CPT] commission errors), vigilance (CPT omission errors), verbal working memory (sentence span, counting span, and forward and backward digit span), spatial working memory (Cambridge Neuropsychological Test Automated Battery), set-shifting (Wisconsin Card Sorting Test [WCST] perseverative errors), and interference control (Stroop task). We also included three measures of what we labeled *executive processing speed* (Trailmaking test, Coding, and Symbol Search). Each of the processing speed tasks also includes an executive component, and all three have been among the strongest predictors of ADHD in our previous analyses *(39,40,44)*. All measures in the battery are described in detail in these previous papers.

The Stroop interference-control score did not load above 0.30 on any obtained factor, and was therefore dropped from the final factor analysis summarized in Table 1. Four factors with eigenvalues greater than 1 were extracted; these factors were labeled Verbal Working Memory, Processing Speed, Response Inhibition/Execution, and Set-Shifting. In combination with previous factor analytic studies, our latest results confirm that it is an oversimplification to describe EF deficits as a unitary construct. Instead, these results provide further evidence that the overarching category of EF is complex and multifactorial, and suggest that it may be important to consider each of these domains separately. In the next section we review studies that tested the EF model of ADHD by examining the relation between ADHD and each of these EF dimensions.

4. ARE EF WEAKNESSES THE CORE DEFICIT IN ADHD?

As noted previously, several authors have suggested that ADHD may be because of a general EF deficit or a core deficit in a specific facet of EF, such as response inhibition *(1,23,26)*. At least four criteria must be satisfied for a neurocognitive weakness to be considered a core deficit:

1. Groups with the disorder must consistently exhibit weaknesses on measures of the putative core deficit. In addition, these weaknesses should ideally remain significant when potential confounding variables, such as age, language, reading ability, symptoms of other psychopathology, and general intelligence are controlled *(45)*.
2. The neurocognitive deficit must explain a large proportion of the variance in symptoms of the disorder.
3. The neurocognitive deficit must be present in most individuals with the disorder.
4. Because ADHD is largely attributable to genetic influences, the neuropsychological weakness should be coheritable with ADHD.

In the following sections we review studies that tested whether EF deficits fulfill each of these four criteria necessary to be considered the core deficit in ADHD.

4.1. Criterion 1: Is ADHD Associated With EF Deficits?

In 1996, Pennington and Ozonoff *(2)* completed a meta-analytic review that systematically examined the neuropsychological correlates of ADHD. Their results suggested that groups with ADHD are characterized by weaknesses in at least a subset of EF domains, but indicated that the effect sizes for most EF measures were relatively small. However, many of the studies were based on small samples, and for several measures only a few studies were available. In contrast, when we searched the literature at the end of 2003 for studies that compared EF performance in groups with and without ADHD, we identified more than 100 papers that were not published at the time of the previous literature review.

This vast new literature suggests that an updated review is warranted to examine the implications of these new data and to identify remaining questions for future research. For this chapter we conducted a targeted meta-analysis of studies that compared groups with and without ADHD on several key EF measures. Our goal was to examine the validity of the EF hypothesis and to illustrate the most prominent unresolved issues regarding the neuropsychology of ADHD. Therefore, as a result of space constraints and the expansive literature on the relation between EF and ADHD, we did not attempt to include all previous neuropsychological studies of ADHD, nor all possible EF tasks. Instead, we chose the measure of each EF dimension that has been used most frequently in previous studies of ADHD, and summarized results from all published studies that included at least one of these measures.

The measure of response inhibition we selected was SSRT as derived from the stop-signal task *(46)*. This task was included in 25 published studies for which sufficient data were provided to allow us to calculate an effect size for the difference between groups with and without ADHD. Perseverative errors on the WCST *(47)* were selected as the representative measure of the ability to shift cognitive set (25 studies), and the Tower of Hanoi *(48)* and Tower of London *(49)* were included as measures of planning (12 studies). Because fewer previous studies administered measures of verbal working memory, we included both studies of working memory sentence span *(50)* and six studies of digit span backward *(51)*. The measure of interference control we selected was the Stroop *(52)*; however, we included only studies that calculated an interference control score that controlled for group differences in word and color naming speed (nine studies). Finally, although measures of processing speed have not always been included within the construct of EF, we included part B of the Trailmaking test *(53)* as a measure of executive processing speed because it cross-loaded on the processing speed and set-shifting factors (13 studies).

The procedure described by Cohen *(54)* was used to compute a standardized effect size (*d*) for the mean difference between groups with and without ADHD on each measure administered in each study (Table 2). The mean effect size across all studies that administered each measure and the corresponding 95% confidence interval were then calculated using the method described by Hedges and Olkin *(55)*. This procedure weights the effect size from each study by its corresponding sample size to obtain the best estimate of the true population parameter *(56)*.

The meta-analysis revealed significant differences between groups with and without ADHD on measures of most EF domains (Table 2). However, a comparison of the mean effect size and consistency of these results across studies suggests that some facets of EF are more strongly associated with ADHD than others. Specifically, mean SSRT was significantly higher in the group with ADHD than the group without ADHD in 84% of studies, and the mean effect size across all of these studies was at the low end of the range typically considered indicative of a large effect ($d = 0.63$). Similarly, 77% of the studies reported a significant group difference on part B of the Trailmaking test, and the mean effect size ($d = 0.72$) was slightly larger than the mean effect size for SSRT. In contrast, significant differences between groups with and without ADHD were obtained somewhat less consistently on measures of planning (58% of studies, $d = 0.54$) and verbal working memory (56% of studies, $d = 0.53$), and only a minority of studies reported a significant group difference on the measures of set-shifting (40% of studies, $d = 0.36$) and interference control (22% of studies, $d = 0.17$).

The overall results of this meta-analysis clearly support the hypothesis that ADHD is associated with significant impairment on EF tasks *(1,2,96,109,110)*, and suggest that these EF weaknesses may be most pronounced on measures of response inhibition and processing speed. Moreover, weaknesses on EF tasks have been demonstrated in both children and adults with ADHD *(111)*, and results from our laboratory and others suggest that the ADHD group deficit on measures of response inhibition, processing speed, and planning remains significant when group differences in intelligence, reading ability, symptoms of other disorders, age, and sex are controlled *(39,40,59,80,112)*. Taken together, these results indicate that weaknesses on these three dimensions meet the first criterion for a core deficit.

Table 2
Meta-Analysis of Previous Studies of Executive Function Tasks in Groups With and Without ADHD

				Effect size of the difference between groups with and without ADHD[a]					
Study	ADHD criteria	Control *n*	ADHD *n*	Response inhibition (SSRT)	Set-shifting (WCST)	Planning (TOH/TOL)[b]	Verbal working memory[c]	Interference control (Stroop)	Processing speed (Trails B)
33	DSM-IV	29	77	0.69^{d}	—	—	—	—	—
39	DSM-III	121	100	0.64^{d}	0.44^{d}	—	$0.44^{d,SS}$	0.00	0.34^{d}
40[e]	DSM-IV	177	151	0.57^{d}	0.43^{d}	—	$0.71^{d,f}$	0.07	0.53^{d}
42	DSM-IV	15	15	—	—	$0.48^{d,TOL}$	—	—	—
57	DSM-III-R	22	22	1.20^{d}	—	1.29^{*TOH}	—	—	—
58	DSM-III	12	24[g]	—	0.46	—	—	—	0.72^{d}
59	DSM-IV	39	101	—	—	—	0.22^{DB}		
60	DSM-IV	59	59	0.57^{d}	—	—	—	—	—
61	DSM-III	28	28	—	0.78^{d}	—	—	—	1.16^{d}
62	DSM-III-R	20	20	—	0.63^{d}	—	—	—	—
63	DSM-III	24	24	—	0.68^{d}	—	—	—	—
64	DSM-III-R	56	99	—	—	$0.94^{d,TOL}$			
65	DSM-IV	13	13	1.31^{d}	—	—	—	—	—
66	DSM-III-R	60	100	—	0.42	—	—	—	—
67	DSM-III	26	21	—	0.66^{*}	—	—	—	1.02^{d}
68[h]	DSM-III-R	64	66	—	0.16	—	—	—	0.32
69	DSM-IV	28	94	—	0.31	0.15^{TOL}	—	0.17	0.56
70	DSM-III-R	27	31	—	—	—	0.49^{DB}	—	—
71	DSM-IV	28	299	—	0.07	No $SD^{d,TOH}$	—	—	—
72	DSM-IV	21	16	1.15^{d}	—	—	—	—	—
73	Conners	119	51	0.22	—	—	$0.50^{d,SS}$	—	—
74	DSM-III-R	20	20	—	0.16	—	—	—	—
75	DSM-III-R	20	29	—	—	—	—	0.70^{d}	—
76	DSM-III-R	16	30	0.17	—	—	—	—	—
77	DSM-III-R	19	11	—	0.35	0.19^{TOH}	—	—	0.80
78	DSM-III	62	25	—	0.12	—	—	—	0.57^{d}

(Continued)

Table 2
(Continued)

Study	Control ADHD criteria	ADHD *n*	Response inhibition *n*	Effect size of the difference between groups with and without ADHD[a] Set-shifting (SSRT)	Planning (WCST)	Verbal working (TOH/TOL)[b]	Interference control memory[c]	Processing speed (Stroop)	(Trails B)
79	DSM-IV	19	39	—	—	—	1.73[dDB]	—	—
80	DSM-IV	25	25	0.88[d]	—	—	—	—	—
81	DSM-IV	41	64	0.80[d]	—	0.70[dTOL]	—	0.05	0.53[d,i]
82	CTRS/CBCL	17	15	0.64[d]	—	—	—	—	
83	CTRS/CBCL	21	12	0.77[d]	—	—	—	—	—
84	DSM-III-R	16	16	0.92[d]	—	—	—	—	—
85	Conners	33	31	—	–0.21	0.39[TOH]	—	—	—
86	DSM-III-R	23	32	—	0.60	0.65[dTOH]	—	—	—
87	DSM-III-R	72	100	—	0.65[d]	—	—	—	—
88	DSM-III-R	14	13	1.36[d]	—	—	—	—	—
89	DSM-IV	10	10	0.75[d]	—	—	—	—	—
90	DSM-III-R	17	34	0.61[d]	—	—	—	—	—
91	CBCL	11	11	1.31[d]	—	—	—	—	—
92	DSM-IV	23	16	0.50	—	—	—	—	—
93	DSM-IV	37	59	0.72[d]	—	—	0.65[dDB]	0.30	—
94	DSM-III-R	19	20	—	0.10	—	—	—	1.65[d]
95	DSM-III	10	27	0.72[d]	—	—	—	—	—
96	DSM-IV	119	33	0.42[d]	—	—	—	—	—
97	DSM-III-R	16	40	0.64[d]	—	—	—	—	—
98	DSM-III-R	22	14	0.60[d]	—	—	—	—	—
99	DSM-IV	41	51	0.18[d]	—	—	—	—	—
100	Clinician	76	76	—	–0.15	—	—	—	—
101	DSM-III-R	36	43	—	0.21	—	—	0.15	—
102	DSM-III-R	99	118	—	0.53[d]	—	—	0.31[d]	—
103	DSM-III	11	10	—	0.54	—	—	—	—
104	DSM-III-R	24	24	—	0.88[d]	—	–0.42[DB]	—	0.72[d]

105	DSM-IV	28	28	—	0.70[d]	—	—	—	0.47[d]
106	DSM-III-R	45	36	—	0.09	0.69[d]TOH	—	—	—
107	DSM-IV	34	28	—	—	0.33TOL	—	—	—
108	DSM-IV	29	83	—	—	0.13TOL	0.53DB	0.42	—
Weighted mean effect size ± 95% confidence interval[k]				0.63 ± 0.09	0.36 ± 0.08	0.54 ± 0.15	0.53 ± 0.13	0.17 ± 0.11	0.72 ± 0.11
Number of studies finding a significant group difference				21/25	10/25	7/12	5/9	2/9	10/13

CBCL, Child Behavior Checklist; CTRS, SSRT, stop-signal reaction time; WCST, Wisconsin Card Sorting Test; TOH, Tower of Hanoi; TOL, Tower of London.

[a]Effect size = Cohen's *d* (e.g., Cohen, 1988): (ADHD *M* - Comparison *M*) / pooled SD. All scores are scaled so that a positive effect size indicates greater impairment in the ADHD group regardless of the original scaling of the measure.

[b]TOH indicates Tower of Hanoi; TOL superscript indicates Tower of London.

[c]Verbal working memory measures: DB, digits backward, SS, working memory sentence span.

[d]indicates significant difference between ADHD and comparison groups; — indicates measure not included in the study.

[e]A subset of this dataset was also presented in ref. *44*.

[f]Mean effect size for digits backward ($d = 0.81$) and sentence span ($d = 0.61$).

[g]Pooled effect size for 12 children with DSM-III attention deficit disorder with hyperactivity and 12 children with attention deficit disorder without hyperactivity.

[h]pooled ES for younger and older samples.

[i]Only significant for the DSM-IV inattentive type.

[j]Mean effect size for 2-, 4-, and 8-s interstimulus intervals.

[k]Weighted mean effect size and confidence interval *(56)* across all studies of each measure.

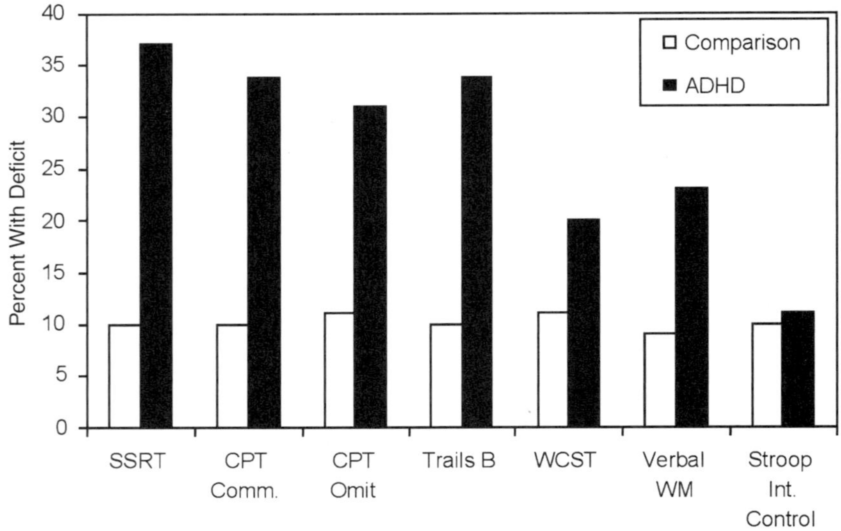

Fig. 1. Percentage of individuals with and without Attention Deficit Hyperactivity Disorder who scored above the 90th percentile of the comparison sample on each executive function measure. WM, working memory.

4.2. Criterion 2: Are EF Deficits Sufficiently Large to Account for the Behavioral Symptoms of ADHD?

The magnitude of the mean difference between groups with and without ADHD on EF measures ($d = 0.2$–0.7) is much smaller than the group difference in ADHD symptoms ($d = 2.5$–4.0 in the studies included in the meta-analysis). Similarly, dimensional analyses *(39,112)* indicate that the correlations between behavioral ratings of ADHD symptoms and performance on EF tasks are typically significant but small in magnitude (relative risk [r] = 0.15–0.35), suggesting that EF performance explains a relatively small proportion of the total variance in ADHD symptoms. These moderate effect sizes and low to medium correlations suggest that EF weaknesses as measured in previous studies cannot fully explain the behavioral symptoms used to define ADHD, and therefore do not meet the second criterion for a core deficit.

4.3. Criterion 3: Are EF Deficits Present in Most Individuals With ADHD?

Comparisons of group means on a continuous measure of EF performance provide greater statistical power than categorical comparisons of the proportion of individuals with significant EF impairment. However, the implications of a significant mean difference between groups must be interpreted with caution. For example, although the means of groups with and without ADHD on EF measures are often significantly different, the moderate effect size of the group difference suggests that the distributions of scores in the two groups overlap substantially *(113)*. Therefore, for any given measure many children with ADHD score in the normal range, and only a subset score in a range that indicates clinically meaningful impairment.

Because few studies have directly tested what proportion of individuals with ADHD exhibit EF deficits, we examined the proportion of individuals with ADHD who scored above the 90th percentile of the comparison sample on each EF task in our battery (Fig. 1). Although some measures were more strongly associated with ADHD than others (i.e., SSRT vs Stroop interference control), only a minority of the individuals in the ADHD group exhibited a deficit on any of the specific EF tasks. Therefore, whereas the presence of a significant EF deficit is associated with significantly increased risk for ADHD (for measures other than the Stroop interference score), the absence of an EF deficit clearly cannot be used to rule out ADHD *(114)*.

This pattern of results is consistent with results in other samples *(115)*, and provides further evidence against the hypothesis that a single EF deficit is the primary neuropsychological weakness in all individuals with ADHD. Instead, these results suggest that a more comprehensive model that incorporates additional neurocognitive weaknesses is necessary to fully explain the neuropsychology of ADHD.

4.4 Criterion 4: Are EF Deficits Coheritable With ADHD?

4.4.1. *Twin Studies*

Because ADHD symptoms are highly heritable *(116,117)*, a putative core deficit must also be heritable, and should be attributable to many of the same genetic influences that lead to the behavioral symptoms of ADHD. Two population-based twin studies estimated the bivariate heritability of elevations of ADHD symptoms and performance on EF measures *(118,119)*. Bivariate heritability estimates (h^2_g) range from 0 to 1, and provide an index of the extent to which extreme ADHD scores are attributable to genetic influences that also lead to deficits on EF tasks.

The first twin study did not find significant bivariate heritability for hyperactivity scores and any specific EF task *(119)*, although a marginally significant result suggested that common genes may contribute to elevations of hyperactivity and commission errors on a continuous performance test ($h^2_g = 0.60$). In contrast, bivariate heritability estimates were significant for a measure of response variability ($h^2_g = 0.64$) and an overall discriminant function score that included the measure of response variability as well as measures of vigilance, reaction time, and verbal IQ.

In the second twin study *(118)*, we examined the etiology of the relation between ADHD and neurocognitive functioning in a larger sample of twins selected for DSM-IV ADHD. The neurocognitive test battery included measures of response inhibition (SSRT and commission errors on a CPT), working memory (sentence span and counting span), vigilance (omission errors on a continuous performance test), set-shifting (WCST Perseverative errors), and processing speed (Wechsler Intelligence Scale for Children-Revised [WISC-R] Coding and Trailmaking test). Estimates of bivariate heritability ($h^2_g = 0.20–0.38$) were somewhat lower than those obtained by Kuntsi and Stevenson *(119)*, but owing to the larger sample size these estimates were significant for all neurocognitive variables with the exception of WCST perseverative errors. Moreover, similar to the results obtained by Kuntsi and Stevenson, the highest bivariate heritability estimate ($h^2_g = 0.52$) was obtained for a discriminant function score that included measures of processing speed, vigilance, working memory, and response inhibition.

4.4.2. *Candidate Gene Studies*

The four studies that examined the relation between a specific candidate gene, ADHD, and EF deficits revealed mixed results. Based on the finding that ADHD is associated with the 7-repeat allele of the DA D4 receptor gene *(20)*, three studies tested if this risk allele is also associated with impairment on EF tasks *(121–123)*. Contrary to this prediction, two studies

(121,122) found that the group with ADHD *without* the 7-repeat allele exhibited EF weaknesses and slower and more variable reaction times. In contrast, a more recent study found that the group with the 7-repeat DRD4 allele exhibited EF deficits in comparison to the group without this allele *(120)*, and another study found that a specific allele of the *monoamine oxidase A* gene was associated with both increased levels of ADHD symptoms and significant neuropsychological impairment *(123)*. The samples in all of these studies were relatively small, suggesting that additional research is needed before any definitive conclusions can be drawn regarding the discrepancies in these results.

4.4.3. Conclusions From Twin and Candidate Gene Studies

Although these results should be interpreted with caution until additional studies with larger samples are available, initial twin and candidate gene studies underscore two important points regarding the relation between ADHD and EF. First, the twin studies and two of the four candidate gene studies suggest that common genes may influence ADHD and at least some aspects of EF. Specifically, although the phenotypic correlations between ADHD symptoms and EF performance are low, these correlations appear to be attributable to common genetic influences *(118)*. On the other hand, the results of the twin studies also indicate that a substantial proportion of the genetic variance associated with ADHD is independent from the genetic influences that lead to EF deficits, and this finding is supported by the counterintuitive results obtained in two studies of the *DRD4* receptor gene *(121,122)*.

4.5. Initial Conclusions Regarding EF Deficit Hypothesis

In summary, the existing data reviewed in this section clearly indicate that ADHD is associated with multiple EF weaknesses. In contrast, these results reject the hypothesis that EF deficits are the core deficit that is necessary and sufficient to cause ADHD. In the next section we examine several possible explanations for the failure to find a core EF deficit in ADHD, and in the final section of the chapter we describe directions for future research that will be useful to test these competing explanations and provide a comprehensive account of the neuropsychology of ADHD.

5. POSSIBLE EXPLANATIONS FOR ABSENCE OF CORE EF DEFICIT

Numerous explanations could account for the failure to find a core deficit on measures of response inhibition, verbal working memory, and other EF domains. In this section we examine five possible explanations in detail. The first hypothesis suggests that the association between ADHD and EF is an artifact, such that ADHD and EF are not associated in the general population. The second and third explanations suggest that EF effect sizes are relatively modest because of weak psychometric properties of EF measures or a low correlation between these measures and the underlying neurocognitive processes they are attempting to measure. The fourth explanation examines the impact of diagnostic heterogeneity, and the final model suggests that EF deficits are one important aspect of the multifactorial neurocognitive etiology of ADHD.

5.1. Explanation 1: EF Hypothesis Is Wrong

Before moving to other more complex explanations, it is important to first rule out the possibility that the relation between ADHD and EF weaknesses is an artifact. This hypothesis suggests that the significant EF weaknesses obtained in groups with ADHD are false-positive results that are attributable to sampling error or clinic-referral bias, whereas in the general population there is no relation between ADHD and EF weaknesses. The results of the meta-analysis clearly reject this hypothesis; several EF weaknesses are consistently associated with ADHD, and the effect sizes for group differences on these measures are medium to large. Moreover, EF weaknesses are present in both population-based samples *(40)* and samples ascertained through clinics *(33)*. Therefore, although neither general EF deficits nor weaknesses in specific EF domains appear to represent a single core deficit, EF weaknesses play a significant role in the complex neuropsychology of ADHD.

5.2. Explanation 2: Weak Psychometric Properties of EF Tasks

Relatively few studies have examined the reliability of EF tasks in children. The studies that have been conducted revealed low to moderate test–retest reliability for WCST perseverative errors (r = 0.30–0.61) and verbal working memory span tasks *(124,125)*. Similarly, Kuntsi et al. *(125)* reported low test-retest reliability for SSRT (intraclass correlation = 0.21) as computed by the algorithm used in their study, although reliability estimates were higher in another study that used an improved algorithm *(46)*. The modest reliability of these measures constrains the range of effect sizes that it will be possible to obtain in group comparisons. Although measurement weaknesses are unlikely to fully explain the failure to find a core EF or response inhibition deficit in ADHD, these results suggest that future neuropsychological studies should carefully assess the reliability of each measure and use available statistical techniques to minimize the impact of the psychometric weaknesses of each task.

5.3. Explanation 3: Putative EF Measures Are Weakly Correlated With Core Deficit in Executive Control

To demonstrate that a neuropsychological weakness is a core deficit, the behavioral tasks used to measure the deficit must be both sensitive and specific to the underlying neurocognitive function. The putative EF measures used in studies of ADHD appear to be reasonably sensitive to the executive control weaknesses that they are designed to measure *(114,126)*. In contrast, the specificity of most of these EF measures is much less clear. This is illustrated by a closer analysis of the stop-signal task and the Trailmaking test, the measures which yielded the largest mean effect size in the meta-analysis.

Part B of the Trailmaking test requires the participant to connect in ascending order a series of circles containing a number or letter, alternating between numbers and letters (i.e., 1, A, 2, B, 3, C,...). Groups with ADHD consistently complete this task more slowly than groups without ADHD, and this group deficit has frequently been interpreted as a weakness in set-shifting *(81)* or executive processing speed *(40)*. However, in addition to these two possible interpretations, poor performance could also be attributable to a weakness in working memory that leads to difficulty monitoring the position in the number and letter sequences to identify the next target, an inefficient visual search strategy to locate the next target stimulus, or even difficulties with the rapid fine motor movements required to connect the circles.

SSRT is a putative measure of the speed of the inhibitory process that occurs when a tone indicates that a response that has already been initiated should be terminated. This task is based on a strong cognitive theory of response inhibition *(46)*, and groups with and without ADHD consistently differ on SSRT. However, similar to the Trailmaking test, other neuropsychological weaknesses could explain the slower SSRT in groups with ADHD. For example, longer SSRTs could be attributable to the slower and more variable responses of

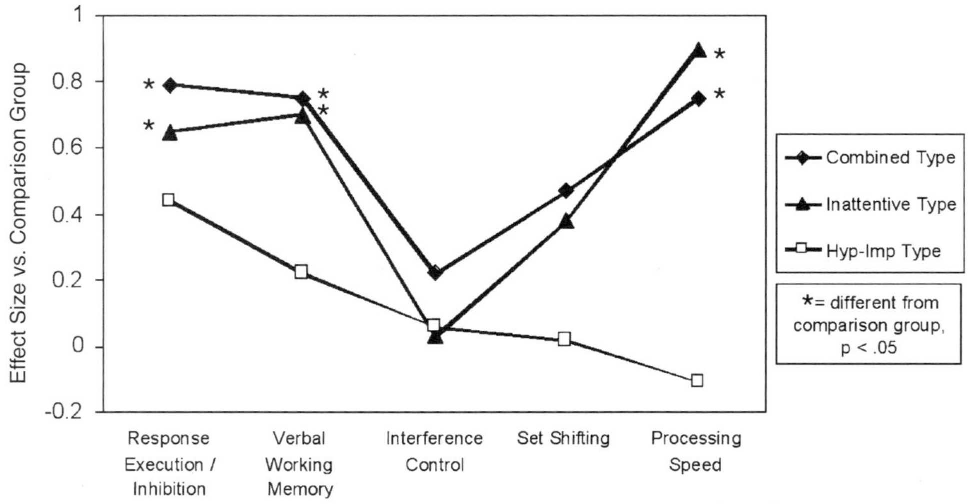

Fig. 2. EF scores of groups with the *Diagnostic and Statistical Manual of Mental Disorders,* 4th ed. Attention Deficit Hyperactivity Disorder. Hyp-Imp, hyperactive–impulsive subtypes.

individuals with ADHD on both stop-signal trials and primary task trials without a stop signal, or may reflect group differences in strategies employed to avoid responding on stop-signal trials *(41)*.

In summary, EF measures that have been used in previous studies are multifactorial, and may correlate only moderately with dysfunctional executive control processes in the brain. Because ADHD group deficits in non-EF domains have also been replicated across studies *(32,33,127)*, it is unlikely that EF measures with improved specificity will reveal a core EF deficit in ADHD. Nonetheless, the development and refinement of more specific measures will provide important clarification regarding the specific facets of EF that are impaired in individuals with ADHD. We return to these issues in more detail when we summarize directions for future research at the end of the chapter.

5.4. Explanation 4: Diagnostic Heterogeneity

As noted previously, ADHD is a complex disorder that may include meaningful diagnostic subtypes *(128,129)*. If these subtypes are characterized by different neuropsychological correlates, studies that include all subtypes in the same group could inadvertently mask effects that are primarily associated with only one of the subtypes. Conversely, neuropsychological deficits could be misattributed to a subgroup in which these weaknesses are not present.

The most recent results from our twin sample illustrate the potential impact of diagnostic heterogeneity (Fig. 2). These results and data from other studies generally suggest that the combined and inattentive types are associated with similar neuropsychological weaknesses *(44,130,131)*, whereas the hyperactive–impulsive type is associated with few neuropsychological weaknesses in comparison to groups without ADHD. Moreover, twin studies suggest that the hyperactive–impulsive type is much less heritable than the other subtypes *(116,132)*, and a recent multisite study of 14 different samples found that the association between ADHD and a polymorphism in the *DRD5* receptor gene is restricted to the inattentive and combined subtypes *(133)*.

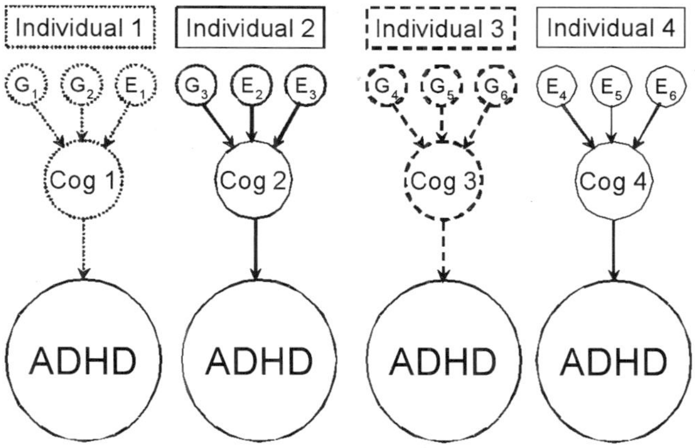

Fig. 3. A hypothetical independent pathway model of the neuropsychology of ADHD. Specific genetic (G) and environmental (E) influences lead to specific neuropsychological weaknesses (Cog 1–Cog 4), and each weakness is sufficient to cause ADHD in that subset of individuals.

Taken together, these results suggest that it may be useful to separate individuals with the hyperactive–impulsive type from those with the combined or inattentive types for neuropsychological analyses. The effect sizes for the group deficits of the inattentive and combined types are still too small to represent a core deficit even when these subtypes are analyzed separately (Fig. 2), suggesting that the inclusion of the hyperactive–impulsive type in analyses of the overall ADHD group does not explain the failure to find a primary EF deficit in the other subtypes. However, these results underscore the need to test for subtype-specific effects in future studies so that the neurocognitive correlates of all subtypes can be accurately described.

5.5. Explanation 5: Multifactorial Models of ADHD

Multifactorial models explicitly hypothesize that ADHD is a complex, neuropsychologically heterogeneous disorder with no core neurocognitive weakness that is sufficient to explain all cases. These models suggest that EF deficits comprise one aspect of the overall neuropsychology of ADHD, but that other neurocognitive weaknesses also increase susceptibility in at least some individuals. To illustrate alternative ways that a multifactorial model could be conceptualized, we next describe two multifactorial models that make different predictions regarding the neuropsychology of ADHD.

5.5.1. Independent Pathway Models

These models suggest that ADHD is a neuropsychologically heterogeneous disorder *(32,113)*. Disruption in any one of two or more pathophysiological substrates can independently lead to the same final behavioral manifestation of ADHD (Fig. 3). Therefore, this type of model describes neuropsychological *subtypes* of ADHD.

The dual-pathway model proposed by Sonuga-Barke et al. *(32,134)* is an excellent example of an independent pathway model. The dual-pathway model suggests that distinct etiological pathways lead to dysfunction in two brain circuits involving DA. The first neural network involves mesolimbic brain circuits that are responsible for signaling availability of reinforcement and maintaining active representations of potential reward to guide decisions *(32)*. Disturbances in this substrate cause an individual to discount the value of future rewards, and are manifest behaviorally as an aversion to delay *(33,34,73,135)*. The second pathway involves EF deficits that are attributable to dysfunction in the prefrontal–basal ganglia–thalamus circuit described earlier in this chapter.

The predictions of the dual-pathway model have been supported by several recent studies. Solanto et al. *(33)* administered the stop-signal task and a measure of delay aversion to a subset of children from the (NIMH) multimodal treatment study *(136,137)*, the largest treatment study ever conducted for a childhood mental disorder. Two critical results emerged from this direct comparison of the inhibition and delay aversion hypotheses. First, the effect size of the difference between groups was larger for the delay aversion task ($d = 0.91$) than for SSRT ($d = 0.69$). More importantly, the two tasks independently predicted ADHD status when they were included in the same model.

Sonuga-Barke et al. subsequently replicated and extended this result in an unselected community sample of preschool children *(127)*. An exploratory factor analysis demonstrated that EF and delay aversion measures loaded on different factors, and both factors independently predicted elevations of ADHD symptoms. Taken together, these provocative results provide the strongest support to date for independent pathophysiological pathways to ADHD, and suggest that a comprehensive neuropsychological model of ADHD must include both delay aversion and EF weaknesses.

5.5.2. *Quantitative Trait Models*

The quantitative trait model *(17)* suggests that multiple genetic and environmental influences comprise a general pool of risk factors for ADHD. Each of these risk factors is associated with a small decrement in some aspect of neuropsychological functioning and a small increase in susceptibility to ADHD. Different combinations of risk and protective factors then lead to individual differences in neurocognitive functioning and symptoms of ADHD, and individuals with a sufficient number of risk factors from the overall pool cross the diagnostic threshold and meet criteria for ADHD. Therefore, rather than conceptualizing ADHD as a categorical diagnosis that is qualitatively distinct from the rest of the population, the quantitative trait model suggests that the threshold for ADHD identifies the extreme tail of a continuous distribution of activity level, attentional functioning, and impulse control.

Several findings support the quantitative trait model of ADHD. First, whereas numerous studies suggest the DSM-IV inattention and hyperactivity–impulsivity symptom dimensions are reliable and externally valid *(5)*, these studies reveal little evidence of a natural threshold between ADHD and "normal" behavior *(114,116)*. The distributions of inattention and hyperactivity–impulsivity symptoms in the general population are not bimodal, associations between the number of ADHD symptoms and degree of functional impairment are linear rather than curvilinear *(8)*, the latent structure of ADHD symptoms appears to be similar in the population at large and in clinically extreme samples *(138)*, and twin studies have found little evidence of a natural diagnostic threshold based on differential heritability *(15,116)*. Thus, similar to most other mental disorders *(139,140)*, it seems probable that there is no natural boundary for the diagnostic category of ADHD.

Candidate gene and linkage studies provide a second strong source of support for the quantitative trait model. As described in more detail earlier in this chapter and elsewhere *(11)*, these studies suggest that ADHD is associated with multiple genetic and environment risk factors. Each of these risk factors has a relatively small effect on symptoms of ADHD (i.e., 1–3 % of the total variance in the behavioral symptoms of ADHD), suggesting that few if any of these specific risk factors are necessary or sufficient to cause ADHD in isolation. Instead, each risk factor must act in combination with other risk factors to cause an individual to develop ADHD.

The fact that ADHD is the extreme end of a continuous trait with a multifactorial etiology does not rule out the possibility that EF deficits could still be the primary cause of ADHD. For example, ADHD could reflect the extreme tail of a distribution of highly heritable individual differences in executive control. However, in addition to multiple EF weaknesses, other studies indicate that ADHD is associated with weaknesses in several non-EF domains *(32,40,45,126)*. Moreover, many of these neuropsychological functions are correlated with one another, and none appears to be necessary or sufficient to cause ADHD. Therefore, rather than a specific primary deficit, this complex pattern of neuropsychological weaknesses is more consistent with a multifactorial quantitative trait model in which some genetic or environmental influences lead to general impairment across all neuropsychological tasks, some etiological factors influence a more specific subset of neural processes or a cluster of functions, such as EF, and still others have a distinct effect on a specific neural function.

6. CONCLUSIONS REGARDING EF DEFICIT HYPOTHESIS AND NEUROPSYCHOLOGY OF ADHD

Existing data argue strongly against a primary deficit model of ADHD. Instead, the models that best fit the data conceptualize EF deficits as one of several important neurocognitive weaknesses that comprise the overall neuropsychology of ADHD. In addition to EF weaknesses, a comprehensive model must also explain the shortened delay gradient described by the dual-pathway model *(32)*, slower and more variable reaction times on individual trials and slower processing speed across entire tasks *(40,93)*, weaknesses in temporal discrimination of stimuli of short duration *(41)* and time estimation/reproduction of longer temporal intervals *(59)*, and deficits in motor control *(141)*. Moreover, even models that are able to explain these multiple deficits will also need to account for neuropsychological heterogeneity in ADHD *(113)*, developmental changes in ADHD symptoms and associated neurocognitive processes *(142)*, and the neuropsychological implications of comorbidity between ADHD and other disorders *(40,128)*.

The correct neurocognitive model of ADHD is likely to involve multiple neural networks distributed across many locations in the brain. Further research is needed to test whether dysfunction in these different networks leads to distinct neuropsychological subtypes within the overall group of individuals with ADHD, or if dysfunctional processes in multiple networks act in combination to increase susceptibility to ADHD. Perhaps the most likely scenario is that both of these models may be partially correct. For example, some cases of ADHD may be attributable to a primary deficit in a relatively specific neurocognitive process, whereas other cases may be caused by the combined effects of dysfunctional processes in multiple neural substrates.

7. DIRECTIONS FOR FUTURE RESEARCH

The transition from models positing a single core deficit to multiple-deficit models represents a paradigm shift in the way that the neuropsychology of ADHD is conceptualized *(32)*. Therefore, in this final section we describe recommendations for future studies of the neurocognitive correlates of ADHD that are conducted within a multifactorial framework. These recommendations are summarized in Table 3 and described in more detail in the text.

Table 3
Suggested Guidelines for Future Studies of the Neuropsychology of ADHD

I. Neuropsychological weaknesses that should be assessed in a comprehensive test battery
  A) Delay aversion *(32)*
  B) Executive functions
    1. Response inhibition *(1,26,96,110)*
    2. Planning *(81)*
    3. Verbal working memory *(79)*
    4. Spatial working memory *(42)*
    5. Vigilance *(146)*
  C) Temporal processing
    1. Intervals longer than two seconds *(59)*
    2. Intervals less than one second *(41)*
  D) Naming/processing speed *(40,93)*
  E) State regulation/response variability *(43,144)*
  F) Motor control *(1)*
  G) Intelligence

II. Comorbidities that may influence the neuropsychological correlates of ADHD
  A) Learning disabilities *(39,40,145)*
  B) Anxiety disorders *(147)*
  C) Conduct disorder/aggression *(148)*

III. Diagnostic procedures and descriptive characteristics of the sample that should be described
  A) Procedures used to diagnose ADHD
    1. Diagnostic criteria (e.g., DSM-IV vs ICD-10 vs normative cutoff scores)
    2. Reporters/measures used
    3. Algorithm to combine information from multiple informants
  B) Descriptive characteristics
    1. Proportion with each diagnostic subtype
    2. Severity of ADHD symptoms
    3. Age
    4. Proportion male and female
    5. Ethnicity
    6. Socioeconomic status
    7. Medication (treatment vs medication naïve, status on the day of testing)
  C) Exclusion criteria
  D) Other potential markers of neuropsychological heterogeneity
    1. Atypical etiology (e.g., head injury, chromosome disorder, traumatic event)
    2. Familial vs nonfamilial ADHD

IV. Characteristics of the task and experimental design that should be described
  A) Task parameters
    1. Task specifications
    2. Computer system/software
    3. Specific instructions
    4. Procedures for data cleaning/adjustment of outliers
    5. Event rate
    6. Reinforcement contingencies within the task

(Continued)

Table 3
(Continued)

B) Characteristics of the experimental environment
   1. Presence of the experimenter
   2. Time of day of the testing
   3. Duration of the session
   4. Order of the task in the session
   5. Compensation for the participant

7.1. Use Theory to Guide Task Development and Refinement

As noted previously, the EF tasks used in previous studies of ADHD are typically complex and multifactorial. As a result, it is often difficult to determine whether poor performance on a task is attributable to a specific EF weakness or to dysfunction in one of the other cognitive processes that is required to complete the task successfully. This lack of specificity could potentially lead to the erroneous conclusion that EF weaknesses are associated with ADHD, when poor performance is, in fact a result of dysfunction in another neurocognitive domain. Alternatively, if the poor performance of the ADHD group on a multifactorial task is explained primarily by a specific EF weakness, the effect size associated with this weakness may be underestimated because of the noise introduced by individual differences in the other processes necessary to complete the task.

Rather than continuing to administer EF measures of convenience borrowed from the adult brain injury literature or from neuropsychological studies of other disorders, future studies should incorporate EF tasks that are carefully constructed to isolate specific parameters of interest. Theoretical models of ADHD can be used to guide the development of within-task manipulations that isolate the function of interest by controlling other functions that might otherwise explain the results *(43)*. In addition to increasing the specificity of each neuropsychological measure, these within-task controls will facilitate direct tests of competing neuropsychological models of ADHD.

7.2. Directly Test Competing Neuropsychological Models

Until recently, most studies have examined the neuropsychological correlates of ADHD from a single theoretical perspective. For example, although several previous studies included a range of EF measures *(44,69,81,93)*, few of these studies also included measures of delay aversion, naming speed, temporal processing, state regulation, and motor output. Moreover, only a handful of studies have tested whether EF performance varies as a function of task parameters, such as the duration of the interstimulus interval *(144)* or the presence of reinforcement contingencies *(82)*.

Future studies are needed that pit the competing theories of ADHD against one another *(43)*. This could be accomplished by administering the optimal measure of each theoretical domain to the same sample of individuals *(33,127)*. The first section of Table 3 lists the neuropsychological weaknesses that have been replicated most consistently in studies that compared groups with and without ADHD. Although it may not be feasible for a single study to include all these measures, this list provides a summary of the neuropsychological domains that should be taken into consideration in future studies.

Alternatively, an experimental manipulation or additional condition could be added to the key measure of each theory to test whether the ADHD group deficit can be better explained by another process. For example, Scheres et al. found that the response speed of individuals with ADHD varied as a function of event rate *(99)*, consistent with the hypothesis that ADHD is partially attributable to difficulties with arousal regulation. In contrast, Oosterlaan and Sergeant found that ADHD was associated with slower SSRT even in the presence of reward or response–cost contingencies *(82)*, arguing against the hypothesis that ADHD is a result of motivational dysfunction. Future studies with similar designs will help to clarify the relations among the key neurocognitive processes described by each theory, as well as their relative contributions to the overall neuropsychology of ADHD.

7.3. Use Statistical Techniques to Reduce Measurement Error

As described previously, the predictive power of EF and other neuropsychological measures may be constrained by the relatively modest reliability of these tasks in children. One method to reduce measurement error is to administer multiple measures that reflect a common latent trait of interest. Because a latent trait represents the shared variance among the tasks, it eliminates error variance that is specific to each task and provides a more reliable measure of the underlying construct of interest.

The potential utility of this approach is illustrated by our most recent results *(40)*. Comparisons between groups with and without ADHD revealed a substantially larger effect size for the response inhibition/execution factor score ($d = 1.19$) than for any individual measure that loaded on this factor ($d = 0.50–0.89$); similar results were obtained for measures that loaded on the processing speed and verbal working memory factors. These results suggest that in addition to carefully assessing the reliability of each individual task, it may be useful for future studies to administer multiple measures of each neuropsychological domain to minimize the impact of the psychometric weaknesses of any individual task.

7.4. Clarify Implications of Diagnostic and Neuropsychological Heterogeneity

Existing data clearly indicate that ADHD is a heterogeneous disorder at both the level of the behavioral phenotype and the underlying neuropsychological correlates *(33,113,134)*. The most obvious example of behavioral heterogeneity is the inclusion of three distinct diagnostic subtypes of ADHD in DSM-IV. In addition, previous studies have reported significant differences in the neuropsychological correlates of subgroups of individuals with ADHD as a function of situational and reporter differences in symptoms *(96)*, comorbid disorders *(144–148)*, and specific genetic risk factors *(120–123)*.

Heterogeneity in groups with ADHD may partially reflect measurement error or minor differences in sampling procedures or symptom severity. Alternatively, diagnostic heterogeneity may be a marker for meaningful variation in the pathophysiology of different subgroups within the overall ADHD diagnosis *(32,113)*, or could even demarcate a subgroup of individuals who exhibit attentional difficulties as a secondary consequence of an atypical etiology, such as a brain injury *(149)* or severe traumatic experience *(150)*. Therefore, to facilitate the development of a comprehensive neuropsychological model of ADHD, future studies are needed to clarify the implications of this heterogeneity.

One approach to address diagnostic heterogeneity is to apply stringent exclusionary criteria at the beginning of the study to maximize the homogeneity of the ADHD sample. However, the a priori exclusion of a subset of individuals with ADHD makes extremely strong assumptions about the meaning of heterogeneity that are not easily justified based on existing knowledge. For example, a procedure that excluded all individuals with a comorbid learning disability is likely to eliminate the subset of individuals with ADHD with the most severe neuropsychological impairment *(39,40,145)*. If this greater severity is simply a secondary consequence of the comorbid learning difficulties the decision to exclude these individuals from the study might be justified. However, because comorbidity between reading disability and ADHD is primarily attributable to common genetic influences *(117,151,152)*, the comorbid group may exhibit the greatest neuropsychological impairment because this subset has the strongest loading of these shared genes. If this turns out to be the case, the decision to exclude individuals with a comorbid learning disability might inadvertently eliminate the group that would be most useful for analyses of the neuropsychological correlates of ADHD.

Therefore, for most purposes, the best strategy may be to include all participants who meet full diagnostic criteria for ADHD, then to carefully measure potential markers of meaningful heterogeneity. (Sections 2 and 3 of Table 3 list some of the variables that may be useful to consider). This procedure avoids any sampling biases that could be produced by a priori exclusionary criteria, and facilitates a direct test whether each type of heterogeneity significantly mediates or moderates the neuropsychological correlates of ADHD.

7.5. Describe Study Characteristics and Task Parameters Sufficiently to Facilitate Comparisons Across Studies

In addition to the complexity introduced by heterogeneity among individuals with ADHD, interpretation of neuropsychological studies of ADHD is complicated by differences across laboratories in specific task parameters and experimental environments. For example, the magnitude of the difference between groups with and without ADHD may be influenced by differences in stimulus presentation rate *(144,153)*, the presence of reward or punishment contingencies *(43,154)*, and the specific procedures used to clean and adjust the data *(41)*. Although it is not realistic to suggest standardization of these parameters across all laboratories, future studies should sufficiently describe both the overall experimental environment and the specific parameters of each task to enable comparisons between studies (we provide an initial list of characteristics in Section 4 of Table 3). Along the same lines, all studies should report group means and standard deviations for each dependent measure to facilitate future meta-analyses.

8. CONCLUSIONS

EF weaknesses are neither necessary, nor sufficient to cause most cases of ADHD. Nonetheless, specific aspects of EF such as response inhibition, planning, and executive processing speed play an important role in the complex multifactorial neuropsychology of ADHD. Additional research is needed to assess the impact of diagnostic and neuropsychological heterogeneity on the neurocognitive correlates of ADHD, and to clarify the relation between EF weaknesses and weaknesses in domains, such as delay aversion, state regulation, and response to reinforcement contingencies.

ACKNOWLEDGMENTS

The authors were supported in part during the preparation of this manuscript by National Institute of Health grants MH 62120 and MH 63941 (Erik Willcutt) and MH 38820 and MH

04024 (Bruce Pennington). Funding for the Colorado Learning Disabilities Research Center is provided by National Institute of Child Health and Human Development Center Grant HD 27802 (Center Director: John C. DeFries). The authors thank John C. DeFries and Richard K. Olson for sharing a portion of the data presented in this chapter.

REFERENCES

1. Barkley RA. ADHD and the nature of self-control. New York: Guilford Press, 1998.
2. Pennington BF, Ozonoff S. Executive functions and developmental psychopathology. J Child Psychol Psychiatry 1996;37:51–87.
3. American Psychiatric Association. Diagnostic and statistical manual of mental disorders, 4th ed. Washington, DC: American Psychiatric Association, 1994.
4. Angold A, Erkanli A, Farmer EMZ, et al. Psychiatric disorder, impairment, and service use in rural African American and white youth. Arch Gen Psychiatry 2002;59:893–901.
5. Willoughby MT, Curran PJ, Costello EJ, Angold A. Implications of early versus late onset of attention-deficit/hyperactivity disorder symptoms. J Amer Acad Child Adolesc Psychiatry 2000;39:1512–1519.
6. DuPaul GJ, Anastopoulos AD, McGoey KE, Power TJ, Reid R, Ikeda MJ. Teacher ratings of attention deficit hyperactivity disorder symptoms: factor structure and normative data. Psychol Assess 1997;9:436–444.
7. DuPaul GJ, Anastopoulos AD, Power TJ, Reid R, Ikeda MJ, McGoey KE. Parent ratings of attention deficit/hyperactivity disorder symptoms: factor structure and normative data. J Psychopathol Behav Assess 1998;20:83–102.
8. Lahey BB, Applegate B, McBurnett K, et al. DSM-IV field trials for attention deficit hyperactivity disorder in children and adolescents. Amer J Psychiatry 1994;151:1673–1685.
9. DeFries JC, Filipek PA, Fulker DF, et al. Colorado Learning Disabilities Research Center. Learn Disabil 1997;8:7–19.
10. Maher BS, Marazita ML, Ferrell RE, Vanyukov MM. Dopamine system genes and attention deficit hyperactivity disorder: a meta-analysis. Psychiatr Genet 2002;12:207–215.
11. Willcutt EG. Genetics of ADHD. In: Barch D, ed. Cognitive and affective neuroscience of psychopathology. Oxford: Oxford University Press. In press, 2004.
12. Faraone SV, Biederman J, Friedman D. Validity of DSM-IV subtypes of attention-deficit/hyperactivity disorder: a family study perspective. J Amer Acad Child Adolesc Psychiatry 2000;39: 300–307.
13. Friedman M, Chhabildas N, Budhiraja N, Willcutt EG, Pennington BF. Etiology of comorbidity between ADHD and reading disability: exploration of the assortative mating hypothesis. Am J Med Genet (Neuropsychiatr Genet) 2003;120B:109–115.
14. Eaves L, Silberg J, Meyer J, et al. Genetics and developmental psychopathology: 2. The main effects of genes and environment on behavioral problems in the Virginia Twin Study of Adolescent Behavioral Development. J Child Psychol Psychiatry 1997;38:965–980.
15. Levy F, Hay D, McStephen M, Wood C, Waldman I. Attention-deficit hyperactivity disorder: a category or a continuum? A genetic analysis of a large-scale twin study. J Amer Acad Child Adolesc Psychiatry 1997;36:737–744.
16. Faraone SV, Tsuang MT, Tsuang DW. Genetics of mental disorders. New York: Guilford Press, 1999.
17. Plomin R, DeFries JC, McClearn GE, McGuffin P. Behavioral Genetics, 4th Ed. New York: Freeman Press, 2001.
18. Comings DE, Gade-Andavolu R, Gonzales N, et al. Multivariate analyses of associations of 42 genes in ADHD, ODD, and conduct disorder. Clin Genet 2000;58:31–40.
19. Volkow ND, Wang GJ, Fowler JS, et al. Dopamine transporter occupancies in the human brain induced by therapeutic doses of methylphenidate. Amer J Psychiatry 1998;155: 1325–1331.

20. Faraone SV, Doyle AE, Mick E, Biederman J. Meta-analysis of the association between the 7-repeat allele of the dopamine D4 receptor gene and attention deficit hyperactivity disorder. Amer J Psychiatry 2001;158:1052–1057.
21. Bakker SC, van der Meulen EM, Buitelaar JK, et al. A whole-genome scan in 164 Dutch sib pairs with attention-deficit/hyperactivity disorder: suggestive evidence for linkage on chromosomes 7p and 15q. Amer J Hum Genet 2003;72:1251–1260.
22. Ogdie MN, MacPhie IL, Minassian SL, et al. A genomewide scan for attention-deficit/hyperactivity disorder in an extended sample: suggestive linkage on 17p11. Amer J Hum Genet; 72:1268–1279.
23. Pennington BF. The development of psychopathology. New York: Guilford Press, 2002.
24. Welsh MC, Pennington BF. Assessing frontal lobe functioning in children: views from developmental psychology. Devel Neuropsychol 1988;4:199–230.
25. Casey BJ, Durston S, Fossella JA. Towards a mechanistic model of cognitive control. Clin Neurosci Res 2001;1:267–282.
26. Barkley RA. Behavioral inhibition, sustained attention, and executive function: constructing a unified theory of ADHD. Psychol Bull 1997;121:65–94.
27. Douglas VI. Attentional and cognitive problems. In: Rutter M, ed. Developmental neuropsychiatry. New York: Guilford Press, 1983:280–332.
28. Fuster JM. The prefrontal cortex: Anatomy, physiology and neuropsychology of the frontal lobe (2nd ed.). New York: Raven Press, 1989.
29. Levin HS, Eisenberg HM, Benton AL. Frontal lobe function and dysfunction. New York: Oxford University Press, 1991.
30. Stuss DT, Benson DF. The frontal lobes. New York: Raven Press, 1986.
31. Rolls ET. The brain and emotion. New York: Oxford University Press, 1999.
32. Sonuga-Barke EJS. The dual pathway model of ADHD: an elaboration of neuro-developmental characteristics. Neurosc Biobehav Rev 2003;27:593–604.
33. Solanto MV, Abikoff H, Sonuga-Barke E, et al. The ecological validity of delay aversion and response inhibition as measures of impulsivity in AD/HD: a supplement to the NIMH multimodal treatment study of AD/HD. J Abnorm Child Psychol 2001;29:215–228.
34. Sonuga-Barke EJS, Taylor E, Sembi S, Smith J. Hyperactivity and delay aversion—I. The effect of delay on choice. J Child Psychol Psychiatry 1992;33:387–398.
35. Pennington BF. Dimensions of executive functions in normal and abnormal development. In: Krasnegor NA, Lyon GR, eds. Development of the prefrontal cortex: evolution, neurobiology, and behavior. Baltimore, MD: Paul H. Brookes, 1997:265–281.
36. Barkley RA, Edwards G, Laneri M, Fletcher K, Metevia L. Executive functioning, temporal discounting, and sense of time in adolescents with attention deficit hyperactivity disorder (ADHD) and oppositional defiant disorder (ODD). J Abnorm Child Psychol 2001;29:541–556.
37. Mariani MA, Barkley RA. Neuropsychological and academic functioning in preschool boys with attention deficit hyperactivity disorder. Devel Neuropsychol 1997;13:111–129.
38. Miyake A, Friedman NP, Emerson MJ, Witzki AH, Howerter A. The unity and diversity of executive functions and their contributions to complex frontal lobe tasks: a latent variable analysis. Cog Psychol 2000;41:49–100.
39. Willcutt EG, Pennington BF, Boada R, et al. A comparison of the cognitive deficits in reading disability and attention-deficit/hyperactivity disorder. J Abnorm Psychol 2001;110:157–172.
40. Willcutt EG, Pennington BF, Chhabildas NA, Olson RK, Hulslander JL. Neuropsychological analyses of comorbidity between RD and ADHD: in search of the common deficit. Devel Neuropsychol. In press, 2004.
41. Castellanos FX, Tannock R. Neuroscience of attention-deficit/hyperactivity disorder: the search for endophenotypes. Nat Rev Neurosci 2002;3:617–628.
42. Kempton S, Vance A, Maruff P, Luk E, Costin J, Pantelis C. Executive function and attention deficit hyperactivity disorder: stimulant medication and better executive function performance in children. Psychol Med 1999;29:527–538.

43. Sergeant JA, Geurts H, Huijbregts S, Scheres A, Oosterlaan J. The top and bottom of ADHD: a neuropsychological perspective. Neurosc Biobehav Rev 2003;27:583–592.
44. Chhabildas N, Pennington BF, Willcutt EG. A comparison of the cognitive deficits in the DSM-IV subtypes of ADHD. J Abnorm Child Psychol 2001;29:529–540.
45. Sergeant JA, Guerts H, Oosterlaan J. How specific is a deficit of executive functioning for attention-deficit/hyperactivity disorder? Behav Brain Res 2002;130:3–28.
46. Logan GD, Schachar RJ, Tannock R. Impulsivity and inhibitory control. Psychol Sci 1997;8:60–64.
47. Heaton RK. Wisconsin Card Sorting Test Manual. Odessa, FL: Psychological Assessment Resources, 1981.
48. Borys SV, Spitz HH, Dorans BA. Tower of Hanoi performance of retarded young adults and nonretarded children as a function of solution length and goal state. J Exp Child Psychol 1982; 33:87–110.
49. Shallice T. Specific impairments of planning. Phil Trans Roy Soc London 1982;298:199–209.
50. Siegel LS, Ryan EB. The development of working memory in normally achieving and subtypes of learning disabled children. Child Devel 1989;60:973–980.
51. Wechsler D. Manual for the Wechsler Intelligence Scale for Children, 3rd ed. San Antonio, TX: The Psychological Corporation, 1991.
52. Golden JC. Stroop Color and Word Test. Chicago: Stoelting Company, 1978.
53. Reitan R, Wolfson D. The Halstead-Reitan Neuropsychological Test Battery: theory and clinical interpretation. Tucson: Neuropsychology Press, 1985.
54. Cohen J. Statistical power analysis for the behavioral sciences. Hillsdale, NJ: Lawrence Erlbaum Associates, 1988.
55. Hedges LV, Olkin I. Statistical methods for meta-analysis. Orlando, FL: Academic Press, 1985.
56. Cooper H. Synthesizing research (3rd ed.). Thousand Oaks, CA: Sage, 1998.
57. Aman CJ, Roberts RJ, Pennington BF. A neuropsychological examination of the underlying deficit in attention deficit hyperactivity disorder: Frontal lobe versus right parietal lobe theories. Devel Psychol 1988;34:956–969.
58. Barkley RA, Grodzinsky G, DuPaul GJ. Frontal lobe functions in attention deficit disorder with and without hyperactivity: a review and research report. J Abnorm Child Psychol 1992;20: 163–188.
59. Barkley RA, Murphy KR, Bush T. Time perception and reproduction in young adults with attention deficit hyperactivity disorder. Neuropsychol 2001;15:351–360.
60. Bedard A, Ickowicz A, Logan GD, Hogg-Johnson S, Schachar R, Tannock R. Selective inhibition in children with attention-deficit hyperactivity disorder off and on stimulant medication. J Abnorm Child Psychol 2003;31:315–327.
61. Boucugnani LL, Jones RW. Behaviors analogous to frontal lobe dysfunction in children with attention deficit hyperactivity disorder. Arch Clin Neuropsychol 1989;4:161–173.
62. Carter CS, Krener P, Chaderjian M, Northcutt C, Wolfe V. Abnormal processing of irrelevant information in attention deficit hyperactivity disorder. Psychiatry Res 1995;56:59–70.
63. Chelune GJ, Ferguson W, Koon R, Dickey TO. Frontal lobe disinhibition in attention deficit disorder. Child Psychiatry Hum Devel 1986;16:221–234.
64. Culbertson WC, Zillmer EA. The Tower of London^{DX}: a standardized approach to assessing executive function in children. Arch Clin Neuropsychol 1998;13:285–301.
65. Dimoska A, Johnstone SJ, Barry RJ, Clarke AR. Inhibitory motor control in children with attention-deficit/hyperactivity disorder: Event-related potentials in the stop-signal paradigm. Biol Psychiatry 2003;54:1345–1354.
66. Fischer M, Barkley RA, Edelbrock CS, Smallish L. The adolescent outcome of hyperactive children diagnosed by research criteria: II. Academic, attentional, and neuropsychological status. J Cons Clin Psychol 1990;58:580–588.
67. Gorenstein EE, Mammato CA, Sandy JM. Performance of inattentive-overactive children on selected measures of prefrontal-type function. J Clin Psychol 1989;45:619–632.

68. Grodzinsky GM, Diamond R. Frontal lobe functioning in boys with attention deficit hyperactivity disorder. Devel Neuropsychol 1992;8:427–445.
69. Houghton S, Douglas G, West J, et al. Differential patterns of executive function in children with attention-deficit hyperactivity disorder according to gender and subtype. J Child Neurol 1999;14:801–805.
70. Karatekin C, Asarnow RF. Working memory in childhood-onset schizophrenia and attention deficit/hyperactivity disorder. Psychiatry Res 1998;80:165–176.
71. Klorman R, Hazel-Fernandez LA, Shaywitz SE, et al. Executive functioning deficits in attention-deficit/hyperactivity disorder are independent of oppositional defiant or reading disorder. J Amer Acad Child Adolesc Psychiatry 1999;27:163–170.
72. Konrad K, Gauggel S, Manz A, Schöll M. Lack of inhibition: a motivational deficit in children with attention deficit/hyperactivity disorder and children with traumatic brain injury. Child Neuropsychol;6:286–296.
73. Kuntsi J, Oosterlaan J, Stevenson J. Psychological mechanisms in hyperactivity: I. Response inhibition deficit, working memory impairment, delay aversion, or something else? J Child Psychol Psychiatry 2001;42:199–210.
74. Loge D, Staton D, Beatty W. Performance of children with ADHD on tests of frontal lobe dysfunction. J Amer Acad Child Adolesc Psychiatry 1990;29:540–545.
75. Lufi D, Cohen A, Parish-Plass J. Identifying attention deficit hyperactivity disorder with the WISC-R and the Stroop color and word test. Psychol in the Schools 1990;27:28–34.
76. Manassis K, Tannock R, Barbosa J. Dichotic listening and response inhibition in children with comorbid anxiety disorders and ADHD. J Amer Acad Child Adolesc Psychiatry 2000;39:1152–1159.
77. Mataró M, Garcia-Sánchez C, Junqué C, Estévez-González A, Pujol J. Magnetic resonance imaging measurement of the caudate nucleus in adolescents with attention-deficit hyperactivity disorder and its relationship with neuropsychological and behavioral measures. Arch Neurol 1997;54:963–967.
78. McGee R, Williams S, Moffitt T, Anderson J. A comparison of 13-year-old boys with attention deficit and/or reading disorder on neuropsychological measures. J Abnorm Child Psychol 1989;17:37–53.
79. McInnes A, Humphries T, Hogg-Johnson S, Tannock R. Listening comprehension and working memory are impaired in attention-deficit/hyperactivity disorder irrespective of language impairment. J Abnorm Child Psychol 2003;31:427–443.
80. Nigg JT. The ADHD response-inhibition deficit as measured by the stop task: replication with DSM-IV combined type, extension, and qualification. J Abnorm Child Psychol 1999;27: 393–402.
81. Nigg JT, Blaskey LG, Huang-Pollock CL, Rappley MD. Neuropsychological executive functions and DSM-IV ADHD subtypes. J Amer Acad Child Adolesc Psychiatry 2002;41:59–66.
82. Oosterlaan J, Sergeant JA. Effects of reward and response cost on response inhibition in AD/HD, disruptive, anxious, and normal children. J Abnorm Child Psychol 1998;26:161–174.
83. Oosterlaan J, Sergeant JA. Inhibition in ADHD, aggressive, and anxious children: a biologically-based model of child psychopathology. J Abnorm Child Psychol 1996;24:19–36.
84. Overtoom CCE, Kenemans JL, Verbaten MN, et al. 2002. Inhibition in children with attention-deficit/hyperactivity disorder: a psychophysiological study of the stop task. Biol Psychiatry 2002;51:668–676.
85. Ozonoff S, Jensen J. Brief report: specific executive function profiles in three neurodevelopmental disorders. J Aut Devel Disord;29:171–177.
86. Pennington BF, Groisser D, Welsh MC. Contrasting cognitive deficits in attention deficit hyperactivity disorder versus reading disability. Dev Psychol 1993;29:511–523.
87. Pineda D, Ardila A, Rosselli M. Neuropsychological and behavioural assessment of ADHD in seven- and 12-year-old children: a discriminant analysis. J Learn Disabil 1999;32:159–173.

88. Pliszka SR, Borcherding SH, Spratley K, Leon S, Irick S. Measuring inhibitory control in children. J Devel Behav Ped 1997;18:254–259.
89. Pliszka SR, Liotti M, Woldorff MG. Inhibitory control in children with attention-deficit/hyperactivity disorder: event related potentials identify the processing component and timing of an impaired right-frontal response-inhibition mechanism. Biol Psychiatry 2000;48:238–246.
90. Purvis K, Tannock RT. Phonological processing, not inhibitory control, differentiates ADHD and reading disorder. J Amer Acad Child Adolesc Psychiatry 2000;39:485–494.
91. Rubia K, Oosterlaan J, Sergeant JA, Brandeis D, Leeuwen TV. Inhibitory dysfunction in hyperactive boys. Behav Brain Res 1998;94:25–32.
92. Rubia K, Taylor E, Smith AB, Oksannen H, Overmeyer S, Newman S. Neuropsychological analyses of impulsiveness in childhood hyperactivity. B J Psychiatry 2001;179:138–143.
93. Rucklidge JJ, Tannock R. Neuropsychological profiles of adolescents with ADHD: effects of reading difficulties and gender. J Child Psychol Psychiatry 2002;43:988–1003.
94. Sartory G, Heine A, Müller BW, Elvermann-Hallner A. Event- and motor-related potentials during the continuous performance task in attention-deficit/hyperactivity disorder. J Psychophys 2002;16:97–106.
95. Schachar R, Logan G. Are hyperactive children deficient in attentional capacity? J Abnorm Child Psychol 1990;18:493–513.
96. Schachar R, Mota VL, Logan GD, Tannock R, Klim P. Confirmation of an inhibitory control deficit in attention-deficit/hyperactivity disorder. J Abnorm Child Psychol 2000;28:227–235.
97. Schachar R, Tannock R. Test of four hypotheses for the comorbidity of attention deficit hyperactivity disorder and conduct disorder. J Amer Acad Child Adolesc Psychiatry 1995;34:639–648.
98. Schachar RJ, Tannock R, Marriott M, Logan G. Control of response processes in attention deficit hyperactivity disorder. J Abnorm Child Psychol 1995;23:411–437.
99. Scheres A, Oosterlaan J, Sergeant JA. Response execution and inhibition in children with AD/HD and other disruptive disorders: The role of behavioural activation. J Child Psychol Psychiatry 2001;42:347–357.
100. Schmitz M, Cadore L, Paczko M, et al. Neuropsychological performance in DSM-IV ADHD subtypes: An exploratory study with untreated adolescents. Can J Psychiatry 2002;47:863–869.
101. Seidman LJ, Biederman J, Faraone SV, Weber W, Mennin D, Jones J. A pilot study of neuropsychological functioning in girls with ADHD. J Amer Acad Child Adolesc Psychiatry 1997;36:366–373.
102. Seidman LJ, Biederman J, Faraone SV, Weber W, Ouellette C. Toward defining a neuropsychology of attention deficit hyperactivity disorder: performance of children and adolescents from a large clinically referred sample. J Cons Clin Psychol 1997;65:150–160.
103. Semrud-Clikeman M, Steingard RJ, Filipek P, Biederman J, Bekken K, Renshaw P. Using MRI to examine brain-behavior relationships in males with attention deficit hyperactivity disorder. J Amer Acad Child Adolesc Psychiatry 2000;39:477–484.
104. Shue K, Douglas VI. Attention deficit hyperactivity disorder and the frontal lobe syndrome. Brain Cog 1992;20:104–124.
105. Tripp G, Ryan J, Peace K. Neuropsychological functioning in children with DSM-IV combined type attention deficit hyperactivity disorder. Aust N Zeal J Psychiatry 2002;36:771–779.
106. Weyandt LL, Willis WG. Executive functions in school-aged children: potential efficacy of tasks in discriminating clinical groups. Devel Neuropsychol 1994;10:1697–1713.
107. Wiers RW, Gunning WB, Sergeant JA. Is a mild deficit in executive functions in boys related to childhood ADHD or to multigenerational alcoholism? J Abnorm Child Psychol 1998;26:415–430.
108. Wu KK, Anderson V, Castiello U. Neuropsychological evaluation of deficits in executive functioning for ADHD children with or without learning disabilities. Devel Neuropsychol 2002;22:501–531.
109. Nigg JT. Is ADHD a disinhibitory disorder? Psychol Bull 2001;127:571–598.
110. Nigg JT. On inhibition/disinhibition in developmental psychopathology: views from cognitive and personality psychology and a working inhibition taxonomy. Psychol Bull 2000;126:1–27.
111. Nigg JT, Butler KM, Huang-Pollock CL, Henderson JM. Inhibitory processes in adults with persistent childhood onset ADHD. J Cons Clin Psychol 2002;70:153–157.

112. Nigg JT, Hinshaw SP, Carte E, Treuting J. Neuropsychological correlates of childhood attention-deficit/hyperactivity disorder: explainable by comorbid disruptive behavior or reading problems? J Abnorm Psychol;107:468–480.
113. Nigg JT, Willcutt EG, Doyle AE, Sonuga-Barke EJS. Heterogeneous causality in ADHD: The need for a neuropsychologically impaired subtype for research purposes. Biol Psychiatry. In press, 2004.
114. Barkley RA. Attention-deficit hyperactivity disorder: a handbook for diagnosis and treatment (2nd ed.). New York: Guilford Press, 1998.
115. Doyle AE, Biederman J, Seidman LJ, Weber W, Faraone SV. Diagnostic efficiency of neuropsychological test scores for discriminating boys with and without attention deficit-hyperactivity disorder. J Cons Clin Psychol 2000;68:477–488.
116. Willcutt EG, Pennington BF, DeFries JC. Etiology of inattention and hyperactivity/impulsivity in a community sample of twins with learning difficulties. J Abnorm Child Psychol 2000;28: 149–159.
117. Willcutt EG, DeFries JC, Pennington BF, Olson RK, Smith SD, Cardon LR. Comorbidity of reading difficulties and ADHD. In: Plomin R, DeFries JC, McGuffin P, Craig I, eds. Behavioral genetics in a postgenomic era. Washington, DC: American Psychiatric Association 2003; 227–246.
118. Chhabildas N. A twin study of the validity of the executive function theory of ADHD. Denver, CO: University of Denver, 2003.
119. Kuntsi J, Stevenson J. Psychological mechanisms in hyperactivity: II. The role of genetic factors. J Child Psychol Psychiatry 2001;42:211–219.
120. Langley K, Marshall L, van den Bree M, et al. Association of the dopamine D_4 receptor gene 7-repeat allele with neuropsychological test performance of children with ADHD. Amer J Psychiatry 2004;161:133–138.
121. Manor I, Tyano S, Eisenberg J, Bachner-Melman R, Kotler M, Ebstein RP. The short DRD4 repeats confer risk to attention deficit hyperactivity disorder in a family-based design and impair performance on a continuous performance test (TOVA). Mol Psychiatry 2002;7: 790–794.
122. Swanson J, Oosterlaan J, Murias M, et al. Attention deficit/hyperactivity disorder children with a 7-repeat allele of the dopamine receptor D4 gene have extreme behavior but normal performance on critical neuropsychological tests of attention. Proc Nat Acad Sci 2000;97:4754–4759.
123. Manor I, Tyano S, Mel E, et al. Family-based and association studies of monoamine oxidase A and attention deficit hyperactivity disorder (ADHD): preferential transmission of the long promoter-region repeat and its association with impaired performance on a continuous performance test. Mol Psychiatry 2002b;7:626–632.
124. Pennington BF, Bennetto L, McAleer OK, Roberts RJ. Executive functions and working memory: Theoretical measurement issues. In: Lyon GR, Krasnegor NA, eds. Attention, memory and executive function. Baltimore, MD: Paul H. Brookes, 1995;327–348.
125. Kuntsi J, Stevenson J, Oosterlaan J, Sonuga-Barke EJS. Test-retest reliability of a new delay aversion task and executive function measures. Br J Devel Psychol 2001;19:339–348.
126. Nigg JT. Status of activation and inhibition theories of ADHD. In: Barch D, ed. Cognitive and affective neuroscience of psychopathology. Oxford University Press; In press, 2004.
127. Sonuga-Barke EJS, Dalen L, Remington B. Do executive deficits and delay aversion make independent contributions to preschool attention-deficit/hyperactivity disorder symptoms? J Amer Acad Child Adolesc Psychiatry 2003;42:1335–1342.
128. Barkley RA, DuPaul GJ, McMurray MB. Comprehensive evaluation of attention deficit disorder with and without hyperactivity as defined by research criteria. J Cons Clin Psychol 1990;58: 775–789.
129. Lahey BB, Willcutt E. Validity of the diagnosis and dimensions of attention deficit hyperactivity disorder. In: Jensen PS, Cooper JR, eds. Attention deficit hyperactivity disorder: state of the science. New York: Civic Research Institute, 2003;1–23.

130. Faraone SV, Biederman J, Weber W, Russell RL. Psychiatric, neuropsychological, and psychosocial features of DSM-IV subtypes of attention-deficit/hyperactivity disorder: results from a clinically-referred sample. J Amer Acad Child Adolesc Psychiatry 1998;37:185–193.
131. Todd RD, Sitdhiraska N, Reich W, et al. Discrimination of DSM-IV and latent class attention-deficit/hyperactivity disorder subtypes by educational and cognitive performance in a population-based sample of child and adolescent twins. J Amer Acad Child Adolesc Psychiatry 2002;41:820–828.
132. Todd RD, Rasmussen ER, Neuman RJ, et al. Familiality and heritability of subtypes of attention deficit hyperactivity disorder in a population sample of adolescent female twins. Amer J Psychiatry 2001;158:1891–1898.
133. Lowe, N, Kirley, A, Hawi, Z, et al. Joint analysis of the DRD5 marker concludes association with attention-deficit/hyperactivity disorder confined to the predominantly inattentive and combined subtypes. Am J Hum Genet 2004;74:348–356.
134. Sonuga-Barke EJS. Psychological heterogeneity in AD/HD-a dual pathway model of behavior and cognition. Behav Brain Res 2002;130:29–36.
135. Tripp G, Alsop B. Sensitivity to reward delay in children with attention deficit hyperactivity disorder. J Child Psychol Psychiatry 2001;42:691–698.
136. Arnold LE, Abikoff HB, Cantwell DP, et al. National Institute of Mental Health collaborative multimodal treatment study of children with ADHD (the MTA). Arch Gen Psychiatry 1997;54: 865–870.
137. MTA Cooperative Group. A 14-month randomized clinical trial of treatment strategies for attention deficit hyperactivity disorder (ADHD). Arch Gen Psychiatry 1999;56:1073–1086.
138. Eaves LJ, Silberg JL, Hewitt JK, et al. Genes, personality, and psychopathology: A latent class analysis of liability to attention-deficit hyperactivity symptoms in twins. In: Plomin R, MacLean G, eds. Nature, nurture, and human behavior. Washington, DC: American Psychological Association, 1993.
139. Nigg JT, Goldsmith HH. Genetics of personality disorders: perspectives from personality and psychopathology research. Psychol Bull 1994;115:346–380.
140. Widiger TA, Clark LA. Toward DSM-V and the classification of psychopathology. Psychol Bull 2000;126:946–963.
141. Hinshaw SP, Carte ET, Sami N, Treuting JJ, Zupan BA. Preadolescent girls with attention-deficit/hyperactivity disorder: II. Neuropsychological performance in relation to subtypes and individual classification. J Cons Clin Psychol 2002;70:1099–1111.
142. Nigg JT, Goldsmith HH, Sachek J. Temperament and attention deficit hyperactivity disorder: the development of a multiple pathway model. J Clin Child Adolesc Psychol 2004;33:42–53.
143. Losier B, McGrath P, Klein R. Error patterns on the continuous performance test in non-medicated and medicated samples of children with and without ADHD: a meta-analytic review. J Child Psychol Psychiatry 1996;37:971–987.
144. Van der Meere JJ, Stemerdink N, Gunning B. Effects of presentation rate of stimuli on response inhibition in ADHD children with and without tics. Perceptual and Motor Skills 1995;81: 259–262.
145. Seidman LJ, Biederman J, Monuteaux MC, Doyle AE, Faraone SV. Learning disabilities and executive dysfunction in boys with attention-deficit/hyperactivity disorder. Neuropsychol 2001;15:544–556.
146. Halperin JM, O'Brien JD, Newcorn JH, et al. Validation of hyperactive, aggressive, and mixed hyperactive/aggressive childhood disorders: a research note. J Child Psychol Psychiatry 1990;31:455–459.
147. Pliszka, S.R. Comorbidity of attention deficit hyperactivity disorder and overanxious disorder. J Amer Acad Child Adolesc Psychiatry 1992;31:197–209.
148. Waschbusch DA. A meta-analytic examination of comorbid hyperactive-impulsive-attention problems and conduct problems. Psychol Bull 2002;128:118–150.
149. Pennington BF. Diagnosing learning disabilities. New York: Guilford Press, 1991.

150. Famularo R, Kintscherff R, Fenton T. Psychiatric diagnosis of maltreated children: preliminary findings. J Amer Acad Child Adolesc Psychiatry 1992;31:836–867.
151. Willcutt EG, Pennington BF, DeFries JC. A twin study of the etiology of comorbidity between reading disability and attention-deficit/hyperactivity disorder. Amer J Med Genet (Neuropsychiatric Genet) 2000;96:293–301.
152. Willcutt EG, Pennington BF, Olson RK, DeFries JC. Understanding comorbidity: a twin study of reading disability and attention-deficit/hyperactivity disorder. Amer J Med Genet (Neuropsychiatric Genet). In press, 2004.
153. Sergeant J, Oosterlaan J, van der Meere J. Information processing and energetic factors in attention-deficit/hyperactivity disorder. In: Quay HC, Hogan AE, (eds.). Handbook of disruptive behavior disorders. New York: Kluwer Academic Plenum Publishing, 1999;75–104.
154. Sagvolden T, Johansen EB, Aase H, Russell VA. A dynamic developmental theory of attention-deficit/hyperactivity disorder (ADHD) predominantly hyperactive/impulsive and combined subtypes. Behav Brain Sci. In press, 2004.

10
Attention Deficit Hyperactivity Disorder and Learning Disabilities

Stephen R. Hooper and Emily A. Williams

1. INTRODUCTION

Attention deficit hyperactivity disorder (ADHD) and learning disabilities (LD) are the most commonly used diagnoses for children who experience academic and behavioral difficulties. Not only do questions concerning ADHD and LD comprise the majority of referrals made to psychologists, psychiatrists, and other professionals, but many children diagnosed with one of these disorders also meet diagnostic criteria for the other disorder *(1)*. Educators, other professionals, and parents often ask questions such as: What are the differences between ADHD and LD? Why do ADHD and LD co-occur so frequently? What impact do the similarities and differences between these disorders have on developing and implementing effective interventions for these children? Although many of the current answers and debates regarding these questions can be examined within many of the chapters contained in this book, this chapter focuses on a unique aspect of ADHD—i.e., the co-occurrence of ADHD and LD. This chapter provides an overview of the definitional issues presented by ADHD and LD, and discusses the notion of comorbidity and co-occurrence of these two disorders. A major portion of this chapter is devoted to reviewing many of the key studies in which the overlap between ADHD and LD has been examined, with a particular focus on ADHD and reading disabilities (RD), ADHD and writing disabilities (WD), and ADHD and math disabilities (MD). The chapter concludes with evidence-based directions for the field based on the available literature.

2. DEFINITIONAL ISSUES

Because ADHD and LD reportedly co-occur in a substantial number of children, it is important to differentiate these two diagnostic labels in order to begin to understand how they might co-occur and mutually affect each other. One key facet of the notion of co-occurrence relates to how these disorders are conceptualized and defined. Generally speaking, LD are neurologically based disorders that influence the cognitive processes necessary for learning. ADHD, on the other hand, is a neurologically based disorder that can cause behaviors, such as hyperactivity–impulsivity and/or inattention, thus potentially interfering with an individual's ability to sit still, concentrate, and think before responding. Behaviors associated with ADHD also can result in secondary emotional, social, and family problems that

From: *Attention Deficit Hyperactivity Disorder: From Genes to Patients*
Edited by: D.Gozal and D. L. Molfese © Humana Press Inc., Totowa, NJ

do not affect a student's *ability* to learn but, rather, can affect his or her availability to learn *(2)*.

Historically, children with learning difficulties and those with attention deficits have been thought of as fitting the same profile. These diagnostic terms are frequently confused in the lay world as well as in some professional circles, perhaps because these two disorders co-occur in so many children, often presenting with similar issues (e.g., underachievement, poor school performance, inattention, overactivity, impulsivity, and social-behavioral challenges and difficulties). Although LD and ADHD often co-occur in children, it is helpful for professionals and parents to understand that ADHD is not a type of learning disability but, instead, and as detailed in this chapter, a distinct and often associated disorder. In order to demonstrate a clear distinction between LD and ADHD, it is helpful to first understand how the definitions of each disorder have evolved to fit into the diagnostic classification systems we use today. Although the bulk of this chapter is devoted to various issues and aspects of the ADHD definition, the following section will focus on definitional issues in LD.

2.1. Definitional Foundations in LD

Throughout the early decades of the 20th century in the United States, children who had difficulty learning were considered to have emotional problems, or mental retardation, or were assumed to be culturally disadvantaged *(2)*. It was not until the 1940s that researchers began to consider that learning difficulties were possibly a neurologically based disorder. Early research concluded that children's learning problems were caused by brain damage, yet these children appeared to be physically normal, indicating that the brain damage must be minimal; thus, the label *minimal brain damage* was employed *(3)*. Because further research revealed no evidence of frank brain damage in children with learning difficulties, this label was changed to *minimal brain dysfunction*, emphasizing a difference in brain function rather than brain damage *(2)*. At that time, the label minimal brain dysfunction was given to children who today would be most likely classified as having a learning disability, difficulties with hyperactivity, inattention, and impulsivity, as well as those with social and emotional problems *(2)*.

During the 1960s researchers began focusing on the various problems of children labeled as having minimal brain dysfunction. Soon, terms like dyslexia (an RD), dyscalculia (an MD), and dysgraphia (a WD) became more popular to describe specific deficits in children's learning. In 1963, Professor Samuel Kirk coined the term *learning disabilities*, and was one of the first to describe these problems from an educational perspective *(4)*. In 1975, the Education for All Handicapped Children Act (Public Law 94–142) provided a definition for "specific learning disabilities," stating that "all handicapped children have available to them...a free appropriate education" *(5)*. In 1990, Public Law 94–142 was renamed the Individuals with Disabilities Education Act (IDEA) and included a definition similar to the original one to determine eligibility for LD services in public schools. While the *Diagnostic and Statistical Manual,* 3rd Edition, (DSM-III) *(6)* and the DSM-III-Revised *(7)* provided a definition for *specific reading disorder*, neither identified the degree of performance deficit required for diagnosis *(3)*. Currently, because neither the DSM-IV *(8)* nor the most current reauthorization of IDEA *(9)* defines how far behind a child must be academically to qualify as having an LD, research is fraught with inconsistencies with regard to diagnosing children with LD. Needless to say, for years researchers have disagreed about the best way to determine whether a child has an LD.

2.1.1. Definition of LD

Definitional issues have confronted the field of LD since the term entered the vocabulary of professionals working with these problems about 40 yr ago *(10)*. Kirk originally described learning disabilities as "unexpected underachievement." This underachievement, by federal definition, should be manifested in one or more of seven core skills: oral expression, listening comprehension, written expression, basic reading skills, reading comprehension, mathematics calculation, and mathematics reasoning. The "unexpected" part of the definition typically relates to some type of ability–achievement discrepancy—even after being provided with learning experiences appropriate to the child's chronological age and ability levels. This aspect of the operationalization of LD, however, has been highly controversial since its introduction in 1977 *(11–13)*. There have been significant concerns raised about the utility of such an operationalization, particularly with respect to who actually may be identified as requiring services, the lack of sensitivity to younger children—including preschool children—who may be at risk, the limited linkages provided for understanding the underlying problems for the academic underachievement, and the poor relationship to treatment response.

Unfortunately, despite much rhetoric, many of the same issues continue to confront clinicians and researchers. The earlier definitions of learning disabilities, such as the one asserted by the Education for All Handicapped Children Act *(14)*, provided little guidance with respect to operational criteria for identification and diagnosis. These earlier definitions also did little to improve our knowledge with respect to specific outcomes, and they served to hinder communication among professionals—especially professionals representing different disciplines. The most recent reauthorization of the IDEA legislation has continued this legacy. The current federal definition of LD in IDEA, which has remained virtually unchanged since 1977, defines LD as follows:

> The term "specific learning disability" means a disorder in one or more of the basic psychological processes involved in understanding or in using language, spoken or written, which may manifest itself in an imperfect ability to listen, think, speak, read, write, spell, or to do mathematical calculations. The term includes such conditions as perceptual disabilities, brain injury, minimal brain dysfunction, dyslexia, and developmental aphasia. The term does not include a learning problem that is primarily the result of visual, hearing, or motor disabilities, of mental retardation, of emotional disturbance, or of environmental, cultural, or economic disadvantage (Individual With Disabilities Education Act, June 4, 1997, p. 602.26a).

Despite the difficulties posed by our federal definition of LD, there have been some notable efforts to improve on the definitional conceptualization. Specifically, the National Joint Committee on Learning Disabilities *(15)* and the Interagency Committee on Learning Disabilities *(16)* did provide more detailed definitions that acknowledged the generic nature of the term *learning disabilities*, the extreme heterogeneity of this population of individuals, and the suspicion of neurological dysfunction. These definitions also adopted a life-span approach to learning problems, and permitted concomitant conditions (e.g., social and emotional disturbance) to be present. Even these definitions, however, did not provide operational guidelines for identification strategies and, consequently, they remained definitions of an exclusionary nature.

More recent research evidence has driven the reemergence of Kirk's original conceptualization of LD as "unexpected underachievement;" however, an increased emphasis on research-based criteria has been asserted. For example, over a decade ago Shaywitz and colleagues *(17)* found that reading disability does not represent a "hump" at the lower end of the normal distribution. Rather than a categorical grouping for individuals with RD, these investigators suggested that reading problems merely represent the lower end of the normal distribution of reading abilities. In fact, their work *(18)*, and that of others *(19)*, demonstrated that a discrepancy definition of RD fares no better than using a simple low-achievement criterion (e.g., standard score <90 on a standardized achievement test); however, where to draw this cut-off criterion will remain a challenge, particularly with respect to uncovering specific subtypes that might manifest in this population or focusing on domain-specific academic disabilities. Perhaps the pending reauthorization of the IDEA legislation will provide the field with more research-based operational criteria for defining LD.

2.2. Co-Occurring Characteristics of ADHD and LD

Throughout the literature focusing on LD and ADHD, the terms *comorbidity* and *co-occurrence* are generally used interchangeably to indicate the overlapping of symptoms and diagnoses in children with both disorders. Recently, however, Kaplan et al. *(20)* argued that the term comorbidity does not accurately represent the overlapping nature of these disorders. The word *comorbid* is a term originally used in the medical field indicating that a patient exhibits the symptoms of two or more distinct disorders simultaneously, whereas the term co-occurring refers to symptoms that appear together but are characteristic of the same disorder *(20)*. For instance, a patient suffering from a cold may exhibit co-occurring symptoms of a sore throat and a fever, yet these symptoms are characteristic of the same medical condition. Although diagnostic criteria and significant evidence from neuropsychological, genetic, and neurobiological studies distinguish LD and ADHD as different disorders *(21)*, research studying both acknowledges the fact that these disorders often have overlapping symptoms. Given the continued debate as to whether LD and ADHD should be viewed as independent disorders or variants of similar symptoms, Kaplan et al. *(20)* suggested using either the term co-occurrence or *overlap* rather than comorbidity to describe the presence of both disorders in children.

2.2.1. Rates of Co-Occurrence

Overall prevalence rates for children with ADHD who also have LD range from 25% *(22,23)* to 50% *(24)*, with the lower estimates being derived from studies in which more stringent diagnostic criteria for both ADHD and LD were employed. Conversely, studies using nonreferred children with heterogeneous learning disorders show that approx 17% meet research diagnostic criteria for ADHD *(1)*. Mayes et al. *(25)* also found that in a clinical sample of 86 children with ADHD, 26.7% had a disability in reading, 31.4% exhibited a disability in math, 30.2% in spelling and, most significantly, 65.1% of the sample had LD in written expression. Furthermore, in a study of 126 children, Kaplan et al. *(20)* found that 63 children in their sample who met criteria for RD also met diagnostic criteria for ADHD.

Currently, our understanding of the association between LD and ADHD is hindered by the fact that research has used various definitions to classify these two disorders. Despite the definitional issues regarding LD, research has consistently shown a relationship between ADHD and academic difficulties in many children diagnosed with ADHD *(21)*. The magnitude of this relationship is greater than what might be predicted from chance alone, particularly given the relative prevalence rates of either LD (i.e., about 3 to 15%) or ADHD (i.e., about 6 to 10%), and raises significant questions as to possible reasons for the co-occurrence of ADHD and LD.

2.2.2. Possible Reasons for Co-Occurrence of ADHD and LD

Perhaps the most difficult feat for researchers is not defining LD and ADHD independently, but trying to discover why each co-occurs so often and just how significant this overlap of symptoms is to children diagnosed with both disorders. As mentioned previously in this chapter, the term minimum brain dysfunction was previously used to classify both learning difficulties and attention deficits in children. Beginning in the DSM-III *(6)*, however, LD were classified as "*specific developmental disabilities*," whereas attention deficit disorders were defined as "disruptive disorders of children," making a major diagnostic distinction between the two disorders *(27)*. Although some findings question the notion that ADHD and LD represent independent disorders, given the overlap of many of their respective features, others conclude that both disorders are indeed independent yet can frequently overlap in some individuals *(21,23,27)*. Although research appears to be inconclusive as to the degree to which ADHD and LD are related, it is important to become familiar with different perspectives on investigating the relationship of both disorders. Two main views concerning the relationship of LD and ADHD include heredity and the notion of causal directions.

2.2.3. Heredity and Co-Occurrence of ADHD and LD

Although many researchers have argued that LD and ADHD are distinct yet co-occurring disorders, some have focused on investigating the question of whether the linkage is may be attributed to genetics. Prevalence rates defined by many studies provide support for a genetic linkage between ADHD and LD. In a study of 3000 children where ADHD was present in approx 5% of the sample, Tirosh and Cohen *(28)* found language impairment in about 45% of children with ADHD. Kaplan et al. *(20)* also found that in a sample of 179 children with various diagnoses, such as ADHD, RD, oppositional defiant disorder, and conduct disorder, 61 children manifested "pure" dyslexia (i.e., only symptoms of reading disorder) and 21 exhibited a "pure" form of ADHD (i.e., only ADHD symptoms). Thus, results from this study indicated that 51.6% of the children with RD had another co-occurring disorder, but that more than 80% of children with ADHD had a co-occurring disorder *(20)*.

In addition to prevalence rates, Light et al. *(29)* discovered that in a sample of 61 identical twins and 43 same-gender fraternal twins diagnosed with co-occurring ADHD and RD, 45% of deficits in reading were the result of genetic factors that also influenced hyperactivity. These findings point to a strong etiological basis for the overlapping of symptoms from these two disorders, and directly supports a genetic-based co-occurrence model.

2.2.4. Causal Direction of the Co-Occurrence of ADHD and LD

2.2.4.1. Does Inattention Cause Low Achievement?

Although the classification systems we use today separate ADHD and LD as two different disorders, it is not uncommon that children with ADHD also demonstrate academic underachievement *(30)*. A crucial question for researchers interested in learning more about designing interventions for this population of children is: does having ADHD lead to exhibiting symptoms of LD or does having LD lead to a diagnosis of ADHD? The most obvious relationship between LD and ADHD in the classroom refers to the assumption that symptoms, such as inattention, hyperactivity, and impulsivity, are likely to interfere with learning (or the availability to learn) and, thus, lead to low academic achievement *(30)*. Although the argument that improving symptoms associated with ADHD could improve academic achievement makes intuitive sense, there is no empirical evidence suggesting that

ADHD directly causes learning difficulties to the extent manifested by those diagnosed with a learning disability *(31)*.

2.2.4.2. Does Low Achievement Cause ADHD?

Researchers have investigated the possibility that academic failure may lead to symptoms of inattention and distractibility *(32)*. It seems logical that a child with reading difficulties may become frustrated if he or she cannot complete the task at hand and, in reaction to these academic demands, may appear distracted or even exhibit behavior problems *(30)*. Also, children with LD who exhibit attention difficulties and associated conduct problems are at a higher risk for displaying achievement deficits throughout their schooling *(33)*. Educators and parents who take this view of causality may be more inclined to design interventions around the learning problems than the ADHD symptoms *(30)*. It is important to recognize the full range of deficits challenging each child and design interventions according to the most significant academic, emotional, and behavioral needs across environments.

2.2.4.3. Do Reciprocal Relationships Exist?

There is also the possibility of a reciprocal relationship between LD and ADHD. In this regard, Pennington et al. *(34)* found that inattention had a negative effect on reading achievement, attitude toward reading, and reading at home with parents. The direction of the relationship was found to flow from reading achievement to attention, noting that a positive attitude toward reading and high reading achievement boosted attention toward reading in school and seemed to encourage reading at home *(34)*.

Whereas the diagnostic criteria for LD and ADHD are distinctly different in the classification nomenclature, the co-occurrence of symptoms among children causes much confusion for health professionals who assess, diagnose, and treat individuals with such difficulties. Regardless of the diagnostic terms used to refer to an individual's learning difficulties or attention deficits, it is clear that interventions for both LD and ADHD should be designed based on each child's independent needs in the classroom and at home. It is important for professionals and parents to understand the effects that co-occurring symptoms have on children with reading, math, and writing disabilities who also have been diagnosed with ADHD. Academic difficulties and attention deficits not only can have an impact on a student's performance in the classroom, but they can also negatively affect peer and family relationships as well as a student's self-efficacy in the classroom, home, and other settings.

3. STUDIES EXAMINING CO-OCCURRENCE OF ADHD AND LD

A review of the literature since 1980, when DSM-III introduced attention deficit disorder (ADD) as a diagnostic option for clinicians and researchers, produced approx 100 studies that have examined various nuances of the co-occurring nature of ADHD and LD. For purposes of this chapter, we have chosen to focus on three primary LD: Reading, spelling/written language, and mathematics. In addition, much of the earlier literature examining this issue focused on heterogeneous groups of children with LD, and these studies are reviewed as well.

3.1. Studies Examining ADHD and Heterogeneous LD

As can be seen in Table 1, about 38 of the studies to date have focused on examining the presence of any kind of LD in children with ADHD. While many of these studies have employed stringent diagnostic criteria for ascertaining children's ADHD, most of the studies

Table 1
Studies Examining Co-Occurrence of ADD/ADHD and Heterogeneous LDS

Author (year)	Sample	Diagnostic procedures	Findings
Tarnowski, Prinz, and Nay (1986)	$n = 14$ (ages 7–9) ADD + H, $n = 12$ LD, $n = 12$ ADDH-LD, $n = 13$ normal boys	DSM-III criteria for ADD + H	ADD + H subjects with and without LD exhibited sustained attention deficits; LD subjects exhibited selective attention deficits; LD and ADD + H-LD subjects exhibited recall difficulties on paired association tasks; all three experimental groups performed more poorly than normal group; attentional deficits were more pervasive for ADD + H-LD
Tarnowski and Nay (1989)	$n = 51$ boys (ages 7–9)	DSM-III criteria for ADD + H	Boys with ADD + H and LD demonstrated the most external locus of control, whereas boys classified as LD-only or ADD/H- only were the lowest
Aylward, Verhulst, and Bell (1990)	$n = 235$ (ages 5.2–14) with ADD and/or LD, or neither	DSM-III criteria, IQ and achievement scores, parent rating scales, Gordon Diagnostic System(GDS)	Performance on the GDS was affected primarily by the presence of ADD and ADD-H and not LD or ADD/ADD-H and LD
Bickett and Milich (1990)	$n = 201$ 4th and 5th graders; subgroups included boys with ADD, LD, ADD/LD.	DSM-III criteria; peer ratings of videotapes of groups interacting with a nondisabled peer	Boys with either ADD/LD, ADD, or LD were devalued relative to controls on measures of popularity
Cantwell and Baker (1991)	$n = 600$ follow-up on students (ages 1–16) who were previously diagnosed as speech-language impaired	DSM-III diagnostic criteria	Increased prevalence of both ADHD and LD among children with early speech-language impairments; LD was strongly associated with ADHD
Robins (1992)	$n = 18$ ADHD; $n = 25$ LD, $n = 25$ ADHD/LD	Standardized rating scales; neuropsychological tests	The construct of self-regulation differentiated the three groups, although sustained attention did not; results support that ADHD is a diagnostic entity separate from LD and suggested that poor self-regulation and inhibition may be the hallmark of ADHD

(Continued)

Table 1 ***(Continued)***

Author (year)	Sample	Diagnostic procedures	Findings
Flicek (1992)	$n = 249$ 2nd–6th graders ($n = 18$ ADHD/LD, $n = 19$ ADHD/LA, $n = 33$ ADHD, $n = 34$ LD, $n = 29$ LA, $n = 116$ control)	Each subject that contained a mean per-item of 1.5 or greater on the five-item inattention/overactivity factor of the Iowa Conners Teacher Rating Scale was considered ADHD; LD was determined by school classification	Serious problems with peer rejection, peer popularity, and social behavior were the most strongly related to the combination of ADHD/LD
Semrud-Clikeman, Bierman, Sprich-Buchminster, Lehman, et al. (1992)	$n = 60$ ADHD, $n = 30$ academic problems, $n = 30$ controls	DSM-III, WISC-R, WRAT-R, Gilmore Reading Test scores determined LD	Among ADHD, 38% had LD; among academic problems, 43% had LD; and among controls, 8% had LD.
Faraone et al. (1993)	$n = 140$ ADHD, $n = 120$ control, $n = 822$ 1st degree relatives	Schedule for Affective Disorders and Schizophrenia for School-Age Children-Epidemiologic with mothers and participants over age 12; parents of participants under age 12 were interviewed with the Structured Clinical Interview for DSM-III-R; academic achievement was assessed by the WRAT and Gilmore Oral Reading Test, and IQ by the WISC and WAIS; LD was determined using a regression model	Risk for LD was highest among relatives of probands with both ADHD and LD; two disorders are transmitted independently in families and co-occurrence may be the result of nonrandom mating; ADHD is likely to be etiologically independent from LD
Korkman and Pesonen (1994)	$n = 21$ (ADHD) 8-yr-olds, $n = 12$ (LD, $n = 27$ (ADHD/LD)	NEPSY	Children with ADHD were impaired in inhibition of impulses; children with LD in phonological awareness, verbal memory span, storytelling, and verbal IQ, and children with ADHD/LD in all of these areas; had more pervasive inattention and more visual–motor problems than the other groups.

Hengenstein and Kelling (1995)	$n = 42$ college students	Through chart review ADHD diagnoses were made using the draft of the DSM-IV, the University of Massachusetts diagnostic criteria, and the Brown Attention Activation Disorder Scale-self report	33% of participants had been evaluated for academic or behavior problems as children; childhood histories showed educational struggles, LD, and behavior problems
Seidman, Biederman, Faraone, and Milberger (1995)	$n = 65$ boys (ages 9–20) with ADHD; $n = 45$ controls	Schedule for Affective Disorders and Schizophrenia for School-Age Children-Epidemiologic with mothers and participants over age 12; parents of participants under age 12 were interviewed using the Structured Clinical Interview for DSM-III-R; academic achievement was assessed by the WRAT and Gilmore Oral Reading Test and cognitive ability by the WISC and WAIS; LD was determined using a regression model.	Participants with ADHD were significantly impaired on neurological functions compared with controls, regardless of comorbidity status; those with a family history of ADHD were most impaired; subjects with ADHD/LD showed reduced motor dominance and slow reading speed; results indicated that neuropsychological performance in ADHD is significantly affected by familial status and presence of LD
Casey, Rourke, and Del-Dotto (1996)	$n = 62$ (ADD + H) and $n = 22$ (ADD–H), ages 6–12	Children referred to a neuropsychology clinic qualified for the study if they met the following criteria: *(1)* complaints of problems related to disruptive behaviors as reported by a parent at the time of referral; *(2)* these problems present for at least 6 mo; *(3)* onset of problems prior to age 7; and *(4)* a score greater than the 93rd percentile on both the Inattention and Overactivity Scales of the Child Attention Problems scale (CAP; Barkley, 1990); participants were grouped based on scores on the CAP; LD was defined as *(1)* a score less than or equal to 1 SD below the normative mean on one or more achievement tests (e.g., WRAT-R, PIAT, PPVT-R) and *(2)* a discrepancy of 15 standard score	The ADD subgroups did not differ significantly on academic performance as rated by teachers using the CBCL; ADD groups did not differ in frequency of LD, regardless of method used to define LD (by IQ-achievement discrepancy, discrepancy from normative mean, considering deficits on neuropsychological measures); however, children in the ADD+H group were 1.5–2 times more likely to have LD in reading and spelling than those in the ADD-H group; overall, these results do not support the notion that there is a stronger association between ADD-H and LD than between ADD + H and LD

(Continued)

Table 1 *(Continued)*

Author (year)	Sample	Diagnostic procedures	Findings
		points between WISC-R FSIQ and achievement	
Javorsky (1996)	$n = 96$ ages 6–17 (hospitalized in a psychiatric hospital), some with ADHD, language LD (LLD), and both	DSM-III-R diagnostic criteria using the Diagnostic Interview Schedule for Children	Those with ADHD + LLD performed similarly to those with LLD-only, but more poorly than those with ADHD-only on measures of phonology and syntax; no differences were noted on semantics.
Webster, Raymond, et al. (1996)	$n = 50$ ADHD/LD and ADHD-only (ages 6–15)	Learning Efficiency Test-II	Both groups struggled with auditory ordered recall; ADHD/LD group had more trouble transferring information into short-term memory and long-term memory stores than ADHD-only group; results indicate that ADHD-only presented significant problems with information processing, but ADHD/LD intensifies the negative impact of ADHD
Nielsen (1997)	Senior undergraduate and graduate students with LD and/or ADHD (number not specified)	LD was diagnosed by a "pronounced difference between seeming potential and tangible achievement"	Three women and all four male participants reported having reading and/or writing difficulties; one woman and two men reported having problems with mathematics; two women and two men reported difficulty with attention
Bussing, Zima, Belin and Forness (1998)	$n = 499$ screened for ADHD (ages 7–12); $n = 148$ at-risk for ADHD all who were also being served in school as LD ($n = 90$) or serious emotional disturbance (SED) ($n = 58$)	LD was classified using discrepancy criteria and by differences of standard deviations; ADHD was screened via parent and teacher interviews using the Abbreviated Symptom Questionnaire and the Attention Deficit Disorders Evaluation Scale; diagnosis of ADHD was made using the Diagnostic Interview Schedule for Children based on the DSM-IV	Children at high risk for ADHD did not differ in symptomology or comorbidity by special education program; children within both LD and SED programs who met diagnostic criteria for ADHD generally had more severe impairments than children who met only the initial screening for ADHD.

Sprouse, Hall, Webster, Raymond, and Bolen (1998)	$n = 57$ (ages 6–10), LD, ADHD/LD, and control	Diagnostic Analysis of Nonverbal Accuracy test (DANVA); Social Perception Behavior Rating Scale (SPBRS) to measure social perception; school placement classified students into groups	On the facial expression subtest, LD students had more difficulty accurately perceiving cues than control or ADHD/LD group; the ADHD/LD group was rated by teachers as significantly less socially perceptive than the control group
Lazar and Frank (1998)	$n = 26$ (ADHD/LD), $n = 22$ (LD, $n = 10$ (ADHD) ages 6–13	Tests of attention, inhibition, working memory, motor learning, and problem solving	Significantly higher impaired scores on attention, inhibition, cueing, working memory, and problem solving were found for children in the ADHD/LD and LD-only groups; results indicated frontal lobe abnormalities are not exclusive to ADHD characteristics and are present in LD children
Tirosh, Berger, Cohen-Ophir, Davidovitch, and Cohen (1998)	$n = 50$ ADHD/LD and $n = 50$ LD-only (ages 6–11)	Parent and teacher questionnaires	ADHD/LD children had lower achievement compared to LD-only children; ADHD appears to be an associated comorbidity and not a specific learning deficit; children with ADHD/LD have a different neurocognitive pattern from LD-only
Marcotte, Thatcher, Butters, Bortz, Acebo, and Carskadon (1998)	$n = 43$ (ADHD), $n = 11$ (LD), $n = 25$ (ADHD/LD) $n = 86$ (normal)	Parent reports of child's sleeping problems	Parents of all three groups reported more sleeping problems than parents of normal children; sleeping problems were the same across ADHD, LD, and ADHD/LD groups
Aro, Ahonen, Tolvanen, Lyytinen, and Todd-de-Barra (1999)	$n = 110$ LD (mean age 8) with and without symptoms of ADHD	DSM-IV diagnostic criteria	Children with ADHD symptoms improved as well as children with no symptoms in a homework support group; improvements of attention were associated with improvement in reading and writing; initial hyperactivity was associated with improvement in mathematics; results indicated that hyperactivity and inattention are differentially associated with treatment outcome among children with ADHD symptoms

(Continued)

Table 1 *(Continued)*

Author (year)	Sample	Diagnostic procedures	Findings
Gomez and Condon (1999)	$n = 15$ (ADHD, ADHD/LD, and normal)	Parent and teacher ratings using an ADHD Rating Scale; hearing test; IQ; reading; central auditory processing battery	Results indicated lower central auditory processing ability and a significant correlation between reading and ADHD symptoms in ADHD/LD group; suggested that central auditory processing deficits more related to LD than ADHD
Hall, Peterson, Webster, Raymond, Bolen, and Brown (1999)	$n = 45$ (ages 7–10) ADHD/LD, ADHD-only, control	Teacher ratings of students' social perceptions; DANVA and the SPBRS	ADHD/LD children demonstrated significant difficulty in comparison to their peers in perceiving paralinguistic cues; improvement noted during the medication trial
Hazell, Carr, Lewin, Dewis, Heathcote, and Brucki (1999)	$n = 50$ boys (ADHD), $n = 45$ (LD), $n = 25$ (ADHD/LD), $n = 50$ controls	Effortful and automatic processing tasks	ADHD and ADHD/LD subjects did not differ from controls at baseline or under reward conditions, and showed similar levels of mental effort; the LD group had superior performance on the effortful task and an inferior performance on the automatic task compared to other groups; results suggest distinctions between LD and ADHD/LD groups
Shimabukuro, Prater, Jenkins, and Edelen-Smith (1999)	$n = 3$ (ADHD/LD) male (ages 12–13)	All participants were identified by a "multidisciplinary team" as having LD and were diagnosed "medically" as having ADHD	When self-monitoring, these students made gains in their productivity, accuracy, and on-task behaviors across all academic areas
Wilcutt, Pennington, Chabildas, Friedman, and Alexander (1999)	$n = 105$ (ages 8–18) twins with ADHD, $n = 95$ twins without ADHD	Comorbidity was assessed by structured interviews of the parent and child; behavior rating scales completed by the teacher	Symptoms of inattention were associated with lower IQ and higher levels of depression; symptoms of hyperactivity and impulsivity were associated with ODD and CD; clinicians

			should screen for comorbid disorders as a part of a comprehensive assessment of ADHD.
Mangina, Beuzeron-Mangina and Grizenko (2000)	*n* = 20 pre-adolescents (10 with LD + ADHD + co-existing behavioral disorders such as CD or ODD and 10 normal controls)	DSM-IV criteria for LD, ADHD, and behavioral disorders; ERPs	Results indicated a significant memory load effect for the P450 latency and amplitude to be present for normal preadolescents but absent in pathological preadolescents; enhanced N450 ERP amplitudes related to the working memory paradigm in the prefrontal and frontal regions and differentiated the controls from those with LD, ADHD, and behavioral disorders
Mayes, Calhoun, and Crowell (2000)	*n* = 119 (ages 8–16), ADHD/LD, ADHD-only, LD-only	WISC-III, WIAT, GDS, and DSM-IV criteria	LD was present in 70% of children with ADHD, with WD twice as common as RD, MD, or spelling; ADHD/LD children had more severe learning problems than LD-only children, and ADHD/LD children had more severe attention problems than ADHD-only children
Willcutt, Pennington, and DeFries (2000)	*n* = 373 (ages 8–18) twin pairs—at least one exhibited learning difficulties	DSM-III-R (ADHD)	Extreme ADHD scores were almost entirely attributable to genetic influences, as were extreme inattention scores; hyperactivity and impulsivity may be attributed to different etiological influences
Faraone, Biederman, Monuteaux, Doyle, and Seidman (2001)	*n* = 260 boys (ages 6–17) of which 140 referred for ADHD and *n* = 120 controls	DSM-III-R structured interviews; cognitive functioning and LD were assessed using subtests from the WISC-R, WRAT-R, and Gilmore Oral Reading Test	A 4-yr follow-up study showed that ADHD/LD children had higher rates of grade retention, in-school tutoring, and placement in special education; psychiatric and psychosocial outcomes were comparable for ADHD/LD and ADHD-only groups

(Continued)

Table 1 *(Continued)*

Author (year)	Sample	Diagnostic procedures	Findings
Seidman, Biederman, Monuteaux, Doyle, and Faraone (2001)	Males (ADHD/LD, ADHD-only, controls)	LD defined by combined regression-based and low-achievement classifications	ADHD/LD children were significantly more impaired on executive and nonexecutive functions than ADHD-only children; neuropsychological performance was impaired for children with ADHD/RD and ADHD/MD
Doyle, Faraone, DuPre, and Biederman (2001)	*n* = 679 first-degree relatives of three groups of girls ages 6–18: girls with ADHD/LD; girls with ADHD-only, and control group of girls	Children over age 12 were interviewed using the Schedule for Affective Disorders and Schizophrenia for School-age—Epidemiologic Version; parent interviews were conducted for children younger than 12 using the Structured Clinical Interview for DSM-III-R; WISC-R and WRAT-R were used to determine the diagnosis of LD via a regression model	Families of girls with ADHD/LD and ADHD-only had significantly higher rates of ADHD than did families of control girls; only among relatives of girls with ADHD/LD was there a higher risk for LD; the comorbidity of ADHD and LD in girls is related to shared familial risk factors
Molina and Pelham (2001)	*n* = 109 adolescents with ADHD	DSM-III-R or DSM-IV (depending on participants' time of diagnosis)	Results indicated that having LD-only did not predict drug use in adolescence; children with ADHD were more likely to smoke and try alcohol at a younger age; children with ADHD and higher reading achievement were less likely to have later alcohol use disorder; it seems that level of cognitive functioning, not an LD, predicts later substance abuse

Zwart and Kallemeyn (2001)	$n = 50$, 72% ADHD, 9% ADHD/LD, and 22% LD, 6% no diagnosis but struggled academically	DSM-IV diagnostic criteria; LD was documented following the guidelines of the Association on Higher Education and Disability	Findings suggested that peer-based support may be an effective means for enhancing general self-efficacy, learning strategies, and study skills for college students with ADHD/LD
Barry, Lyman, and Klinger (2002)	$n = 66$ (ages 8–14)	DSM-IV diagnostic criteria	Participants scored significantly below prediction in reading, writing, and math skills; the more severe the behavioral symptoms, the better the prediction of underachievement in reading, writing, and math
Marks, Nichols, Blasey, Kato and Huffman (2002)	$n = 40$ girls, $n = 55$ boys	CBCL	Girls with ADHD/LD had few behavioral symptoms compared to ADHD/LD boys
Tabassam and Grainger (2002)	$n = 172 - n = 44$ (LD), $n = 42$ (ADHD/LD), $n = 86$ (controls)	WISC-III, WRAT-R, Conners Teacher Rating Scale, Conners Parent Rating Scale, ADHD-Teacher Rating Scale (DuPaul, 1990)	Students with LD and ADHD/LD had significantly lower scores on academic self-concept, academic attributional style, and academic self-efficacy than controls; ADHD/LD students reported poorer peer-relation self-concept

ADHD, attention deficit hyperactivity disorder; ADD, attention deficit disorder; WISC-R, Wechster Intelligence Scale for Children, Revised; WAIS, Wechster Adult Intelligence Scale; SED, serious emotional disturbance; WIAT, Wechster Individual Achievement Test; CBCL, children's Behavior checklist; DSM-III, *Diagnostic and Statistical Manual of Mental Disorders,* 3rd Edition; DSM-IV, DSM-4th Edition; DSM-III-R, DSM-3rd Edition, Revised; LD, learning disabilities; WRAT-R, Wide Range Achievement Test Revised; CBCC, Child Behavior Checklist; MD, math disabilities; CD, conduct disorder; ODD, oppositional defiant disorder; WD, writing disabilities; RD, reading disabilities; ERP, event-related potential; LA, low achievement; NEPSY, neuropsychological battery; FSIQ, Full-Scale IQ; H, hyperactive; PIAT, Peabody Individual Achievement Test; PPVT-R, Peabody Picture Vocabulary Test-Revised.

did not use stringent criteria for the diagnosis or presence of the LD and, instead, tended to use school-based classifications to identify the presence of learning problems. One exception to this was the work by Wilcutt et al. *(35)* who employed structured interviews for all diagnoses and suggested the need for screening for comorbid disorders as part of a comprehensive ADHD assessment.

Many of the studies showed that ADHD in the presence of LD generally reflected more impairment on motor *(36)*, attention and disinhibition *(37)*, language-based functions *(38,39)*, working memory *(37)*, memory *(40,41)*, executive functions *(36,37)*, and overall neuropsychological performance *(42,43)* than either children with ADHD-only, LD-only, or typical controls. Increased electrophysiological abnormalities also were present in frontal and prefrontal regions *(44)*.

Further, consistent with the neurocognitive findings in children with co-occurring ADHD and LD, these studies documented the presence of more frequent and severe academic deficits *(23,25,36,45–47)*; however, there was a lack of clarity on the issue of whether children with ADD/ADHD with hyperactivity performed more poorly on academic tasks than children with ADD/ADHD without hyperactivity *(48)*. Further, upon follow-up, ADHD/LD children have been shown to have higher rates of grade retention, in-school tutoring, and placement in special education services *(56)*.

Within the social–behavioral realm, children with ADHD/LD were reported as having more external locus of control *(49)*, lower academic self-concept and academic self-efficacy *(50)*, more peer rejections and peer popularity *(51)*, and poorer social perception than typically developing children *(52,53)*. They also were described as being at increased risk for substance abuse *(54)* than ADHD-only, LD-only, or typically developing comparison groups. Gender differences have emerged in the social-behavioral arena, with ADHD/LD boys showing more difficulties than ADHD/LD girls *(55)*. In the social–behavioral and academic realms, and many children with ADHD/LD continue to struggle into adulthood *(57–59)*.

3.2. Studies Examining Co-Occurrence of ADHD and RD

Although the studies described in Subheading 3.1. clearly point to the significance and magnitude of the overlap between ADHD and LD, a more precise examination of the nature of this overlap can be obtained from studies using more precise definitions of LD within domain-specific academic areas. In this regard, when research diagnostic criteria are employed for both ADHD and RD, studies ascertaining subjects clinically *(23)* or epidemiologically *(17)* suggest a co-occurrence of anywhere between 15 and 30%. More recently, Mayes et al. *(25)* found that in a sample of 86 children with ADHD, 26.7% also had a disability in reading. Most of the studies over the past 20 yr have focused on the overlap between ADHD and RD.

As can be seen in Table 2, there have been approx 46 studies conducted examining some aspect of the co-occurrence of ADHD and RD, and it has been the findings from many of these studies that have supported the existence of ADHD and LD as separate diagnostic entities *(34,60–63)*. Findings from these studies also have implicated different behavioral manifestations, different electrophysiology patterns—with a signature associated more with RD than ADHD *(64)*—different physiological functioning *(65,66)*, and, perhaps, different developmental trajectories, in children with ADHD/RD compared with those with ADHD only or RD only *(34)*. Further, these findings have suggested similar genetic contributions of both ADHD and RD in children with ADHD/RD *(67,68)*.

Earlier studies using DSM-III and DSM-III-R diagnostic criteria have documented the presence of RD more frequently in children with ADD without hyperactivity *(24,69)*. Studies using these diagnostic formulations also noted that children with ADD/RD manifested greater problems than children with ADD only, RD only, and controls on phonological processing *(70,71)*, memory *(72)*, and language-related functions *(72)*. Similar findings showing deficits in verbal working memory and verbal retrieval speed *(73)* and general memory *(74)* have been reported for studies using DSM-IV criteria.

The preponderance of evidence has shown that children with co-occurring ADHD and RD show symptoms specific to both disorders. Specifically, children with ADHD/RD demonstrate problems with executive dysfunctions and general inhibitory control as well as deficits in the phonological processing functions tied to reading *(34,63,75,76)*. Further, while some studies have shown greater problems in math for the ADHD-inattentive type *(77)*, others have continued to show the presence of RD as being related more to inattention than to hyperactivity–impulsivity *(78,79)*, with information-processing speed recently being identified as a critical contributor to the distinction between children with RD only vs those with ADHD/RD. In one of the few studies to examine the neurobehavioral functioning of preschool children (ages 3–5 yr), Pisecco et al. *(80)* found that boys with RD only performed poorly on measures of receptive and expressive language, whereas boys with ADHD/RD performed poorly on measures of receptive language, and exhibited more behavior problems. Pisecco et al. *(81)* also demonstrated that children with ADHD/RD showed more hyperactivity and antisocial behaviors than controls—even after controlling for oppositional defiant disorder *(82)*. Despite these findings, Rashid et al. *(83)* found that adults with ADHD or RD did not differ from each other on measures of verbal naming and verbal memory.

Pennington et al. *(34)* also provided some counter-evidence that children with ADHD/RD demonstrated similarities with children with RD only, but not with ADHD only. Specifically, they noted that their ADHD/RD group was similar to the RD-only group in terms of deficits in phonological processing; however, they did not show the expected deficits in executive functioning that would align them with the ADHD-only group. These investigators noted that the problems with reading actually may be the primary contributor to many of the symptoms of ADHD seen in this population. Although this finding is supportive of a "phenocopy" hypothesis, where one disorder (RD) contributes to some, but not all, of the symptoms of a second disorder (ADHD), it has not received universal support *(84,85)*.

The inheritability of the two disorders also provides some clues as to their makeup. Specifically, Light et al. *(29)* have demonstrated a 45% heritable pattern between measures of reading and hyperactivity. Interestingly, Kaplan et al. *(20)* also found that children with ADHD were at higher risk of having at least one additional disorder compared to those with RD.

3.3. Studies Examining Co-Occurrence of ADHD and Writing Disabilities

Closely linked to the area of RD is the literacy domain of WD; however, as can be seen in Table 3, there is a relative paucity of studies that have studied children with ADHD and WD. To date, there are only about four studies that have examined this co-occurrence directly, although the high rate of co-occurrence between ADHD and RD might suggest a similar degree of overlap for ADHD and WD. Indeed, recent work by Mayes et al. *(25)* employing a clinical sample actually documented an extraordinarily high rate of overlap

Table 2
Studies Examining Co-Occurrence of ADD/ADHD and RDs

Author (year)	Sample	Diagnostic procedures	Findings
Halperin et al. (1984)	$n = 22$ (mixed group) "hyperactive reading-disabled children" (ages 6–12), $n = 62$ ("pure" group) "hyperactive children" (ages 6–22)	RD diagnosed by low achievement scores, diagnosis of hyperactivity, not defined	Results indicated that "pure" hyperactive and mixed hyperactive RD constitute distinct subgroups of ADD+H
Richardson, Kupietz, and Maitinsky (1986)	$n = 42$ ADD-H and developmental reading disorder (DRD)	DSM-III	Special reading instruction improved achievement of both groups; degree to which the methylphenidate decreased the symptoms of ADD-H was crucial factor in determining a child's response to DRD intervention
Felton et al. (1987)	$n = 45$ (ages 8–12) RD, $n = 53$ control (with and without ADD)	WISC-R, previously diagnosed as LD by school system; Diagnostic Interview for Children and Adolescents (DICA)	Deficits in learning and memory for recently acquired information manifested as a function of ADD rather than RD; deficits in naming specific to RD rather than ADD; ADD seems to be a major source of additional, but separate cognitive morbidity in RD children
Harter, Diering, and Wood (1988)	$n = 52$ (ages 8–12) boys with ADD/RD, RD-only, ADD-only, controls	Event related potentials (ERPs)	RD subjects showed a smaller amplitude wave over the left and right central hemispheres, a larger wave over the left and right occipital hemispheres, and a smaller variability of ERP waveform; the effects of ADD and RD appear to not interact; selective neural processing due to stimulus relevance was reduced in RD subjects and was greater in ADD subjects, indicating that these disorders involve different underlying brain deficits

McGee, Williams, Moffitt, and Anderson (1989)	$n = 13$ (13-yr old boys) ADD-only, $n = 13$ ADD/RD, $n = 62$ controls	Battery of verbal and nonverbal neuropsychological measures	No measures differentiated ADD-only boys from the controls; the only deficit associated with ADD was slightly lower IQ; RD was associated with deficits in memory and verbal skills
Ackerman, Dykman, and Gardner (1990)	$n = 82$ ADD and dyslexia, $n = 83$ ADD, $n = 52$ "nonproblem" children	DSM-III	ADD/dyslexic children made significantly more errors than ADD only children on a simple auditory test of phonological sensitivity to rhyme and alliteration
August and Garfinkel (1990)	$n = 115$ boys with ADHD (ages 7–17) ADHD, 39% of ADHD also RD, and $n = 43$ controls	DSM-III-R diagnostic criteria; RD was defined as a score of ≤85 on the reading or spelling subtest on the WRAT and at least 15 points below IQ as measured by the PPVT	Both ADHD subgroups performed worse than controls on measures of sequential memory, impulse control, and planful organization; only ADHD/RD differed from controls on measures of rapid word naming and vocabulary
Kupietz (1990)	$n = 11$ DRD, $n = 13$ DRD/ADDH, $n = 11$ controls (all ages 7–12)	Continuous performance task	All groups showed a decline in sustained attention over the course of the task; DRD subjects made more correct detections with increased age, but not when they had ADD-H; ADD-H and DRD/ADD-H subjects were associated with impulsive responding; DRD subjects showed problems associated with inattention or short-term memory deficits that diminished with age
Dykman and Ackerman (1991)	$n = 182$ (ages 7–11) ADD; Three subgroups identified: ADD with hyperactivity; ADD with hyperactivity and aggressivity; and ADD without hyperactivity or aggressivity	DSM-III-R, teacher ratings	More girls were in the ADD-only subgroup; 82 subjects met the criteria for RD; more boys than girls met RD criteria

(Continued)

Table 2
(Continued)

Author (year)	Sample	Diagnostic procedures	Findings
Gilger, Pennington, and DeFries (1992)	$n = 81$ mono twins, $n = 52$ dizyg twins (ages 8–20), at least one member of twin pair had RD	RD was diagnosed by a discriminant function that used weighted scores from the Reading Recognition, Reading Comprehension, and Spelling subtests of the Peabody Individual Achievement Test; ADHD was diagnosed using parent DICA.	RD/ADHD diagnosis was higher for monozygotic than for dizygotic twins, although not significant; RD and ADHD may be genetically independent, however, in some cases, RD and ADHD may co-occur because of a shared genetic etiology
Gillis, Gilger, Pennington, and DeFries (1992)	$n = 37$ identical twins, $n = 37$ fraternal twins–ages 8–20 (ADHD, at least one twin had a reading disability)	DICA; multiple regression model fit to DICA to assess inheritability of ADHD	High inheritability of ADHD noted; adjusting DICA scores for reading performance did not show a change in parameter estimates
Elbert (1993)	$n = 115$ ADD (ages 6–12), ADD+H (72%), ADD-H (28%); all participants were clinic referrals.	Child Behavior Checklist (CBCL); Teacher ratings on Child Attention Profile; reading and writing were measured by the WJ-R and the WRAT-R	54% of sample met public school criteria for LD; achievement on most measure was globally poorer than normative group; ADHD + H performed more poorly on a non-word reading task than ADHD-H; subgroups did not differ on other reading/writing measures; 29% of sample showed poorer performance on spelling/written language relative to reading
Halperin et al. (1993)	$n = 24$ boys (ages 7–11)	CBCL, WISC-R, WRAT	ADHD/RD had significantly higher level of plasma 3-mathoxy-4-hydroxyphenylglycol (MHPG), the metabolite of norepinephrine, but the groups did not differ on the dopamine metabolite homovanillic acid

Pennington, Groisser, and Welsh (1993)	*n* = 70 boys of early school age	DSM-III-R diagnostic criteria; CBCL; Home Situations Questionnaire	RD-only and ADHD-RD were significantly impaired compared with both the control and ADHD-only groups on the phonological processing composite, but performed the same on the EF composite score; the ADHD-only group was significantly different from all other groups on EF; the comorbid group resembled the RD-only group, indicating that their ADHD symptoms are secondary to RD; evidence for the separability of phonological processing and executive functions
Light, Pennington, Gilger, and DeFries (1995)	*n* = 61 identical twin pairs, *n* = 43 same-sex fraternal twin pairs (ages 8–20), at least one had RD and all had ADHD	Parent reports of interests, health, and behavior	Genetic factors substantially contributed to the comorbidity of hyperactivity and spelling deficits; 45% of the proband deficits were the result of genetic factors that influenced hyperactivity; heritable variation accounted for 70% of the observed covariance between reading and hyperactivity measures; heritable influences partly explained the comorbidity of RD and ADHD
Naerhi and Ahonen (1995)	*n* = 21 RD, n = 25 ADHD/RD, *n* = 17 ADHD, *n* = 10 controls (ages 8–12)	Measures of rapid naming and executive functions	Executive tasks failed to differentiate the clinical groups from each other; rapid naming was equally impaired in the ADHD/RD group and RD-only group suggesting that problems with reading acquisition are related to RD and not attention deficits
Shaywitz et al. (1995)	*n* = 186 (ages 7–9)	Comprehensive assessment of academic ability, language, and cognitive skills	When RD and ADHD children are compared, both the linguistic deficits associated with RD and the behavioral characteristics associated with ADHD are apparent, but these deficits are not synergistic; ADHD and RD are separate disorders that frequently co-occur

(Continued)

Table 2
(Continued)

Author (year)	Sample	Diagnostic procedures	Findings
Belfiore, Grskovic, Murphy, Anita, and Zentall (1996)	$n = 3$ (ages 10–11) ADHD/LD	Physician's diagnosis of ADHD; Conners Teacher Rating Scale; a "severe discrepancy" between students' achievement and potential	When presented with reading passages in black and white vs a bright color, ADHD/LD had better reading comprehension in the color condition; color may enhance attention duration for ADHD/LD
Pisecco, Baker, Silva, and Brooke (1996)	RD, ADHD/RD, ADHD-only and controls (ages 5–15)	Parent and teacher ratings of hyperactive and antisocial behaviors	At home ADHD-only and ADHD/RD exhibited more hyperactivity than RD-only and controls; at school RD-only, ADHD-only, and ADHD/RD showed more hyperactivity and antisocial behaviors than controls; ADHD/RD subjects exhibited more antisocial behaviors than any other group
Hall, Halperin, Schwartz, and Newcorn (1997)	$n = 70$ psychiatric outpatients (ages 6–13), ADHD/RD, ADHD-only, RD-only	Continuous Performance Test; solid-state actigraph; Response Incompatibility Task	Children with ADHD, RD and ADHD/RD have partially distinct underlying cognitive and neuropsychological disturbances, and executive dysfunction may be present primarily in ADHD-only
Halperin, Newcorn, Koda, Pick, McKay, and Knott (1997)	ADHD/RD and ADHD-only children	Parent and teacher rating of behavior	Plasma levels of MHPG were significantly lower in ADHD-only, replicating the previous finding; levels of plasma MHPG were inversely related to measures of academic achievement and verbal processing
Purvis and Tannock (1997)	$n = 50$ males (ages 7–11) ADHD-only, ADHD/RD, RD-only, and controls	DSM-III-R diagnostic criteria; Parent Interview for Child Symptoms-Revised; RD was diagnosed by an achievement score at least 1.5 SD below the mean for age, plus a discrepancy of at least 1 SD between that achievement score and the child's WISC-R IQ.	ADHD-only had difficulty with organizing and monitoring their story telling; RD-only had deficits in receptive and expressive semantic language abilities; ADHD/RD exhibited deficits of both ADHD and RD groups

Kaplan, Crawford, Fisher, and Dewey (1998)	$n = 248$ (parents of school-age children) $n = 49$ ADHD, $n = 59$ RD, $n = 50$ ADHD/RD, $n = 90$ controls	General Function Scale from the McMaster Family Assessment Device	35 children met the criteria for ODD; ADHD-only and ADHD/RD was associated with significantly more family dysfunction, even after children with ODD were excluded from the analyses
Kaplan, Dewey, Crawford, and Fisher (1998)	$n = 53$ ADHD, $n = 63$ RD, $n = 63$ ADHD/RD, $n = 112$ controls	Each participant and his/her parents were interviewed using the Diagnostic Interview Schedule for Children (DISC) and DSM-III-R criteria to diagnose ADHD; RD was defined as a scoring ≤ the 24th percentile on the WJ-R Word Attack subtest and scoring ≤ the 16th percentile on the WRAT or WJ-R Spelling subtest and scoring ≤17 on the Auditory Analysis Test; for higher level reading deficits, children were classified as RD if they scored ≤ the 16th percentile on the WJ-R Basic Reading or Reading Comprehension subtest	RD children were impaired in their ability to remember previously learned material, unless repeated over four trials; children with ADHD performed as well as controls for material presented only once; children with ADHD performed poorly on three subtests stressing attention/concentration; ADHD is associated with impaired initial learning owing to attentional deficits, but long-term retention of learned material is commensurate with control group
Nigg, Hinshaw, Carte, and Treuting (1998)	$n = 171$ 6–12 $n = 37$ ADHD/ODD, $n = 21$ ADHD/CD, $n = 16$ ADHD/RD, and $n = 71$ normal controls	DSM-III-R criteria for ADHD, ODD, and CD; a reading quotient was computed from the WJ total reading score and the VIQ, and RD was diagnosed when the reading quotient on the WJ-R was <0.85 and the reading percentile was <25.	Boys with ADHD/RD exhibited impairment on linguistic output tasks and attempts at simultaneous control of reading and behavior problems; results indicated that difficulties on effortful tasks that require planning and controlled motor output pertain at least to ADHD, and may not be accounted for by comorbid conditions
Klorman et al. (1999)	$n = 359$ (ages 7–13) ADHD (combined and inattentive type) with and without ODD, RD	Wisconsin Card Sorting Test; Tower of Hanoi	Executive dysfunction was found only in ADHD/CT children and was independent of comorbidity with RD or ODD

(Continued)

Table 2
(Continued)

Author (year)	Sample	Diagnostic procedures	Findings
Johnson, Altmaier, and Richman (1999)	*n* = 40 (ages 7–13) ADHD, *n* = 40 undifferentiated ADD (UADD), then subgroups according to an LD in reading	Pediatrician diagnosis of ADHD	Children with ADHD/RD had greater memory deficits, suggesting that RD had an additive effect; children with ADHD had significantly more memory deficits than children with UADD
Bonafina, Newcorn, McKay, Koda, and Halperin (2000)	*n* = 54 (ages 7–11) ADHD divided by FSIQ and reading ability	CBCL, Iowa Conners Teacher Questionnaire, DISC; DSM-III-R diagnostic criteria; WISC-R; WRAT-R Reading Recognition	Cluster 1: average FSIQ and reading score; Cluster 2: average FSIQ and impaired reading score; Cluster 3: high FSIQ and reading scores; and Cluster 4: low FSIQ and reading scores; findings reflect variability in academic performance of ADHD
Kaplan, Crawford, Dewey, and Fisher (2000)	*n* = 63 ADHD, *n* = 69 RD, *n* = 68 ADHD/RD	WISC-III Vocab and Block Design subtests	No significant differences were found between any of the groups
Kroese, Hynd, Knight, Hall, and Hiemenz (2000)	*n* = 78 (ages 8–12) *n* = 34 (RD), *n* = 31 (ADHD), *n* = 13 (control)	Comprehensive neuropsychological evaluation consisting of cognitive, linguistic, academic, visual processing, visual–motor, and behavioral measures; RD was defined as a 20-point discrepancy between scores on both reading recognition and reading comprehension from the Woodcock Reading Mastery Test-Revised and the WRAT-3, and WISC-III FSIQ; ADHD was diagnosed as via parent and teacher rating scales and was consistent with DSM-IV criteria	The RD group was found to produce more errors that were phonetically inaccurate than the other two groups; spelling "error" words beyond the RD students' achievement level appeared to elicit greater weaknesses in their phonological recoding abilities than in those of the ADHD or controls

Purvis and Tannock (2000)	$n = 68$: 17 (ADHD/RD), 17 (ADHD-only), 17 (RD-only), 17 (controls), all ages 7–11	DSM-III-R diagnostic criteria via parent and teacher interviews; classification of RD was based on a score of at least 1.5 SD below the mean for age on either the Reading subtest of the WRAT or the PIAT Reading Recognition subtest	ADHD/RD and RD-only groups were significantly impaired relative to controls and ADHD-only groups in all phonological processing measures; ADHD/RD and ADHD-only groups were significantly impaired on simple go/no-go task responding relative to non-ADHD groups; the ADHD/RD groups exhibited deficits of both ADHD-only and RD-only groups; results question inhibition control as a unique marker for ADHD and suggest that there may be true comorbidity in children with ADHD/RD
Rabiner and Coie (2000)	$n = 387$ followed from K-5	Reading achievement was collected from kindergarten through fifth grade using the WJ-R; attention and hyperactivity were assessed using the Children Attention Problems Scale; WISC-R; Teacher Report Form of the CBCL	Attention problems predicted reading achievement even after controlling for prior reading achievement, IQ, and behavioral difficulties; inattentive 1st graders with normal reading scores were at risk for poor reading outcomes; screening for attention problems may help identify those at risk for reading problems
Tannock, Martinussen, and Frijters (2000)	$n = 67$ ADHD-only, $n = 21$ ADHD/RD, $n = 27$ controls	DSM-IV diagnostic criteria for ADHD; a low achievement cutoff score on the WRAT-III Reading subtest was used to define RD	Both ADHD groups were lower in color naming than controls, but did not differ from one another; methylphenidate selectively improved color-naming speed, but had no effect on the speed of naming letters or digits
Wilcutt and Pennington (2000)	$n = 494$ twins with RD (ages 8–18), $n = 373$ twins without RD	Parent and teacher behavior reports	Individuals with RD were more likely to meet the criteria for ADHD than individuals without RD; the association between RD and ADHD is stronger for inattention than for hyperactivity–impulsivity; boys and girls equally exhibit inattention but only boys were significantly associated with hyperactivity–impulsivity symptoms.

(Continued)

Table 2
(Continued)

Author (year)	Sample	Diagnostic procedures	Findings
Weiler, Holmes-Bernstein, Bellinger, and Waber (2000)	$n = 82$ (ages 7–12): $n = 25$ ADHD, $n = 52$ RD, $n = 9$ ADHD/RD (only ADHD-Inattentive-type was included in this study)	ADHD was diagnosed based on teacher and parent ratings on the Diagnostic Rating Scale, which is based on the DSM-IV; RD was classified by scores on the Basic Reading subtest of the WIAT using either a regression-discrepancy definition or a low-achievement definition	ADHD-only children performed poorly on measures of information processing speed, ADHD/RD children were distinguishable from RD-only children on only speed of processing measures; information processing deficits may be at the root of behavioral manifestations of ADHD
Breier, Gray, Fletcher, Diehl, Klass, Foorman, and Molis (2001)	$n = 38$ RD, $n = 29$ ADHD, $n = 32$ ADHD/RD, $n = 43$ controls (ages 7–14)	RD diagnosed by scores on the Basic Reading cluster of the Woodcock Reading Mastery Test-R, Spelling subtest on the WIAT, and the Test of Word Reading Efficiency; ADHD was diagnosed by a licensed psychologists using DSM-IV criteria	RD children had difficulty processing speech and nonspeech stimuli containing similar auditory temporal cues; results were independent of the presence of ADHD, suggesting that children with RD have a deficit in phoneme perception that correlates with reading and phonological processing ability
Kaplan, Dewey, Crawford, and Wilson (2001)	$n = 179$ (ages 8–16) with learning or attention problems	Parents were interviewed using the Diagnostic Interview Schedule for Children; CBCL; Abbreviated Symptom Questionnaire; DSM-III-R criteria; RD was defined as scoring ≤ the 24th percentile on the Work Attack subtest of the WJ-R, scoring ≤ the 16th percentile on the Spelling of the WRAT-R, and scoring <17th percentile on the Auditory Analysis Test.	50% of children met the criteria for two disorders (among ADHD, RD, developmental coordination disorder, ODD, CD, depression, and anxiety); children with ADHD were at higher risk of having at least a second disorder compared to those with RD; a common overlapping of deficits supports the idea that comorbidity is an inadequate concept and propose ABD to explain overlap

Piseco, Baker, Silva, and Brooke (2001)	n = 82 (11-yr-old boys) RD-only, ADHD-only, ADHD/RD	DSM-III criteria were used for diagnosis at the beginning of the study 9 yr prior; DISC, Rutter Child Scales; parent, teacher, and self-report; RD was diagnosed if boys obtained a reading score <1 SD below the sample's average	At ages 3 and 5, the RD-only boys performed poorly on measures of receptive and expressive language, whereas ADHD/RD groups performed poorly on measures of receptive language and exhibited more behavior problems
Rashid, Morris, and Morris (2001)	n = 186 (ages 18–54) referred for evaluation of LD or ADHD	Psychologist diagnosis using DSM-IV criteria for ADHD; RD was diagnosed using a regression-based criterion requiring a discrepancy of one standard error between predicted reading ability on the WAIS-R and actual WJ-R reading achievement scores	When compared on naming and verbal memory abilities, adults with ADHD and RD did not significantly differ from each other
Roodenrys, Koloski, and Grainger (2001)	n = 16 ADHD/RD, n = 16 RD, n = 16 normal	ADHD was diagnosed by a 14-item ADHD Rating Scale and the Conners Rating Scale completed by the teacher and parent; RD was defined as a lag of at least 12 mo in reading as measured by the Neale Analysis of Reading Ability-Revised and a clinically significant score on the Learning Problem Index of the Conners Rating Scale	As the involvement of the central executive in tasks increased, ADHD/RD children performed worse than the other groups on measures of controlled information processing, modifying and accommodating new input, and supervisory capacity; results support the efficacy of executive processing tasks in discriminating ADHD from RD
Wilcutt, Pennington, Broada, et al. (2001)	n = 93 RD, n = 52 ADHD, n = 48 ADHD/RD, n = 121 controls	RD was diagnosed by scoring 1.65 SD below the mean on the PIAT; ADHD was diagnosed using the DICA Parent Report based on the DSM-III diagnostic criteria	ADHD was associated with inhibition deficits whereas RD was associated with deficits in phoneme awareness and verbal working memory; the ADHD/RD group was impaired on both executive functions and phoneme awareness
Aaron, Joshi, Palmer, Smith, and Kirby (2002)	n = 50, (grades 2–5) at risk for reading failure	Woodcock Language Proficiency Battery, Stanford Diagnostic Reading Test; Conners' Continuous Performance Test	RD performed more poorly on language-based tasks while ADHD inattentive-type performed more poorly on attention measures

(Continued)

Table 2
(Continued)

Author (year)	Sample	Diagnostic procedures	Findings
Clarke, Barry, McCarthy, and Selikowitz (2002)	$n = 20$ ADHD/RD, $n = 20$ ADHD-only, $n = 20$ controls	ADHD was diagnosed using DSM-IC criteria and Conners Rating Scale; RD was diagnosed based on scores 2 years or more below each participants' chronological age for accuracy and comprehension of reading and having a standard score of ≤75 for spelling using the WISC-III, WRAT-R, and the Neale Analysis of Reading; EEG	Differences found in the ADHD/RD group represented an electrophysiological component associated with the ADHD/RD that is independent of the EEG pattern typically seen in children with ADHD only
Foster, Hynd, Morgan,and Hugdahl (2002)	$n = 9$ dyslexia, $n = 10$ ADHD/dyslexia, $n = 23$ ADHD, $n = 12$ control	Dyslexia was diagnosed by a 20-point discrepancy between WISC-III and WRAT-3 reading subtest, and the Woodcock Reading Mastery Test-R; dichotic listening test; previous diagnosis of ADHD not reassessed.	Results indicated no significant difference between ADHD and dyslexic subjects in regard to ear advantage on the free recall listening task
Rucklidge and Tannock (2002)	Adolescents ages 13–16 females, ADHD, RD, and ADHD/RD	Various methods used to diagnose ADHD; RD was defined using reading tests.	The ADHD and ADHD/RD groups showed deficits in processing speed, naming of objects, poor behavioral inhibition, and greater variability of reaction times; ADHD/RD and RD groups showed verbal working memory deficits and slower verbal retrieval speed; the ADHD/RD group was slower with naming and had slower reaction times; incongruent color naming and variability in reaction time were the best predictors of hyperactivity–impulsivity; variability in go/no-go reaction time and processing speed were the best predictors of inattentive ADHD

Weiler, Bernstien, Bellinger and Waber (2002)	$n = 24$ ADHD, $n = 33$ RD, $n = 9$ ADHD/RD, controls	ADHD-inattentive subtype was diagnosed by parent and teacher versions of the Diagnostic Rating Scale based on the DSM-IV-TR; children who either met the regression-discrepancy definition on the WISC-III and WIAT or had a Basic Reading score <90 were classified as RD	Children with ADHD were characterized by difficulty with a visual search, whereas children with RD had difficulty with auditory processing; children with ADHD demonstrated diminished speed of visual processing not attributable to inattention
Dewey, Crawford, and Kaplan (2003)	$n = 159$ learning and attention problems (ages 8–16)	Parental Ratings of Everyday Cognitive and Academic Abilities (PRECAA); WJ-R; Bruininks-Oseretsky Test of Motor Proficiency-Short Form; WISC-III Vocabulary and Block Design; VMI	The PRECAA was sensitive to group differences between children with RD, ADHD, and ADHD/RD; PRECAA may be a useful aid to clinicians in identifying children with learning and attention problems

ADD, attention deficit disorder; ADHD, attention deficit hyperactivity disorder; RDs, reading disabilities; H, hyperactive; DSM-III, *Diagnostic and Statistical Manual of Mental Disorders,* 3rd Edition; WISC-R, Wechsler Intelligence Scale for Children-Revised; LD, learning disabled; DSM-III-R, DSM-III-revised; WRAT, Wide-Range Achievement Test; PPVT, Peabody Picture Vocabulary Test; ADD-H, attention deficit disorder with hyperactivity; WJ-R, Woodcock–Johnson Revised Test of Cognitive Disorder with Hyperactivity; WJ-R, Woodcock-Johnson Revised Test of Cognitive Ability; EF, executive function; ODD, oppositional defiant disorder; SD, standard deviation; CD, conduct disorder, VIQ; verbal IQ, FSIQ full-scale IQ; CT, combined type.

between ADHD and WD, with 30.2% exhibiting a disability in spelling and, more significantly, 65.1% of the sample showing a disability in written expression. Further, work by Stevenson and colleagues *(86)* also suggested that 75% of the co-occurrence of spelling disability and hyperactivity represented a shared genetic influence. These findings, as well as others *(87)*, suggested a possible mirroring of the ADHD/RD findings; that is, there likely is a double dissociation between ADHD and WD, with the co-occurrence reflecting more of the WD than the ADHD. Finally, Donfrancesco *(90)* documented increased prevalence of writing problems in children with ADHD as reported by teachers.

Elbert *(88)* examined the written language functioning of a clinical sample of children diagnosed with ADD and subdivided them into two groups: children with ADD with hyperactivity (n = 83) and ADD without hyperactivity (n = 32). Elbert reported that both groups demonstrated pervasive deficits in reading, spelling, and written expression; however, they evidenced disproportionate deficits in their writing skills. Further, the children in the ADD-without-hyperactivity group showed more written language deficiencies than their ADD-with-hyperactivity counterparts. Conversely, work by Resta and Eliot *(89)* showed children with ADD with hyperactivity to manifest more difficulties with graphomotor output than children with ADD without hyperactivity, although written language measures were equally poor for both groups.

3.4. Studies Examining Co-Occurrence of ADHD and Math Disabilities

Similar to the examination of the co-occurrence of ADHD and WD, relatively few studies exist with respect to the co-occurrence of ADHD and math disabilities (MD). As can be seen in Table 4, there are approximately five studies that have addressed this clinical overlap. Despite the presence of only a few studies, the work of Mayes et al. *(25)* suggested that this particular co-occurrence would be a fruitful avenue for exploration in that they found about a 31.4% rate of co-occurrence of math problems in their clinical sample of children with ADHD. Other researchers have documented a co-occurrence between ADHD and MD ranging from 10 to 60% in their clinical samples *(22–24)*, with a greater association being made to children with ADD without hyperactivity/ADHD–inattentive type *(69,77,91)*.

Benedetto-Nash and Tannock *(92)* and DuPaul et al. *(93)* reported that children with ADHD exhibited lower mathematical proficiency than a normal comparison group. Specifically, these children showed problems with subtraction processes, accurately reading signs, disruptive behaviors, memory retrieval, and general academic inefficiency. Marshall et al. *(77)*, using elementary school students, and Zentall and Ferkis *(94)* both found that inattention exerted a specific and deleterious effect on the acquisition of arithmetic computation skills. Conversely, Gross-Tsur et al. *(95)*, employing a large sample of fifth-grade students with dyscalculia, found that 25% manifested problems with ADHD as documented from parent and teacher ratings.

In perhaps one of the most well-done studies to date, Klorman et al. *(96)* identified 310 children, ages 7–13 yr, with ADHD/RD and ADHD/MD. Identification of the different ADHD subgroups was completed using structured interviews for DSM-IV criteria, and standardized IQ and achievement testing with an associated regression equation were used to determine the presence of an RD or MD. Results indicated that students with ADHD/MD or who were MD-only manifested significant deficits in their working memory. Both of these groups demonstrated a lower sensitivity to sequence irregularities in their event-related potentials than the other ADHD groups.

3.5. Summary: What Do We Know About Co-Occurrence of ADHD and LD?

The available literature predominantly resides in the ADHD/LD and ADHD/RD domains, with studies scattered across older ADD and more contemporary ADHD terminology. Further, interpreting the bulk of this literature is complicated by the use of small samples, the use of clinical as opposed to epidemiological samples, the use of differing diagnostic strategies across studies for both ADHD and LD, and the changing diagnostic components that have evolved since the inception of DSM-III in 1980. Despite these challenges and concerns, a corpus of nearly 100 studies has examined the co-occurrence of ADHD and LD, albeit stilted toward studying children with ADHD and heterogeneous LD or ADHD/RD. In this regard, a number of trends do emerge.

First, across nearly all the studies there appears to be a high rate of co-occurrence of all core academic domains with ADHD. In fact, children with ADHD and any kind of LD appear to be more severely involved across neuropsychological, academic, and social–behavioral areas. The preponderance of evidence has shown that children with co-occurring ADHD/RD show symptoms specific to both disorders, with academic deficits perhaps presenting a signature for ADHD/LD per the phenocopy hypothesis, although this will require further study. There also is some emergent evidence suggesting that ADHD/LD might be manifested electrophysiologically as well, although more work is needed here in comparing different subgroups of ADHD/LD.

Second, there appears to be a rather high rate of inheritability present such that current findings reflect co-occurrence rates of up to 65% (i.e., ADHD/WD), with reports of 80.4% of children with ADHD having some type of co-occurring disorder *(20)*. Further, in addition to prevalence rates, a study using identical twins and same-gender fraternal twins diagnosed with ADHD/RD showed that 45% of the deficits in reading were due to genetic factors that also influenced hyperactivity *(29)*. Genetic factors clearly are contributory to the type and severity of the co-occurrence of ADHD/RD.

Third, children with ADD without hyperactivity/ADHD–inattentive type appear more vulnerable to academic deficits. On follow-up, ADHD/LD children have presented higher rates of grade retention, in-school tutoring, and placement in special education services *(56)*. Such risk factors clearly have been documented for ADHD/RD, and more work in ADHD/WD and ADHD/MD must be conducted to determine whether these findings generalize to other patterns of co-occurrence.

Fourth, within the social–behavioral realm, children with ADHD/LD were reported as having more external locus of control *(49)*, lower academic self-concept and academic self-efficacy *(50)*, more peer rejections and peer popularity *(51)*, as being less socially perceptive than typically developing children *(52,53)*, and as being at increased risk for substance abuse *(54)* than ADHD-only, LD-only, or typically developing comparison groups. These findings only serve to compromise the overall functioning of children with ADHD/LD to a greater extent, and research needs to take these factors into consideration when examining these subgroups.

Fifth, gender differences also have emerged in this literature, and more work is needed to examine these similarities and differences, particularly from a neurodevelopmental framework. For example, boys with ADHD/LD reportedly show more social and behavioral difficulties than ADHD/LD girls *(55)*.

Table 3
Studies Examining Co-Occurrence of ADD/ADHD and WDS

Author (year)	Sample	Diagnostic procedures	Findings
Elbert (1993)	$n = 115$, all referred for suspected ADHD; WISC-R FSIQ ≥85; no other primary psychiatric disorders; no neurological history; children classified into ADD + H and ADD-H	Teacher Child Attention Profile Scale; WISC-R/WISC-III; WJ-R Tests of Academic Achievement for Reading and Written Expression; Structured Behavioral Observations	Achievement on most WJ-R scales was significantly lower than the respective normative expectations; the ADD+H group performed more poorly on word attack skills, and no other group differences were present; for the total sample, 17% were more than 1.5 SD below the mean in total reading achievement, and 29% were below the mean in total written language
Resta and Eliot (1994)	$n = 32$ boys (ages 8–13): $n = 10$ ADD+H, $n = 11$ ADD, $n = 11$ controls	Teacher and parent rating scales for DSM-III ADD; visual-motor gestalt (VMG), Written Language Assessment, CBCL, WISC-R	ADD+H group produced significantly more errors on the VMG test; both groups with attention deficits had lower scores on written language assessment.
Stevenson et al. (1993)	$n = 190$, $n = 260$ same-sex twin pairs	Measured comorbidity of spelling disability and hyperactivity	Approximately 75% of the co-occurrence of these two conditions was because of shared genetic influence
Donfrancesco (1998)	$n = 38$ school-age children with writing problems (mean age 9)	Teacher ADHD questionnaire	Results indicated that children with other scholastic deficits had a lower verbal IQ; the performance IQ of these children decreases with age; higher prevalence of ADHD in sample

ADD, attention deficit disorder; ADHD, attention deficit hyperactivity disorder; WISC-R, Wechster Intelligence Scale for children, Revised; FSIQ, full-scale IQ; WJ-R, Woodcock–Johnson Revised Test for Cognitive Ability; WD, writing disabilities; ht, hyperactivity, WISC-III, WISC, 3rd Edition, DSM-III, *Diagnostic and Statistical Manual of Mental Disorders*, 3rd Edition, CBCL, Child Behavior Checklist.

Sixth, with respect to developmental continuity, many children with ADHD/LD continue to struggle into adulthood *(57–59)*, and it will be important for diagnostic and treatment planning to ensure that attention is devoted to both areas of concern (i.e., both attention and learning need to receive comprehensive evaluation, treatment, and follow-up).

4. EVIDENCE-BASED DIRECTIONS

Based on the findings from this overview of the literature on the co-occurrence of ADHD and various kinds of LD, there are some clear directions for the field that emerge. These directions should fuel both the research and clinical activities within the area of ADHD and includes the following:

1. Definitional concerns.
2. Developmental patterns.
3. Biological linkages.
4. Clinical assessment.
5. Treatment issues.

4.1. Definitional Concerns

As noted throughout this chapter, the issue of definitions clearly provides a significant challenge to this field. This issue spans not only the ADHD diagnosis, but also how LD is conceptually defined and operationalized. For researchers, the ADHD diagnosis has been a moving target over the past 20 yr or so, moving from the criteria offered by DSM-III, DSM-III-R, and DSM-IV. The DSM is nearing the beginning of its next iteration and undoubtedly the ADHD diagnosis will change again. It is difficult to study a taxon when the criteria shift from one version of a diagnostic system to another. Further, journals that publish studies that employ more dated criteria (e.g., DSM-III and DSM-III-R) also do not offer much to the field in terms of its advancement.

Similarly, the heterogeneous area of LD has long been hindered by these problems and, in fact, likely has been even more confusing given the lack of clear operational criteria for diagnosis. Severity issues notwithstanding, it will be important for future studies in this area to provide clear diagnostic criteria so that, at a minimum, study methodologies could be replicated. Further, given the mixed findings on different outcomes for the current ADHD subtypes, and the lack of studies examining co-occurring WD and MD, future studies would do well to examine specific ADHD subtypes and the co-occurrence of domain-specific academic areas. Few studies have attempted this type of methodology to date.

4.2. Developmental Patterns

One clear line of inquiry that has been lacking in this literature relates to developmental patterns. Few studies have been conducted using follow-up strategies, and even fewer studies have employed longitudinal methodologies. What studies do exist suggest that predictive relationships between early attention problems and later academic problems can be derived *(97)*. Given this, it becomes nearly impossible to track developmental continuity in children with ADHD/LD, or to determine which problem surfaces first and at what developmental epoch. Do they emerge at the same time or at different times? Are there neurodevelopmental, behavioral, academic, or physiological cues to alert clinicians and

Table 4
Studies Examining Co-Occurrence of ADD/ADHD and MDs

Author (year)	Sample	Diagnostic procedures	Findings
Gross-Tsur, Manor, and Shalev (1996)	*n* = 555 5th graders tested (ages 11–12); *n* = 188 with dyscalculia; *n* = 143 of these students participated	Participants were diagnosed with dyscalculia if score on arithmetic battery was ≤ mean score for normal children two grades younger (3rd grade); ADHD was diagnosed using the Conners Ratings Scales for parents and teachers	IQ's ranged from 80–129; 26% had symptoms of ADHD; 17% had dyslexia; significantly lower socioeconomic status than rest of cohort; 42% had first degree relative with LD; prevalence of dyscalculia in cohort was 6.5% and similar to dyslexia and ADHD; no gender differences
Benedetto-Nash and Tannock (1999)	*n* = 14 ADHD, *n* = 15 normal (ages 7–11)	DSM-IV diagnostic criteria	Children with ADHD had lower levels of academic efficiency, used more immature computation strategies, made more errors in subtraction, and exhibited increased levels of inattention and disruptive behavior
Marshall, Schafer, O'Donnell, Elliot, and Handwerk (1999)	*n* = 40 elementary students	DSM-IV diagnostic criteria	Results showed that inattention exerts a specific and deleterious effect on the acquisition of arithmetic-computation skills
Klorman et al. (2002)	*n* = 310 (ages 7–13) ADHD (all subtypes) with/without RD and MD	DSM-IV diagnoses of ADHD were done using the DICA parent interviews; RD was defined by <1.5 SD below prediction from IQ by a regression equation (WJ, letter–word ID and word attack) and < 25th percentile for published norms; MD was defined similarly (Calculation subtest on the WJ)	Mismatch with preceding trials more greatly reduced MD and RD/MD children's speed and accuracy; MD and MD/RD children's lower sensitivity to sequence irregularity in their event-related potentials, along with greater disruption of performance, suggest working memory deficits that adversely affects response selection

DICA, Diagnostic Interview for Children and Adolescents; SD; standard deviation WJ; Woodcock–Johnson Test for Cognitive Ability.

researchers to the impending co-occurrence of ADHD and a learning problem? Can we predict which will manifest first? What do these children look like across the developmental age span into adulthood? The literature provides some clues as to these possibilities (e.g., adults still struggle), but future research needs to tackle these concerns from a developmental perspective.

4.3. *Neurobiological Linkages*

The literature provided a number of enticing findings suggestive of possible electrophysiological signatures for ADHD/LD, differences in physiological functioning, and important genetic findings. Indeed, although the evidence is suggestive of a common genetic etiology for ADHD/RD, there is little evidence suggesting a similar genetic pathway for children with ADHD/WD or ADHD/MD. Gender differences also appear to be present, with boys showing more severe deficits in academics and behavior than girls, but additional work has begun to examine girls exclusively, and this should yield interesting findings in the near future *(98)*. Although not reviewed here, neuroimaging studies also will provide some hints at the neurobiological similarities and differences in ADHD with co-occurring academic disorders *(99)*, and the imaging work in the area of ADHD is rapidly moving forward *(26)*. Additional studies need to be conducted to followup on these important neurobiological findings, with future studies using more refined operational definitions and, it is hoped, epidemiologically ascertained samples.

4.4. *Clinical Assessment*

What is clear from this literature is that there tends to be a high rate of LD in children with ADHD. Regardless of when the studies were conducted or what diagnostic criteria were employed, nearly every study showed some type of learning problems in many children with ADHD. For clinicians, this creates a "when there's smoke, there's fire" phenomenon, and it becomes critical for clinicians to obtain a comprehensive assessment of any child diagnosed with ADHD. This should include, at a minimum, a subtyping of the ADHD according to contemporary diagnostic criteria, an assessment of cognitive functioning, and an in-depth appraisal of academic and learning functions. This would be consistent with the earlier assertion by Wilcutt et al. *(35)*. Other assessment strategies should be employed as needed (e.g., EEG). While this type of recommendation goes against current strategies employed by many insurance companies and managed care organizations, it truly represents an evidence-based best practice for the clinical assessment of children with ADHD. Further, this strategy should be implemented across the age span—including preschool children—and routine developmental surveillance should ensue whenever feasible.

4.5. *Treatment Issues*

Finally, with a thorough assessment of the possible co-occurring conditions, clinicians will be in a better position to provide treatment to children, adolescents, and adults with ADHD/LD. In this regard, the current literature suggests that symptoms from both ADHD and LD should be treated, and treating only one set of problems and not the other will provide ongoing and unnecessary challenges for the child and the family.

5. CONCLUSIONS

This chapter has provided an overview of the co-occurrence of LD in individuals with ADHD. We have discussed the importance of understanding this area, particularly from a definitional perspective, and we have provided a thorough overview of the literature examining ADHD/LD. Specific attention in this chapter was devoted to evidence-based findings in domain-specific academic areas, and to providing some initial considerations for what we know about the co-occurrence of ADHD and LD. Evidence-based directions were offered for both the clinician and researcher, with an eye toward moving the field forward with respect to advancing this complex area of investigation.

ACKNOWLEDGMENTS

This work was conducted with grant support from the Maternal Child Health Bureau (#MCJ379154A) and the Administration on Developmental Disabilities (#90DD043003).

REFERENCES

1. Shaywitz BA, Fletcher JM, Shaywitz SE. Defining and classifying learning disabilities and attention-deficit/hyperactivity disorder. Ch Neuro 1995;10;S50–S57.
2. Silver LB. Attention deficit-hyperactivity disorder: is it a learning disability or a related disorder? J Learn Dis 1990;23:394–397.
3. Cantwell DP, Baker L. Association between attention deficit-hyperactivity disorder and learning disorders. J Learn Dis 1991;24:88–95.
4. Smith DD, Luckasson R. Introduction to special education: teaching in an age of challenge. Needham Heights, MA: Allyn and Bacon, 1992.
5. Jacob-Timm S, Hartshorne TS. Ethics and law for school psychologists (3rd ed). New York: John Wiley & Sons, 1998.
6. American Psychiatric Association. Diagnostic and statistical manual of mental disorders-third edition. Washington, DC: American Psychiatric Association, 1980.
7. American Psychiatric Association. Diagnostic and statistical manual of mental disorders-third edition-revised. Washington, DC: American Psychiatric Association, 1987.
8. American Psychiatric Association. Diagnostic and statistical manual of mental disorders-fourth edition. Washington, DC: American Psychiatric Association, 1994.
9. IDEA Legislation (1997).
10. Kirk SA. Behavioral diagnosis and remediation of learning disabilities. In: Proceedings of the Conference on Exploration into the Problems of the Perceptually Handicapped Child. Chicago: Perceptually Handicapped Children, 1963.
11. Gresham F. Responsiveness to intervention: an alternative approach to the identification of learning disabilities. In: Bradley R, Danielson L, Hallahan, DP, eds. Identification of learning disabilities: research to practice. Mahwah, NJ: Lawrence Erlbaum Associates, 2002:
12. Kavale K. Discrepancy models in the identifications of learning disability. In: Bradley R, Danielson L, Hallahan, DP, eds. Identification of learning disabilities: research to practice. Mahwah, NJ: Lawrence Erlbaum Associates, 2002:
13. Lyon GR, Fletcher JM, Shaywitz SE, Shaywitz BA, Torgesen JK, Wood FB, et al. Rethinking learning disabilities. In: Finn CE Jr., Rotherham AJ, Hokanson CR Jr., eds. Rethinking special education for a new century. Washington, DC: Thomas B. Fordham Foundation, 2001:.
14. US Office of Education. Public Law 94–142 regulations: proposed rulemaking. Fed Reg 41:52404–52407, 1977.
15. Hammill DD, Leigh J, McNutt G, Larsen S. The new definition of learning disabilities. Learn Dis Quart 1981;4:336–42.
16. Interagency Committee on Learning Disabilities: Learning disabilities: a report to the US Congress. Bethesda, MD: National Institutes of Health (ERIC Document Reproduction Service No. ED 294 358), 1987.
17. Shaywitz SE, Escobar MD, Shaywitz BA, Fletcher JM, Makush R. Distribution and temporal stability of dyslexia in an epidemiological sample of 414 children followed longitudinally. N Engl J Med 1992;326:145–150.

18. Fletcher JM, Shaywitz SE, Shakweiler DP, et al. Cognitive profiles of reading disability: comparisons of discrepancy and low achievement definitions. J Ed Psych 1994;85:1–18.
19. Siegel LS, Metsala J. An alternative to the food processor approach to subtypes of learning disabilities. In: Singh NN, Beale IL, eds. Learning disabilities. Nature, theory, and treatment. New York: Springer-Verlag, 1992:44–60.
20. Kaplan BJ, Dewey DM, Crawford SG, Wilson BN. The term comorbidity is of questionable value in reference to developmental disorders: data and theory. J Learn Dis 2001;34: 555–565.
21. DuPaul GJ, Stoner G. ADHD in the schools: assessment and intervention strategies. New York: Guilford Press, 1994.
22. Frick P, Kamphaus, RW, Lahey, BB, et al. Academic underachievement and the disruptive behavior disorders. J Consult Clin Psychol 1991;59:289–294.
23. Semrud-Clikeman M, Biederman J, Sprich-Buckminster S, Lehman BK, Faraone SV, Norman D. Comorbidity between ADDH and learning disability: a review and report in a clinically referred sample. J Am Acad Child Adolesc Psychiatry 1992;31:439–448.
24. Barkley RA. What to look for in a school for a child with ADHD. ADHD Report 1994;2:1–3.
25. Mayes SD, Calhoun SL, Crowell EW. Learning disabilities and ADHD: overlapping spectrum disorders. J Learn Dis 2000;33:417–424.
26. Pineda DA, Restrepo MA, Sarmiento RJ, et al. Statistical analyses of structural magnetic resonance imaging of the head of the caudate nucleus in Colombian children with attention-deficit hyperactivity disorder. J Child Neurol 2002;17:97–105.
27. Riccio CA, Gonzalez JJ, Hynd GW. Attention-deficit hyperactivity disorder (ADHD) and learning disabilities. Learn Dis Q 1994;17:311–322.
28. Tirosh E Cohen A. Language deficit with attention deficit disorder: prevalent comorbidity. J child Neurol 1998;13:493–497.
29. Light JG, Pennington BF, Gilger JW, DeFries JC. Reading disability and hyperactivity disorder: Evidence for a common genetic etiology. Dev Neuropsychol 1995;11:323–335.
30. Riccio CA, Jemison. ADHD and emergent literacy: Influence of language factors. Read Writ Q 1998;14:43–55.
31. Baker L, Cantwell DP. Attention deficit disorder and speech/language disorders. Comp Ment Health Care 1990;2:3–16.
32. Maynard J, Tyler JL, Arnold M. Co-occurrence of attention-deficit disorder and learning disability: an overview of research. J Instruct Psych 1999;26:183–187.
33. Hinshaw SP. Academic underachievement, attention deficits, and aggression: Comorbidity and implications for intervention. J Consult Clin Psych 1992;60:893–903.
34. Pennington BF, Grossier D, Welsh MC. Contrasting cognitive deficits in attention deficit hyperactivity disorder versus reading disability. Dev Psychol 1993;29:511–523.
35. Willcutt EG, Pennington BF, Chabildas NA, Friedman MC, Alexander J. Psychiatric comorbidity associated with DSM-IV ADHD in a nonreferred sample of twins. J Am Acad Child Adolesc Psychiatry 1999;38:1355–1362.
36. Seidman LJ, Biederman J, Faraone SV, et al. Effects of family history and comorbidity on the neuropsychological performance of children with ADHD: Preliminary findings. J Am Acad Child Adolesc Psychiatry 1995;34:1015–1024.
37. Lazar JM, Frank Y. Frontal systems dysfunction in children with attention-deficit/hyperactivity disorder and learning disabilities. J Neuropsychol 1998;10:160–167.
38. Gomez R, Condon M. Central auditory processing ability in children with ADHD with and without learning disabilities. J Learn Dis 1999;32:150–158.
39. Javorsky J. An examination of youth with attention-deficit/hyperactivity disorder and language learning disabilities: a clinical study. J Learn Dis 1996;29:247–258.
40. Tarnowski KJ, Prinz RJ, Nay SM. Comparative analysis of attentional deficits in hyperactive and learning-disabled children. J Abnorm Psychol 1986;95:341–345.
41. Webster RE, Hal, CW, Brown MB, Bolen LM. Memory modality differences in children with attention deficit hyperactivity disorder with and without learning disabilities. Psych Sch 1996;33:193–201.

42. Robins PM. A comparison of behavioral and attentional functioning in children diagnosed as hyperactive or learning-disabled. J Abnorm Child Psych 1992;20:65–82.
43. Korkman M, Pesonen AE. A comparison of neuropsychological test profiles of children with attention deficit-hyperactivity disorder and/or learning disability. J Learn Dis 1994;27:383–392.
44. Mangina CA, Beuzeron-Mangina JH, Grizenko N. Event-related potentials, bilateral electrodermal activity and Mangina-test performance in learning disabled/ADHD pre-adolescents with severe behavioral disorders as compared to age-matched normal controls. Intl J Psychophys 2000;37: 71–85.
45. Barry TD, Lyman RD, Klinger LG. Academic underachievement and attention-deficit/hyperactivity disorder: the negative impact of symptom severity on school performance. J Sch Psych 2002;40:259–283.
46. Bussing R, Zima BT, Belin TR, Forness SR. Children who qualify for LD and SED programs: do they differ in level of ADHD symptoms and comorbid psychiatric conditions? Behav Dis 1998;23:85–97.
47. Tirosh E, Berger J, Cohen-Ophir, M, Davidovitch M, Cohen A. Learning disabilities with and without attention-deficit hyperactivity disorder: parents' and teachers' perspectives. J Child Neurol 1998;13:270–276.
48. Casey JE, Rourke BP, Del Dotto JE. Learning disabilities in children with attention deficit disorder with and without hyperactivity. Child Neuropsych 1996;2:83–98.
49. Tarnowski KJ, Nay SM. Locus control in children with learning disabilities and hyperactivity: a subgroup analysis. J Learn Dis 1989;22:381–383.
50. Tabassam W, Grainger J. Self-concept, attributional style and self-efficacy beliefs of students with learning disabilities with and without attention deficit hyperactivity disorder. Learn Dis Q 2002;25:141–151.
51. Flicek M. Social status of boys with both academic problems and attention-deficit hyperactivity disorder. J Abnorm Child Psych 1992;20:353–366.
52. Hall CW, Peterson AD, Webster RE, Bolen LM, Brown MB. Perception of nonverbal social cues by regular education, ADHD, and ADHD/LD students. Psych Sch 1999;36:505–514.
53. Sprouse CA, Hall CW, Webster RE, Bolen LM. Social perception in students with learning disabilities and attention-deficit/hyperactivity disorder. J Nonverb Behav 1998;22:125–134.
54. Molina BSG, Pelham WE. Substance use, substance, abuse, and LD among adolescents with a childhood history of ADHD. J Learn Dis 2001;34:333–342.
55. Marks A, Nicholas M, Blasey C, Koto PM, Huffman L. Girls with ADHD and associated behavioral problems: patterns of comorbidity. N Am J Psychol 2002;4:321–332.
56. Faraone SV, Biederman J, Montuneaux MC, Doyle AE, Seidman LJ. A psychometric measure of learning disability predicts educational failure four years later in boys with attention-deficit/hyperactivity disorder. J Att Dis 2001;4:220–230.
57. Heiligenstein E, Keeling RP. Presentation of unrecognized attention deficit hyperactivity disorder in college students. J Am Coll Health 1995;43:226–228.
58. Neilsen JA. Increasing awareness of learning disabilities. Alberta J Ed Res 1997;43:169–72.
59. Zwart LM, Kallemeyn LM, College C. Peer-based coaching for college students with ADHD and learning disabilities. J Postsecond Ed Dis 2001;15:1–15.
60. Felton RH, Wood FB, Brown IS, Campbell SK. Separate verbal memory and naming deficits in attention deficit disorder and reading disability. Br Lang 1987;31:171–184.
61. Halperin JM, Gittelman R, Klein DF, Rudel RG. Reading-disabled hyperactive children: A distinct subgroup of attention deficit disorder with hyperactivity? J Abnorm Child Psych 1984;12:1–14.
62. Harter MR, Diering S, Wood FB. Separate brain potential characteristics in children with reading disability and attention deficit hyperactivity disorder. Br Cog 1988;7:54–86.
63. Purvis KL, Tannock R. Language abilities in children with attention deficit hyperactivity disorder, reading disabilities, and normal controls. J Abnorm Child Psych 1997;25:133–144.
64. Clarke AR, Barry RJ, McCarthy R, Selikowitz M. EEG analysis of children with attention-deficit/hyperactivity disorder and comorbid reading disabilities. J Learn Dis 2002;35:276–285.

65. Halperin JM, Newcorn JH, Schwartz ST, McKay KE, Bedi G, Sharma V. Plasma catecholamine metabolite levels in ADHD boys with and without reading disabilities. J Clin Child Psych 1993;22:219–225.
66. Halperin JM, Newcorn JH, Koda VH, Pick L, McKay KE, Knott P. Noradrenergic mechanisms in ADHD children with and without reading disabilities: a replication and extension. J Am Acad Child Adolesc Psychiatry 1997;36:1688–1697.
67. Gilger JW, Pennington BF, DeFries JC. A twin study of the etiology of comorbidity: Attention-deficit hyperactivity disorder and dyslexia. J Am Acad Child Adolesc Psychiatry 1992;31:343–348.
68. Gillis JJ, Gilger JW, Pennington BF, DeFries JC. Attention deficit disorder in reading disabled twins: Evidence for a genetic etiology. J Abnorm Child Psych 1992;29:303–315.
69. Hynd GW, Lorys AR, Semrud-Clikeman M, et al. Attention deficit disorder without hyperactivity: a distinct behavioral and neurocognitive syndrome. J Child Neurol 1991;6:S37–S43.
70. Ackerman PT, Dykman RA, Gardner MY. ADD students with and without dyslexia differ in sensitivity to rhyme and alliteration. J Learn Dis 1990;23:279–83.
71. August GJ, Garfinkel BD. Comorbidity of ADHD and reading disability among clinic referred children. J Abnorm Child Psychol 1990;18:29–45.
72. McGee R, Williams S, Moffitt T, Anderson J. A comparison of 13-year-old boys with attention deficit and/or reading disorder on neuropsychological measures. J Abnorm Child Psychol 1989;17:37–53.
73. Rucklidge JJ, Tannock R. Neuropsychological profiles of adolescents with ADHD: effects of reading difficulties and gender. J Child Psych Psychiatry All Discip 2002;43:988–1003.
74. Johnson BD, Altmaier EM, Richman LC. Attention deficits and reading disabilities: are immediate memory deficits additive? Dev Neuropsych 1999;15:213–226.
75. Roodenrys S, Koloski N, Grainger J. Working memory function in attention deficit hyperactivity disordered and reading disabled children. Br J Dev Psych 2001;19:325–337.
76. Willcutt EG, Pennington BF, Boada R, et al. A comparison of the cognitive deficits in reading disability and attention-deficit/hyperactivity disorder. J Abnorm Psych 2001;110:157–172.
77. Marshall RM, Schafer VA, O'Donnell L, Elliott J, Handwerk ML. Arithmetic disabilities and ADD subtypes: implications for DSM-IV. J Learn Dis 1999;32:239–247.
78. Aaron PG, Joshi RM, Palmer H, Smith N, Kirby E. Separating genuine cases of reading disability from reading deficits caused by predominately inattentive ADHD behavior. J Learn Dis 2002;35:425–435.
79. Willcutt EG, Pennington BF. Comorbidity of reading disability and attention-deficit/hyperactivity disorder: differences by gender and subtype. J Learn Dis 2000;33:179–191.
80. Pisecco S, Baker DB, Silva PA, Brooke M. Boys with reading disabilities and/or ADHD: distinctions in early childhood. J Learn Dis 2001;34:98–106.
81. Pisecco S, Baker DB, Silva PA, Brooke M. Behavioral distinctions in children with reading disabilities and/or ADHD. J Am Acad Child Adolesc Psychiatry 1996;35:1477–1484.
82. Kaplan BJ, Dewey D, Crawford SG, Fisher GC. Deficits in long-term memory are not characteristic of ADHD. J Clin Exp Neuropsych 1998;20:518–528.
83. Rashid FL, Morris MK, Morris R. Naming and verbal memory skills in adults with attention deficit hyperactivity disorder and reading disability. J Clin Psych 2001;57:829–838.
84. Narhi V, Ahonen T. Reading disability with or without attention deficit hyperactivity disorder: do attentional problems make a difference? Dev Neuropsych 1995;11:337–349.
85. Purvis KL, Tannock R. Phonological processing, not inhibitory control, differentiates ADHD and reading disability. J Am Acad Child Adolesc Psychiatry 2000;39:485–494.
86. Stevenson J, Pennington BF, Gilger JW, DeFries JC, Gillis JJ. Hyperactivity and spelling disability: Testing for shared genetic aetiology. J Child Psych Psychiatry 1993;34:1137–1152.
87. Kroese JM, Hynd GW, Knight DF, Hiemenz JR, Hall J. Clinical appraisal of spelling ability and its relationship to phonemic awareness (blending, segmenting, elision, and reversal), phonological memory, and reading in reading disabled, ADHD, and normal children. Read Writ: Interdisciplin J 2000;13:105–131.

88. Elbert JC. Occurrence and pattern of impaired reading and written language in children with attention deficit disorders. Ann Dys 1993;43:26–43.
89. Resta SP, Eliot J. Written expression in boys with attention deficit disorder. Percep Mot Sk 1994;79:1131–1138.
90. Donfrancesco R. Distinctive features between isolated and associated disease in writing disorder. Psichiatria dell' Infancia e dell' Adolescenza 1998;65:753–766.
91. Faraone SV, Biederman J, Lehman BK, et al. Evidence for the independent familial transmission of attention deficit hyperactivity disorder and learning disabilities: results from a family genetic study. Am J Psych 1993;150:891–895.
92. Benedetto-Nash E, Tannock R. Math calculation, error patterns and stimulant effects in children with attention deficit hyperactivity disorder. J Atten Dis 1999;3:212–134.
93. DuPaul GJ, Rapport MD, Perriello LM. Teacher ratings of academic skills: the development of the Academic Performance Rating Scale. Sch Psychol Rev 1991;20:284–300.
94. Zentall, SS, Ferkis MA. Mathematical problem solving for youth with ADHD, with and without learning disabilities. Learn Dis Q 1993;16:6–18.
95. Gross-Tsur V, Manor O, Shalev RS. Developmental dyscalculia: Prevalence and demographic features. Dev Med Child Neuro 1996;38:25–33.
96. Klorman R, Thatcher JE, Shaywitz SE, et al. Effects of event probability and sequence on children with attention-deficit/hyperactivity, reading and math disorder. Bio Psych 2002;52:795–804.
97. Rabiner D, Coie JD. Early attention problems and children's reading achievement: A longitudinal investigation. J Am Acad Child Adolesc Psychiatry 2000;39:859–867.
98. Doyle AE, Faraone SV, DuPre EP, Biederman J. Separating attention deficit hyperactivity disorder and learning disabilities in girls: a familial risk analysis. Am J Psych 2001;158:1666–1672.
99. Semrud-Clikeman M, Hooper SR, Hynd GW, Hern K, Presley R, Watson T. Prediction of group membership in developmental dyslexia, attention deficit-hyperactivity disorder, and normal controls using brain morphometric analysis of magnetic resonance imaging. Arch Clin Neuropsych 1996;11:521–528.

11

Selective Attention Deficits in Children With Attention Deficit Hyperactivity Disorder

A Review of Behavioral and Electrophysiological Studies

Lisa M. Jonkman

1. INTRODUCTION

The definition of attention deficit hyperactivity disorder (ADHD) has undergone a major transition from the time it was discovered to the present date. As previously discussed, ADHD is a disorder that is accompanied by many neuropsychological, academic, and cognitive deficits. With the introduction of the Diagnostic and Statistical Manual of Mental Disorders, Third Edition (DSM-III) and subsequent research *(1)* the importance of *attentional* problems in ADHD has been established. Most neuropsychological evidence for attentional problems in ADHD comes from studies using the continuous performance test (CPT) that was originally designed to measure brief attention lapses in brain-injured soldiers *(2)*. Seidel and Joschko *(3)* and Corkum and Siegel *(4)* reviewed a huge number of ADHD–CPT studies and concluded that ADHD children are disturbed in sustained-attention processes.

The past decade's research interests have, however, increasingly shifted to ADHD being considered as primarily an inhibition disorder thought to be caused by deficits in frontostriatal brain circuits and dopamine neurotransmission *(5–9)*. As a consequence, research has specifically focused on executive functions and behavioral inhibition and mainly in the Diagnostic and Statistical Manual of Mental Disorders, 4th edition (DSM-IV) combined subtype (ADHD-C). Although this research has undoubtedly demonstrated behavioral inhibition problems in these ADHD children (for an elaborate review, *see* ref. *9*), attention research has been neglected and it is as yet unclear which relationships exist between attention and inhibition. This is an important issue as recently it has been suggested that combined and inattentive DSM-IV subtypes suffer from a related disorder: both display deficits in vigilance (sustaining attention) and maintaining effort on neuropsychological tasks *(10)*. In another neuropsychological study *(11)* it even appeared that symptoms of inattention, rather than hyperactivity/impulsivity, predicted neuropsychological impairment in vigilance, as well as inhibition.

As recently recognized by researchers in the field *(12)*, the problem with most neuropsychological tests measuring executive functions or attention is that they are rather nonspecific in the sense that they address many different cognitive processes at the same time, making it impossible to identify involved neural circuits. By applying more specific task paradigms, the cognitive neuroscience approach has in recent years yielded important information concerning the

From: *Attention Deficit Hyperactivity Disorder: From Genes to Patients*
Edited by: D. Gozal and D. L. Molfese © Humana Press Inc., Totowa, NJ

neuroanatomical structures underlying behavioral function in laboratory attention tasks in normal adults. Unfortunately, this knowledge has as yet not been applied to ADHD.

The above facts indicate that there is a need for a renewed interest in studies focusing on attention as being a core symptom in ADHD. One of the specific research questions that still needs to be answered is whether ADHD children have deficits only in controlled attentional processing, like sustaining attention, or whether deficits occur already at a very early, more automatic processing level. This requires the use of carefully controlled task paradigms, each measuring different aspects of selective attention, such as filtering, orienting, response selection or attention shifting. Two of these aspects, filtering and orientation, have been studied somewhat more elaborately in ADHD children by application of specific task paradigms. The aim of the present chapter is to give an overview of these specific attention studies that were performed in ADHD children in order to get a clearer picture on deficits in early bottom-up and later-occurring top-down attention processes in filtering and orientation of attention. In the next sections, first the filtering and orienting paradigms and the application and interpretation of event-related brain potentials (ERPs) within such paradigms will be explained. This is followed by a review of the results from behavioral and electrophysiological studies in which these paradigms were administered to ADHD children. Finally, conclusions will be drawn regarding filtering and orienting deficits and involved neuroanatomical circuits.

2. NEUROCOGNITIVE ATTENTION TASKS AND ERPs

When reviewing the ADHD-attention literature, besides CPT tasks and other neuropsychological tasks, one encounters two attention paradigms that have been used repeatedly and that do allow looking at attention subprocesses and their specific underlying structures. One of these is the two-channel selective attention task, which has been applied in ADHD children in eight studies, and of which the dichotic listening task is a good auditory example. This type of task enables the measurement of nonspatial auditory or visual selective attention on the basis of varying stimulus features such as tone frequency, color, shape, and the like. The second task that is encountered in 10 studies is the so-called Posner cueing task, measuring three subprocesses involved in the orientation of attention in space (visuospatial attention). These two paradigms have been elaborately applied in normal adult subjects and by measuring behavioral parameters, such as percentages of correct detections (hits), false alarms, and reaction times (RTs), one can study attentional performance. However, before the actual response is given, different information processing steps take place in the brain, such as first stimulus selection, further evaluation of the stimulus, the selection of the relevant response, and the execution of the response. These different processing steps are, however, not visible in the performance measures that show only the final outcome of all of them. The most reported response pattern of ADHD children is slow and inaccurate responding, often interpreted as decreased alertness or vigilance. Regarding treatment and therapy it is important to know whether this is because of worse orientation of attention or inefficient early attentional selection processes, to inefficient stimulus evaluation or to later motor-related processes such as worse response selection, inhibition, or initiation. Psychophysiological studies have shown that by measuring event-related brain potentials (ERPs), in addition to performance, more can be said about the course of the different attention processes that precede the response.

2.1. *Event-Related Potentials*

The electrical activity of the brain can be measured from electrodes that are placed on the scalp; this is called an electroencephalogram (EEG). ERPs are short-lasting changes in the electrical activity of the brain that are time-locked to an external event, for example, a stimulus. ERPs can be evoked by stimuli from different modalities (visual, auditory, somatosensory) and are considered as the cortical representations of perceptual and cognitive processes that are involved in the processing of a stimulus. Compared to the spontaneous electrical activity of the brain, ERPs have a very small amplitude and are most often extracted from the EEG by averaging pieces of the EEG that follow stimulus presentations. By using this averaging method, electrical changes in brain activity that are time-locked to the stimulus are amplified with respect to other electrical changes in the EEG that have no relation to the stimulus. The resulting ERP consists of a sequence of positive and negative waves that are mostly defined by their polarity (positive or negative), latency (the time point after stimulus presentation at which the wave occurs), and scalp distribution. A distinction can be made between very early waves that have a latency shorter than 50–100 ms after stimulus presentation and later waves with a latency longer than 50–100 ms; note that latencies are mostly somewhat later in children. The early waves are thought to reflect automatic processing of physical–perceptual characteristics of stimuli and are called "exogenous" because they are less sensitive to psychological manipulations. The later waves are thought to reflect the more consciously controlled processing of cognitive–semantic properties of a stimulus and are called "endogenous" because they are more sensitive to psychological manipulations and task instructions.

2.2. *Two-Channel Selective Attention Paradigm and ERPs*

Although in the neuropsychological ADHD literature, the term "selective attention" is used in a broad sense, applying to attention measured in varying paradigms such as, for example, Stroop and CPT tasks, in cognitive information processing models the term often describes more specific processes. In this chapter nonspatial selective attention is defined as the processes by which one stimulus is selected above another stimulus and thus refers to a filter process by which incoming irrelevant information is filtered out in order to enhance further processing of relevant information. This type of early selective filtering is measured best within a two-channel selective attention task. The dichotic listening task as used by Hillyard et al. *(13)* is the best known example of such a task. In this task, a different series of frequent and infrequent tones is presented to each ear and the subject's task is to direct attention to the tones in only one ear and to respond whenever a deviant tone (a target) appears in this ear. The attended ear is called the relevant channel, while the unattended ear is the irrelevant channel. In the visual modality two-channel tasks consist of a conjunction of two features, for instance color (red, blue) and gratings (vertical, horizontal). The instruction is to attend only to one stimulus attribute, such as, for example, the color red, and to generate a response only to a red stimulus that contains vertical bars (the target). In both auditory and visual versions of the task two different types of selection processes are involved, namely inter- and intrachannel selection. Interchannel selection is needed for distinguishing between the relevant and the irrelevant channel (independent of whether stimuli are targets or nontargets) and these selection processes are referred to as the selective attention processes.

To obtain ERP activity that is evoked by the investment of such selective attention, so-called selection potentials are computed by subtracting ERPs to nontarget unattended (left ear, color blue) stimuli from nontarget attended (right ear, color red) stimuli. The advantage of using ERPs to attended and unattended nontargets, which is possible only in two-channel tasks, is that early attention processes can be studied independently of target evaluation/selection and motor preparation. In the auditory modality, interchannel selection processes (selection between channels) are reflected in an early negative wave, maximal above the frontocentral cortex, called the processing negativity (PN) *(14,15)*. The PN may in some situations overlap with occipital negative (N1 or N2) waves, depending on the length of the interstimulus interval. In the visual modality in normal adults, three different waves can be distinguished in the selection potential:

1. A frontal selection positivity (FSP) *(16)* in adults occurring between 100 and 300 ms.
2. A temporal-occipital selection negativity (OSN) *(17)* starting between 150 and 200 ms.
3. A negative wave (the PN or N2b in visual studies) that, in adults, occurs between 250 and 300 ms and has a central maximum *(18)*.

The FSP, OSN, and PN have been respectively associated with an early filter that encodes only the primary selection features *(19)*, an early filter in the posterior visual system enabling selective analysis of the visual percept (e.g., perceptual analysis in short-term memory, feature integration) *(20)* and a later, more executive process located in anterior cingulate gyrus, involved with stimulus evaluation according to task instructions and response selection *(21)*.

The Intrachannel selection processes refer to the later-occurring attention processes involved in further processing of the target stimulus within the attended channel and the selection of the relevant response. The ERP wave that is associated with such target processing is the P3b, a positive wave occurring between 300 and 800 ms post-stimulus. The P3b amplitude has been found to be larger to target stimuli than to nontarget stimuli and thus manifests target selection/evaluation processes. The P3 is by far the most investigated ERP wave in ADHD children in so-called oddball tasks, of which the CPT task is an example. In such tasks, as opposed to the earlier-described two-channel tasks, stimuli that differ in one feature are presented of which one is designated the target to which a response has to be generated. In standard oddball tasks target stimuli are presented infrequently amongst a series of nontarget stimuli. These one-channel ERP studies will not be discussed in this chapter.

2.3. *Posner Cueing Task and ERPs*

The tasks described in Subheading 12.2. involve filtering on the basis of nonspatial stimulus attributes, such as size, color, or pitch. These processes occur in situations in which it is important to focus attention on one area of the visual field or one information source. Processes involved in the orientation and allocation of attention across space (when detecting something important outside your field of fixation) are called visuospatial attention processes. It has been shown that different neuroanatomical circuits are involved in the selection of an object on the basis of its primary features or on the basis of its location in space *(22,23)*. In order to study processes and neural structures involved in covert visuospatial attention, Posner and colleagues *(24,25)* introduced the Posner cueing task. In this task, target stimuli (letter *X*, for example) are presented with equal probability in left or right peripheral fields and are preceded by a cue. Cues can be valid (by directing attention to the visual field in which the target will appear), invalid (by directing attention to the wrong visual field) or neutral (by not giving any location information). The subjects' assignment depends on the type of task that is used; in a simple detection task the subject must press a button with one hand as fast as possible whenever a target is detected. In a more difficult discrimination task, two different targets are presented (e.g., letters *O* and *X*) and the subject has to respond with the left hand to one target and with the right hand to the other target. By measuring and comparing reaction times to validly, invalidly, and neutrally cued targets one can study the processes of engagement, disengagement, and the movement or allocation of attention across visual space. Subjects have faster reactions times to valid than to neutral or invalid targets because priming of attention at the correct location occurred; these are called benefits or response facilitation. The reaction times to invalid targets are generally longer than to valid and neutral cues (also called costs or inhibition), caused by the fact that attention first has to be disengaged from the cued location and then has to be moved to the correct location, whereas in valid and neutral conditions disengagement is not necessary. During the task, the subjects fixate their eyes on a fixation cross and are instructed not to move their eyes during the experiment. The importance of not making any eye movements is that otherwise one cannot exclude the influence of overt attention mechanisms localized in midbrain structures (superior colliculus) *(26)* on covert attention processes. Therefore, to study pure covert attention, eye movements should be monitored and trials containing eye movements must be rejected.

Another important distinction that can be made is between exogenous and endogenous cueing tasks. In exogenous tasks, attention is pulled more or less automatically to a certain location by pheripherally presented cues. In these tasks, the time interval between the presentation of the cue and the target is mostly short; for example, below 300 ms. When the interval is longer than 400 ms in young adults, a phenomenon called inhibition of return (IOR) occurs, during which the normal reaction time patterns are reversed by showing longer reaction times to valid than to invalid or neutral targets. Rafal et al. *(27)* reported that a necessary condition for the occurrence of an IOR appears to be the programming (not the execution) of an eye movement. The IOR is explained as an inhibition of attention to return to a previously attended location, the function of which has been suggested to be the protection of the individual from missing important other information.

In endogenous cueing tasks symbolic or informative cues (for example, arrows pointing to the right or left field) are presented at a central location of the visual field, requiring the allocation and shifting of attention in a controlled way. In endogenous tasks mostly longer cue-target intervals are used; the longer the interval, the larger the benefits and costs because more time is available for processing of the cue and subsequent engagement of attention. Because attention allocation is under voluntary control, no IOR response occurs in endogenous tasks. Finally, in endogenous tasks the probability of occurrence of valid cues (in comparison with invalid and neutral cues) is often enhanced in order to make them more predictable and thereby ensure that the subject will make use of the cues.

Cognitive neuroscientists have attempted to link the subprocesses of attentional orienting to neuroanatomical structures. ERP studies into visuospatial attention have increased insight into the temporal dynamics of involved neural activity. In normal adults, different ERP responses appear to be evoked in visuospatial attention tasks than in tasks in which stimulus selection is based on nonspatial features *(28)*. In the visual modality, attending to a specific location leads to an enhancement of both occipital positive (P1) and negative (N1) components, occurring between 50 and 200 ms poststimulus, that are largest over the extrastriate visual cortex. This P1–N1 amplitude modulation has been observed in several spatial attention tasks *(29)*. In Posner cueing tasks, benefits have been associated with enhanced P1 or N1 components to validly cued targets. This P1–N1 effect was interpreted as representing a mechanism of early sensory facilitation in extrastriate visual cortex. Furthermore, Luck et al. *(30)* reported that costs associated with invalid cues lead to suppression of evoked activity (smaller P1 amplitude) in response to invalid cues. After having discussed the two paradigms and related ERPs, we will review the results of studies in which the tasks were applied in ADHD children.

3. FILTERING IN TWO-CHANNEL SELECTIVE ATTENTION TASKS IN ADHD

An overview of ERP studies in which two-channel selective attention tasks were used is presented in Table 1. Most studies on selective attention in ADHD children were performed in the auditory modality. A dichotic listening task was administered to normal controls and ADHD subjects in three studies. Prior et al. *(31)* used only performance data to study selective attention processes (not included in table) but did not find a selective attention deficit in ADHD children; these children did not differ from normal control children in the ability to focus attention. ADHD children differed from normal controls only in that they showed lower sensitivity (*d′*) than normal controls, indicative of a reduced ability to detect signals. In two other dichotic listening studies both performance and ERP waves of hyperactive boys were compared with those of normal controls *(32,33)*. The results of both studies showed that hyperactive boys performed worse (lower hit percentages and more false alarms, i.e., errors of commission) than control subjects and also failed to show enhanced N1 amplitudes in response to attended stimuli when compared to nonattended stimuli, whereas controls did show such a "selective attention effect." In these studies the selective attention effect was already found in the N1 time window, which can be explained by the relatively small interstimulus intervals (ISIs) that were used. Hansen and Hillyard *(34)* showed that the PN may in some situations overlap with the N1 or N2 depending on the length of the ISI; the shorter the ISIs, the earlier the PN.

Later, Satterfield et al. *(35,36)* performed two selective attention experiments in which the visual and auditory modalities were the relevant and irrelevant input channels, respectively, and vice versa. Only data from the condition in which auditory stimuli had to be attended were reported, however. In the first study *(35)*, the performance and ERPs of 6-yr-old ADHD subjects were compared with those of normal controls of the same age. It was found that ADHD boys performed worse (lower percentage of hits and more false alarms) than their normal peers. Also, pointing to a deficit in selective attention, ADHD subjects did not show a significant frontal PN (to standard stimuli), whereas normal controls did. In the second study *(36)*, 6- and 8-yr-olds were compared. Both 6- and 8-yr-old controls showed frontal PNs, although ADHD children showed this frontal PN only at age 8, but they did not show a PN with a central maximum, which was present in the 8-yr-old normal controls. In a later study *(37)* with 6-yr-old children, the same paradigm was used but now, ERPs from both attend–auditory and attend–visual conditions were analyzed. It was found that hyperactive children showed significantly lower hit percentages than controls in the visual task, and more false alarms and lower *d′* in the auditory task. In this study, interchannel attention effects were tested only between deviant (and not standard) stimuli and thus no PN was measured. Some interchannel effects were found on other early peaks than the PN but since these effects were measured regarding only deviant, and not standard, stimuli, they do not reflect "classical" selective attention processes and are not discussed in the present section.

From the aforementioned studies it appears that ADHD children have selective filtering deficits in the auditory modality evident from both behavioral and ERP measures. As visual filtering studies were scarce, we performed an electrophysiological study *(38)* to measure selective attention processes in two-channel tasks in both auditory and visual modalities. In agreement with earlier studies, auditory selective attention deficits were evident in both behavior (more false alarms and lower hit percentages) and ERP activity (smaller PN amplitude) of the ADHD children. In the visual task, ADHD children did show a selective attention deficit as evident in behavior (lower hit and higher false-alarm rates), but this was not preceded by a

Table 1
Overview of Two-Channel Selective Attention ERP Studies in ADHD Children

Authors	Type of selective attention task	Subjects	Age	Performance results	ERP results N1 or PN, FSP OSN	P3 results
Zambelli et al., 1977	Dichotic listening task	9 HY 9 controls	Range:12.9–16.1 yr Mean: 14 yr	% hits< % FA >	Controls: N1 attended > N1 nonattended HY: N1 attended = N1 nonattend	Not reported
Loiselle et al., 1980	Dichotic listening task	12 HY 15 controls	Range: 12–14 yr Mean: 12.8 yr	% hits < % FA >	Controls: N1 attended > nonattended HY: N1 attended = N1 nonattended	P3 amplitude < for targets
Satterfield et al., 1988	Channels defined by stimuli from auditory and visual modalities; auditory results	20 ADHD 20 controls	6–7 yr	% hits < % FA >	Controls: frontal PN ADHD: no frontal PN	P3 amplitude =
Satterfield et al., 1990	Channels defined by stimuli from auditory and visual modalities; auditory results	15 ADHD 15 controls	Initial age: 6 yr Follow-up: 8 yr	% hits< d' < % FA >	All controls: frontal PN Controls 8 yr: central PN; ADHD: frontal PN at 8, no central PN	P3 amplitude < in 8-yr-old ADHD subjects
Satterfield et al., 1994	Channels defined by stimuli from auditory and visual modalities; auditory and visual results	36 ADHD 35 controls	6 yr	Visual attend: % hits < Auditory attend: % FA > and d'<	No PN or N1 measured to standards	Auditory attend: P3 amplitude < visual attend: P3 amplitude =
Novak et al., 1995	Channels defined by right and left visual half-fields	17 ADHD 10 controls	11.1 yr 11.6 yr	% hits <	No group difference in N1 attention effects	P3 amplitude = P3 latency =

(Continued)

Table 1
(Continued)

Authors	Type of selective attention task	Subjects	Age	Performance results	ERP results N1 or PN, FSP OSN	P3 results
Jonkman et al., 1997	Auditory task: channels defined by ears visual task: channels defined by color	18 ADHD (DSM-III-R) 18 controls	10.6 yr 10 yr Range 7–13 yr	Auditory task: % hits < and %FA > Visual task: %hits < and %FA <	Auditory: < central PN Visual: no group difference in frontal or central PN attention effects	In both auditory and visual tasks: P3 amplitude < for nontargets
Van der Stelt et al., 2001	Visual task: channels defined by color	24 ADHD (DSM-IV-C) 24 controls	9.1 yr 9.3 yr	< hit rate > FA rate < d'	No OSN in ADHD or control FSP absent in ADHD Frontotemporal N2b/PN =	Parietal P3 : same target-nontarget effects in both groups
Jonkman et al., 2004	Visual task: channels defined by color	18 ADHD (DSM-III-R) 18 controls	10.6 yr 10 yr Range: 7–13 yr	< hit rate > FA rate < d'	OSN= N2b–PN= FSP absent in ADHD	

FA, false alarms; RT, reaction time; HY, hyperactives (no DSM diagnosis); PN, processing negativity; OSN, occipital selection negativity; FSP, frontal selection positivity. <, ADHD < controls; >, ADHD > controls; =, ADHD, controls.

smaller PN amplitude in this group, so in this study the deficit could not be attributed to inefficient early filtering. Because in this study only the frontal PN wave was studied, it might, however, be possible that visual attention deficits occurred in earlier selective attention subprocesses, such as reflected by FSP and OSN (*see* Subheading 2.2.). In a study by van der Stelt et al. *(39)* a similar task as in Jonkman et al. *(38)* was used and behavioral data were indicative of inefficient filtering in ADHD children. Besides the PN, in this study FSP and OSN activity were also measured. No statistically significant OSN was reported for either ADHD or control children and the groups did not differ in PN amplitude, but FSP amplitudes appeared to be absent in the ADHD group as compared to controls. In another study *(40)*, in the same subjects as in the Jonkman et al. study *(38)*, the available data from 32 electrodes were analyzed to study FSP and OSN activity and to compute underlying sources. The results replicated those of van der Stelt et al. *(39)* by showing that ADHD children had lower hit rates and perceptual sensitivity scores accompanied by normal PN amplitudes but absent FSP activity. In contrast to van der Stelt et al. *(39)* significant OSN activity was present in both groups in our study, but was not different between groups. Source localization indicated that exogenous ERP activity that was not modulated by attention (P1) could be reliably localized in the extrastriate visual cortex in both control and ADHD children and there were no group differences in location and dipole strength of these bilateral sources. The source of the FSP in control children was localized in a medial lateral area and because of the absence of FSP activity, no such sources were detected in the ADHD group *(40)*. Interestingly, in a recent event-related functional magnetic resonance imaging (fMRI) study *(41)*, feature-specific areas in left and right fusiform gyri were found to be activated when attention was directed to color, as opposed to motion. This study also investigated which higher-order attention processes were involved in the modulation of this extrastriate activity; a difference was made between areas involved in sustained attention (focusing on one feature) and in transient attention (shifts between attending to color or motion). Sustained activity for color was reported to occur in the medial superior frontal gyrus (SFG), whereas transient activity was reported in the precentral gyrus (PCG), precuneus, and left intraparietal sulcus (IPS). Thus, the results from this study tentatively suggest that extrastriate neural activity in the fusiform gyrus is enhanced when attending to the color-feature of a stimulus and that this enhancement is brought about or regulated by activity in frontal areas (SFG) when sustained attention is required. In light of these findings, the absence of FSP in ADHD children might be an electrophysiological sign of reduced sustained attentional control involved in feature selection tasks in such frontal areas. But note that to properly investigate top-down influences on color selection a paradigm comparable to that of Liu et al. *(41)* is required.

On the basis of these results it is concluded that in all but one of the auditory two-channel selective attention tasks, deficits in ADHD children in behavior, as well as in ERP activity indicative of attentional filtering (PN) is evident. In another study from our lab *(42)*, the sources of the auditory PN were localized in the auditory sensory cortex in both control and ADHD children. Although the source solutions were less reliable in the ADHD group, the PN deficit was visible in the reduced strength of these dipole sources, especially in the right hemisphere. Early exogenous, not attention-related, ERP components (N1 and P2) were localized in both groups in primary and secondary auditory cortex and showed no location or strength differences between groups. Just as in the visual modality, these results tentatively suggest that bottom-up auditory processing is normal in ADHD children, but auditory selective attention (as evidenced by the PN) is disturbed owing to a processing problem in the secondary auditory cortex. Although the involvement of higher-order attentional control from other (frontal or parietal) cortical sources was not evident in this study, this needs further investigation, preferably in combined EEG–fMRI studies in which both temporal and spatial resolution are high. In the visual domain, the discussed results suggest that exogenous, bottom-up visual processing is normal in ADHD children but filtering deficits are present in early FSP, the precise neuroanatomical sources of which have to be further determined but are tentatively suggested to be in the frontal cortex *(40)*. N2b/PN activity appears to be normal in ADHD children in visual tasks. In recent fMRI and ERP studies, in varying visual task paradigms, the generator of the N2b has been localized in the anterior cingulate cortex, and appears to play a role in the process of conflict monitoring *(43–45)*. In a two-channel color selection study with normal adults, the N2b source was also localized near the anterior cingulated cortex and was hypothesized to reflect feature-nonspecific selection mechanisms related to executive attentional and/or motor processes *(21)*. On the basis of this converging information, it might be hypothesized that the absence of PN/N2b differences between control and ADHD groups in visual selection tasks indicates that their behavioral problems are not caused by deficits in top-down control mechanisms in the frontal cortex involved in conflict monitoring and allocation of attention. The fact that an absence of FSP activity in ADHD children occurred in two independent studies *(39,40)*, using comparable tasks is promising and future studies should more precisely localize the sources involved in this early filtering process. Furthermore, because FSP has been described as a color-feature-specific process *(20,21,46)*, the question is raised whether ADHD children have a specific color-filtering deficit or whether it generalizes to other stimulus features or conjunctions of features.

4. OVERT AND COVERT ATTENTIONAL ORIENTING IN ADHD

A summary of covert and overt orienting studies that have been performed in ADHD children is given in Table 2. Only two of the 10 studies combined behavioral with ERP measures. The interpretation of the results from these orienting studies is complicated owing to the different task designs that were used. In different studies, different types of cues were used; in some studies only valid and invalid cues were used, in others neutral cues were included, and in some studies there was a third condition in which no cues were presented. When no neutral cues are included it is difficult to determine whether eventual valid–invalid differences are caused by higher benefits (faster RTs to valid targets) or higher costs (slower RTs to invalid targets). Most studies *(47–52)* used a task design that was neither purely exogenous nor endogenous; peripheral cues were presented by which attention should be drawn automatically, at least in the short (varying from 100 to 300 ms) cue–target intervals, but at the same time the predictability of valid cues was larger than to invalid (or neutral) cues, thereby inducing endogenous strategy (expectancy) effects at longer intervals. Besides this, at longer cue–target intervals the attentional shift is believed to be overt and under voluntary control *(53)*.

When looking at behavioral outcome measures it appears that ADHD subjects made more omission errors in two studies *(47,48)*, had overall higher error levels in one study *(54)*, and had normal percentages of omissions in five other studies *(50–52,55,56)*, and in two studies no omission error information was given. In eight studies, anticipation errors were measured separately as responses to targets occurring before 150–300 ms. The only two studies in which ADHD subjects were reported to make more anticipation errors were the two ERP studies *(52,56)*; in a third study anticipation errors were higher in ADHD children only in an endogenous, but not an exogenous, task *(55)*. Only in the two ERP studies was a single fixed cue–target interval of 500 ms used. Thus, it seems as if ADHD children tend to make more

Table 2
Overview of Visual-Spatial Orienting Studies in ADHD Children

Authors	Type of task	Subjects	Mean age	Performance (and ERP) results
Swanson et al., 1991	Mixed exogenous (cues) and endogenous task (higher predictability valid targets), TT = 240. Cue types: valid (66.7%), invalid (16.7%), and no cue (16.7%). Cue–target interval: random mixed 100 or 800 ms	28 ADHD *(1)* 27 controls	9 yr 9.2 yr	Omissions > Anticipation errors = RT valid = RT invalid faster to LVF targets
Tomporowski et al., 1994	Endogenous cueing task with feedback, TT = 450. Cue types: neutral (50%), valid (40%), and invalid (10%). Cue–target intervals: 50, 150, 300, 500, 1000 ms (separate blocks)	15 ADHD *(3)* 18 controls	10.8 yr 9.7 yr	Anticipation errors = RT benefits/costs = At 1000 ms interval: overall slower RT ADHD Conclusion: difficulty sustaining attention
Carter et al., 1995	Exogenous task (peripheral cues, no predictability valid cues) and endogenous task (central cues, higher predictability valid targets), TT = 192. Cue types exogenous: valid (33%), invalid (33%), neutral (33%). Cue types endogenous: valid (53%), invalid (14%), neutral (33%). Cue–target interval: random mixed 150 or 800 ms	20 ADHD *(1)* 20 controls	10.5 yr 10.7 yr	Exogenous: omissions = anticipation errors =; RT = endogenous: omissions = anticipation errors. At 150 ms: no differences in costs or benefits; at 800 ms: benefits (neutral–valid) = costs (neutral–invalid) : ADHD no costs for LVF targets
Pearson et al., 1995	Four two-choice-reaction time tasks (letters *X* and *O*) varying in target position (far, near) and	20 ADHD *(1)*	10.7 yr	Errors > in ADHD RT: At longer intervals controls had significant benefits (valid–neutral)

(Continued)

Table 2
(Continued)

Authors	Type of task	Subjects	Mean age	Performance (and ERP) results
	cue-type (peripheral or central). In each task: TT = 150. Cue types: valid (66.7%) , invalid (16.7%), neutral (16.7%). Cue–target interval:random mixed 38, 150, 200, 300, 367 ms	20 controls	0.7 yr	and costs (invalid–neutral), whereas ADHD subjects had similar RTs in valid condition but inconsistent RTs to neutral and invalid stimuli across different time intervals (no costs) No differences between peripheral and central cues. Conclusion: problem with reorientation of attention
Novak et al., 1995	Task with simlultaneously presented central and peripheral cues, higher predictability of valid trials.	17 ADHD *(1)*	11.1 yr	Behavioral results: Anticipation errors >, omission =, d' and B =; RT: no differences in validity effect (valid–invalid)
	TT = 450. Cue types: valid (72%), invalid (18%), catch (10%) Cue–target interval: 500 ms	10 controls	11.6 yr	ERP results: Targets: larger P1 validity effect (valid–invalid) in RVF in ADHD, N1 = P3 smaller to invalidly cued RVF targets. No cue ERPs computed
Nigg et al., 1997	Mixed exogenous (peripheral cues) and endogenous (higher predicatability valid targets) task.	27 ADHD *(1)*	9. 8 yr	Omissions >; Anticipatory = RT: no validity differences; In 100 ms delay: no-cue condition
	TT = 240. Cue types: valid (67%), invalid (16.5%), no cue (16.5%). Cue–target interval: random mixed 100 and 800 ms	17 control	9.25 yr	slower responses to LVF targets in ADHD Conclusion: problems generating alertness to detect unwarned stimuli
Aman et al., 1998	Mixed exogenous (peripheral cues) and endogenous (higher valid target probability) task.	22 ADHD (2: 16 C, 4 IA and 2 HI)	12. 1 yr	Errors: not mentioned RT: no group differences, both groups showed equal costs (valid–invalid),
	TT = 240. Cue types: valid (67%), invalid (16.5%), neutral (16.5%).	22 controls	12. 1 yr	neutral cues not considered in analysis

	Cue–target interval: random mixed 100 and 500 ms			
McDonald et al., 1999	Endogenous cueing task (central arrow cues and higher probability of valid and neutral trials). TT = 400. Cue types: valid (32%), invalid (8%), neutral (40%), catch (cue but no target) (20%). Cue–target interval: 800 ms (control of eye movements).	20 ADHD 20 control	8 yr (range 5.7–11 yr) 8 yr (range 6–11 yr)	Omissions = ; Anticipation = RT: Overall slower RTs to LVF targets. Independent of hemisphere: larger benefits (neutral–valid) and larger costs (valid–invalid) in ADHD Costs: neutral–invalid similar
Wood et al., 1999	Mixed exogenous (peripheral cueing) and endogenous (higher predictability valid targets) task. TT = 200. Cue types: valid (72%) and invalid (18%), 10 % catch trials. Cue-target intervals: random mixed 150 and 350 ms (control of eye movements)	15 pure ADHDp *(1)* 24 ADHDc + ODD 39 controls	9.8 yr 9.6 yr 10.4 yr	Omissions =; Anticipation errors = RT: no differences between ADHD groups. At 150 ms: no control-ADHD group differences At 350 ms: invalid cue effect sizes were larger in ADHD groups, RTs of ADHD did not decrease with increasing SOA for invalid trials. Conclusion: problems with disengaging
Perchet et al., 2001	Mixed exogenous (peripheral cueing) and endogenous (higher predictility valid targets) task TT = 120. Cue types: valid (60%), invalid (20%), no cue (20%). Cue–target interval: 500 ms	28 ADHD (2-C) (24 EEG) 22 Control (13 EEG)	6–10.5 yr 5.5–9 yr 7.4 yr	Behavioral results: Omissions: =; Anticipation errors > RT = no differences in validity effect (valid–invalid), but overall faster RTs in ADHD group. ERP results: Targets: P1 validity effect (valid–invalid) smaller in ADHD, N2-P3 amplitude = Cues: P1 and P3 amplitude = CNV amplitude: < in ADHD in no-cue condition.

Cue type percentages are computed on the basis of the total amount of trials in each task. TT, total amount of trials; RT, reaction time; <, ADHD < controls; >, ADHD > controls; = , ADHD = controls; LVF, left visual field. ADHD (1), DSM-III-R; ADHD (2), DSM-IV (C, combined; IA, inattention; HI, hyperactive/impulsive); ADHD (3), TRF and Conners (no DSM) diagnosis.

anticipation (impulsive) errors when stimulus appearance is predictable. It should however be mentioned that in Carter et al. *(55)* anticipation errors were also higher but two intervals were used. Furthermore, in McDonald et al. *(50)* a single fixed cue–target interval was used while no group differences in errors were reported. The latter study is, however, one of the only two studies that reported to have controlled for eye movements, thus assuring the measurement of purely covert attention shifts, especially regarding the long cue–target intervals. Thus, it cannot be excluded that the anticipation errors are related to the programming or execution of eye movements.

Large differences in reaction time results are present between the different studies. In the discussion of these results we will first focus on exogenous and subsequently on endogenous orienting results. In both domains we will focus on the presence of benefits and costs and how these differ between control and ADHD children.

In different studies exogenous covert attention was studied by using peripheral cues but with a larger probability of valid cues, thereby inducing strategy effects at longer cue–target intervals. To study purely exogenous covert attention effects we looked at peripheral cueing studies and only the short cue–target intervals (below 350 ms in children) in which execution of eye movements or strategy influences are less likely to occur. In five of these studies *(43,47–49,51)* significant validity effects were reported to occur at the short intervals of 100 or 150 ms. In one study *(54)* validity effects were reported only at longer intervals of about 300 ms. However, in none of the studies benefit/cost differences between control and ADHD children were reported in short interval conditions, indicating that they have intact covert exogenous orienting responses.

In five studies *(50,54–57)* purely endogenous tasks were used with central, symbolic cues and a higher predictability of validly cued targets. In all studies except one *(54)*, simple target detection was required by pressing a button with one (mostly the dominant) hand. In one detection study *(57)* left and right hand-presses were required depending on the occurrence of the target in right or left visual fields, thereby mixing response speed differences between hands with laterality effects. The cue-target interval also varied in these studies: in two studies, only one longer interval was used *(50,56)*, in another study, short (100 ms) and long (800 ms) intervals were randomly mixed *(55)*, in another study *(54)*, intervals were randomized between 38 and 300 ms, and in the last study, five different intervals between 50 and 1000 ms were administered in separate blocks *(57)*. In only one study *(50)* was a difference in benefits reported; ADHD children had larger benefits than control children independent of the hemifield in which targets were presented. These results imply that attentional priming is not deficient, if not better, in ADHD children. In adult studies it has been shown that an enhancement of the P1-N1 ERP component in the valid condition (as compared to invalid) would be indicative of such attentional priming effects in visual sensory areas. In the only two ERP studies different results were reported; Novak et al. *(56)* did report an *enhanced* P1 validity effect in ADHD children, although in this study this was not accompanied by enlarged behavioral benefits. Perchet et al. *(52)* reported the P1 validity effect to be smaller in ADHD children. These differences might be explained by differences in age of the subjects (*see* Table 2) and differences in diagnoses; in the Perchet et al. study, *(52)* only ADHD subjects of the combined type were included. Furthermore, the number of trials that were included in the invalid and no-cue ERP averages by Perchet et al. *(52)* was unusually small ($n = 24$ before artifact removal), leading to a low signal-to-noise ratio, especially with regard to low-amplitude components such as N1 and P1.

Higher costs (slower RT to invalid than neutral stimuli) were reported to occur in ADHD children in two studies at cue–target intervals of 800 ms *(50)* and 350 ms *(51)*. In both studies it was concluded that ADHD children had problems with disengagement of attention. The difference with other studies is that in these two studies catch trials were included; these are usually included to enhance alertness or vigilance in paradigms in which one fixed cue-target interval is used and the time of appearance of events is completely predictable. Note, however, that no group differences in validity effects were reported by Novak et al. *(56)*, whereas catch trials were also present, but children were also older in this study. Carter et al. *(55)* found no validity differences at the 150 ms interval but at the 800 ms interval ADHD children, compared with controls, appeared to have no costs in response to left visual field (LVF) invalid targets. The same finding was reported earlier by Swanson et al. *(47)*, albeit in a mixed design; the study by Carter et al. *(55)* demonstrated this to be a purely endogenous deficit. Carter et al. *(55)* concluded that ADHD children have problems sustaining attention in the right hemisphere. A similar finding, although no hemisphere differences were reported, occurred in the study by Pearson et al. *(54)*; only at the longest cue–target intervals used in this study (around 300 ms) were costs smaller or absent in ADHD children compared to in the control group. The authors attributed this to a highly variable response pattern in ADHD children since costs varied across the different time intervals in a nonlinear pattern. It was suggested that the variable response pattern in ADHD children was the result of problems with reorienting attention back to the relevant location after they were misled by invalid cues or when no information about where to expect the stimulus was available. Perchet et al. *(52)* derived support for such an hypothesis by the ERP data; in response to the no-cues the amplitude of the CNV wave, indicative of preparatory attention, was smaller in ADHD than in control children.

In a recent event-related fMRI study *(58)* two different circuits were identified to be involved in cue-based shifting of attention and target-based reorienting of attention in an endogenous orienting task. A dorsal frontoparietal network (including the intraparietal and superior frontal cortex) was activated when attention was voluntarily allocated (shifted) to, and maintained on, a location that was indicated by symbolic central cues. A separate ventral network (including the temporal parietal junction [TPJ]) that was lateralized to the right hemisphere was activated when subjects (re)oriented toward unattended target stimuli (invalid targets). The authors hypothesized that two processes might be involved in the activation of the latter, reorienting network; the disengagement of attention from the current location that is necessary to be able to redirect attention, or a more general change in alertness or vigilance established by the infrequent occurrence of invalid targets. When considering the reaction time results from the orienting studies in ADHD children within this theoretical framework, they point primarily in the direction of deficits in the reorienting network and specifically to a deficit in alertness/vigilance rather then to a disengagement deficit. Several findings support this hypothesis. First, ADHD children do not appear to have deficits in attentional priming (they have equal benefits as controls), indicating that attention could be allocated efficiently to a certain spatial location on the basis of cue information. Second, higher costs (representing problems with disengagement of attention) in ADHD children were only reported in two of 10 studies *(50,51)*. Third, RT deficits of ADHD children in orienting tasks appear to be of a more general origin in the sense of slow and variable responding (*see* Table 2), especially in response to unexpected events (invalid, no-cue, or neutral targets). Fourth, in several studies *(47,48,50,55)* deficits were specifically reported in response to LVF targets, indicating the involvement of the right hemisphere that is also activated most during reorienting *(58)*.

A deficit in alertness or vigilance is also likely when considering deficits in other, sustained-attention tasks. The most often reported ERP-deficit in ADHD children is the reduced amplitude of the parietal P3b component in oddball/vigilance tasks, such as the CPT. In several studies it was demonstrated that the P3b, evoked by infrequent events in oddball tasks, was abolished in the case of damage to TPJ and frontal cortex *(59,60)*. In fact, a reduced P3 amplitude in response to invalid targets was reported in ADHD children, albeit in the right hemifield *(56)*. Thus, on the basis of these studies it might be hypothesized that the P3-deficit in ADHD children, and the reaction time deficits of slow and variable responding in the orienting, but also other attention tasks, might be linked to deficits in the ability to reorient attention after the occurrence of unexpected or unattended events. Based on Corbetta et al. *(58)* this deficit might be caused by damage to structures in the ventral route such as in the TPJ. Further imaging research is needed to investigate these hypotheses and the involvement of the TPJ in attention problems in ADHD.

Summarizing the review of orienting studies, ADHD children don't seem to have problems with bottom-up, exogenous orienting. In endogenous tasks, deficits have been reported only when larger cue–target intervals are used. It seems as if ADHD children do not have deficits in attentional priming in primary or secondary visual areas, but mainly have problems concerning costs after invalid or neutral cueing. These conclusions have, however, to be taken with caution because the differences between studies and especially the paradigms that were used were very large (*see* Table 2). To be able to draw more definite conclusions regarding covert exogenous and endogenous orienting in ADHD patients, future studies should incorporate similar designs, using similar stimuli and cue–target intervals. In the study of covert attention it is very important to control for eye movements, to include enough trials in each stimulus category in order to reduce the variance between and within conditions in reaction time and ERPs (even more important in children), and to use only purely exogenous or endogenous manipulations; mixing both in one design makes it impossible to draw unequivocal conclusions.

5. CONCLUSIONS

As illustrated in this chapter, ADHD children ranging in age between 7 and 12 yr clearly have deficits in auditory and, albeit less investigated, in visual attentional filtering. In the visual domain filtering deficits have been demonstrated in behavior (lower perceptual sensitivity), as well as ERPs in tasks where selections were based on color features of a stimulus. In the adult selective attention literature, it has been suggested that color selection is special in the sense that it evokes a specific ERP component, the FSP, that seems, at least in two studies to be absent in ADHD children *(39,40)*. To find out whether this visual selection deficit in ADHD children substantiates to other features, such as shape, or to conjunctions of features, future studies should apply tasks incorporating other features or combinations between them in combination with the measurement of ERPs and/or fMRI (for ERP examples *see* refs. *20,21,46*). The present review further demonstrates that ADHD children clearly have problems with auditory selective attention in dichotic listening tasks. Although this behavioral deficit is accompanied by absent or smaller PN that seems to have its source in the sensory auditory cortex, future studies should focus on identifying the exact neuroanatomical sources underlying the PN and to elucidate the top-down processes involved in this deficit.

With regard to covert or overt orienting, results are less clear. The most consistent findings appear to be that ADHD children do not show deficits in purely exogenous orienting tasks, but show deficits only on endogenous tasks, in cases of longer intervals between cue and target stimuli, and especially in response to neutral and invalid conditions. In both conditions, at the time the stimulus appears, attention is primed or fixated at another location than the target locations, requiring the reorientation of attention. In multiple studies *(47,54,55)* costs appeared to be decreased or absent in ADHD children in only the left or both hemifields. In the present chapter it is suggested that these response patterns can be explained by a more general deficit in the flexibility with which attention can be reoriented or redirected after an unexpected or unattended event, causing reaction times to be highly variable, sometimes being slower to neutral events and sometimes to invalid events. This variability is hypothesized to be caused by a deficit in maintaining a sufficient level of alertness during the task to deal efficiently with such events. This hypothesis is further strengthened by the fact that in several studies ADHD children showed slow responding in response to all stimuli or unexpected events in the left *(48,50)* or in both *(57)* visual fields. The neuroanatomical basis of such a reorienting/alertness deficit might be in structures in the TPJ *(58)*. All conclusions regarding visual orienting must, however, be taken with caution as there were large differences between paradigms used in the studies, the number of trials in some studies was very low, yielding unreliable RT or ERP data, and in many studies using longer intervals eye movements were not monitored.

Finally, it is important to view attentional and other cognitive deficits in ADHD children within existing theories on life-span cognitive development (*see* Plude et al. *[61]* and Brodeur and Enns *[62]* for reviews on lifespan development of selective attention and covert visual orienting). In their study, Brodeur and Enns *(62)* stress the importance of two views on development, the strategy view and the capacity view. The strategy view defines development as changes in the management of cognitive strategies; in this view deficits might be explained as a failure to deploy the right strategy at the right time. The capacity view explains development as changes in some fixed level of energy or resources and explains deficits or developmental delay as insufficient quantities of resources or capacity to adequately perform a task (such as working memory capacity, speed of information transmission, or quality of neural representations) *(62)*. It might be clear that the more attentionally demanding a task, the higher the appeal for strategies or capacity. In an ERP study in our lab *(63)*, the question of whether sustained attention deficits in ADHD children, accompanied by a smaller amplitude of the P3b component, were caused by inefficient allocation (strategy) or shortage of attentional capacity was addressed. For this purpose, a double-task paradigm, in which the primary task varied in working memory load, was administered to ADHD and control children. With the aid of ERPs, even in the absence of performance requirements in the secondary task, capacity trade-offs between primary and secondary tasks could be studied in both groups. The results showed that ADHD children performed worse on the primary task, especially when attentional demands increased, but P3 activity showed that this appeared to be caused by different attention allocation strategies rather than a shortage of attentional capacity. This is in accordance with some theories on ADHD *(64,65)*. In view of these results deficits in selective attention or orientation of attention would be expected especially in more demanding tasks in which allocation of attention to different conditions is required or in which it is difficult to focus because of the presence of many distracting events or because of the unpredictability of events. The present review gives some support for such a view since deficits were reported only in the more demanding endogenous orienting tasks, and only in unexpected conditions (invalid, neutral) in which attention has to be voluntarily reallocated to another location in space. A next step would be to try to elucidate the neural generators involved in such top-down processes by performing combined EEG-fMRI experiments. Last, we would like to stress the importance of studying differences between DSM-IV subtypes in both filtering and orienting tasks. In the currently reviewed studies mainly subjects suffering from the combined disorder (DSM-III-R) were included, not allowing for a conclusion whether such deficits are resulting from inattention or hyperactivity/impulsivity factors. This is especially interesting because there is recent evidence that vigilance disorders are shared by inattentive and combined subtypes *(10,11)*. Future research should focus on studying links between neuroanatomical circuits involved in attention and inhibition functions.

REFERENCES

1. Douglas VI. Attentional and cognitive problems. In: Rutter M, ed. Developmental neuropsychiatry. New York: Guilford Press, 1983:280–329.
2. Rosvold HE, Mirsky AF, Sarason I, Bransome ED, Beck LH. A continuous performance test of brain damage. J Consult Psychol 1956;20:343–350.
3. Seidel WT, Joschko M. Evidence of difficulties in sustained attention in children with ADDH. J Abnorm Child Psychol 1990;18:217–229.
4. Corkum PV, Siegel LS. Is the continuous performance task a valuable research tool for use with children with Attention-Deficit-Hyperactivity Disorder? J Child Psychol Psychiatry 1993;34:1217–1239.
5. Barkley RA. Behavioral inhibition, sustained attention, and executive functions, constructing a unifying theory of ADHD. Psychol Bull 1997;121:65–94.
6. Swanson J, Castellanos FX, Maichels M, LaHoste G, Kennedy J. Cognitive neuroscience of attention deficit hyperactivity disorder and hyperkinetic disorder. Curr Opin Neurobiol 1998;8:263–271.
7. Castellanos FX, Tannock R. Neuroscience of attention-deficit/hyperactivity disorder: the search for endophenotypes. Nat Rev Neurosci 2002;3:617–628.
8. Rubia K. The dynamic approach to neurodevelopmental psychiatric disorders: use of fMRI combined with neuropsychology to elucidate the dynamics of psychiatric disorders, exemplified in ADHD and schizophrenia. Behav Brain Res 2002;130:47–56.
9. Nigg JT. Is ADHD a disinhibitory disorder? Psychol Bull 2001;127:571–598.
10. Nigg JT, Blaskey LG, Huang-Pollock CL, Rappley MD. Neuropsychological executive functions and DSM-IV ADHD subtypes. J Am Acad. Child Adolesc Psychiatry 2002;41:59–66.
11. Chhabildas N, Pennington BF, Willcutt EG. A comparison of the neuropsychological profiles of the DSM-IV subtypes of ADHD. J Abnorm Child Psychol 2001;29:529–540.
12. Sergeant JA, Geurts H, Oosterlaan J. How specific is a deficit of executive functioning for attention-deficit/hyperactivity disorder? Behav Brain Res 2002;130:3–28.
13. Hillyard SA, Hink RF, Schwent VL, Picton TW. Electrical signs of selective attention in the human brain. Science 1973;182:177–180.
14. Alho K, Paavilainen P, Reinkainen K, Sams M, Naatanen R. Separability of different negative components of the event-related potential associated with auditory stimulus processing. Psychophysiology 1986;23:613–623.
15. Alho K. Selective attention in auditory processing as reflected by event-related brain potentials. Psychophysiology 1992;29:247–263.
16. Kenemans JL, Kok A, Smulders FTY. Event-related potentials to conjunctions of spatial frequency and orientation as a function of stimulus parameters and response requirements. Electroencephalogr Clin Neurophysiol 1993;88:51–63.

17. Harter MR, Aine CJ. Brain mechanisms of visual selective attention. In: Parasuraman R, Davies DR, eds. Varieties of attention. New York: Academic Press, 1984;293–321.
18. Wijers AA, Mulder G, Okita T, Mulder LJM Scheffers MK. Attention to color: an ERP-analysis of selection, controlled search and motor activation. Psychophysiology 1989;26:89–109.
19. Kenemans JL, Lijffijt M, Camfferman G, Verbaten MN. Split-second sequential selective activation in human secondary visual cortex. J Cogn Neurosci 2002;14 48–61.
20. Smid HGOM, Jakob A, Heinze HJ. An event-related potential study of visual selective attention to conjunctions of color and shape. Psychophysiology 1999;36:264–279.
21. Lange JJ, Wijers, AA, Mulder JM, Mulder G. Color selection and location selection in ERPs: differences, similarities and neural specificity. Biol Psychiatry 1998;48:153–182.
22. Corbetta M, Miezen FM, Dobmeyer S, Shulman GL, Petersen SE. Selective and divided attention during visual discrimination of shape, color and speed: functional anatomy by positron emission tomography. J Neurosci 1991;11:2382–2402.
23. Corbetta M, Miezen FM, Shulman GL, Petersen SE. A PET study of visuospatial attention. J Neurosci 1993; 13: 1202–1226.
24. Posner MI, Snyder CRR, Davidson BJ. Facilitation and inhibition in the processing of signals. In: Rabbit PMA, ed. Attention and performance. London:Academic Press, 1975:669–682.
25. Posner MI. Orienting of attention. Q J Exp Psychol 1980;32:3–25.
26. Johnson, MH. Cortical maturation and the development of visual attention in early infancy. J Cogn Neurosci 1990, 2:81–95.
27. Rafal, RD, Calabresi P, Brennan, C, Sciolto T. Saccade preparation inhibits reorienting to recently attended location. J Exp Psychol Hum Percept Perform 1989;15:673–683.
28. Eimer M. Mechanisms of visuospatial attention: evidence from event-related brain potentials. Vis Cogn 1998;5:257–286.
29. Hillyard SA, Anllo-Vento L, Clark VP, Heinze HJ, Luck SJ, Mangun GR. In: Kramer AF, Coles MGH, eds. Converging operations in the study of visual spatial attention. Washington, DC: American Psychological Association 1996:107–138.
30. Luck SJ, Hillyard SA, Mouloua M, Woldorff MG, Clark VP, Hawkins HL. Effects of spatial cuingon luminance detectability: psychophysical and electrophysiological evidence for early selection. J Exp Psychol Hum Percept Perform 1994;20:887–904.
31. Prior M, Sanson A, Freethy C, Geffen G. Auditory attentional abilities in hyperactive children. J Child Psychol Psychiatry 1985;26:289–304.
32. Zambelli AJ, Stamm JS, Maitinsky S, Loiselle DL. Auditory evoked potentials and selective attention in formerly hyperactive adolescent boys. Am J Psychiatry 1977;134:742–747.
33. Loiselle D, Stamm JS, Maitinsky S, Whipple SC. Evoked potential and behavioral signs of attentive dysfunctions in hyperactive boys. Psychophysiology 1980;17:193–201.
34. Hansen JC, Hillyard SA. Effects of stimulation rate and attribute cueing on event-related potentials during selective auditory attention. Psychophysiology 1984;21:394–405.
35. Satterfield JH, Schell AM, Nicholas T, Backs RW. Topographic study of auditory event related potentials in normal boys and boys with attention deficit disorder with hyperactivity. Psychophysiology 1988;25:591–606.
36. Satterfield JH, Shell AM, Nicholas TW, Satterfield BT, Freese TH. Ontogeny of selective attention effects on event-related potentials in attention-deficit hyperactivity disorder and normal boys. Biol Psychiatry 1990;28:879–903.
37. Satterfield JH, Schell AM, Nicholas T. Preferential neural processing of attended stimuli in attention-deficit hyperactivity disorder and normal boys. Psychophysiology 1994;31:1–10.
38. Jonkman LM, Kemner C, Verbaten MN, et al. Event-related potentials and performance of attention-deficit hyperactivity disorder children and normal controls in auditory and visual selective attention tasks. Biol Psychiatry 1997;41:595–611.
39. Van der Stelt O, van der Molen M, Gunning B, Kok A. Neurelectrical signs of selective attention to color in boys with attention-deficit hyperactivity disorder. Preliminary results of this study were presented at the 39th meeting of the Society for Psychophysiological Research (SPR), Granada, Spain, October 6–10, 1999. Cogn Brain Res 2001;12:245–264.

40. Jonkman LM, Kenemans, JL, Kemner C, Verbaten MN, van Engeland H. Dipole source localisation of event-related brain activity indicative of an early visual selective attention deficit in ADHD children. Clin Neurophysiol 2004;115:1537–1549.
41. Liu T, Slotnick SD, Serences JT, Yantis S. Cortical mechanisms of feature-based attentional control. Cereb Cortex 2003;13:1334–1343.
42. Kemner C, Jonkman LM, Kenemans JL, Verbaten MN, van Engeland H. Sources of auditory selective attention and the effects of MPH in children with ADHD. Biol Psychiatry 2004;55:776–778.
43. Carter CS, MacDonald AM, Botvinick M, et al. Parsong executive processes: strategic vs. evaluative functions of the anterior cingulated cortex. PNAS 2000;97:1944–1948.
44. Van Veen V, Carter CS. The anterior cingulate as a conflict monitor: fMRI and ERP studies. Physiol Behav 2002;77:477–482.
45. Nieuwenhuis S, Yeung N, van den Wildenberg W, Ridderinkhof R. Electrophysiological correlates of anterior cingulate function in a go/no-go task: effects of response conflict and trial type frequency. Cogn Affect Behav Neurosci 2003;3:17–26.
46. Michie PT, Karayanidis F, Smith GL, et al. An exploration of varieties of visual attention: ERP findings. Cogn Brain Res 1999;7:419–450.
47. Swanson JM, Posner M, Potkin S, et al. Activating tasks for the study of visual-spatial attention in ADHD children: a cognitive anatomic approach. J Child Neurol 1991;6:S119–S127.
48. Nigg JT, Swanson JM, Hinshaw SP. Covert visual spatial attention in boys with attention deficit hyperactivity disorder: lateral effects, methylphenidate response and results for parents. Neuropsychologia 1997;35:165–176.
49. Aman CJ, Roberts RJ, Pennington BF. A neuropsychological examination of the underlying deficit in Attention Deficit Hyperactivity Disorder. Dev Psychol 1998;34:956–969.
50. McDonald S, Bennett KMB, Chambers H, Castiello U. Covert orienting and focusing of attention in children with attention deficit hyperactivity disorder. Neuropsychologia 1999;37: 345–356.
51. Wood C, Maruff P, Levy F, Farrow M, Hay D. Covert orienting of visual spatial attention in attention deficit hyperactivity disorder: does comorbidity make a difference? Arch Clin Neurophysiol 1999;14:179–189.
52. Perchet C, Revol O, Fourneret P, Maugiere F, Garcia-Larrea L. Attention shifts and anticipatory mechanisms in hyperactive children: an ERP study using the Posner paradigm. Biol Psychiatry 2001;50:44–57.
53. Posner MI, Rafal RD. Cognitive theories of attention and the rehabilitation of attentional deficits. In: Meier MJ, Benton AL, Diller L, eds. Neuropsychological rehabilitation. New York: Guilford Press 1987:182–201.
54. Pearson DA, Yaffee LS, Loveland KA, Norton AM. Covert visual attention in children with attention deficit hyperactivity disorder: evidence for developmental immaturity ? Dev Psychopathol 1995;7:351–367.
55. Carter CS, Krener P, Chaderjian M, Northcutt C, Wolfe V. Asymmetrical visual-spatial attentional performance in ADHD: evidence for a right hemisphere deficit. Biol Psychiatry 1995;37:789–797.
56. Novak GP, Solanto M, Abikoff H. Spatial orienting and focused attention in attention deficit hyperactivity disorder. Psychophysiology 1995;32:546–559.
57. Tomporowski PD, Tinsly V, Hager LD. Visuospatial attentional shifts and choice responses of adults and ADHD and non-ADHD children. Percept Mot Skills 1994;79:1479–1490.
58. Corbetta M, Kincade JM, Shulman GL. Neural systems for visual orienting and their relationships to spatial working memory. J Cogn Neurosci 2002;14:508–523.
59. Daffner KR, Mesulam MM, Scinto LF, et al. The central role of the prefrontal cortex in directing attention to novel events. Brain 2000;123: 927–939.
60. Knight RT, Scabini D. Anatomic bases of event-related potentials and their relationship to novelty detection in humans. J Clin Neurophysiol 1998;15:3–13.
61. Plude DJ, Enns JT, Brodeur D. The development of selective attention: a life-span overview. Acta Psychol 1994;86:227–272.

62. Brodeur DA, Enns JT. Covert visual orienting across the lifespan. Can J Exp Psychol 1997;51:20–35.
63. Jonkman LM, Kemner C, Verbaten MN, et al. Attentional capacity, a probe ERP study: differences between children with attention-deficit hyperactivity disorder and normal control children and effects of methylphenidate. Psychophysiology 2000;37:334–346.
64. Sergeant JA, Scholten CA. On resource strategy limitations in hyperactivity: cognitive impulsivity reconsidered. J Child Psychol Psychiatry 1985;26:97–109.
65. Sergeant JA. The cognitive-energetic model: an empirical approach to Attention-Deficit Hyperactivity Disorder. Neurosci Biobehav Rev 2000;24:7–12.

12
Working Memory in Children With ADHD

Jack Stevens

1. INTRODUCTION

Over the past few years, working memory has become one of the hottest topics in regards to the neurocognitive functioning of children with attention deficit hyperactivity disorder (ADHD). Working memory has been recently hypothesized as either a core *(1)* or secondary *(2)* deficit in these children.

The purpose of this chapter is to provide information to the reader regarding the following four key questions:

1. What are the characteristics of working memory?
2. Do children with ADHD have deficits in working memory?
3. Are working memory deficits specific to ADHD?
4. What is the clinical usefulness of this construct and how can we improve its utility in the future?

Each of these questions will be discussed in turn.

2. WHAT ARE THE CHARACTERISTICS OF WORKING MEMORY?

2.1. *Defining Working Memory and Its Relation to Major Theories of ADHD*

Working memory is a psychological construct that has been conceptualized and assessed differently across investigators. An overview of working memory—what it is, what it is not, how it is typically assessed, and how it differs from other prefrontal functions—will hopefully facilitate the critical examination of its potential importance in children with ADHD offered in Sections 3 through 5 of this chapter. Therefore, a nonexhaustive review of working memory is presented here.

Perhaps the most widely cited definition and model of working memory come from the work of Alan Baddeley. Baddeley *(3)* defined this construct as the "simultaneous storage and processing of information." Baddeley's model suggested that working memory is composed of three systems: a phonological loop for verbal and acoustic information, a visuospatial sketchpad for visual and spatial information, and a central executive overseeing the aforementioned systems. Baddeley *(4)* recently added a fourth component called the episodic buffer, which integrates information from the central executive and different modalities. In their recent model of ADHD, Rapport and colleagues *(1)* utilize a very similar definition of working memory—"a set of memory processes that serve to construct, maintain, and manipulate cognitive representations of incoming stimuli." Their theory posits that working memory is a primary deficit in children with ADHD that results in disorganized behavior and a need to seek additional stimulation.

From: *Attention Deficit Hyperactivity Disorder: From Genes to Patients*
Edited by: D. Gozal and D. L. Molfese © Humana Press Inc., Totowa, NJ

Another frequently cited definition of working memory comes from the comprehensive theory of ADHD offered by Russell Barkley *(5)*, who defined working memory as "the capacity to hold information in mind across a delay in time to guide a subsequent response." Barkley suggested that working memory impairments can interfere with one's sense of time, organizational skills, and ability to learn from past mistakes. In contrast to Rapport et al.'s model *(1)*, Barkley's theoretical framework suggested that children with ADHD have a primary deficit in behavioral inhibition, resulting in a failure to utilize other executive functions, such as working memory.

Regardless of how exactly the concept is defined, working memory presumably involves several interrelated processes. To begin with, Fry and Hale *(6)* identified improvements in processing speed as mediating age-enhanced working memory performance. In contrast, Swanson *(7)* concluded that changes in capacity, not processing efficiency, may underlie improvements in working memory performance across age groups. Using a slightly more complicated framework, Roberts et al. *(8)* suggested that working memory depends on "capacity," "inferencing and computation," "maintenance over delays," and "level of moment-to-moment activation." Finally, Stout et al. *(9)* noted two additional processes: information searching and attention shifting between storage and processing demands. Therefore, deficits in working memory performance may exist as a result of any number of factors that affect one's ability to store and process information.

2.2. *How Is Working Memory Different From Other Memory Constructs?*

Researchers have proposed that children with ADHD do not have global memory impairments but rather have selective deficits in working memory, as opposed to other types of memory processes. Working memory is a limited capacity system that can be differentiated from three other major types of memory: sensory memory, short-term memory, and long-term memory.

Working memory holds information longer than sensory memory does. In addition, working memory is more active than short-term memory, which involves only passive storage of information that is to be recalled in an unaltered state *(10)*. That is, working memory describes a more complicated neurocognitive function than short-term memory because working memory requires information to be remembered (storage) while either this information or other information is manipulated in some fashion (processing). Finally, working memory is distinguished from long-term memory, which involves a virtually infinite capacity system for information that can be stored for prolonged time periods.

Working memory differs from other memory constructs not only in terms of capacity, duration of storage, and function, but also regarding its neurobiological basis. In her review of the neuroanatomical basis of working vs short-term memory based on neuroimaging techniques, Gathercole *(11)* concluded that working memory is primarily mediated by the dorsolateral prefrontal cortex, whereas short-term memory is mediated by other portions of the brain (e.g., posterior parietal and inferior prefrontal cortex). Moreover, Siegel *(12)* noted that working memory is mediated primarily by chemical changes between synapses, whereas long-term memory often occurs as a result of changes in the actual structure of synapses.

2.3. *How Is Working Memory Typically Measured by Psychologists and Other Researchers?*

Although a newly developed rating scale (Behavioral Rating Inventory of Executive Function) *(13)* exists that has a subscale titled "Working Memory," working memory has been typically assessed through the use of clinical tests or laboratory tasks. A plethora of these performance-based measures purportedly assess this complex construct. Inconsistency in task requirements across measures is not entirely surprising, given that "working memory" has been defined in different ways across studies, as Hulme and Roodenrys *(14)* have pointed out. Therefore, classifying these numerous tasks is no easy undertaking, given that tasks differ in terms of which aspects of working memory (e.g., capacity, activation, maintenance, information processing) are most involved.

D'Esposito et al. *(15)* proposed one such framework in which tasks that have been labeled as assessing working memory can be placed into two categories: "maintenance plus" and "maintenance only." Maintenance-plus tasks require performing operations on stored information or processing interfering information before recall of the initial information can occur. In contrast, maintenance-only tasks involve just holding information for a short period of time without distraction and without performing any additional tasks.

Span tasks involving reading or counting are among the most recognized measures of working memory and are excellent examples of maintenance-plus tasks. Reading span tasks, based on the work of Daneman and Carpenter *(16)*, often involve showing participants a series of sentences with the last word missing in each sentence. Participants must fill in a missing word at the end of each sentence as it is presented and then recall those missing words at the end of the block. The participant must process each sentence's content in order to determine the correct missing word, store each missing word, and then recall those words at the end of the trial. Counting span tasks similarly require both processing and storage of information. For these tasks, participants are shown of series of cards, asked to count the number of particular stimuli on each card (processing), and then told to recall in order the number of counted stimuli from each card at the end of the block (storage).

Additional examples of maintenance-plus tasks are mental arithmetic and digit backwards. Mental arithmetic tasks (e.g., serial addition) require processing of information (e.g., adding one number to another) while keeping that new number in mind as the next number is being presented. Participants are then asked for a final number at the end of the block based on computations conducted as the numbers were presented. Digit backward involves storage of a series of just-heard numbers and transformation of that stored information by recalling them in reverse order.

What about maintenance-only tasks, the second type of working memory task identified in the framework of D'Esposito *(15)*? These later tasks do not appear to conform to Baddeley's *(3)* definition of working memory because no processing of information is explicitly required. These maintenance-only tasks are sometimes incorrectly identified as being working memory tasks but instead may be best regarded as short-term memory tasks. Examples of maintenance-only tasks include digit span forward, pattern recall, and word recall *(11)*.

Digit span forward requires a participant to repeat just-heard digits ranging in span from two to nine without explicit processing of those numbers and therefore falls outside the domain of working memory. Pattern recall and word recall tasks, in which the only requirement is to retain visuospatial information or a series of words, may not meet Baddeley's standard for working memory either. The reader should be aware that investigators have sometimes identified these maintenance-only tasks as assessing working memory. For instance, Kerns et al. *(17)* and Karatekin and Asarnow *(18)* are two recent examples of using digit span forward to assess working memory. Therefore, if one wishes to adhere to Baddeley's rigorous definition of working memory, a careful examination of what "working memory" tasks are used is warranted.

However, a caveat should be mentioned here. One could argue that these maintenance-only tasks do assess working memory if participants use chunking, mnemonics, or other organization strategies in order to recall the lists of stimuli. That is, trying to find patterns in information to be remembered in order to facilitate recall could be considered processing of information, not just storage. For example, if the word recall task requires the identification and utilization of categories to facilitate recall, this additional processing requirement may make a presumably "short-term memory" task into an actual "working memory" task. However, if the word recall task involves no categorization of words or use of mnemonic strategies, it may be just tapping short-term memory capacity.

In conclusion, it may be quite difficult to identify memory tasks in which absolutely no processing of information occurs. Trying to demarcate memory tasks as assessing either working memory or short-term memory is not easy. In fact, researchers sometimes use the terms "working memory" and "short-term memory" interchangeably. Nevertheless, it should be stressed that investigators not directly studying ADHD have found systematic differences between maintenance-plus and maintenance-only tasks, suggesting that the distinction between working memory and short-term memory is not arbitrary.

Based on previous studies, Swanson and Sachse-Lee *(19)* noted that digit span forward, a classic short-term memory task, loaded onto a different factor than maintenance-plus tasks. Similarly, Cantor et al. *(20)* found that working memory and short-term memory tasks loaded onto different factors. Finally, Hale et al. *(21)* similarly found that digits forward was related to short-term memory, whereas digits backward was related to executive function. Taken together, these studies provided data suggesting that short-term memory and working memory are related but still somewhat independent constructs. Therefore, given that the topic of this chapter is working memory, short-term memory (and hence maintenance-only tasks) in children with ADHD will not be explicitly reviewed in the remaining sections.

2.4. How Is Working Memory Different From Other Higher Level Psychological Constructs?

Just as we can differentiate working memory from other memory constructs, it is important to distinguish between working memory and other related constructs, particularly academic achievement, general intelligence, and executive dysfunction, in order to demonstrate the utility and uniqueness of working memory. This differentiation is particularly important when examining potential deficits in children with ADHD, given that many of these children perform poorly academically, have mildly lower scores on intelligence tests, and exhibit difficulties with executive dysfunction, such as disinhibition, when compared to children without the disorder.

As can be seen in Section 2, which described prototypical working memory tasks, performance on these measures often involves academic skills in math or reading. Performance for serial addition tasks depends not only on storage but also on computational skills. Similarly, performance on reading span tasks depends not only on storage but also on reading comprehension. Not surprisingly, strong correlations have been found between reading span tasks and reading comprehension tasks *(10)*. This may lead one to ask: Can working memory be assessed outside an academic domain?

Two pieces of information suggest that working memory can be separated from performance in individual academic domains. First, empirical data have suggested that working memory is a central executive system that cuts across different academic domains. Swanson *(22)* utilized different working memory tasks—some whose processing component involved reading and some whose processing component involved math. He found similar relationships between individual academic achievement areas (e.g., reading) and working memory measures that required similar processing requirements (e.g., reading) vs different processing requirements (e.g., math). Swanson concluded that "working memory transcends the type of processing required." Dyche and Johnson *(23)* further provide data that working memory and math achievement are related but no so much that they cannot be considered fairly independent constructs.

Second, working memory tasks have been developed that require minimal academic skills. For example, Stevens et al. *(24)* used a color/digit span task in which participants named the color of each digit as it was presented and then recalled the digits at the end of the block. For this task, only the ability to name colors and digits were required—no sophisticated computation skills or reading comprehension abilities were needed. The ability to name colors and digits should have been well within the capabilities of their sample of elementary-school-aged children. Thus, it appears possible to assess working memory outside of academic achievement in an individual subject.

However, working memory and general intelligence may be harder to distinguish from each other. The most recent version of the Wechsler Adult Intelligence Scale-3rd edition (WAIS-III) *(25)* actually identifies working memory as one of its factors. Nevertheless, other factors from the WAIS-III have also been identified as composing general intelligence, such as verbal comprehension and processing speed. Therefore, working memory appears to be an important element of, but not identical to, general intelligence. Stevens et al. *(24)* provided empirical data for this assertion by finding a significant but not overwhelming (0.31) correlation between measures of working memory and general intelligence in a sample of children with and without ADHD. The issue of controlling for general intelligence when examine working memory deficits in children is discussed in greater detail in Subheading 3.1 of this chapter.

Finally, several studies suggest that working memory is not synonymous with other executive functions. Using a sample of normally developing adolescents, Lehto *(26)* found that working memory tasks were sometimes uncorrelated with measures of planning and impulsivity. Moreover, using a sample of adolescents with ADHD, Barkley et al. *(27)* reported that working memory measures loaded onto different factors than inattentive and impulsive factors reflected performance on a continuous performance test. Finally, using a sample of children with ADHD and control children, Wiers et al. *(28)* reported nonsignificant to small relationships among working memory, impulsivity, and planning.

In summary, working memory appears to be a somewhat independent construct that is not completely subsumed by academic achievement, general intelligence, or executive dysfunction. Therefore, working memory deserves independent attention as an area of potential deficit in children with ADHD.

3. DO CHILDREN WITH ADHD HAVE DEFICITS IN WORKING MEMORY?

3.1. Empirical Evidence For and Against Working Memory Deficits in Children With ADHD

Table 1 presents studies *(18,24,28–36)* in which children identified as having ADHD or attention problems differed from normally developing control children on working memory tasks. In contrast, Table 2 presents studies *(18,27,31,35,37–40)* that failed to find group differ-

Table 1
Studies Finding Working Memory Differences Between Children With ADHD and Control Children

Study by	Publication date	Age range	Measure of working memory	Did controlling for IQ alter results?
Shallice et al.	2002	7–12 yr	N-back working memory task	Groups equivalent on IQ
Stevens et al.	2002	7–12 yr	Color/digit dual span task	Controlling removed differences
Kalff et al.	2002	5–6 yr	Kaufman-ABC Word Order	Groups equivalent on IQ
Kuntsi et al.	2001	7–11 yr	Sentence span	Controlling removed differences
		7–11 yr	Delayed response alternation	Controlling removed differences
Barnett et al.	2001	6–12 yr	Spatial working memory task	Controlling did not change results
Cornoldi et al.	2001	8–12 yr	Listening span task	Groups equivalent on IQ
		8–12 yr	Visuospatial working memory task	Groups equivalent on IQ
Karatekin et al.	1998	$\bar{x} = 13$ yr	Dot test of visuospatial working memory	Groups equivalent on IQ
Wiers et al.	1998	7–11 yr	Self-ordered pointing task	Controlling did not change results
Mariani and Barkley	1997	4–5 yr	"Working memory" factor	Controlling did not change results
Shue and Douglas	1992	8–12 yr	Self-ordered pointing task (representational pictures)	Groups equivalent on IQ
Gorenstein et al.	1989	8–12 yrs	Sequential matching memory task	Groups equivalent on IQ

Table 2
Studies Failing to Find Working Memory Differences Between Children With ADHD and Control Children

Study by	Publication date	Age range	Measure of working memory
Rucklidge and Tannock	2002	13–16 yr	Digit span backward
Barkley et al.	2001	12–19 yr	"Working memory" factor (e.g., Digit span backward)
Kuntsi et al.	2001	7–11 yr	Counting span
Adams and Snowling	2001	8–11 yr	Counting span
Willcutt et al.	2001	8–16 yr	"Working memory" factor (e.g., Sentence span, counting span)
Karatekin et al.	1998	$\bar{x} = 13$ yr	Digit span backward
Shue and Douglas	1992	8–12 yr	Self-ordered pointing task (abstract design version)
Siegel and Ryan	1989	7–13 yr	Sentence span and counting span

ences in working memory between these children and normally developing control children. Only those studies that utilized tasks that conform to Baddeley's definition that working memory require both storage and processing of information were included in the tables. Therefore, studies, such as Kerns et al. *(17)*, which involved primarily maintenance-only or short-term memory tasks, were outside the scope of this article and hence were excluded from the tables.

Also excluded from Tables 1 and 2 were results from studies that used the arithmetic or coding subtests of childhood intelligence tests to assess working memory. These studies were excluded because the results from these subtests were thoroughly and recently summarized by Rapport et al. *(41)*, who concluded that children with ADHD performed worse on these tasks than did normally developing children on 75% of the identified studies.

An examination of Table 1 indicates that differences in working memory have been found between ADHD and control groups on several different working memory tasks. However, some of those studies *(24,31)* also reported that statistically controlling for intelligence (IQ) removed those group differences, particular in terms of verbal working memory (e.g., digit span, sentence span). Whether or not to control for IQ in these studies is an unresolved dispute in the field. Those who argue for control of IQ suggest that only then can we find specific impairment in working memory, as opposed to overall intellectual functioning, in children with ADHD. Those who caution against controlling for IQ note the negative association between ADHD symptoms and IQ scores and hence warn that controlling for IQ may remove part of the variance that should be attributed to ADHD itself.

Nevertheless, a review of Table 1 also suggests that controlling for IQ did not remove all group differences, particular in regard to nonverbal working memory tasks, such as the spatial working memory task and the self-ordered pointing task. This finding suggest that nonverbal working memory may be a particular area of impairment in children with ADHD, which may be related to deficits in time perception, as Barkley *(2)* and others have hypothesized.

An examination of Table 2 suggests that several studies have failed to find group differences in working memory. These studies used primarily verbal working memory tasks, such as digit span backward and sentence span. Also, three of these studies used primarily teenagers with ADHD.

3.2. Reconciling Discrepant Results

Explaining the discrepant results across studies is not entirely clear given that working memory impairment has been inconsistently found in children with ADHD. Population characteristics and parameters of working memory tasks are possible candidates to explain the inconsistencies. Two trends are worth noting.

First, when compared to normally developing control children, teens with ADHD were much less likely to exhibit working memory differences compared with elementary-school-aged children with ADHD. This tendency suggests that working memory problems may occur in elementary school ADHD but not in later forms of the disorder. This trend suggests that these working memory problems may be transient in nature, but of course longitudinal studies would be needed to confirm this. Alternatively, working memory measures may not be sensitive enough to capture real deficits in adolescents with ADHD vs normally developing adolescents. Neither explanation appears entirely plausible, as some studies *(42)* have demonstrated working memory deficits in adults with ADHD. Thus, it would be surprising, albeit not impossible, if working memory measures were sensitive enough to detect group differences in childhood and adulthood but not the transition time between those two time periods.

Second, the studies that failed to find group differences mostly require participants to remember verbal information, whereas several of the studies that did find group differences required participants to recall spatial information. This trend suggests that nonverbal working memory, as opposed to verbal working memory, may be a more pronounced problem for those with ADHD. This conclusion is also consistent with the finding of Rapport et al. *(41)*, who found that measures requiring recall of visual material frequently distinguished between ADHD and control groups. However, nonverbal working memory has received less empirical attention than verbal working memory. Moreover, impairment on spatial working memory has been linked to solely storage deficiencies in, as opposed to problems with, manipulating/processing the visual stimuli *(32)*. Hence, the above conclusion should be considered tentative at this time.

Sample size, or lack of power, does not appear to be a likely explanation for the null findings. Although some of the studies from Table 2 utilized sample sizes under 35 of children with ADHD *(18)*, other studies *(18,27,39)* using sample sizes over 50 of children with ADHD have also failed to find group differences. Considering sample size is important, as some theories of ADHD *(2)* postulated that working memory deficits are secondary to more central impairments, such as behavioral inhibition, in this population.

3.3. Evidence for Working Memory Impairments in Conjunction With Other Prefrontal Functions

Besides working memory tasks, a somewhat different way of documenting deficits in this domain for children with ADHD is through the investigation of other tasks that primarily assess another prefrontal function, like behavioral inhibition, but also place significant demands on working memory. In their review of performance measures that reliably distinguish between children with ADHD and normally developing controls, Rapport et al. *(41)* found that the continuous performance test and stop-signal task, two well-known measures of behavioral inhibition, frequently distinguished between ADHD and control groups. Although these tasks are generally assumed to measure primarily inhibitory control, they also may have a working memory component, in that participants must keep storing and utilizing basic task instructions (e.g., how to respond to different types of stimuli). In other words, when children with ADHD are required to demonstrate skills in working memory and inhibitory control simultaneously, a greater likelihood of finding deficient performance compared to control groups may occur. It should be stressed, however, that this interaction may not be unique to children with ADHD. Other investigators *(8)* have found in normal controls that inhibitory control may be at its worst under conditions that place a high demand on working memory.

A rare study that explicitly examined behavioral inhibition under different working memory loads in an ADHD population was that by Lawrence et al. *(43)* Using a novel but yet to be validated methodology involving following a route at a local zoo, the study indicated that these children showed the most pronounced difficulties with inhibitory control when working memory demands were at their greatest. These researchers found that while children with ADHD had no impairment in terms of remembering task instructions, they were more likely to deviate from the assigned route (exhibit inhibitory control problems) than children without ADHD when task instructions were at their most complex. This suggests an interaction effect between working memory and inhibitory control for the ADHD group that was not present for the control sample. Children with ADHD may be more sensitive to working memory load, thereby resulting in behavioral disinhibition when demands on working memory are at their greatest.

3.4. Summary of Evidence for Working Memory Deficits in Children With ADHD

In conclusion, major inconsistencies across studies exist regarding whether or not children with ADHD have difficulties with working memory. The following four factors, however, appear to increase the likelihood of finding working memory differences between children with ADHD and control children:

1. Not statistically controlling for general intelligence.
2. Employing an elementary-school-aged, as opposed to a teenager, sample.
3. Utilizing measures of nonverbal, as opposed to verbal, working memory.
4. Implementing tasks that require not only working memory, but also another executive function, such as behavioral inhibition.

4. ARE WORKING MEMORY DEFICITS UNIQUE TO ADHD?

Working memory has not been just a key concept in regard to the neurocognitive functioning of children with ADHD. H. Lee Swanson and his colleagues have frequently found that children with reading disabilities (RDs) have poorer working memories than same-age children without these academic problems *(19,44,45)*. These findings beg the question: are working memory deficits more or less severe in children with ADHD compared with children with other psychiatric disorders?

Perhaps the most rigorous data regarding this question can be found in studies that compare children with ADHD to children with other conditions on identical measures of working memory, because task characteristics are controlled in these studies. Table 3 provides an overview of studies *(37–40, 46)* that compare working memory in children with ADHD or children with RDs. As can be seen from the results highlighted in that table, children with ADHD generally performed *better* than children with RD did.

Moreover, children with comorbid ADHD and RD sometimes performed worse than children with only ADHD, suggesting that it is reading disabilities, not ADHD, that lead to working memory impairments. One exception to this general finding was Roodenrys et al. *(46)*, who found that children with ADHD + RD performed worse than children with RD on two different working memory tasks. However, all studies involving comorbid groups must be interpreted with caution, as authors sometimes did not state whether comorbid and single-diagnosis groups were equivalent in terms of the severity of the diagnosis both groups shared. For example, although both the RD and ADHD + RD groups in the Roodenrys et al. study *(46)* had reading problems, if the comorbid group had more severe reading impairment than the single-diagnosis group, group differences could be also be attributed to more severe RD, as opposed to ADHD symptomatology.

In addition to RD, other psychiatric conditions have been examined in comparison to ADHD in terms of working memory performance. To begin with, Karatekin and Asarnow *(18)* found that children with early-onset schizophrenia performed comparably to children with ADHD on digit span backward. In addition, Seguin et al. *(47)* found a negative association between working memory and physical aggression even after controlling for ADHD symptoms. Moreover, Bennetto et al. *(48)* found than children with autism performed worse on working memory measures than did children with other clinical conditions, including children

Table 3
Studies Comparing Working Memory Performance in Children With ADHD and Children With Reading Difficulties

Study by	Publication date	Age range	Measure of working memory	Chief finding
Rucklidge and Tannock	2002	13–16 yr	Digit span backwards	ADHD + RD < ADHD
			WISC-III arithmetic	ADHD + RD < ADHD
Willcutt et al.	2001	8–16 yr	Sentence span and counting span	RD, RD + ADHD < ADHD
Roodenrys et al.	2001	$\bar{x}$ = 10 yr	Auditory serial addition task	RD > RD + ADHD
			Memory updating task	RD > RD + ADHD
Adams and Snowling	2001	8–11 yr	Counting span	RD = ADHD = RD + ADHD
Siegel and Ryan	1989	7–13 yr	Sentence span	ADHD > RD
			Counting span	ADHD > RD

RD, reading difficulties; WISC-III, Wechsler Intelligence Scale for Children, 3rd Edition.

with RD or ADHD. Finally, Cohen et al. *(49)* reported that working memory problems were more strongly related to language impairments, based on poor performance on tests of syntax, phonology, or semantics, than to ADHD. Taken together, these four studies, as well as the studies highlighted in Table 3, suggest that working memory deficits are not unique to ADHD. In fact, many of the studies discussed in this section indicate that working memory problems are more severe in children with reading or language problems than in children with ADHD.

5. WHAT IS THE CLINICAL UTILITY OF THIS CONSTRUCT AND HOW CAN WE IMPROVE IN THE FUTURE?

5.1. Diagnostic Utility

Given that differences in working memory are often (but not always) found between ADHD and normal control groups, the practicing psychologist may wonder if such measures should be incorporated into a routine testing battery. First, it should be noted that none of the measures listed in Table 1 have widespread normative data or established cutoff scores. In addition, it remains unclear whether any of those working memory measures appear promising for the classification purposes. Given the small but statistically significant differences in magnitudes reported in the studies outlined in Table 1, the classificatory power of those working memory measures appears doubtful. Although researchers have reported differences in means between groups, they have infrequently reported rates of sensitivity, specificity, or predictive power regarding task performance between these groups using a cutoff criterion.

The most studied clinical measure of working memory in an ADHD population is the Freedom from Distractibility factor from the Wechsler Intelligence Scale for Children 3rd edition (WISC-III). This factor is composed of three working memory measures—arithmetic, digit span, and coding—that sometimes differentiate ADHD and control groups. Given the widespread use of the WISC-III in cognitive assessment, it is not surprising that this factor has received significant attention in regard to ADHD. However, Gordon and Barkley *(50)* reviewed the literature on this factor's utility in the assessment of ADHD and noted a great inconsistency in this factor's ability to differentiate ADHD from learning disabilities (LD) or normal control groups. In fact, Krane and Tannock *(51)* recently provided data indicating that impaired performance on this factor is more strongly related to learning difficulties than to ADHD. These data are consistent with the literature review from Section 4 of this chapter. Working memory impairment often is more severe in children with reading or language problems than it is in children with ADHD.

Therefore, the empirical literature does not yet support the use of working memory measures, including Freedom from Distractibility, in the clinical assessment of ADHD. First, the convergent validity between ADHD and working memory impairment has not been consistently established across studies from either the scientific literature or large normative groups. Second, the discriminant validity of working memory assessment for ADHD appears fuzzy, as children with RD compared to ADHD often perform worse on these measures. In fact, future applied clinical research should explore whether working memory assessment is more valuable in identifying RD than ADHD, especially considering the vastly different evidence-based treatment implications of each diagnosis (e.g., training in phonics versus stimulant medication and/or behavioral therapy). In the meantime, for those clinicians who insist on using working memory measures as part of their ADHD testing batteries, they should be forewarned that deficient performance may be suggestive of several other diagnoses as well, particular learning disorders.

5.2. Treatment Utility

Just because working memory measures may not have diagnostic utility does not automatically imply that they cannot be useful for treatment purposes. In this section, the potential usefulness of working memory in predicting medication response and serving as an important area for remediation in children with ADHD is discussed.

Predicting medication response in children with ADHD is very challenging. Although the majority of children with ADHD demonstrate improvements in activity level and attention on stimulant medication, the response of an individual child to a particular type and dose of medication is largely idiosyncratic. Reliable *a priori* prediction of medication response has yet to be achieved for individual children with ADHD. However, some general trends across groups of children with ADHD have been reported. In their review of articles examining predictors of response to methylphenidate (Ritalin™), Gray and Kagan *(52)* recently concluded that older children, children with less symptomatology, and children with concurring anxiety often do not respond as well to methylphenidate. In contrast, they concluded that co-occurring oppositional defiant disorder or conduct disorder symptoms, gender, socioeconomic status, and ethnicity often do not predict medication response. In addition, Fischer et al. *(53)* reported that children with ADHD who performed in the normal range on a continuous performance test were less likely to benefit from stimulants than did children with ADHD who performed in the deviant range. This study suggested that the continuous performance test may predict medication response, independent of this test's diagnostic utility.

However, to my knowledge, no study has utilized working memory assessment to predict medication response in an ADHD sample. This may be a worthwhile area to explore, as stimulants often affect dopamine levels, and dopamine function has been linked to working memory. In one of the only studies examining working memory as a predictor of medication response, Mehta et al. *(54)* found that methylphenidate produced the largest improvement in working memory performance in participants with the poorest working memory performance at baseline. However, those researchers utilized adults without ADHD and used working memory as its sole psychological outcome measure. Therefore, it remains unclear if baseline working memory performance would predict response to methylphenidate in a domain outside of working memory (e.g., parent and teacher ratings) in children with ADHD. Given the dearth of psychological tests available to predict medication response, it would be interesting to see whether working memory measures could have any incremental utility in this area.

Besides predicting medication response, there is some small preliminary evidence that working memory may be a useful area for remediation in children with ADHD. Klingberg et al. *(55)* found that seven children with ADHD who received approx 3.5 wk of computerized instruction in working memory tasks demonstrated mild improvements in spatial working memory relative to seven children with ADHD who received much less intensive computerized instruction. Moreover, these researchers found that the treatment group outperformed the control group on a nonworking memory task as well. However intriguing this study may be, it must be interpreted with extreme caution given the small sample size, the differential amount of time spent with children in the treatment vs control conditions, and the lack of substantial additional ADHD studies demonstrating beneficial outcomes for computerized training.

5.3. Conclusions and Future Research Directions

Working memory can be differentiated from other memory constructs, as well as other higher level psychological constructs. Nevertheless, four key future directions for working memory research, based in part on the major conclusions of this chapter, are as follows:

1. Given the inconsistent results across studies of working memory in children with ADHD, future research should focus on delineating more clearly which population (e.g., age), and task (e.g., spatial vs verbal) characteristics are most strongly related to finding group differences.
2. Given that working memory deficits have been found in several different clinical populations, exploring the use of working memory tasks as screening measures for reading problems or general psychopathology, as opposed to ADHD, may be warranted.
3. Given that several authors have noted that working memory measures frequently have demonstrated poor reliability *(31,56)* and the lack of normative data, future research should concentrate on establishing more firmly the psychometric characteristics of these measures.
4. Given that this construct's treatment utility remains largely unexplored by ADHD researchers, determining the malleability of working memory performance and its ability to predict medication response may be fruitful avenues to consider.

REFERENCES

1. Rapport MD, Chung KM, Shore G, Isaacs P. A conceptual model of child psychopathology: implications for understanding attention deficit hyperactivity disorder and treatment efficacy. J Clin Child Psychol 2001;30:48–58.
2. Barkley RA. Behavioral inhibition, sustained attention, and executive functions: constructing a unifying theory of ADHD. Psychol Bull 1997;121:65–94.
3. Baddeley A. Working memory. Sci 1992;255:556–559.
4. Baddeley A. The episodic buffer: a new component of working memory? Trends Cogn Sci 2000;4:417–423.
5. Barkley RA. Associated problems. In: Barkley RA, ed. Attention-deficit hyperactivity disorder: a handbook for diagnosis and treatment. New York: Guilford Press, 1998, pp. 97–138.
6. Fry AF, Hale S. Processing speed, working memory, and fluid intelligence: evidence for a developmental cascade. Psychol Sci 1996;7:237–241.
7. Swanson HL. What develops in working memory? A life span perspective. Dev Psychol 1999;35:986–1000.
8. Roberts RJ, Hager LD, Heron C. Prefrontal cognitive processes: working memory and inhibition in the antisaccade task. J Exp Psychol Gen 1994;123:374–393.
9. Stout JC, Salmon DP, Butters N, et al. Decline in working memory associated with HIV infection. Psychol Med 1995;25:1221–1232.
10. Swanson HL. Using the Cognitive Processing Test to assess ability: development of a dynamic assessment measure. Sch Psychol Rev 1995;24:672–693.
11. Gathercole SE. Cognitive approaches to the development of short-term memory. Trends Cogn Sci 1999;3:410–419.
12. Siegel DJ. Memory: an overview, with emphasis on developmental, interpersonal, and neurobiological aspects. J Am Acad Child Adolesc Psychiatry 2001;40:997–1011.
13. Gioia GA, Isquith PK, Guy SC, Kenworthy L. Behavior Rating Inventory of Executive Function. Child Neuropsychol 2000;6:235–238.
14. Hulme C, Roodenrys S. Verbal working memory development and its disorders. J Child Psychol Psychiatry Allied Disciplines 1995;36:373–398.

15. D'Esposito M, Aguirre GK, Zarahn E, Ballard D, Shin RK, Lease J. Functional MRI studies of spatial and nonspatial working memory. Cogn Brain Res 1998;7:1–13.
16. Daneman M, Carpenter PA. Individual differences in working memory and reading. J Verbal Learning Verbal Behav 1980;19:450–466.
17. Kerns KA, McInerney RJ, Wilde NJ. Time reproduction, working memory, and behavioral inhibition in children with ADHD. Child Neuropsychol 2001;7:21–31.
18. Karatekin C, Asarnow RF. Working memory in childhood-onset schizophrenia and attention-deficit/hyperactivity disorder. Psychiatry Res 1998;80:165–176.
19. Swanson HL, Sachse-Lee C. Mathematical problem solving and working memory in children with learning disabilities: both executive and phonological processes are important. J Exp Child Psychol 2001;79:294–321.
20. Cantor J, Engle RW, Hamilton G. Short-term memory, working memory, and verbal abilities: how do they relate? Intelligence 1991;15:229–246.
21. Hale JB, Hoeppner J-AB, Fiorello CA. Analyzing digit span components for assessment of attention processes. J Psychoeduc Assess 2002;20:128–143.
22. Swanson HL. Generality and modifiability of working memory among skilled and less skilled readers. J Educ Psychol 1992;84:473–488.
23. Dyche GM, Johnson DA. Development and evaluation of CHIPASAT, an attention test for children: II. Test-retest reliability and practice effect for a normal sample. Percept Motor Skills 1991;72:563–572.
24. Stevens J, Quittner AL, Zuckerman JB, Moore S. Behavioral inhibition, self-regulation of motivation, and working memory in children with attention deficit hyperactivity disorder. Dev Neuropsychol 2002;21:117–140.
25. Wechsler D. Wechsler Adult Intelligence Scale-Third Edition. San Antonio, TX: The Psychological Corporation, 1997.
26. Lehto J. Are executive function tests dependent on working memory capacity? Special Issue: Working Memory 1996;49:29–50.
27. Barkley RA, Edwards G, Laneri M, Fletcher K, Metevia L. Executive functioning, temporal discounting, and sense of time in adolescents with attention deficit hyperactivity disorder (ADHD) and oppositional defiant disorder (ODD). J Abnorm Child Psychol 2001;29:541–556.
28. Wiers RW, Gunning WB, Sergeant JA. Is a mild deficit in executive functions in boys related to childhood ADHD or to parental multigenerational alcoholism? J Abnorm Child Psychol 1998;26:415–430.
29. Shallice T, Marzocchi GM, Coser S, Del Savio M, Meuter RF, Rumiati RI. Executive function profile of children with attention deficit hyperactivity disorder. Dev Neuropsychol 2002;21: 43–71.
30. Kalff AC, Hendriksen JGM, Kroes M, et al. Neurocognitive performance of 5- and 6-year-old children who met criteria for attention deficit/hyperactivity disorder at 18 months follow-up: results from a prospective population study. J Abnorm Child Psychol 2002;30:589–598.
31. Kuntsi J, Oosterlaan J, Stevenson J. Psychological mechanisms in hyperactivity: I Response inhibition deficit, working memory impairment, delay aversion, or something else? J Child Psychol Psychiatry Allied Disciplines 2001;42:199–210.
32. Barnett R, Maruff P, Vance A, et al. Abnormal execution function in attention deficit hyperactivity disorder: The effect of stimulant medication and age on spatial working memory. Psychol Med 2001;31:1107–1115.
33. Cornoldi C, Marzocchi GM, Belotti M, Caroli MG, De Meo T, Braga C. Working memory interference control deficit in children referred by teachers by ADHD symptoms. Child Neuropsychol 2001;7:230–240.
34. Mariani MA, Barkley RA. Neuropsychological and academic functioning in preschool boys with attention deficit hyperactivity disorder. Dev Neuropsychol 1997;13:111–129.
35. Shue KL, Douglas VI. Attention deficit hyperactivity disorder and the frontal lobe syndrome. Special Issue: the role of frontal lobe maturation in cognitive and social development 1992;20:104–124.

36. Gorenstein EE, Mammato CA, Sandy JM. Performance of inattentive-overactive children on selected measures of prefrontal-type function. J Clin Psychol 1989;45:619–632.
37. Rucklidge JJ, Tannock R. Neuropsychological profiles of adolescents with ADHD: effects of reading difficulties and gender. J Child Psychol Psychiatry Allied Disciplines 2002;43:988–1003.
38. Adams JW, Snowling MJ. Executive function and reading impairments in children reported by their teachers as "hyperactive." Bri J Dev Psychol 2001;19:293–306.
39. Willcutt EG, Pennington BF, Boada R, et al. A comparison of the cognitive deficits in reading disability and attention-deficit/hyperactivity disorder. J Abnorm Psychol 2001;110:157–172.
40. Siegel LS, Ryan EB. The development of working memory in normally achieving and subtypes of learning disabled children. Child Dev 1989;60:973–980.
41. Rapport MD, Chung K-M, Shore G, Denney CB, Isaacs P. Upgrading the science and technology of assessment and diagnosis: laboratory and clinic-based assessment of children with ADHD. J Clini Child Psychol 2000;29:555–568.
42. Schweitzer JB, Faber TL, Grafton ST, Tune LE, Hoffman JM, Kilts CD. Alterations in the functional anatomy of working memory in adult attention deficit hyperactivity disorder. Am J Psychiatry 2000;157:278–280.
43. Lawrence V, Houghton S, Tannock R, Douglas G, Durkin K, Whiting K. ADHD outside the laboratory: boys' executive function performance on tasks in videogame play and on a visit to the zoo. J Abnorm Child Psychol 2002;30:447–462.
44. Swanson HL. Working memory in learning disability subgroups. J Exp Child Psychol 1993;56:87–114.
45. Swanson HL, Ashbaker MH, Lee C. Learning-disabled readers' working memory as a function of processing demands. J Exp Child Psychol 1996;61:242–275.
46. Roodenrys S, Koloski N, Grainger J. Working memory function in attention deficit hyperactivity disordered and reading disabled children. Bri J Dev Psychol 2001;19:325–337.
47. Seguin JR, Boulerice B, Harden PW, Tremblay RE, Pihl RO. Executive functions and physical aggression after controlling for attention deficit hyperactivity disorder, general memory and IQ. J Child Psychol Psychiatry Allied Disciplines 1999;40:1197–1208.
48. Bennetto L, Pennington BF, Rogers SJ. Intact and impaired memory functions in autism. Child Dev 1996;67:1816–1835.
49. Cohen NJ, Vallance DD, Barwick M, et al. The interface between ADHD and language impairment: An examination of language, achievement, and cognitive processing. J Child Psychol Psychiatry Allied Disciplines 2000;41:353–362.
50. Gordon M, Barkley, RA. Tests and observational measures. In: Barkley RA, ed. Attention-deficit hyperactivity disorder: a handbook for diagnosis and treatment. New York: Guilford Press, 1998, pp. 294–311.
51. Krane E, Tannock R. WISC-III third factor indexes learning problems but not attention deficit/hyperactivity disorder. J Attention Dis 2001;5:69–78.
52. Gray JR, Kagan J. The challenge of predicting which children with attention deficit-hyperactivity disorder will respond positively to methylphenidate. J Applied Dev Psychol 2000;21:471–489.
53. Fischer M, Newby RF, Gordon M. Who are the false negatives on continuous performance tests? J Clin Child Psychol 1995;24:427–433.
54. Mehta MA, Owen AM, Sahakian BJ, Mavaddat N, Pickard JD, Robbins TW. Methylphenidate enhances working memory by modulating discrete frontal and parietal lobe regions in the human brain. J Neurosci 2000;20:RC65.
55. Klingberg T, Forssberg H, Westerberg H. Training of working memory in children with ADHD. J Clin Exp Neuropsychol 2002;24:781–791.
56. Waters GS, Caplan D. The measurement of verbal working memory capacity and its relation to reading comprehension. Special Issue: Working Memory 1996;49:51–79.

13

Developmental Underpinnings of the Association of Attention Deficit Hyperactivity Disorder and Its Subtypes to Neuropsychological and Academic Weaknesses

Tuija Aro, Margaret Semrud-Clikeman, Anne-Mari Lapveteläinen, and Heikki Lyytinen

1. INTRODUCTION

Caron and Rutter *(1)* and Pennington *(2)* recently published excellent conceptual and methodological reviews and analyses of comorbidity in child psychopathology, and a special issue of *Developmental Neuropsychology (3)* reviewed attention deficit hyperactivity disorder (ADHD)-learning disabilities (LD) comorbidity in particular. None of these reviews, however, focused on the association of dimensions of ADHD and cognitive development, which are included in this chapter. Moreover, relatively little empirical data exist from early development. It is very likely that language-related impairments and extreme temperament traits contribute to the emergence of developmental problems and/or the accumulation of difficulties. To understand the nature of the association between attention disorders and LD we introduce results in this chapter from our studies from infants and kindergarten-age and school-age children. The dimensions of ADHD, inattention and hyperactivity, are evaluated separately in this chapter. In addition, neuropsychological correlates and the developmental history of ADHD are reviewed to explore possible associations to the acquisition of academic achievements.

We introduce data from several studies involving different sociocultural environments (United States, Chile, and Finland). The data are used to illustrate the associations among early temperament, cognitive development, LD, and ADHD. First, we review the state of art concerning the comorbidity of ADHD and LD for school age children. Second, we introduce results based on a US sample collected by Margaret Semrud-Clikeman and her colleagues at the University of Texas at Austin. Tuija Aro (earlier Lamminmäki) and her colleagues similarly examined the co-occurrence of the attention disorders with learning disorders among school-age children in Chile.

The Finnish data, not previously published, are used to evaluate empirically the specific relation that inattention and hyperactivity have in relation to reading accuracy and reading fluency in the first grade. The Finnish data are also used to examine the relation of early (at ages 1 and 2 yr) individual variation of attentional style (hyperactivity) and shyness to later (at 5 yr) cognitive development. These data are based on the 8-yr follow-up of Finnish children from birth in the Jyväskylä Longitudinal Study of Dyslexia (JLD). In the JLD, children

From: *Attention Deficit Hyperactivity Disorder: From Genes to Patients*
Edited by: D. Gozal and D. L. Molfese © Humana Press Inc., Totowa, NJ

with and without familial risk for dyslexia were assessed yearly in many domains to provide observations relevant to this context *(4,5)*. This follow-up includes not only attention and development of cognitive skills, language, reading, and math skills, but also the previously mentioned early assessment of temperament.

2. ATTENTION AND ACHIEVEMENT

2.1. Perspectives on Comorbidity of ADHD and LD

ADHD has been conceptually associated with difficulties in learning and these difficulties are thought to continue throughout the school experience *(6)*. The comorbidity of ADHD and learning problems is widely documented *(7–20)*. These studies tend to indicate that there is a significant overlap between LDs and ADHD at school age. For example, Shaywitz and Shaywitz *(21)* found that 11% of children with ADHD also had dyslexia, whereas 33% of children with LD had ADHD. As a clear exception to this study, Halperin et al. *(22)* found that the rate of dyslexia in an ADHD population was similar to population expectations (9–10%). They also found that 15% of the ADHD sample were excellent readers and scored one standard deviation above age expectations in reading. Most of the studies have not, however, separated the possible differential role of activity level and attentional difficulties associated with ADHD to the issue of comorbidity. The consequences of this separation are discussed later in this chapter.

Indications of even more overlap have been reported between attention and language problems. About 20–50% of the children having language difficulties also have attention deficit disorders *(23)*. Tirosh and Cohen *(24)* showed that among 5.2% of children who had attention-related problems in a large random sample, 42% had language problems. These findings are particularly interesting when the close relation between language deficits and reading disabilities (RD) is considered. Although the reason for comorbidity commonly has been thought to be related to early neural development *(25)*, other kinds of explanations are also plausible. For example, Stevenson *(26)* has speculated that the high comorbidity between these disorders may be owing to the fewer opportunities for children with inattentive, impulsive, or distracted behavior to gain from social interactions fostering language development. This possibility is assessed from the JLD data later in this chapter.

Longitudinal studies have indicated that approx 40% of children with ADHD in the United States are placed in special education programs, with 25% of those experiencing difficulties learning to read *(6,27)*. For adolescents, those with attentional difficulties show academic difficulties with 58% retained in at least one grade, 10% dropping out of school and showing below-ability performance in reading and mathematics *(6,28,29)*. These difficulties have been found to continue into adulthood with approx 30% dropping out of college *(30)*; this difficulty occurs despite average to superior ability.

Semrud-Clikeman et al. *(16)* evaluated different methods of determining comorbidity of ADHD and LD in a sample of children. Three groups were present in this sample: those with ADHD, those with academic difficulties, and a group of controls. Using the more stringent diagnostic methods, 15–23% of the ADHD sample was found to have a reading difficulty. A new finding in this study was that a significant number of the children with ADHD also showed difficulties in mathematics. In the sample of ADHD children using the two most stringent methods, Semrud-Clikeman et al. *(16)* found that 30–33% of the sample had significant difficulties with mathematics. A review of other studies by Semrud-Clikeman et al. *(16)* found that when children with severe conduct problems were included in a study, the rates of learning disability increased dramatically. Thus, it may be that the level of severity of externalizing behavior exacerbates learning problems. Additional studies using participants with conduct disorder and ADHD have found significant difficulties with information processing of verbal information and lower cognitive ability *(31,32)*. An alternative explanation is that such behavior decreases the on-task time at school and hence may also affect learning of academic skills.

Pennington *(33)* suggests that ADHD is best understood using a four-part model that attempts to separate out correlated from primary symptoms. He states that inattention, impulsivity, and hyperactivity are the hallmarks for ADHD with academic problems being secondary. Thus, not all children with ADHD show learning deficits but may show learning problems because of difficulties with attention and executive functioning. However, the higher incidence of ADHD in samples of children with a learning disability may in turn show that there is a separate subtype of LD children.

Learning problems, Pennington *(33)* suggests, may also cause attentional difficulties as school failure prompts less attention to task. Poskiparta et al. *(34)* have shown recently that soon after school-entry children who had difficulties in acquisition of reading skills and who did not differ in task orientation before school were highly likely starting to use avoiding behaviors in the face of challenging tasks through inattentive behavior. Studies by Pennington *(33)* in the Boulder dyslexic sample suggest that these effects increase with age as more and more school failure is experienced. Similarly observations from the Finnish context (JLD) reveal that very few of those children whose reading acquisition is clearly slower than classmates in the first grade are able to keep their attention, motivation, and interest optimal for the challenging tasks at school. These results indicate how attention and learning difficulties intertwine in a complex manner with motivational factors and the child's self-efficacy and self-concepts.

The genetic correlation between the two disorders has also been studied *(2,9,12)*. The Boulder study found an elevated rate of ADHD in twins who were also diagnosed with dyslexia, with ADHD found to be significantly heritable. For monozygotic and dizygotic twins, the concordance rates of ADHD and LD were higher than would be expected, and monozygotic rates were substantially higher than the dizygotic rates. Thus, Gilger et al. *(9)* suggest that there is a subtype in which ADHD and LD share a common genetic etiology. There was also evidence that the family environment may contribute to the expression of ADHD in the twin pairs.

To better understand the comorbidity between ADHD and LDs several studies have focused on the possible differential neurocognitive features or core-deficits of ADHD and LD and related these to comorbid ADHD and LD. These studies have provided contrasting results. Pennington et al. *(13)* found that a group of children with comorbid ADHD and RD showed deficits in phonological processes similar to those with pure RD, but did not have deficits in executive functions, which were evident in children with pure ADHD. Based on their results Pennington et al. concluded that attention–hyperactivity problems of children with comorbid ADHD and RD are secondary. When trying to replicate this result, Närhi and Ahonen *(35)* found that their comorbid group was impaired on a rapid naming task to the same degree as the pure RD group, but had also deficits in executive functions. Similarly, Willcutt and colleagues *(36)* studied a nonreferred sample of twins to evaluate the performance of individuals with RD, ADHD, RD and ADHD, and neither RD nor ADHD on measures of phoneme awareness and executive functioning. They found that ADHD was associated with inhibition deficits, whereas RD was associated with deficits on measures of phonological awareness and verbal working memory. The RD and ADHD group was most impaired on all measures. At this point it seems likely that children with comorbid ADHD and RD have deficits characteristic for both ADHD and RD *(36)*. Using groups of children with sole diagnoses of ADHD and RD, Semrud-Clikeman et al. *(37)* found that the ADHD sample performed more poorly in rapid automatized naming because of timing and slower response, whereas the LD group had difficulty with automaticity owing to increased numbers of errors.

In a recent study, Rucklidge and Tannock *(38)* found a dissociation of deficits between ADHD and RD adolescents after controlling for socioeconomic status (SES), IQ, and comorbid diagnoses. The ADHD children demonstrated slower processing speed and deficits in object naming, for example, regardless of their RD status. The RD groups showed deficits in verbal working memory and were slower in letter naming and naming color words regardless of their ADHD status. Only the comorbid group showed severe impairment in number and color naming, as well as slower response times and less accurate responses. On the basis of their results, the authors raise the question whether ADHD + RD is a specific subtype with unique cognitive profile.

Based on the several studies focusing on ADHD and LDs we can be fairly confident that there is rather high comorbidity between these difficulties. The nature and etiology of this comorbidity are, however, far from clear. Most of the studies have used samples with diagnosed children, and the emphasis has been on the deficits, especially RDs. There is, though, interesting evidence indicating that not all children with ADHD have learning difficulties, but instead, some might have average or even above-average performance.

2.2. *Reading and Mathematics in ADHD*

In order to further understand the comorbidity of ADHD and LDs, a sample of children with ADHD without diagnosed learning problems and control children were evaluated by one of us recently through a study in a southwestern US university research program. There were 53 children who met criteria for ADHD: combined type and 35 control children without identified learning disabilities and ADHD. Reading and mathematics skills were both evaluated and compared with behavioral ratings of inattention, activity level, as well as results from a structured clinical interview. Teacher and parent behavioral rating scales were obtained using the Behavioral Assessment System for Children (BASC) *(39)*. Parents were all interviewed using the Structured Interview for Diagnosis Assessment of Children (SIDAC) *(40)*, a semistructured clinical interview adapted from the children's version of the Schedule for Affective Disorders and Schizophrenia (SADS) *(41)*, using the ADHD module.

Participants ranged in age from age 8 to 14 similarly with mean of 10.25 for the ADHD group and 10.42 for the control group ($p = 0.52$). All children were administered the vocabulary and block design subtests from the Wechsler Intelligence Scale for Children III (WISC-III) *(42)*. Sattler's *(43)* method of computing the full-scale IQ using this abbreviated test was utilized. A one-way analysis of variance (ANOVA) found no significant difference between the two groups on IQ ($p = 0.22$) with the mean for the ADHD group being 103.8 and for the control group 107.1 (*see* Table 1).

The basic reading, mathematics calculation, and mathematics reasoning tests were utilized from the Wechsler Individual Achievement Test (WIAT-III) *(44)*. There was no difference between the groups on any of these measures (Table 1). As expected, a one-way ANOVA found significant differences on the teacher and parent BASC for these groups. The ADHD group scored significantly more poorly on the parent hyperactivity ($p < 0.0001$) and inattention ($p < 0.0001$) scales. Similarly, significant group differences were present on the teacher BASC on the hyperactivity scale ($p = 0.0004$) and inattention scales ($p < 0.0001$).

Table 1
Results From Demographic and Behavioral Measures for Two Groups

	ADHD	Control	*F* statistic	*p* value
Age (in months)	123.2 (21.4)	125.8 (21.8)	0.412	0.522
FSIQ	103.8 (14.7)	107.1 (14.3)	1.553	0.215
Basic Reading	99.02 (17.9)	192.7 (15.7)	1.38	0.24
Math calculation	113.9 (13.2)	103.86 (16.6)	.32	0.573
Math reasoning	102.6 (20.7)	109.29 (16.9)	3.712	0.0565
BASC-P Hyperactivity	69.18 (13.9)	53.76 (12.67)	39.1	<0.0001
BASC-P Attention	67.96 (10.3)	56.9 (11.4)	29.662	<0.0001
BASC-T Hyperactivity	59.2 (13.1)	51.03 (9.7)	13.499	0.0004
BASC-T Attention	63.27 (8.9)	53.7 (10.7)	22.64	<0.0001

FSIQ, full-scale IQ; BASC-T, Behavior Assessment System for Children, Teacher form; BASC-P, BASC Parent form.

When the full-scale IQ (FSIQ) and WIAT achievement scores were compared using a 20 standard score point difference to determine the presence of a LD (a conservative estimate), the total sample showed an incidence of 4.5% deficits in reading recognition, 5.6% in arithmetic calculation, and 13.6% in mathematical reasoning. For the ADHD group 6.6% were found to show significant learning difficulties in reading recognition, 5% in mathematics calculation, and 15% in mathematics reasoning. The control group showed an incidence of 2.9% reading recognition difficulties, 5.8% mathematics calculation, and 5.8% mathematics reasoning. The same two children in the control sample had difficulties in mathematics in both calculation and reasoning.

For the ADHD group 15% showed one SD or more above ability level achievement in reading, 5.6% in mathematics calculation, and 15% in mathematics reasoning. For the control group 28.5% showed above-expectations performance on the reading recognition test, 5.7% on both the mathematics calculation and mathematics reasoning subtests.

Correlations were computed to evaluate the relationship between dimensions of ADHD and achievement in this sample. Parent and teacher scores of inattention ($r = -0.085, -0.09$ respectively) and hyperactivity ($r = -0.115, -0.076$) on the BASC did not show a significant relationship to word recognition ($p > 0.05$). However, there was a significant relationship between mathematics calculation and parent ratings of inattention ($r = -0.323, p = 0.001$) and hyperactivity ($r = -0.283, p = 0.007$). Similarly, mathematics reasoning and parent ratings of inattention was also found to be significantly correlated ($r = -0.272, p = 0.008$). Parent ratings of hyperactivity and mathematics reasoning were not significantly related ($r = -0.19, p > 0.07$). The number of inattention symptoms was also significantly related to mathematics performance for both mathematics calculation ($r = -0.21, p = 0$) and mathematics reasoning ($r = -0.26; p = 0.01$). Similarly, teacher ratings of inattention were found to be related to both mathematics calculation ($r = -0.28, p = 0.01$) and mathematics reasoning ($r = -0.21, p = 0.008$) but not to hyperactivity ($r = -0.026$, ns). An area that was also evaluated was the relationship between written language and attention and hyperactivity. Significant correlations were found between parent ratings of inattention and written language ($r = -0.29, p = 0.005$) and hyperactivity ($r = -0.28, p = 0.009$). Similarly, teacher ratings of inattention were significantly correlated with written language ($r = -0.24, p = 0.02$) but not hyperactivity ($r = -0.10$, ns).

These findings indicate that there is a small but important number of children with ADHD who show learning difficulties particularly in mathematics and written language. There were more pronounced difficulties in mathematics reasoning than in reading recognition. Mathematics may not be as readily reported as an area of difficulty as reading but should certainly be evaluated in children with ADHD given these findings. Further evaluation of mathematics skills is sorely needed. Previously reported results by Schnoebelen and Semrud-Clikeman *(45)* found poorer performance in the ADHD group on measures of fluid reasoning compared to control groups. We are continuing to evaluate the relationship between fluid reasoning, executive functioning, and arithmetic skills in our groups of ADHD children. Written language subtests on the WIAT require planning and organization and likely relate to difficulties with fluid reasoning and with executive functions. Further evaluation of this area is required.

The mathematics difficulties found in the present sample appeared related more to difficulties in inattention than to problems with activity level or impulsivity. Thus, the relationship between learning and inattention continue to be an area that requires additional study. Studies that carefully control attentional deficits in samples of children with learning problems or conversely those that control learning deficits in children with ADHD—and preferably in a longitudinal design—are needed to more fully understand the relationship between these two disorders. A further need is for a more specific understanding of the contribution of inattention in relation to learning.

3. ADHD SUBTYPES AND LEARNING DISORDERS

3.1. Specific Meaning of Inattention

Lahey and colleagues *(46)* noted a long time ago: "No term in the history of childhood psychopathology has been subject to as many reconceptualizations, redefinitions, and renamings" as hyperactivity. The diagnostic nomenclature changed again in 1995 when the *Diagnostic and Statistical Manual of Mental Disorders,* 4th edition (DSM-IV) was published. Ongoing discussions have explored whether or not there are different subtypes of ADHD, and how these subtypes actually differ from each other and from other clinical populations. Even though a rather unanimous consensus has been reached on multifaceted nature of the ADHD syndrome, the distinctive and specific nature of the subtypes is not clear. Research evidence for the distinctive nature has been searched studying cognitive *(47–49)*, behavioral *(18,50,51)*, and neuropsychological *(48)* differences between the subtypes. We believe that the distinction between hyperactivity dimension and inattention is relevant when we try to evaluate how attentional behavior is related to the development of cognition or acquisition of academic skills.

Results regarding comorbidity of LDs with ADHD have been summarized above. Although the many changes in the DSM diagnostic criteria complicate the interpretation of the results regarding ADHD subtypes, there is some evidence showing that children with inattention are particularly prone to having academic problems. The studies of academic performance using the DSM-III criteria for attention deficit disorder have not found conclusive results. For example, Hynd et al. *(40)* compared attention deficit disorder with hyperactivity (ADD/h) and attention deficit disorder without hyperactivity (ADD/wo) on several cognitive and academic measures and found that ADD/wo children had somewhat lower scores in reading and spelling tests but the difference was not significant. Carlson et al. *(47)* found that both ADD/h and ADD/wo groups performed poorer that the controls on reading and spelling achievement test. Barkley et al. *(52)* compared ADD children with hyperactivity to those without hyperactivity, as well as with LD and control children. They found that the three clinical groups performed worse than the control group on measures of reading and spelling but did not differ from each other.

The diagnostic criteria proposed in the DSM-III-R *(53)* did not differentiate dimensions of ADHD, whereas DSM-IV *(54)* has provided better opportunity to study the differential effects of inattention and hyperactivity–impulsivity on academic achievement. For example, we examined how academic problems are associated with three different subtypes of ADHD using a sample of 110 Chilean school-age children referred to a local remediation center for their learning difficulties *(11)*. Three ADHD subtype groups (predominantly inattentive, $n = 20$; predominantly hyperactive, $n = 8$; combined, $n = 17$ defined on the basis of the DSM-IV) and a clinical control group ($n = 22$) with no ADHD symptoms were formed on the basis of the ADD-H Comprehensive Teacher's Rating Scale *(55)*. Children's academic problems were determined by their performance of the Woodcock Spanish Psycho-Educational Battery *(56)*.

There were no significant differences in the age or FSIQ of the groups. However, notable differences were found in the percentages of children with academic problems. Children belonging to the predominantly inattentive subtype and the combined type showed most problems among the groups. The percentage of reading problems was highest among the inattentive subgroup, and the percentage of mathematic difficulties was highest in the combined subgroup. A logit model analysis indicated that inattention had a significant main effect for the presence of academic problems. When the children were reevaluated after treatment, it was found that changes in the levels of inattention and hyperactivity were differentially associated also with treatment outcomes *(57)*. Improvement of attention was associated with improvement in reading and writing skills among the ADHD children. Treatment was not, however, sufficiently highly focused to allow separation of the causal relations.

Similar results concerning inattention and learning disabilities have also been reported from the DSM-IV field trials for ADHD *(58)* and by Baumgaertel et al. *(59)*. More recently, Willcutt and Pennington *(20)* studied a sample selected for RD and found that children with RD were more likely to meet the criteria for ADHD than children without RD. They also reported that the association between RD and ADHD was stronger for symptoms of inattention than for symptoms of hyperactivity–impulsivity. Thus, it can be concluded that empirical studies on the nature of comorbidity between different ADHD dimensions and LD support the hypothesis of differential clinical meaning of inattention and hyperactivity. Table 2 summarizes the studies focusing on the association between inattention and academic outcome, especially reading ability.

The few longitudinal studies conducted so far have given evidence of a specific, but yet not understood, association between inattention and reading. The direction of the association between attention and reading skills development has been the focus of much discussion. Rowe and Rowe *(15)* found a reciprocal association between inattention and reading within their Australian sample. Using longitudinal data from 5 to 15 yr, McGee et al. *(60)* also found evidence for pathways from inattention to later literacy. Fergusson and Horwood *(8)* found that attention deficit influenced reading, but evidence suggesting that reading achievement influenced attention deficit level was not found. Velting and Whitehurst *(19)* used structural equation modeling to study how preschool inattention–hyperactivity was related to elementary school reading achievement among low-SES children. They found no significant path between inattention–hyperactivity and prereading skills, but found significant association between inattention–hyperactivity level and first-grade reading skills. Rabiner and Coie *(14)* studied whether attention problems predict development of reading difficulties. Their results

Table 2
Summary of Studies Focusing on Association Between Inattention and Academic Outcome

Investigators	Independent variable	Dependent variable	Age	Results
McGee, Prior, Williams, Smart, and Sanson, (2002)	Hyperactive–inattentive behaviors	Reading ability	Longitudinal data: 5–15 yr	Hyperactivity, and especially inattention component, have a significant influence on later levels of literacy.
Willcutt and Pennington, (2000)	Reading disability (RD)	ADHD: inattention, hyperactivity-impulsivity (DSM-III/-IV)	8–18 yr	Individuals with RD were more likely than individuals without RD to meet criteria for ADHD. Association between RD and ADHD was stronger for symptoms of inattention than for symptoms of hyperactivity–impulsivity.
Rabiner and Coie, (2000)	Inattention	Reading achievement	Longitudinal data: kindergarten 1st grade 2nd grade 5th grade	Attention problems predicted reading achievement: Inattentive first graders (normal reading scores after kindergarten) were at risk for poor reading outcomes.
Velting and Whitehurst, (1997)	Inattention–hyperactivity	Reading achievement	Longitudinal data: 4–5 yr–1st grade	No significant relationship between the prereading skills and inattention–hyperactivity before school age. Significant relationship between first grade inattention–hyperactivity and poor reading achievement.
Baumgaertel, Wolraich, Dietrich, (1995)	ADHD subtypes (DSM-III/-IIIR/-IV)	Academic performance	5–12 yr	Inattention was associated with academic problems.
Lamminmäki, Ahonen, Närhi, Todd de Barra and Lyytinen, (1995)	ADHD subtypes (DSM-IV)	Reading, mathematics, writing	8.6–9.8 yr	Academic problems are related to inattention: the percentage of reading problems was highest in the ADHD/inattention group and mathematic problems in the ADHD/combined group.

(Continued)

Table 2
(Continued)

Investigators	Independent variable	Dependent variable	Age	Results
Ferguson and Horwood, (1992)	ADHD (DSM-IIIR)	Reading achievement	12 yr	At age 12 attention deficits causally influence reading achievement and there is no evidence that reading achievement influenced attention deficit levels.
Rowe and Rowe, (1992)	Inattentiveness	Reading achievement	5–14 yr	A strong reciprocal association between inattentiveness and reading achievement: in attentiveness has a strong negative effects on reading achievement and vice versa.

DSM-III-R, *Diagnostic and Statistical Manual of Mental Disorders*, 3rd edition revised.

indicated that attention problems predicted reading achievement even after controlling for prior reading achievement, IQ, and parental involvement. With regard to the predictive value of the presence of inattention, they found that children who had normal reading scores after kindergarten but who were highly inattentive in first grade were at risk for poor reading outcomes in the fifth grade. Thus, longitudinal studies indicate that presence of inattention might have predictive value in terms of the child's academic performance.

Neuroimaging has been used to validate the existence of the specific subtypes. Posner *(61)* suggests that there are three attentional networks. The first network allows for orienting and shifting attention from the previous stimuli. This area is thought to involve the posterior part of the brain. Schaughency and Hynd *(62)* hypothesized that this area may be most important in directing attention to needed targets and that children with ADD/wo may have difficulty associated with posterior functions. Subsequent neuroimaging results tend to support this assumption. Filipek et al. *(63)* found that children with more symptoms of inattention than problems in activity level had smaller right-matter volumes bilaterally in the retrocallosal (posterior to the corpus callosum) than did those with more activity than inattention-related difficulties. These children also showed relatively poorer scores on reading and mathematics measures, although within the low average range for their age.

The second attentional network involves the executive function networks and allows the child to detect an object that is occurring and bring it to conscious processing. This area is thought to involve the limbic system (anterior cingulate) and caudate *(64)*. Neuroimaging results have also supported this system in children with significant difficulties in overactivity. Semrud-Clikeman and colleagues *(65–67)* analyzed magnetic resonance imaging scans of boys with ADHD with hyperactivity and found a relationship between reversed asymmetry of the caudate and difficulties with inhibition and activity level.

Posner's third attentional network involves vigilance and is believed to include the right frontal lobe and is responsible for sustained attention. Accordingly, children with ADHD-combined type would show deficits in this area. Neuroimaging results have supported this

Table 3
The BASC and the Reading Test Means and SDs

Measure	Mean	SD
Attention problems		
4 yr	6.2	2.4
$n = 162^a$		
5 yr	6.1	2.8
$n = 172$		
6 yr	6.3	2.8
$n = 166$		
Hyperactivity		
4 yr	16.5	5.2
$n = 162$		
5 yr	14.1	5.3
$n = 172$		
6 yr	12.9	5.4
$n = 166$		
Reading		
Fluency (ms)	2709	1476
$n = 172$		
Accuracy (percent)	91.9	11.6
$n = 171$		

[a] Note that *n* varies because of missing data.

hypothesis with the finding of smaller white matter volume in the right frontal lobes in children with ADHD with hyperactivity and attentional difficulties.

In summary, the studies on differential association between learning disabilities and ADHD dimensions (hyperactivity and inattention) are not conclusive. All together these, however, suggest that inattention might be more strongly associated with LDs than hyperactivity. Most of the studies have been conducted with clinical samples of school-aged children, and there is an obvious need for studies with epidemiological and developmental samples including younger participants.

3.2. *Early Inattention and Hyperactivity as Predictors of Later Reading Acquisition and Cognitive Skills*

The association between reading acquisition and developmental history of inattention and hyperactivity was studied with 172 children (78 girls and 94 boys who had ended the first grade at the time of writing this chapter, from the whole number of 200 participants of the JLD). Reading skills were assessed at the end of the first grade (at age 7). A recent study of Holopainen et al. *(68)* reveals that at this stage most Finnish children are accurate decoders, assuring that the reading accuracy scores do not have floor values any more. The reading acquisition test utilized for this study consisted of nine bisyllabic and nine complex nonwords. The words were presented on a computer display one item at a time. Reaction time and reading duration as well as percentage of correctly read items were recorded to measure reading fluency and accuracy. Inattention and hyperactivity were assessed repeatedly with the parental BASC–Parent Rating Scale *(39)* before school entry at the ages of 4, 5, and 6 yr. For the

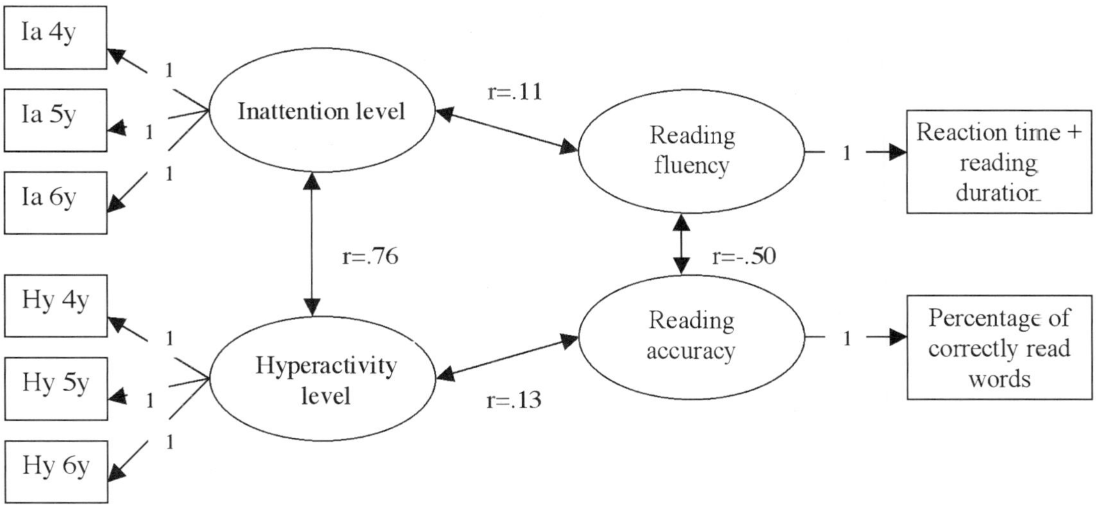

Fig. 1. Structural equation model. Association between hyperactivity, inattention, and reading acquisition measures. $\chi^2(20) = 19.60$, $p = 0.48$, RMSEA = 0.

means and standard deviations *see* Table 3. The mean (and SD) verbal and performance IQ (WPPSI-R *[69]*) were 108 *(15)* and 102 *(14)*, respectively.

The structural equation modeling (*see* Fig. 1) indicated interesting but mild associations between developmental inattention and hyperactivity and early reading acquisition. Preschool inattention level was significantly ($r = 0.11$) associated with poor results in reading fluency. The higher the child's inattention level was during the preschool years, the slower was his or her reading speed at the age of 7 yr. Preschool hyperactivity level was significantly ($r = 0.13$) associated with reading accuracy showing that the lower the child's hyperactivity level was at preschool ages, the less accurately he or she read at the end of the first grade. This finding was rather surprising. Close inspection of the data indicated that there were eight children with high hyperactivity scores and good reading accuracy. There were also seven children with especially poor reading accuracy scores and especially low hyperactivity scores. Thus, it might be, that by chance, the seven children with low hyperactivity scores (all coming from families with familial dyslexia) were identified. It is also plausible that they form some kind of subgroup within the children with familial risk for dyslexia.

Our findings on inattention, hyperactivity, and reading add a level of dimension to the earlier studies and show that hyperactivity was not detrimentally associated with beginning reading. Instead, inattention was associated with lower early reading fluency, but not with reading accuracy. Most of the studies concerning reading have assessed only reading accuracy. The separation of accuracy and fluency is especially relevant in the Finnish language. In the shallow orthographies, of which Finnish is an extreme example, children learn basic alphabetical reading processes quite easily and reading difficulties are typically seen in reading fluency, as has been recently shown by Aro and Wimmer *(70)* (*see also* ref. *71*, and for more details of the reading acquisition in Finnish, ref. *72*). Still in adulthood reading-related problems, which hinder reading Finnish, comprise not only reading or spelling inaccuracy but also dysfluency of reading *(73)*.

Schoot et al. *(74)* studied association between reading subtypes (guessers and spellers, meaning inaccurate fast readers vs accurate slow ones, respectively) and attention-related inhibitory deficits, and found that those children who read fast and inaccurately were impaired in their ability to inhibit inappropriate responding. The authors speculated whether the specific reading disorder of guessers might be linked to the executive deficits underlying ADHD. They concluded that executive function deficit in guessers led to both poor behavioral and cognitive inhibition, whereas spellers (slow and accurate) showed superior behavioral inhibition. The authors assumed that this "may be a burden to slow and accurate readers when speeding up reading, that is, they may have overactive inhibition system, which slows down the mechanism of word recognition."

The interpretation of the aforementioned results from the JLD data is complicated by the usage of computers in the reading assessment. It is plausible that children with inattention were possibly more distracted than they would have been in the more typical reading situation at the moment the word was presented, thereby delaying their reaction time. Similarly, distraction during the reading process would have made the reading duration longer. To control for this effect, we used an additional reading fluency measure of the JLD that indicated how many words the child read per minute in a story reading situation. The correlation between parent rating of inattention and this reading fluency measure also reached significance ($r = 0.17$; $p = 0.03$; $n = 164$), and was thus very comparable with the results based on reading from the computer display. Therefore, one can safely conclude that the association found between inattention and reading fluency was not because of usage of the computer.

The finding of an association between inattention and fluency raises further questions about the general relationship between inattention and processing speed. Earlier studies on the cognitive performance and inattention symptoms have found that children with attention deficits disorder may have deficits in automaticity *(49,75)*. Children with inattention symptoms have been characterized as having sluggish cognitive tempo *(40,46,76)* or problems with perceptual-motor processing and speed *(38,77)*. However, several studies have failed to find cognitive differences between ADHD subtypes *(47,78)*.

In a recent study Chhabildas et al. *(48)* evaluated neuropsychological differences between ADHD subtypes and found that the symptoms of inattention were associated with reduced performance on tasks assessing processing speed, vigilance, and inhibition. The symptoms of hyperactivity–impulsivity did not predict performance in any of these domains. They concluded that the symptoms of inattention are associated with significant neuropsychological deficits, whereas symptoms of hyperactivity–impulsivity are not. To test the hypothesis that inattention, rather than hyperactivity–impulsivity, would be associated with neuropsychological deficit in the JLD data, we examined correlations between the neuropsychological test results at the age of 5 yr and the BASC attention-related results at the age of 6 yr (*see* Table 4).

As one can see from Table 4, this analysis of the JLD data indicated that most of the significant correlations were found between inattention and neuropsychological tests supporting the hypothesis that inattention, especially, is associated with cognitive performance. Several of the correlations could be expected on the basis of the literature, e.g., executive functions, working memory, and attention. With regard to the Chhabildas et al. *(48)* and Rucklidge and Tannock *(38)* findings that processing speed is particularly associated with inattention, we also found that many of the tests correlating with inattention were time-sensitive.

The possibility that inattention compromises cognitive performance may be a confounding factor when interpreting the results from the reading measures. DeShazo et al. *(79)* found that severity of ADHD symptoms reported by parents predicted academic underachievement even after controlling for executive functions and diagnosed LDs. They concluded that impairment in academic functioning of children diagnosed as having ADHD could not be

Table 4
Correlations Between Inattention, Hyperactivity, and Neuropsychological Tests

NEPSY domain at 5 yr, 6 mo	Attention problems at 6 yr	Hyperactivity at 6 yr
Attention		
Tower $n = 162^a$	-0.20^b	0.01
Visual attention $n = 125$	–0.15	–0.04
Design copying $n = 162$	-0.29^b	–0.06
Knock and tap $n = 155$	-0.32^b	-0.19^c
Language		
Phonological processing $n = 181$	-0.27^b	-0.15^c
Comprehension of instructions $n = 179$	-0.19^c	-0.17^c
Reproduction of nonsense words $n = 163$	–0.12	-0.16^c
Verbal fluency (food + drink) $n = 174$	-0.24^b	–0.13
Motor functions		
Visuo-motor precision $n = 141$	-0.25^b	–0.08
Memory		
Memory for names $n = 165$	-0.24^b	–0.14
Memory for faces $n = 132$	-0.28^b	-0.18^c
Sentence repetition $n = 162$	-0.19^c	-0.18^c
Narrative $n = 173$	-0.16^c	–0.06

[a]Note that *n* varies because of missing data.
[b]$p < 0.07$.
[c]$p < 0.05$.

accounted for by cognitive deficits associated with executive functioning. Our data imply that a more comprehensive battery of neurocognitive tests should be used to understand the associations between cognitive development, behavioral symptoms of inattention, hyperactivity, and impulsivity, as well as academic performance.

It is still possible that failure experiences in the cognitive domain, at least during the early years of schooling (possibly including kindergarten), initiate developmental processes and psychological dynamics, which tend to affect learning-related attentive behavior *(80)*. As described above, this type of phenomenon has been experimentally documented recently by Poskiparta et al. *(34)*. It is important to observe the developmental proceedings from an earlier stage to learn to understand whether and how comorbid problems emerge during the life span. One way to accomplish this goal is to begin follow-ups from birth and examine groups whose members are genetically vulnerable to one of the difficulties belonging to the comorbid patterns. In the JLD we have had an opportunity to follow prospectively children born to families which have several dyslexic members. Below we make an attempt to also follow attentive behavior from a very early age among these at-risk children and their nonaffected controls.

4. CORRELATIONS OF EARLY TEMPERAMENT AND ATTENTION TO LATER COGNITIVE SKILLS

4.1. Temperamental Correlates of Attention-Related Behavioral Styles

Attention-related behaviors show variation both by content and by age. The content variation associated with problems in attention has been widely discussed, resulting in a consensus about diagnostic labels. The age-related variation is poorly known. In the following section an attempt is made to shed some light on the expressions of attention at the early ages and its possible association with the development of cognitive skills. Very early attentive behavior is evaluated on the basis of assessments of temperamental features most close to the diagnostic categories hyperactivity and inattention. The time window is from infancy (1–3 yr of age) where temperament was assessed to 5 yr of age when cognitive skills were tested using a neuropsychological battery (NEPSY) *(81)*. The data come from the JLD.

Very little is known about the developmental beginning of attention-related behavioral deviation. One could speculate that it may be related to characteristics assessed as temperamental features that can be identified soon after birth. This hypothesis is compatible with the present belief that ADHD is based on genetic atypicalities *(82,83)* and that a similar and related background affects temperament *(84)*. It is still unclear whether the temperamental feature of the shy, inhibited child *(85,86)* has any relation to later ADHD-inattention problems *(87)*. Robinson et al. have observed that 10–15% of 1–3-yr-olds are consistently shy and avoidant in facing new people or events and that this extreme shyness seems to have a genetic background *(88,89)*.

Temperamental observations from infancy may provide, in the present context, an answer to a type of question such as: is a pervasive behavioral feature that affects selection of behavior (avoidance of social contacts in shyness or avoidance of challenging cognitive efforts in a situation characterizing "defensive" inattention demonstrated by Poskiparta et al. *[34]*) an important determinant of the attention-related behavior and associated with learning difficulties or cognitive ability, e.g., resulting from compromised openness to benefit from learning opportunities during early development? Logically it might be, but we do not have empirical proof showing that this is really the case. But the observed comorbidity might suggest a causal connection between the time when one difficulty starts and another during the developmental course.

Shyness and overactivity as temperamental features are expressed in everyday behavior and in exposure to learning in such a way that they could be reflected in the development of cognitive skills. It is apparent that only overactivity is directly connected to the kind of behavior typical in children with ADHD. But data from children who are very shy may also provide interesting indirect evidence about the association of behavioral style *(90)* and cognitive development.

Activity is a temperamental characteristic identified practically in all theoretical categorizations of temperament. The most extensive body of literature exists from temperamental-type hyperactivity expressed in motor activity *(85)* and energy consumption *(91)*, as well as tempo, vigor, and endurance *(92)*. It has been widely thought to have a genetic background *(93,94)*, and the possible connection (when appearing in an extreme form) to ADHD-hyperactivity has at least some face validity. In our data illustrated below, the correlations between temperamental overactivity during the first years and BASC overactivity and impulsivity scores at 4–6 yr varied between 0.15 and 0.34 ($n = 105–109$; thus at best, $p = 0$), showing that a significant relationship exists between the variables.

A possible association between temperament (or extreme behavioral style factor such as hyperactivity) and cognitive development (and its specific but extreme impairment such as a learning disability) can be found by considering the differential mediation of environmental effects on the learning skills. Shy and inattentive children may have lower or nonoptimal exposure to learning opportunities because of their likely avoidance of social activities or defensiveness concerning new or challenging situations. Similarly, a hyperactive or impulsive child may also have less time to concentrate in a task-oriented way on the challenging learning situations owing to distractibility and inability to main attention in a goal-directed way.

If the attention and cognition related vulnerabilities—such as ADHD and specific language impairment (SLI)—co-occur, the likelihood of cumulative effects on the development of cognitive and academic skills is very high. One may be interested in knowing whether the overlap of milder temperamental traits—such as shy or hyperactive temperament and familial risk for dyslexia—are a potential risk for developmental delay or difficulties in the acquisition of cognitive and academic skills. It is apparent that unwanted developmental consequences may be higher if early vulnerabilities in these two domains co-occur. Co-occurrence may be more likely than expected based on independent occurrence. We know that psychological characteristics and even ADHD-related characteristics tend to show normal variation *(95)* and thus even milder expression of characteristics may show similar associations compared to the extreme ones. It has been shown convincingly that ADHD and SLI show a tendency to overlap *(7,23,96–99)*. This type of comorbidity is more likely affected by biological factors if it can be observed at an earlier age.

4.2. Association Between Temperamental Shyness and Overactivity During Infancy and Cognitive Skills at 5 Yr of Age

To test these hypotheses we compared children identified as shy using the Strange Situation method *(88)* and shy or overactive identified in repeated parental assessments during ages 1–3 yr. The consistent position in shyness or hyperactivity across repeated tests and types of assessment (questionnaire and behavioral observations) comprised the criterion of the group memberships. The groups of the most stably shy or overactive thirds ($n = 32$ and 34, respectively) for each temperament group, from the first 109 children born among the JLD infant participants, were compared with the rest (77 and 75 of the group) on the NEPSY for children *(79)* at 5.5 yr of age.

The results revealed no consistent differences in test profiles between the shy children and the others. There was a slight nonsignificant tendency ($p < 0.1$) for lower scores in the sentence

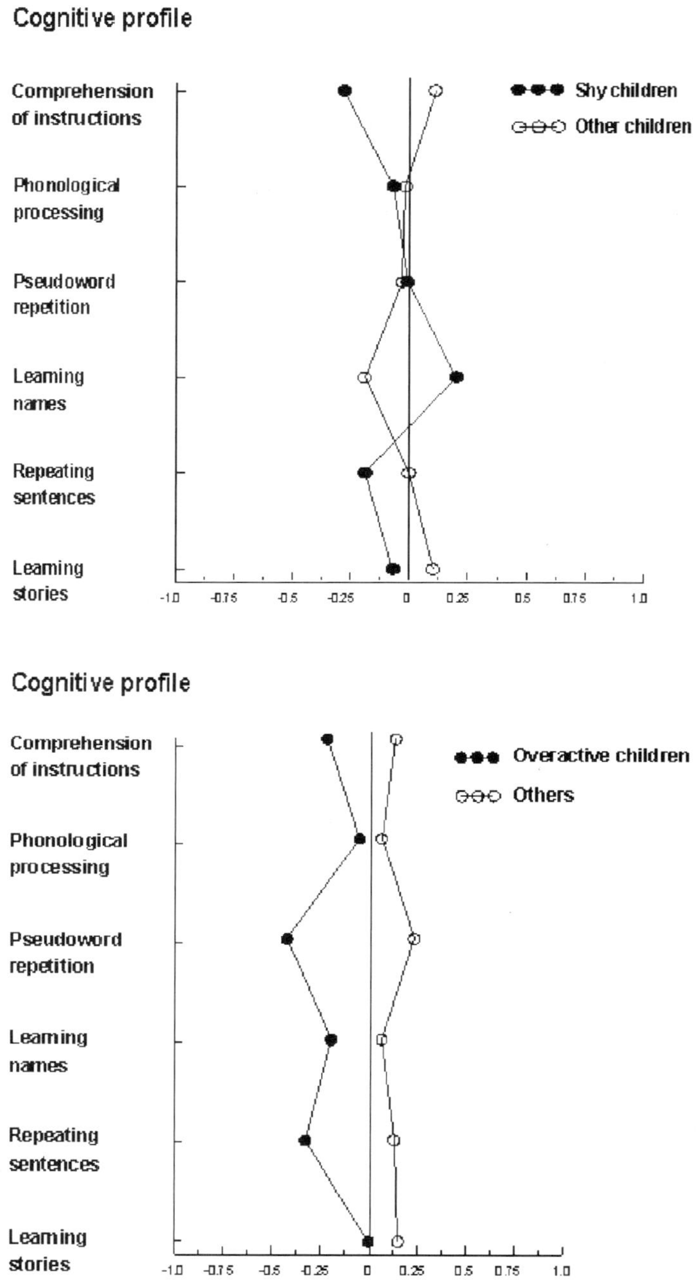

Fig. 2. Neuropsychological battery profiles at 5 yr of age from shy and overactive children identified during the first years of life.

repetition task among shy children who, in contrast, had higher scores on the name learning task (*see* Fig. 2). The overactive children achieved reliably lower scores in the repeating pseudowords and in the comprehension of instructions. Because the pseudoword repetition is usually predicting reading acquisition and discriminating for children with reading problems *(68,100)*, the group status (whether the child belonged to the group with a familial risk for dyslexia or not) was included as a covariate. It is worth noting first that the memberships in temperamental characteristics did not discriminate between the risk groups. Overactive children were poorer in pseudoword repetition only if they belonged to the at-risk group for dyslexia. We wanted, however, to elaborate our interpretation of this difference and used two additional covariates to find out whether the rated (by the tester) behavior in the test situation could explain this finding. Both of the differences disappeared when the ratings of the activity level and cooperation during the test situation were used as covariates. The first affected the difference in the pseudoword repetition and the co-operation in the scores of the comprehension of instructions so that no significant group difference between overactive and other children was found any more. This means that it may be the test behavior that is affected by the temperamental feature to such an extent that no significant variation is left to be explained by any accumulative developmental effects of overactivity feature of temperament. This is an interesting observation—e.g., by raising the question to what extent the test scores of academic skills are affected by overactive behavior in the test situation in the comorbidity studies.

We concluded that according to these results attention-related early temperament has at best a small effect on the development of cognitive skills, which probably has no or little clinical value. Our data do not allow conclusions concerning effects of extreme deviations corresponding to clinical expressions of the attention or language problem. Language delays were, however, more common than in a random sample in our data because many children among the index group (at familial risk for dyslexia, to which belonged a little bit more than half of the members of the overactive group) in the JLD sample were clearly delayed in many language skills at the critical age of 5 yr of the present comparison *(4,101,102)*. Because the subgroups representing those children among the at-risk group who belonged to the most shy/hyperactive third of the whole group were not significantly different from the rest in any of the NEPSY measures, we can be quite safe in our beliefs that early temperamental expressions of deviation in attention-related behavior do not add the risk for a cognitive delay possibly related to that for familial dyslexia. The results also fail to support an assumption that dyslexia-related familial risk has any reliable early association with comorbidities which had been reflected in the assessed features of infant temperament.

5. CONCLUDING REMARKS

Based on the studies conducted during the past two decades, we can conclude that there is a unanimous consensus that attention and learning deficit have a fairly high comorbidity. This clinically and empirically compelling conceptualization is also reflected in the several diagnostic concepts used during the years. The historical Minimal Brain Dysfunction and the more modern Deficits in Attention, Motor Control, and Perception *(103)* and the Atypical Brain Development *(25)* have been used to describe that is the co-occurrence of developmental deficits or they even more rule than exception. These conceptualizations also incorporate the idea that comorbity is not only common, but also that there is some shared etiology behind the comorbid deficits or they even may have a genetic basis *(12)*.

Consideration of the same results from another perspective shows us that there is a vast number of children diagnosed with ADHD who do not demonstrate LDs or who have above-average performance in academic tests, both reading and mathematics. These children have commonly been called "pure ADHD." Moreover, it is plausible to think that children demonstrating ADHD + LD form a subgroup (or group of their own), which might have a distinctive neuropsychological profile *(104)* and etiology *(9)*. Thus, children with uncomplicated ADHD and children with comorbid LD + ADHD may have features or core deficits that are unique to that subtype, explaining why cognitive deficits typical to ADHD have been so difficult to find. It is very possible that the ADHD diagnosis as such is not specific enough to form homogeneous groups. Moreover, using behavioral symptoms of ADHD as a basis to form groups may lose some crucial information needed for appropriate intervention and programming. This situation may be one reason why the findings of several ADHD studies continue to be equivocal or even divergent—even though ADHD is one of the most researched developmental deficits. (Note: in this context, the other likely reason why results differ is the variations of comorbidities connected via artifactual instead of genuine causal relations *[2]*.) In the future, more emphasis is needed on features other than those observed via sole behavioral ratings concerning attention issues. Two lines of research that are required include longitudinal studies to identify the possible behavioral origins of the co-occurrence of other disorders with ADHD, and neuropsychological, genetic, and cognitive studies to assess the origins of the comorbidity.

Most research to date has focused on the co-occurrence of attention and reading deficits giving mathematical difficulties lesser attention. This chapter as well as the earlier studies conducted by Semrud-Clikeman have shown that mathematics is also an essential area of both empirical and clinical research. Findings that mathematics and visual-spatial reasoning may be interlinked, at least in children with nonverbal LDs, appears to be a promising area of research. Many children with mathematics difficulties also appear to have ADHD and they may have more difficulties with attention than with activity level *(66)*. Difficulties in fluid reasoning in these children may also contribute to problems in social cognition, executive functions, and subsequently, mathematics achievement *(105)*. Further work is sorely needed in this area.

The literature has shown that inattention, particularly, may be associated with learning deficits. This is also confirmed by the present data using developmental longitudinal data. The finding that indicates an association between inattention and neuropsychological tests warrants the speculation that inattention should be considered as a separate feature from hyperactivity, and that inattention might be connected to cognitive deficits, which accumulate to produce learning deficits. Based on the recent findings demonstrating that inattention might be especially associated with reading fluency and speed-related cognitive processes, the notion of sluggish cognitive tempo seems to have more validity than has recently been acknowledged. We also may not want to forget the possibility that in some children the tendency to inattentive behavior may be triggered, maintained, or even generalized to nonchallenging contexts by relatively specific but serious failure experiences at school, such as perception of problems in reading acquisition during the early school years. This psychologically motivated defensive response to school challenges however, requires an apparently, different treatment than does a biologically originated atypical attention.

A finding that inattention is concurrently associated with reading difficulty may not always refer to genuine comorbidity, but may be a result of diagnostic procedures. Teacher and parent observations are used to diagnose the presence of inattention, while tests are usually used to evaluate child's reading skills. One could speculate that if experiences of academic difficulties have continued for some time, and if a child's concept of himself or herself has been affected by the continuous failures, this manifests itself in the child's classroom behavior because of "defensive" attention disorder. Behavioral traits associated with lack of learning motivation, mild depression, anxiety, or poor self-esteem could be interpreted by both teachers and parents as inattention. This problem is encountered particularly in the studies using clinical samples, and thus, population-based studies using developmental data, and preferably longitudinal designs, would help us to determine the causal connections and define design related artifacts.

To learn to understand the whole nature of comorbidity we had to be able to observe the developmental beginnings of route(s) to or earliest expressions of co-occurrence of two or more neurocognitive disorders in the same way prospective studies of more narrow disorders, which are known to have familial backgrounds, are done. A potential focus of study to approach this goal is to investigate the relationship between early temperament and attention in large-scale follow-up studies of dyslexia or attention disorders. To utilize observations of early behaviors for study, we had to learn more about the early expression of attention and its normal and atypical developmental variations. The development of attention is an important milestone for infants and very young children. Studies searching for developmental antecedents of attention deficits from early temperament and other developmental factors have not found strong predictors *(106)*. Our own data extended these findings, indicating at best only a weak connection between early temperamental hyperactivity and later skills, meaning that a small portion of attention-related individuality may affect the development of skills.

Clinically and pedagogically, it is essential to differentiate the reasons for a child's learning deficits. In theory, remedial programs are based on careful diagnosis and a deep understanding of the nature of the child's difficulties, as well as possible remedial processes and expected outcome. In practice, however, we often have to settle for a "sophisticated guess." In order to improve clinical services and practices to children with these types of needs, we require tools that would help us to better understand the cognitive strengths and deficits that children with ADHD experience. Comprehensive neuropsychological test batteries and methods similar to those commonly used in laboratories would perhaps help clinicians better differentiate between different features and cognitive dimensions of ADHD, which are essential for learning, teaching, and remediation—even as essential as the features captured by behavioral assessment. The development of psychometrically sound and clinically useful neuropsychological tests for children at very young ages through adolescence would be very helpful in our study of the neuropsychological underpinnings of the development of constructs, such as attention and memory in children with and without difficulty.

ACKNOWLEDGMENTS

We would like to express our thanks to the personnel and families collaborating with the Jyväskylä Longitudinal Study of Dyslexia, as well as with our study in Santiago de Chile. We also thank Lic. Sc. Asko Tolvanen for his statistical advice. We would also like to thank the many families participating in the study at the University of Texas at Austin, as well as the many hours volunteered by school psychology doctoral students to support our project.

REFERENCES

1. Caron C, Rutter M. Comorbidity in child psychopathology: concepts, issues and research strategies. J Child Psychol Psychiatry 1991;32:1063–1080.
2. Pennington BF. The development of psychopathology. Nature and nurture. New York: Guilford Press, 2002.
3. Lyytinen H. Comorbidity and developmental neurocognitive disorders. Dev Neuropsychol 1995;11:269–273.

4. Lyytinen H. In search of precursors of dyslexia: a prospective study of children at risk for reading problems. In: Snowling M, ed. Dyslexia: biology, cognition and intervention London: Whurr Publishers, 1997:97–107.
5. Lyytinen H, Ahonen T, Eklund K, et al. Developmental pathways of children with and without familial risk for dyslexia during the first years of life. Dev Neuropsychol 2001;20:535–554.
6. Teeter PA. Interventions for ADHD. New York: Guilford Press, 1998.
7. August GJ, Garfinkel MD. Comorbidity of ADHD and reading disability among clinic-referred children. J Abnorm Child Psychol 1990;18:29–45.
8. Fergusson DM, Horwood LJ. Attention deficit and reading achievement. J Child Psychol Psychiatry 1992;33:375–385.
9. Gilger J, Pennington BF, DeFries JC. A twin study of the etiology of comorbidity: attention deficit hyperactivity disorder and dyslexia. J Am Acad Child Adolesc Psychiatry 1992;31:343–348.
10. Hynd GW, Lorys AR, Semrud-Clikeman M, Nieves N, Huettner MI, Lahey BB. Attention deficit disorder without hyperactivity: a distinct behavioral and neurocognitive syndrome. J Child Neurol 1991;6;37–43.
11. Lamminmäki T, Ahonen T, Närhi V, Todd de Barra H, Lyytinen H. Attention-deficit/hyperactivity disorder subtypes: are there differences in academic problems? Dev Neuropsychol 1995;11: 297–310.
12. Light JG, Pennington BF, Gilger JW, DeFries JC. Reading disability and hyperactivity disorder: Evidence for a common genetic etiology. Dev Neuropsychol 1995;11:323–336.
13. Pennington BF, Groisser D, Welsh MC. Contrasting cognitive deficits in attention deficit-hyperactivity disorder versus reading disability. Dev Neuropsychol 1993;29:511–523.
14. Rabiner D, Coie D. Early attention problems and children's reading achievement: a longitudal investigation. J Am Acad Child Adolesc Psychiatry 2000;39:859–867.
15. Rowe KJ, Rowe KS. The relationship between inattentiveness in the classroom and reading achievement (Part B): an explanatory study. J Am Acad Child Adolesc Psychiatry 1992;31:357–368.
16. Semrud-Clikeman M, Biederman J, Sprich-Buckminster S, Krifcher B. Lehman BK, Faraone SV, Norman D. The incidence of ADDH and concurrent learning disabilities. J Am Acad Child Adolesc Psychiatry 1992;31:439–448.
17. Shaywitz SD, Shaywiz BA. Critical issues in attention deficit disorder. In: Sagvolden T, Archer T, eds. Attention-deficit disorder: clinical and basic research. Hillsdale, NJ: Lawrence Erlbaum, 1989:53–70.
18. Stanford LD, Hynd GW. Congruence of behavioral symptomatology in children with ADD/H, ADD/WO, and learning disabilities. J Learn Disabil 1994;27:243–253.
19. Velting ON, Whitehurst GJ. Inattention-hyperactivity and reading achievement in children from low-income families: a longitudinal model. J Abnorm Child Psychol 1997;25:321–331.
20. Willcutt EG, Pennington BF. Comorbidity of reading disability and attention–deficit/ hyperactivity disorder: differences by gender and subtype. J Learn Disabil 2000;33:179–191.
21. Shaywitz SD, Shaywitz BA. Attention deficit disorder comes of age. Austin, TX: Pro-Ed, 1992.
22. Halperin JM, Gittelman R, Klein DF, Rudel RG. Reading-disabled hyperactive children: a distinct subgroup of attention deficit dsorder with hyperactivity? J Abnorm Child Psychol 1984;12:1–14.
23. Riccio CA, Hynd GW. Developmental language disorders and attention deficit hyperactivity disorder. In: Scruggs TE, Mastropieri MA, eds. Advances in learning and behavioral disabilities. New York: Elsevier, 1995:9:1–20.
24. Tirosh E, Cohen A. Language deficit with attention-deficit disorders: a prevalent comorbidity. J Child Neurol 1998;13:493–497.
25. Gilger J, Kaplan BJ. Atypical brain development: a conceptual framework for understanding developmental learning disabilities. J Dev Neurol 2001;20:465–481.
26. Stevenson J. Developmental changes in the mechanisms linking language disabilities and behavior disorders. In: Beitchman JH, Cohen NJ, Konstantareas MM, Tannock R, eds. Language, learning, and behavior disorders. New York: Cambridge University Press, 1996:78–99.

27. Barkley R. Behavioral inhibition, sustained attention and executive functions: constructing a unifying theory of ADHD. Psychol Bull 1997;121:65–94.
28. Barkley RA, Fisher M, Edelbreock CS, Smallish L. The adolescent outcome of hyperactive children diagnosed by research criteria: I. An 8- year prospective follow-up study. J Am Acad Child Adolesc Psychiatry 1990;29:546–557.
29. DuPaul GJ, Stoner G. ADHD in the schools: assessment and intervention strategies. New York: Guilford Press, 1994.
30. Barkley R. Attention-deficit hyperactivity disorder: a handbook for diagnosis and treatment. New York: Guilford Press, 1990.
31. Nieves N. Childhood psychopathology and learning disabilities: neuropsychological relationships. In: Obzrut JE, Hynd GW, eds. Neuropsychological foundations of learning disabilities. San Diego, CA: Academic Press, 1991:113–146.
32. Schachar RJ, Rutter M, Smith A. The characteristics of situationally and pervasively hyperactive children: implications for syndrome definition. J Child Psychol Psychiatry 1981;22:375–392.
33. Pennington BF. Diagnosing learning disabilities. New York: Guilford Press, 1990.
34. Poskiparta E, Niemi P, Lepola J, Ahtola A, Laine P-L. Motivational-emotional vulnerability and difficulties in learning to read and spell. Br J Edu Psychol 2003;73:187–206.
35. Närhi V, Ahonen T. Reading disability with or without attention deficit hyperactivity disorder: do attentional problems make a difference? Dev Neuropsychol 1995;11:337–350.
36. Willcutt EG, Pennington BF, Boada R, et al. A comparison of the cognitive deficits in reading disability and attention-deficit/hyperactivity disorder. J Abnorm Psychol 2001;110:157–172.
37. Semrud-Clikeman M, Guy KA, Griffin JD. Rapid automatized naming in children with reading disabilities and attention deficit hyperactivity disorder. Brain Lang 2000;74:70–83.
38. Rucklidge J, Tannock R. Neuropsychological profiles of adolescents with ADHD: effects of reading difficulties and gender. J Child Psychol Psychiatry 2002;43;998–1003.
39. Reynolds CR, Kamphaus RW. BASC. Behavioral Assessment System for Children. Manual. Circle Pines, MN: American Guidance Services, Inc., 1992.
40. Hynd GW, Lorys AR, Semrud-Clikeman M, Nieves N, Huettner M, Lahey BB. Attention deficit disorder without hyperactivity (ADD/WO): a distinct behavioral and neurocognitive syndrome. J Child Neurol 1991;6:37–43.
41. Puig-Antich J, Chambers W. The schedule for affective disorders and schizophrenia for schoolage children. New York: New York State Psychiatric Institute, 1978.
42. Wechsler D. Wechsler Intelligence Scale for Children. 3rd ed. San Antonio, TX: Psychological Corporation, 1991.
43. Sattler, J. Assessment of children. San Diego: Jerome Sattler Publishers, 2000.
44. Wechsler Individual Achievement Test. San Antonio, TX: Psychological Corporation, 1992.
45. Schnoebelen S, Semrud-Clikeman M, Guli L, Corlett M. Planning and organization in children with learning disabilities. Paper presented at the annual conference of the American Psychological Association, August 2002.
46. Lahey BB, Pelham WE, Schaughency EA, et al. Dimensions and types of attention deficit disorder. J Am Acad Child Adolesc Psychiatry 1988;27:330–335.
47. Carlson C, Lahey B, Neeper R. Direct assessment of the cognitive correlates of attention deficit disorder with and without hyperactivity. J Psychopathol Behav Assess 1986;8:69–86.
48. Chhabildas N, Pennington BF, Willcutt EG. A comparison of the neuropsychological profiles of the DSM-IV subtypes of ADHD. J Abnorm Child Psychol 2001;29:529–540.
49. Goodyear P, Hynd G. Attention-deficit disorder with (ADD/H) and without (ADD/WO) hyperactivity: behavioral and neuropsychological differentiation. J Clin Child Psychol 1992;21:273–305.
50. Cantwell DP, Baker L. Association between attention deficit-hyperactivity disorder and learning disabilities. J Learn Disabil 1992;24:88–95.
51. Dykman RA, Ackerman PT. Cluster versus dimensional analysis of attentional deficit disorder. In: Matson J, ed. Handbook of hyperactivity in children. Massachusetts: Allyn and Bacon, 1993:11–34.

52. Barkley RA, DuPaul G, McMurray M. Comprehensive evaluation of attention deficit disorder with and without hyperactivity as defined by research criteria. J Consult Clin Psychol 1990;58:775–789.
53. American Psychiatric Association. Diagnostic and statistical manual of mental disorders, 3rd ed. Washington, DC: American Psychiatric Association, 1980.
54. American Psychiatric Association. Diagnostic and statistical manual of mental disorders, 4th ed. Washington, DC: American Psychiatric Association, 1994.
55. Ullman RK, Sleator EK, Sprague RL. ADD-H Comprehensive Teacher's Rating Scale. Champaign, IL: MetriTech, 1988.
56. Woodcock RW. Bateria Woodcock Psico-Educativa en Español. Allen, TX: DLM Teaching Resources, 1982.
57. Aro T, Ahonen T, Tolvanen A, Lyytinen H. Contribution of ADHD characteristics to the academic treatment outcome of children with academic difficulties. Dev Neuropsychol 1999;15:291–305.
58. Lahey B, Applegate B, McBurnett K, et al. DSM-IV field trial for attention deficit/hyperactivity disorder in children and adolescents. Am J Psychiatry 1994;151:1673–1685.
59. Baumgaertel A, Wolreich M, Dietrich M. Comparison of diagnostic criteria for attention deficit disorders in a German elementary school sample. J Am Acad Child Adolesc Psychiatry 1995;34:629–638.
60. McGee R, Prior M, Williams S, Smart D, Sanson A. The long-term significance of teacher-rated hyperactivity and reading ability in childhood: findings from two longitudinal studies. J Child Psychol Psychiatry 2002;43:1004–1017.
61. Posner M. Attention: the mechanisms of consciousness. Proc Natl Acad Sci USA 1994;91: 7398–7403.
62. Schaughency EA, Hynd GW. Attention an impulse control in attention deficit disorder (ADD): neural control systems. Learn Indiv Diff 1989;1:423–449.
63. Filipek PA, Semrud-Clikeman M, Steingard RJ, Renshaw PF, Kennedy DN, Biederman J. Volumetric MRI analysis comparing subjects having attention deficit hyperactivity disorder with normal controls. Neurology 1997;48:589–601.
64. Gazzaniga MS. Ivry RB. Mangun GR. Cognitive neuroscience: the biology of the mind, 2nd edition. New York: WW Norton & Co. 2002.
65. Semrud-Clikeman M, Hooper S, Hynd GW, Hern K. The ability of brain morphological measures to discriminate between clinical groups. Arch Clin Neuropsychol 1996;11:521–528.
66. Semrud-Clikeman M, Shaefer V. Social competence in developmental disorders. J Psychother Ind Practice 2000;4;3–20.
67. Semrud-Clikeman M, Steingard R, Filipek PA, Bekken K, Biederman J, Renshaw P. Neuroanatomical-neuropsychological correlates of ADHD. J Am Acad Child Adolesc Psychiatry 2000;39:477–484.
68. Holopainen L, Ahonen T, Lyytinen H. Predicting delay in reading achievement in a highly transparent language. J Learn Disabil 2001;34:401–413.
69. Wechsler D. Wechsler Preschool and Primary Scale of Intelligence-Revised. San Antonio, TX: Psychological Corporation, 1989.
70. Aro M, Wimmer H. Learning to read: English in comparison to six more regular orthographies. Appl Psycholinguistics 2003;24:619–634.
71. Seymour P, Aro M, Erskine J. Foundation literacy acquisition in European orthographies. Br J Psychol 2003;94:143–174.
72. Lyytinen H, Aro M, Holopainen L. Dyslexia in highly orthographically regular Finnish. In: Smith I, ed. International handbook of dyslexia. West Sussex, UK: Wiley, 2003:81–91.
73. Leinonen S, Müller K, Leppänen PHT, Aro M, Ahonen T, Lyytinen H. Heterogeneity in adult dyslexic readers: relating processing skills to the speed and accuracy of oral text reading. Reading and Writing: an Interdisciplinary Journal, 2001;14:265–296.
74. Schoot M, Licht R, Horsley TM, Seargeant JA. Inhibitory deficits in reading disability depend on subtype: guessers but not spellers. Child Neuropsychol 2001;6:297–312.

75. Ackerman PT, Anhalt JM, Holcomb PJ, Dykman RA. Presumably innate and acquired automatic processes in children with attention and/or reading disorders. J Child Psychol Psychiatry 1986;4:513–529.
76. McBurnett K, Pfiffner LJ, Frick PJ. Symptom properties as a function of ADHD type: an argument for continued study of sluggish cognitive tempo. J Abnorm Child Psychol 2001;29:207–213.
77. Barkley RA, Grodzinsky G, DuPaul G. Frontal lobe functions in attention deficit disorder with and without hyperactivity: a review and research report. J Abnorm Child Psychol 1992;2:163–187.
78. Hynd GW, Nieves N, Connor RT, et al. Attention deficit disorderwith and without hyperactivity: reaction time and speed of cognitive processing. J Learn Disabil 1989;22:573–580.
79. Kemp S, Kirk U, Korkman M. Essentials of NEPSY Assessment. New York: John Wiley 2001.
80. DeShazo BT, Lyman RD, Klinger LG. Academic underachievement and attention-deficit/hyperactivity disorder: the negative impact of symptom severity on school performance. J Sch Psychol 2002;40:259–283.
81. Douglas VI, Peters KG. Toward a clearer definition of the attentional deficit of hyperactive children. In: Hale GA, Lewis M, eds. Attention and cognitive development. New York: Plenum Press, 1979;173–247.
82. Tannock R. Attention deficit hyperactivity disorder: advances in cognitive, neurobiological, and genetic research. J Child Psychol Psychiatry 1998;39:65–99.
83. Wilens TE, Biederman J, Spencer T. Attention deficit/ hyperactivity disorder across the lifespan. Annu Rev Med 2002;53:113–131.
84. Schmidt LA, Fox N, Rubin KH, Hu S, Hamer DH. Molecular genetics of shyness and aggression in preschoolers. Personality and Individual Differences 2002;32:227–238.
85. Rothbart MK. Measurement of temperament in infancy. Child Dev 1981;52:569–578.
86. Kagan J. Behavioral inhibition in young children. Child Dev 1984;55:1005–1019.
87. Lahey BB, Carlson CL. Validity of the diagnostic category of attention deficit disorder without hyperactivity: a review of the literature. J Learn Disabil 1991;24:110–20.
88. Robinson JL, Kagan J, Reznick JS, Corley R. The heritability of inhibited and uninhibited behavior: a twin study. Dev Psychol 1992;28:1030–1037.
89. DiLalla LF, Jones S. Genetic and environmental influences on temperament in preschoolers. In: Molfese VJ, Molfese DL, eds. Temperament and personality development across the life span. Hillsdale, NJ: Lawrence Erlbaum 2000:33–55.
90. Kinsbourne M. Kaplan PJ. Children's learning and attention problems. Boston, MA: Little Brown, 1979.
91. Eaton WO. Temperament, development, and the five-factor model: Lessons from activity level. In: Halverson CF, Kohnstamm GA, Martin RP, eds. The developing structure of temperament and personality from infancy to adulthood. Hillsdale, NJ: Lawrence Erlbaum, 1994:173–187.
92. Buss A. Temperament as personality traits. In: Kohnstamm GA, Bates JE, Rothbart MK, eds. Temperament in childhood. New York: John Wiley, 1989:49–58.
93. Emde RN, Plomin R, Robinson JA, et al. Temperament, emotion and cognition at fourteen months: the MacArthur Longitudal Twin Study. Child Dev 1992;63:1437–1455.
94. Goldsmith HH, Lemery KS, Buss KA, Campos JJ. Genetic analyses of focal aspects of infant temperament. Dev Psychol 1999;35:972–85.
95. Levy F, Hay D, McStephen M, Wood C, Waldman I. Attention-deficit hyperactivity disorder: a category or a continuum? Genetic analysis of a large-scale twin study. J Am Acad Child Adolesc Psychiatry 1997;36:737–744.
96. Baker L. Cantwell DP. Factors associated with the development of psychiatric illness in children with early speech/language problems. J Autism Dev Disord 1987;17:499–510.
97. Cohen MJ. Riccio CA. Gonzalez JJ. Methodological differences in the diagnosis of attention-deficit hyperactivity disorder: impact on prevalence. J Emotional Behav Disord 1994;2:31–38.
98. Silva PA, Williams S, McGee R. A longitudinal study of children with developmental language delay at age three: later intelligence, reading and behaviour problems. Dev Med Child Neurol 1987;29:630–640.

99. Weimberg WA, Emslie GJ, Attention deficit hyperactivity disorder: the differential diagnosis J Child Neurol 1991;6:23–36.
100. Berninger, VW, Abbott RD. Modeling developmental and individual variability in reading and writing acquitision: a developmental neuropsychological perspective. In: Molfese DL, Kirk U, eds. Developmental variations in learning: applications to social, executive function, language, and reading skills. Hillsdale, NJ:Erlbaum. 2001:275–308.
101. Lyytinen P, Eklund K, Lyytinen H. The play and language behavior of mothers with and without dyslexia and its association to their toddlers' language development. J Learn Disabil 2003;36:74–86.
102. Lyytinen P, Poikkeus A-M, Laakso M-L, Eklund K, Lyytinen H. Language development and symbolic play in children with and without familial risk for dyslexia. J Speech Lang Hear Res 2001;44:873–885.
103. Gillberg C, Rasmussen P, Carlström G, Svenson B, Waldenström E. Perceptual, motor and attentional deficits in six-year-old children: epidemiological aspects. J Child Psychol Psychiatry 1982;23:131–134.
104. Tirosh E, Berger J, Cohen-Ophir M, Dadovitch M, Cohen A. Learning disabilities with and without attention-deficit hyperactivity disorder: parents' and teachers' perspective. J Child Neurol 1998;13:270–276.
105. Semrud-Clikeman M. Executive function and social communication disorders. Perspectives 2003;29:20–22.
106. Olson S. Bates J. Sandy J. Schilling E. Early developmental precursors of impulsive and inattentive behavior: from infancy to middle childhood. J Child Psychiatry Psychother 2002;43:435–447.

14

Social Functioning of Children With Attention Deficit Hyperactivity Disorder

Hana Tur-Kaspa

1. INTRODUCTION

Children with attention deficit hyperactivity disorder (ADHD) experience pervasive interpersonal difficulties and peer disapproval that go beyond the diagnostic criteria. ADHD occurs in approx 3–5% of the school-aged population, with male to female ratios ranging from 4:1 to 9:1, depending on the setting *(1)*. The disorder persists into adolescence in about 50–80% of cases clinically diagnosed in childhood *(2)*. Core characteristics of the disorder include inattention, hyperactivity, and impulsivity. The current clinical view of ADHD *(1)* offers three subtypes of the disorder: predominantly inattentive, predominantly hyperactive–impulsive, and the combined type. This chapter refers to the hyperactive–impulsive and combined types of ADHD.

The salient symptoms of ADHD (i.e., inattention, hyperactivity, and impulsivity) can be expected to interfere with the child's social functioning and social adjustment. Indeed, extensive research has documented that many children with ADHD experience serious difficulties in the social domain *(3–6)*. As they develop, children with ADHD are at greater risk for poor school performance, poor peer relations, anxiety and depression, aggression, conduct problems and delinquency, early substance use, as well as difficulties in social and personal relations during adulthood *(7)*.

Concerns have been raised pertaining to the social difficulties experienced by children with ADHD, and the role these difficulties have in putting these children at heightened risk for future social maladjustment *(8–10)*. Thus, the problems of children with ADHD in their social interactions and peer relations are a crucial target for intervention *(11)*.

This chapter reviews the research relevant to the social functioning of children with ADHD including social status, social interactions with peers, social skills and behavior problems, and social–cognitive skills. The chapter also discusses the major findings pertaining to these children's social functioning. Suggestions for future research are proposed.

2. SOCIAL STATUS OF CHILDREN WITH ADHD

A host of studies have demonstrated that many children with ADHD are less accepted and often socially rejected by their peers. This finding is independent of whether peers, teachers, or parents complete the sociometric ratings *(3,4,6)*. Measurement of social status has been

From: *Attention Deficit Hyperactivity Disorder: From Genes to Patients*
Edited by: D. Gozal and D. L. Molfese © Humana Press Inc., Totowa, NJ

shown to provide unique and potentially vital information in predicting children's success within peer relationships *(12)*.

Research indicated that the social status problems of children with ADHD emerge rapidly within a new group of peers *(13)* and are resistant to reversal thereafter *(14)*. Pelham and Bender *(15)* investigated the behavioral correlates of negative peer status of children with ADHD in comparison to non-ADHD controls, all of whom were initially unfamiliar with each other. They found that children with ADHD quickly attained social rejection status, which was related to high rates of aggressive, destructive, and noncompliant behaviors in group play situations.

Research attempts to examine various predictors of sociometric status of children with ADHD documented externalizing behavior patterns (i.e., aggression and noncompliance) to be key predictors of negative peer status *(13)*. This was even after a very short period (i.e., after 1–3 d) of social interactions among children with and without ADHD who attended a 5-wk summer camp and did not know each other before attending the camp. Interestingly, non-behavioral variables, such as intelligence, academic achievement, physical attractiveness, and athletic skills did not predict sociometric status. In another study *(16)*, the predictive power of antisocial behavior, internalizing, and familial variables with respect to peer status in boys (aged 6–12 yr) with and without ADHD were examined. Results indicated that aggression predicted peer rejection more strongly for non-ADHD comparisons than for boys with ADHD, whereas authoritative parenting beliefs (i.e., involving clear, firm structuring and limit setting in the presence of warmth and responsiveness) were stronger predictors in the ADHD group than in comparison boys.

Results of a study *(17)* that examined the relative contributions of low achievement, learning disabilities, and ADHD to problems in social status and social behavior among second- through sixth-grade boys, revealed that the combination of ADHD and learning disabilities was associated with the greatest risk of social status problems (i.e., significantly higher on social rejection and lower on popularity) and of social behavior problems.

A recent study *(18)* that compared the social functioning of ADHD subgroups (i.e., combined type and predominantly inattentive type) and controls without ADHD revealed that children with ADHD-combined type were judged by parents and teachers to be less popular than controls, whereas children with ADHD-inattentive type were not rated as evidencing impaired social status. Regardless of group, social performance, emotional regulation, and to a lesser extent, social knowledge appeared to be predictive of social status.

Taken together, the results of these studies highlight the complexity of the concomitants and the underlying bases for social status difficulties of children with ADHD. Thus, it is essential to consider both internal (e.g., child's characteristic and behavior patterns) and external (e.g., parents' functioning, school environment) factors in the attempt to better understand the social status and functioning of these children.

3. SOCIAL INTERACTIONS AND PEER RELATIONS

Research has documented that more than 50% of children with ADHD have problems in interactions with peers *(15)*. The interpersonal interactions of children with ADHD with their parents, siblings, teachers, and—the focus of this chapter—peers are frequently characterized as being negative and conflicting *(6,19,20)*. According to Whalen and Henker's review *(20)*, children with ADHD are described by peer as annoying, boisterous, irritating, and intrusive. When compared to boys with learning disabilities or low-achieving comparisons, boys with

ADHD were seen by peers as disruptive and by teachers as oppositional/defiant, and as deficient on cooperation and self-control *(17)*.

The interpersonal problems of children with ADHD manifest during early childhood, even before the children enter school. For instance, preschool children with ADHD were found to be less competent with peers than non-ADHD preschoolers, and were less attentive and cooperative during group activities *(21)*.

Observations of school-aged children with ADHD during structured and unstructured playgroup interactions with non-ADHD peers revealed that children with ADHD displayed "bossy, aggressive, and bothersome interpersonal style" *(15)*. They were more talkative, engaged in more frequent high-rate activity, and used more negative verbal and nonverbal behavior and less neutral nonverbal behavior than their non-ADHD peers.

In more detailed observations of dyadic peer interactions, a comparison was made between mixed dyads (i.e., composed of a boy with ADHD and a boy with no ADHD) and "normal" dyads (i.e., composed of two boys with no ADHD) during free-play, cooperative task, and simulated classroom situations *(22)*. The children were unfamiliar with one another and uninformed as to the ADHD child's diagnostic status. Mixed dyads engaged in more controlling interaction than "normal" dyads in both free-play and simulated classroom settings. In the simulated classroom, mixed dyads completed fewer math problems and were less compliant with the commands of peers. The results suggested that children with ADHD prompt a more controlling, less cooperative pattern of responses from non-ADHD peers.

Using similar methodology, the frequency and patterns of play activity and verbal behavior of previously unacquainted mixed dyads and "normal" dyads were analyzed during their initial social encounter *(23)*. The mixed dyads engaged in more solitary play and less associative play than the "normal" dyads during their initial encounter. In addition, the interactions in the mixed dyads were marked by lower levels of affective expression and by less verbal reciprocity than were those of the children in the "normal" dyads. The mixed dyads' social interactions suggested that children with ADHD have difficulties in the development of acquaintanceship, and are at greater risk for losing socialization opportunities with peers.

In sum, children with ADHD have difficulties establishing and maintaining satisfying interpersonal relationships with peers. They tend to be bossy, disruptive, and easily frustrated when in the playgroup *(24)*. It is not surprising, therefore, that they have few, if any, friends.

4. SOCIAL SKILLS AND BEHAVIOR PROBLEMS

Children with ADHD begin having problems with social skills at an early age. Researchers *(25)* have assessed whether preschool children can successfully identify externalizing symptomatic behaviors (i.e., hyperactivity and aggression) in their male classmates, and whether these perceptions were associated with peer-rated popularity and rejection. Results indicated that preschool children's nominations of externalizing behavior correlated significantly with teacher ratings of the same behavior. Furthermore, peer nominations of rejection correlated significantly with both teacher ratings and peer nominations of hyperactivity and aggression. Boys nominated as aggressive were more often rejected by their classmates; whereas boys nominated as hyperactive were either more popular or more rejected.

In a more recent study, Merrell and Wolfe *(26)* examined the relationship of teacher-rated social skills deficits and ADHD characteristics among kindergarten-aged (5–6 yr) children. Findings indicated that young children with ADHD characteristics (i.e., not formally diagnosed) were rated as having significantly poorer social skills than matched children with no ADHD. Although young children with ADHD exhibited comparative deficits in virtually all areas of social competence, they were especially lacking in social cooperation skills (e.g., following directions from adults, cooperating and compromising with peers, sharing toys and other belongings, taking turns). Furthermore, children in the ADHD group were between five and six times as likely as children in the non-ADHD group to be rated by their teachers as having significant deficits in overall social skills. The fact that more than half of the participants in the ADHD group showed significant social skills deficits indicates a strong co-occurrence of these problems.

Social skills deficits of children with ADHD have been found to persist from early childhood into the elementary school years and adolescence and to have negative effects on social and emotional adjustment *(7)*. By virtue of the diagnostic criteria, children with ADHD show patterns of hyperactivity and impulsivity. In addition, aggression has been strongly associated with ADHD. These characteristics are likely to play a role in sharpening the social difficulties of these children *(4,27)*.

4.1. Hyperactivity and Impulsivity

Hyperactivity involves motor excess or overactivity, which is considered to be one of the hallmark characteristics of the disorder. It can take many forms but is especially apparent as excessive motor and verbal behaviors *(7)*. Research *(28)* has shown that children rated as being more hyperactive–impulsive or those who were clinically diagnosed as ADHD displayed a higher activity level than those children with no ADHD. In the context of social interactions, children with ADHD are often overactive and ceaselessly talkative, which may have a negative effect on peer relations *(24)*.

Impulsivity represents the child's difficulty in withholding or inhibiting his/her response in certain situations *(29)*. According to Barkley's *(29)* unifying theory of ADHD, the essential impairment in the combined and hyperactive–impulsive types of ADHD is a deficit involving basic inhabitation processes, such as those related to inhibition of the initial prepotent response to an event.

Impulsivity has been hypothesized to serve as a powerful interfering response in social behavior *(30)*, and may influence peer interactions and account for some of the unpopularity experienced by children with ADHD *(27,31)*. For example, impulsivity may impair the social interactions of children with ADHD by causing them to act without considering all alternatives and the long-term consequences of their actions, and to have a difficult time waiting their turn in line or in games. This behavioral style is likely to be met with peer rebuff and subsequent dislike *(27)*.

4.2. Aggression

One of the most pervasive social problems for children with ADHD is the development of aggressive behavior *(6)*. Early aggressive behavior is a prominent predictor of future problem behavior *(32)*, and aggressive acts are significantly associated with peer rejection *(33)*.

Furthermore, the combination of both hyperactivity and aggression has been associated with negative social outcomes *(6,18)*. Research *(34)* has documented that young children who had high ratings in kindergarten of hyperactivity and aggression were more likely than children who had average or low ratings of these measures to have third- and fourth-grade outcomes of peer-ratings of aggression and self-reports of delinquency.

Similarly, children with ADHD and learning disabilities, as well as children with "pure" ADHD without learning disabilities, significantly differed from children with "pure" learning disabilities with respect to their performance on behavioral and neuropsychological measures sensitive to deficit in self-regulation, classroom functioning, and aggression. Those in the ADHD or combined ADHD/learning disabilities samples were more impulsive, less accurate when response speed was required, worked less well independently, and were rated by their parents and teachers as exhibiting greater behavioral concerns (e.g., more aggressive, less compliant, and more oppositional) than the learning disabilities sample *(35)*.

In sum, children with ADHD exhibit significantly poorer social adaptive skills from an early age compared with their peers. Hyperactivity and impulsivity are likely to play a role in sharpening the social difficulties of these children. Children with the combination of both hyperactivity and aggression, however, seem to be at most risk for negative social outcomes.

5. SOCIAL–COGNITIVE SKILLS

Several researchers *(36,37)* have suggested that deficient and/or biased perception and interpretation of social cues may account for the difficulties children with ADHD experience in social situations. This kind of inquiry has been based on the premise that social cognition constitutes the mechanisms leading to social behaviors, which, in turn, form the basis of social adjustment *(36,38,39)*.

Dodge and his colleagues developed a model that postulates a comprehensive assessment of multiple social–cognitive processes involved in a child's processing of social information *(36,38)*. According to Crick and Dodge's model *(36)*, a child comes to a particular situation or task with a biologically determined set of response capabilities and a database that includes a memory store of past experience and a set of goals. Then, he or she receives a set of social cues as input from the environment. The child's response to those cues occurs as a function of the way he or she processes the social information. The model presumes that this processing occurs in sequential stages of steps: the encoding of social cues, interpretation of cues, clarification of goals and selection of a goal or desired outcome for the situation, access or construction of behavioral response to the situation, response decision, and behavioral enactment of the selected response.

The model describes competent processing of social information. A deviant outcome may be a function of any step or any combination of steps. The processing and interpretation of information from each of these steps will determine the nature of the response. If performance at some point in the progression is unskilled, either because of deficits in cognitive ability or biases in perception and interpretation of environmental stimuli, then the outcome will be maladaptive behavior.

Studies have demonstrated that children with ADHD differ from comparison children on various measures of the steps suggested in Crick and Dodge's model. With respect to the encoding step, children and adolescents with ADHD were found to have deficits in their ability to accurately recognize facial expressions of emotions, which is a vital component of social information processing *(40)*. Another study *(41)* examined developmental and individual differences in children's online encoding and representations of positive and negative social interactions among hypothetical peers. Results indicated that boys with ADHD generated less-integrated online representation networks than did non-ADHD boys, and they were profoundly impaired in their tendency to represent online the other's inner needs, cognitions, and affective states. The online representation of older boys with ADHD was found to be similar to that of younger non-ADHD controls; however, they engaged in a qualitatively different process of online representation.

Recently, Tur-Kaspa and Michal *(42)* examined two social information-processing skills; response access or construction, and response decision of diagnosed children (i.e., second- to fourth-graders) and adolescents (i.e., seventh- to ninth-graders) with ADHD compared to those children without ADHD, utilizing Crick and Dodge's model *(36)* as a theoretical framework. Moreover, children's motivations to respond in certain ways to resolve everyday situations they encounter were examined. Results indicated that students with ADHD displayed lower social information-processing skills in comparison to controls, in both the response access or construction and the response decision processes. Age differences in social-information processing skills were demonstrated across the two groups, although group differences remained. In addition, children with ADHD were likely to be driven by a will to control and to exercise power in their social interactions with peers.

In an earlier study *(43)*, three kinds of social information processing (i.e., encoding and utilization of cues, interpretation of social cues, and response decision) were examined among five diagnosed groups: hyperactive–aggressive, exclusively hyperactive, exclusively aggressive, psychiatric control, and normal control boys. Hyperactive–aggressive boys were found to be deficient in all three areas assessed, relative to the normal controls. They were also deficient in response decisions and cue utilization, relative to the other three groups of psychiatrically referred boys. Hyperactive–aggressive boys were more likely than normal controls to attribute hostile intentions to peers, following an ambiguous provocation by the peer, and were also more likely to expect that the peer would continue to behave in a hostile manner in the future. In comparison to normal controls and other psychiatrically referred boys, they were more likely to decide that they would retaliate aggressively against the peer instigator of the provocation. Murphy et al. study *(44)*, however, failed to find significant differences between subgroups of high-aggressive and low-aggressive boys with ADHD on several social information processing measures (i.e., encoding, attributional bias, and response decision bias).

Social information-processing skills of children with ADHD were also examined under automatic and controlled conditions *(45)*. In a condition designed to elicit automatic processing, children with hyperactivity and aggression did not differ in identifying the components of a social problem or in the number of solutions generated to solve a problem, but were more likely to show a bias toward aggressive solutions in handling the situations, as compared to nonhyperactive–nonaggressive children. Furthermore, in a condition designed to elicit controlled processing, children with hyperactivity and aggression did not differ in identifying problem components, generating solutions, or in anticipating outcomes for solutions, but were less able to anticipate consequences of aggressive solutions, and were more aggressive in choosing the best solution to solve a problem, as compared to the control.

Recent research interest *(46,47)* has focused on goals for social interactions of children with ADHD, suggesting that those decisions about which interpersonal outcomes to pursue may be the foundation of their social behavior. In Melnick and Hinshaw's study *(46)*, children with ADHD-high-aggressive were found to hold less appropriate goals for social interactions. Examination of the social goals of children with ADHD for a competitive interaction task (i.e., foosball game) revealed that boys diagnosed with ADHD-high-aggressive prioritized trouble-seeking, domination, and disruption goals for the social interaction to a greater extent than ADHD-low-aggressive and comparison boys. Furthermore, children's goal endorsements in the pre-game interview, particularly those pertaining to trouble-seeking and cooperation, predicted children's social acceptance at the end of the 5-wk summer camp, even when the effects of children's interactive behaviors and subgroup status were controlled statistically. Results of a recent study *(47)* indicated, however, that girls with and without ADHD responded to hypothetical vignettes with similar goals (i.e., instrumental and relational goals) but differed with respect to selection of social behaviors to attain their goals.

Children with ADHD also appear to possess less knowledge of how to maintain relationships and handle interpersonal conflicts than do controls *(31)*. They offered less-friendly solutions, showed less impulse control, and were less effective than controls in situations that required relationship maintenance and conflict resolution skills. Similar findings were reported by Thomeer *(48)*, who investigated the social knowledge and peer relations of children with ADHD and found that they exhibited strategies that were more impulsive and less relationship-enhancing, effective, and friendly than those of the comparison non-ADHD children.

In sum, the reviewed studies (*see* Table 1) have demonstrated that children with ADHD have difficulties in various aspects of social cognition, as well as in social knowledge. Social-cognitive skills were found to underlie differences in social behaviors that, in turn, led to children's social adjustment. This might shed light on the social maladjustment exhibited by children with ADHD, especially of those who are initially disposed toward aggression *(33)*.

6. DISCUSSION AND SUGGESTIONS FOR FUTURE RESEARCH

The literature is quite clear about the social functioning of children with ADHD. As a group, these children are less accepted and often socially rejected by their peers, have difficulties in establishing and maintaining satisfying social relationships with peers, and have social-skills deficits and interfering problem behaviors *(3,4,6)*. Furthermore, researchers *(20)* have suggested that children with ADHD serve as negative social catalysts, eliciting negative behaviors from those around them.

When considering the social–behavioral difficulties of children with ADHD, a useful distinction would be between acquisition and performance deficits *(30)*. Social skills acquisition deficits refer to the absence of knowledge required for executing particular social skills even under optimal conditions. Social performance deficits refer to the failure to perform social skills, which are present in a behavioral repertoire, at acceptable levels in given situations. Moreover, children may have social skill acquisition or performance deficits with or without interfering problem behaviors. Interfering behaviors refer to internalizing (e.g., anxiety, social withdrawal, depression) and/or externalizing (e.g., impulsivity, hyperactivity, aggression) behaviors that prevent either the acquisition or the performance of particular social skills *(49)*.

The distinction between these deficit types is important as it may delineate the nature of the social difficulties of children with ADHD and thus may suggest different intervention approaches and different settings for the implementation of these interventions. Accordingly, a central question would be whether children with ADHD have more trouble knowing what to do (i.e., acquisition deficits) than doing what they know (i.e., performance deficits). Another question is whether they have a behavioral problem that is interfering with the acquisition of what to do or with the execution of what they had already acquired (i.e., an interfering problem behavior).

According to Wheeler and Carlson's *(27)* research review, there is evidence to support the notion that children with ADHD possess the appropriate social knowledge, but exhibit performance deficits. They engage frequently in peer interactions, and seem to have the opportunities to learn appropriate social behaviors. Thus, the social difficulties of children with ADHD appear to be owing more to deficits in performance than to lack of appropriate

Table 1
Summary of Research on Social Functioning of Children With ADHD

Ref.	Authors	Year	Participants	Age	Instruments (response measured)	Main results
21	Alessandri	1992	20 ADHD (17 males, 3 females)	4–5 yr	1. Videotape recordings of free play (quality of social participation, and level of cognitive play)	ADHD, relative to non-ADHD, engaged in less mature (both cognitively and socially) play patterns.
			20 matched non-ADHD (17 males, 3 females)	4–5 yr	2. Observations of group activities (child's attention and cooperative behavior)	ADHD, relative to non-ADHD, were less competent with peers, and were less attentive and cooperative during group activities.
45	Bloomquist et al.	1997	70 hyperactive–aggressive (HA) (58 males, 25 females)	9.3 yr ± 1.2	1. CPSM (social problem-solving in automatic and controlled conditions) 2. BASC (Teachers' and parents' ratings of behavioral problems and social adjustment)	In automatic condition, HA were more aggressive in their generated solutions than non-HA. In the controlled condition, HA were less able to anticipate consequences, and were more aggressive in choosing best solutions than non-HA. Groups did not differ in the identification of problem or in the number of solutions generated. Significant relation between problem-solving and child's overall adjustment was found.
			40 non-HA (30 males, 10 females)	9.0 yr ± 1.2	3. RCP (social adjustment)	
22	Cunnigham and Siegel	1987	30 ADHD boys	2 age levels:	1. Videotapes of dyad's interactions during free play, cooperative task, and classroom activity (dyad's interaction patterns, child's social behavior, activity level, simulated school performance, on-task behavior)	The ADHD/normal dyads engaged in more controlling interaction than the normal/normal dyads in both free-play and simulated classroom settings. In the simulated classroom, mixed dyads completed fewer math problems and were less compliant with the commands of peers.
			90 normal (non-ADHD) boys	5–8 yr 9–12 yr		

13	Erhardt and Hinshaw	1994	25 ADHD boys 24 comparison (non-ADHD) boys	6–12 yr	1. Physical attractiveness 2. Intelligence test (verbal IQ) 3. Psychoeducational battery (reading and math achievements) 4. Motor skills competence 5. Behavior observations in classroom and playground (noncompliance, aggression, prosocial actions, and isolation)	Boys with ADHD and comparisons displayed clear differences in social behaviors, and ADHD youngsters were overwhelmingly rejected. Boys' aggression strongly predicted negative nominations, independent of diagnostic status.
17	Flicek	1992	18 boys/with ADHD/learning disabilities (LD) 19 ADHD/LA boys 33 ADHD boys 34 LD boys 29 LA (low achv) 116 control boys	Grades 2 to 6	1. SSRS-T (teachers' ratings of social behaviors) 2. Peer nominations and ratings (peer popularity and ratings of social behaviors)	Serious social problems were the most strongly related to the combination of ADHD and LD.
50	Gaub and Carlson	1997	123 ADHD-IA IT 47 ADHD-HI HT 51 ADHD-C CT 221 Controls (gender ratio range in four groups: 2.3 to 4.1 M:1F)	7.6 yr ± 1.9 7.5 yr ± 1.6 7.6 yr ± 1.6 7.6 yr ± 1.7	1. TRF (teachers' evaluations of children's functioning and impairment in behavioral and emotional realms) 2. Teachers' perception of the child's level of social functioning	The IA group was impaired in all areas, but were rated as displaying more appropriate behavior and fewer externalizing problems that HI or C groups. The HI group displayed externalizing and social problems, but was rated as no different than controls in learning or internalizing problems. The C group demonstrated severe and pervasive difficulties across domains.

(Continued)

Table 1
(Continued)

Ref.	Authors	Year	Participants	Age	Instruments (response measured)	Main results
31	Grenell et al.	1987	15 HI boys 15 control boys	7–11 yr $M = 9.4$	1. SKI interview (social knowledge) 2. Videotapes of free play, cooperative puzzle and persuasion task (peer interaction behaviors, and persuasion strategies) 3. Judges' global ratings (physical appearance and academic potential) 4. Peer ratings (partner for work)	HI boys exhibited knowledge deficits of how to maintain relationships and to handle interpersonal conflicts, and demonstrated more negative behavior in the cooperative puzzle tasks than controls. Significant correlation between social knowledge and performance with peers was found.
16	Hinshaw et al.	1997	73 ADHD boys 60 comparison boys	6–12 yr	1. Observations (social interactions) 2. Laboratory measure (covert antisocial behavior) 3. Child Depression Inventory 4. IAP (parents' ideas about parenting) 5. Peer sociometric	Aggression, covert behavior, and authoritative parenting beliefs were the independent predictors of both negative peer status and peer social preference.
23	Hubbard and Newcomb	1991	8 medicated ADHD boys 24 normal (non-ADHD) boys	8.6–9.2 yr	1. Videotapes of free play (frequency and patterns of play, play duration, verbal content of dyad's interaction)	The ADHD/normal dyads engaged in more solitary play and less associative play, and exhibited lower levels of verbal reciprocity and affective expression than the normal/normal dyads

(Continued)

19	Mash and Johnston	1983	40 families with HI child (16 younger 24 older children) 51 families with normal child (26 younger 25 older children)	2 age levels: 5 and 8.5 yr 5 and 8.5 yr	1. CBCL (child's behavior and hyperactivity level) 2. PSOC (parenting self-esteem) 3. PSI (stress degree in mother–child relations)	Parenting self-esteem was lower in parents of HI than those of normal children. Mothers of HI children, especially younger ones, reported higher levels of stress associated with both child characteristics and with their own feelings (depression, self-blame, and social isolation). Ratings of child disturbance and maternal stress were positively correlated.
46	Melnick and Hinshaw	1996	27 ADHD (14 high aggressive and 13 low aggressive) boys 18 control boys	2 age levels: 6–8.5 yr 9–12 yr	1. Child self-report (social goals) 2. Adult observer ratings (inferred importance of achieving goals) 3. Behavior observations (social behavior during football game) 4. Peer sociometric nominations	ADHD-high-aggressive boys prioritized trouble seeking and fun at the expense of rules to a greater extent than did ADHD and control boys. Observers judged ADHD boys to seek attention more strongly and seek fairness less strongly than the other two groups.
26	Merrell and Wolfe	1998	95 ADHD (not diagnosed) (72 males, 23 females) 95 non-ADHD (72 males, 23 females)	5–6 yr	1. PKBS scales (preschool and kindergarten children' social skills and problem behaviors)	Children with ADHD were rated by their teachers as having significantly poorer social skills than were comparisons. They were especially lacking in social cooperation skills, the ability to follow rules, structure, and important social expectations of both peers and adults.

(Continued)

Table 1
(Continued)

Ref.	Authors	Year	Participants	Age	Instruments (response measured)	Main results
41	Milch-Reich et al.	1999	38 ADHD boys 41 non-ADHD boys	5.9–10.3 yr ($M = 8.3 \pm 1.33$)	1. Structured interview (children's prior social schemes, online representation, free recall, and social reasoning)	Younger boys and boys with ADHD showed less integrated online representations of social information, accounting for poorer recall and social reasoning.
43	Milich and Dodge	1984	24 HA boys 14 HI boys 14 aggressive boys 23 psychiatric control boys 60 normal controls	6–12 yr	1. Hypothetical attribution task (hostile attribution biases) 2. Recall task (cue utilization) 3. Detective decision task (response decision biases)	The HA group was found to be deficient in all three information-processing skills assessed, relative to the normal control group. They were also deficient in response decision and cue utilization, relative to the other three groups.
25	Milich et al.	1982	86 preschool boys	3.25 –6.67 yr $M = 5$	1. Conners Teacher Rating scale (children's inattention/ overactivity, aggression, and sociability) 2. SNAP checklist (to identify ADD children) 3. Peer nominations (popularity, rejection, aggression, and sociability)	Preschool children were capable of providing stable nominations of popularity, rejection, and aggression. Teachers' and peer's ratings of hyperactivity and aggression were correlated. Teachers' ratings of peer problems correlated with actual peer popularity and rejection. Boys nominated as aggressive were more rejected, whereas boys nominated as HI were either more popular or more rejected.

(Continued)

44	Murphy et al.	1992	14 ADHD-high-aggressive boys (medicated) 12 ADHD-low-aggressive boys (medicated)	8 yr ± 1.6 7.9 yr ± 1.7	1. Naturalistic observations in recreation periods (verbal and nonverbal aggressive behaviors) 2. Laboratory provocation task (aggressive responding) 3. Hypothetical stories interview (social information processing: recall, attribution bias, and decision bias)	The high-aggressive group showed more aggression than the low-aggressive group during naturalistic observations and the laboratory provocation task. There were no high-aggressive–low-aggressive differences on the social information processing measures. Methylphenidate decreased aggression for both subgroups, and had an effect on only two recall information-processing measures.
35	Robins	1992	18 ADHD (17 males, 1 female) 25 LD (19 males, 6 females) 25 ADHD/LD (20 males, 5 females)	95.9 mo ± 15.7 112.6 mo ± 22.4 100.8 mo ± 26.5	1. A battery of standardized neuropsychological tests (WISC-R, Visual-Motor Integration, Trail Making, Matching Familiar Figures, Rey Auditory-Verbal Learning, Gordon Diagnostic System) 2. ACTeRS (teacher's ratings of child's behavior and social skills) 3. CBCL (parents' ratings of child's behavior)	Those in the ADHD or combined ADHD/LD samples were more impulsive, less accurate when response speed was required, worked less well independently, and were rated by their parents and teachers as exhibiting greater behavioral concerns (e.g., more aggressive, less compliant, and more oppositional) than the LD sample.
40	Singh et al.	1998	50 ADHD (34 males, 16 females)	5–13 yr $M = 8.6$	1. Sets of six photographs of faces and their associated sets of stories (recognition of facial expressions of emotions)	In comparison to children in the general population, children with ADHD have deficits in their ability to accurately recognize facial expressions of emotion.

(Continued)

Table 1
(Continued)

Ref.	Authors	Year	Participants	Age	Instruments (response measured)	Main results
18	Wheeler et al.	2000	16 ADHD-C (12 males, 4 females) 14 ADHD-IA (9 males, 5 females) 17 nondiagnosed controls (12 males, 5 females)	119.5 mo ± 13.85 125.4 mo ± 12.18 122.4 mo ± 9.47	1. Parents' and teachers' ratings of CABS (children's social skills—passive and aggressive —in social situations) 2. Parents' and teachers' ratings of child's social status 3. Child ratings of CABS (social knowledge and performance) 4. Emotion regulation task (child's self-ratings of affect) 5. Videotaped behavioral observations (child's facial and nonfacial expressive behavior during disappointing and nondisap pointing conditions)	ADHD subtypes exhibited difficulties in social functioning relative to controls, but the nature of their social deficits was different. Children with ADHD-C were rated as showing more aggressive behavior and displayed emotional dysregulation. In contrast, children with ADHD-IA were perceived as displaying social passivity and showed deficits in social knowledge but did not evidence problems in emotion regulation. Regardless of group, social performance, emotional regulation, and to a lesser extent, social knowledge appeared to be predictive of social status.
48	Thomeer	1996	28 ADHD (17 males, 11 females) 29 controls (15 males, 14 females)	N/A	1. Children's strategies and goals for initiating a relationship, maintaining a relationship, and resolving a conflict 2. Children's social behavior 3. Children's self-report of social anxiety 4. Knowledge of game rules	Relative to controls, children with ADHD presented strategies that were more impulsive and less relationship-enhancing, effective, and friendly. Children with ADHD also reported goals that were less positive, more negative, and more rule-oriented. The ADHD group presented more inappropriate social skills and exhibited a tendency to report more social anxiety. They also knew fewer game rules than controls.

(Continued)

Table 1
(Continued)

Ref.	Authors	Year	Participants	Age	Instruments (response measured)	Main results
47	Thurber et al.	2002	49 ADHD girls 30 non-ADHD comparison girls	115.8 mo ± 19.6 112.3 mo ± 19.4	1. Social goals interview (stated goals, self-described actions, and predicted peer thoughts in response to behaviors) 2. Peer nominations (negative and positive peer nominations) 3. Behavior observations (noncompliance, verbal aggression, and physical aggression)	No group differences found on stated social goals. Girls with ADHD generated higher rates of aggressive responses to the hypothetical vignettes than comparison girls, whereas comparison girls generated a larger number of negotiating behaviors than did the ADHD group. ADHD anticipated negative peer responses, whereas comparisons predicted positive reactions from peers. Perceived peer responses were correlated with girls' social behavior and sociometric status.
42	Tur-Kaspa and Michal	2003	48 ADHD (36 males, 12 females) 52 non-ADHD (31 males, 21 females)	Two grade levels: 2nd–4th (7–10 yr) and 7th–9th 12–14yr	1. Social information-processing interview (response access or construction and response decision processes, and the participants' internal motives for their response decisions)	ADHD in comparison to controls displayed lower social information-processing skills, in both the response access and the response decision processes. Age differences in social information-processing skills were demonstrated across the two groups, although group differences remained. Children with ADHD were likely to be driven by a will to control and to exercise power in their social interactions.

(Continued)

Table 1
(Continued)

Ref.	Authors	Year	Participants	Age	Instruments (response measured)	Main results
34	Vitaro et al.	1994	178 high-risk kindergarten boys	6 yr ± 0.2	1. Peer sociometric 2. PSBQ (teacher's ratings of child's aggressiveness and hyperactivity) 3. Pupil Evaluation Inventory (aggression, social withdrawal, and popularity) 4. SPPC (children's self-perceptions of scholastic competence, social acceptance, physical appearance, and behavior conduct) 5. Child's self-report delinquency 6. Academic performance in grades 3 and/or 4 (math and French scores) 7. Child's abstract, nonverbal cognitive abilities 8. Socio-familial adversity index (family structure, educational level, parents' occupation, mother's age)	Children who had high teacher's ratings in kindergarten of hyperactivity and aggression were more likely than children who had average or low ratings of these measures to have third- and fourth-grade outcomes of peer-ratings of aggression and self-reports of delinquency.

IT, inattentive type; HT, hyperactive type; CT, combined type.

social skills. In contrast, children with attention deficit disorder without hyperactivity, owing to their isolation and withdrawal, have fewer opportunities for social interactions with peers, and thus do not appear to acquire appropriate social knowledge. Other researchers have suggested that children with ADHD exhibit social knowledge deficits and biases, as well as social performance deficits *(6,31)*.

Presently, the existing literature is equivocal in terms of whether the social difficulties of children with ADHD are the result of social knowledge, performance deficits, or to social skills acquisition and/or performance deficits that are accompanied by interfering problem behaviors. It is more plausible to conclude that the social problems of children with ADHD are complex and multifaceted. Clearly, longitudinal studies are needed that address the complexity of the social and emotional developmental paths of children with ADHD.

Moreover, in light of growing evidence that children with ADHD are not a homogeneous group with respect to their psychological characteristics; an unanswered question is whether the documented social skills deficits are specific to certain ADHD subtypes or whether they are consistent across subtypes. Findings of a study *(50)* that explored behavioral correlates of the three *Diagnostic and Statistical Manual of Mental Disorders*, 4th edition diagnosed subtypes of ADHD in a school-based population revealed that all three ADHD subtypes exhibited poorer social functioning relative to non-ADHD controls, but showed different patterns of behavioral characteristics. Future research is needed to further investigate the social skills of ADHD children and their relation to social behavior and adjustment among the three subtypes of the disorder. In addition, the findings that an increased risk is associated with the combination of ADHD and learning disabilities, and either aggression or withdrawal *(17)* emphasize the importance of identifying appropriate behavioral and academic subgroups when investigating social status and behavior problems of these children.

Finally, recent concern has been expressed about the social-behavioral characteristics of females vs males with ADHD *(51,52)*. Gaub and Carlson's meta-analysis *(51)* revealed no significant gender differences on measures of impulsivity and social functioning among clinic-referred populations. Both boys and girls with ADHD were found to be significantly more aggressive with peers than their same-sex counterparts. However, among children with ADHD identified from nonreferred populations, girls with ADHD displayed greater intellectual impairment, lower levels of hyperactivity, and lower rates of peer aggression in comparison with boys with ADHD. Recently, similar findings were reported for young (ranging in age from 3:10 to 7:0 yr) girls and boys who met the *Diagnostic and Statistical Manual of Mental Disorders*, 4th edition criteria for ADHD, showing that they are more alike than different, with the exception that boys tend to display more symptoms of ADHD (i.e., inattention, hyperactivity/ impulsive), particularly in school *(52)*. Relatively, few studies have examined gender-based differences among children with ADHD, leaving unanswered many questions pertaining to the nature of ADHD in girls. Additional research relevant to this issue is strongly warranted.

In conclusion, the social problems of children with ADHD are obvious and pervasive and should be targeted for systematic interventions. Future research should utilize multidimensional models that will capture the complexities of the reciprocal and interactive effects of various individual and environmental factors and how they relate to social and affective characteristics of children with ADHD. This kind of research will offer an important contribution to our understanding of the social functioning of these children, and would allow us to develop effective intervention programs addressing the specific needs of children with ADHD.

REFERENCES

1. American Psychiatric Association. Diagnostic and statistical manual of mental Disorders. 4th ed. Washington DC: American Psychiatric Association, 1994.
2. Weiss G, Hechtman L. Hyperactive children grown up. New York: Guilford Press, 1993.
3. Frederick BP, Olmi, JD. Children with attention-deficit/hyperactivity disorder: A review of the literature on social skills deficits. Psychol Sch 1994;31:288–296.
4. Landau S, Moore LA. Social skill deficits in children with attention-deficit hyperactivity disorder. Psych Rev 1991;20:235–251.
5. Saunders B, Chambers SM. A review of the literature of attention-deficit hyperactivity disorder children: Peer interactions and collaborative learning. Psychol Sch 1996;33:333–340.
6. Stormont M. Social outcomes of children with AD/HD: contributing factors and implications for practice. Psychol Sch 2001;38:521–531.
7. Barkley RA. Attention-deficit hyperactivity disorder: a handbook for diagnosis and treatment. 2nd ed. New York: Guilford Press, 1998.
8. Kupersmidt JB, Coie JD, Dodge KA. The role of poor peer relationships in the development of disorder. In: Asher SR, Coie JD, eds. Peer rejection in childhood. New York: Cambridge University Press, 1990; 274–305.
9. Parker JG, Asher SR. Peer relations and later personal relations: a meta-analytic review. Psychol Bull 1987;117:306–347.
10. Wallander JL, Hubert NC. Peer social dysfunction in children with developmental disabilities: empirical basis and conceptual model. Clin Psychol Rev 1987;7:205–221.
11. Hinshaw SP, Zalecki C. Attention-deficit hyperactivity disorder. In: Orvaschel H, Faust J, Hersen M, eds. Handbook of conceptualization and treatment of child psychopathology. London: Pergamon, 2001:77–104.
12. Coie JD, Dodge KA. Continuities and changes in children's social status: a five-year longitudinal study. Merrill-Palmer Q 1983;29:261–282.
13. Erhardt D, Hinshaw SP. Initial sociometric impressions of attention-deficit hyperactivity disorder and comparison boys: prediction from social behaviors and from nonbehavioral variables. J Consult Clin Psychol 1994;62:833–842.
14. Hinshaw SP, Melnick SM. Peer relationships in boys with attention-deficit hyperactivity disorder and comparison with and without co-morbid aggression. Dev Psychopathol 1995;7:627–647.
15. Pelham WE, Bender ME. Peer relationships in hyperactive children: Description and treatment. In: Gadow KD, Bialer I, eds. Advances in learning and behavioral disabilities: a research annual.Vol. 1. Greenwich, CT: JAI Press, 1982:365–436.
16. Hinshaw SP, Zupan BA, Simmel C, Nigg JT, Melnick S. Peer status in boys with and without attention-deficit hyperactivity disorder: Predictions from overt and covert antisocial behavior, social isolation, and authoritative parenting beliefs. Child Dev 1997;68:880–896.
17. Flicek M. Social status of boys with both academic problems and attention-deficit hyperactivity disorder. J Abnorm Child Psychol 1992;20:353–366.
18. Wheeler Maedgen J, Carlson CL. Social functioning and emotional regulation in the attention deficit hyperactivity disorder subtypes. J Clin Child Psychol 2000;29:30–42.
19. Mash EJ, Johnston C. Sibling interactions of hyperactive and normal children and their relationship to reports of maternal stress and self-esteem. J Consult Clin Psychol 1983;51:86–98.
20. Whalen CK, Henker B. The social worlds of hyperactive (ADHD) children. Clin Psychol Rev 1985;5:447–478.
21. Alessandri SM . Attention, play, and social behavior in ADHD preschoolers. J Abnorm Child Psychol 1992;20:353–366.
22. Cunningham CE, Siegel LS. Peer interactions of normal and attention-deficit hyperactivity disordered boys during free-play, cooperative task, and simulated classroom situations. J Abnorm Child Psychol 1987;15:247–268.
23. Hubbard JA, Newcomb AF. Initial dyadic peer interactions of attention deficit-hyperactivity disorder and normal boys. J Abnorm Child Psychol 1991;19:179–195.

24. Landau S, McAninch C. Young children with attention deficits. Young Child 1983;48:49–58.
25. Milich R, Landau S, Kilby G, Whitten P. Preschool peer perceptions of the behavior of hyperactive and aggressive children. J Abnorm Child Psychol 1982;10:497–510.
26. Merrell KW, Wolfe TM. The relationship of teacher-rated social skills deficits and ADHD characteristics among kindergarten-age children. Psychol Sch 1998;35:101–109.
27. Wheeler J, Carlson CL. The social functioning of children with ADD with hyperactivity and ADD without hyperactivity: a comparison of their peer relations and social deficits. J Emotion Behav Disord 1994;2:2–11.
28. Luk S. Direct observations studies of hyperactive behaviors. J Am Acad Child Adolesc Psychiatry 1985;24:338–344.
29. Barkley RA. Behavioral inhibition, sustained attention, and executive functions:Constructing a unifying theory of ADHD. Psychol Bull 1997;121:265–294.
30. Gresham FM. Social skills: conceptual and applied aspects of assessment, training, and social validation. In Witt JC, Elliot SN, Gresham FM, eds. Handbook of behavior therapy in education. New York: Plenum, 1988:523–546.
31. Grenell MM, Glass CR, Katz KS. Hyperactive children and peer interaction: knowledge and performance of social skills. J Abnorm Child Psychol 1987;15:1–13.
32. Campbell SB, Ewing LJ. Follow-up of hard to manage preschoolers: adjustment at age 9 and predictors of continuing symptoms. J Child Psychol Psychiatr 1990;31:871–889.
33. Dodge KA, Lansford JE, Salzer Burks V, et al. Peer rejection and social information-processing factors in the development of aggressive behavior in children. Child Dev 2003;74:374–393.
34. Vitaro F, Tremblay RE, Gagnon C, Pelletier D. Predictive accuracy of behavioral and sociometric assessments of high-risk kindergarten children. J Clin Child Psychol 1994;23:272–282.
35. Robins PM. A comparison of behavioral and attentional functioning in children diagnosed as hyperactive or learning-disabled. J Abnorm Child Psychol 1992;20:65–82.
36. Crick NR, Dodge KA. A review and reformulation of social information-processing mechanisms in children's social adjustment. Psychol Bull 1994;115:74–101.
37. Dodge KA, Richard BA. Peer perceptions, aggression and the development of peer relations. In: Pryor JB, Day JD, eds. Social developmental perspectives of social cognition. New York: Springer Verlag, 1985:35–38.
38. Dodge KA. A social information processing model of social competence in children. In: Perlmutter M, ed. Cognitive perspective on children's social and behavioral development: The Minnesota Symposia on Child Psychology. Vol. 18. Hillsdale, NJ: Lawrence Erlbaum, 1986:77–125.
39. Ladd GW, Mize J. A cognitive-social learning model of social skills training. Psychol Rev 1983;90:127–157.
40. Singh SD, Ellis CR, Winton ASW, Singh NN, Leung JP, Oswald DP. Recognition of facial expressions of emotion by children with attention-deficit hyperactivity disorder. Behav Modif 1998;22:128–142.
41. Milch-Reich S, Campbell SB, Pelham WE, Connelly LM, Geva D. Developmental and individual differences in children's on-line representations of dynamic social events. Child Dev 1999;70:413–431.
42. Tur-Kaspa H, Michal Y. Social information-processing skills of students with ADHD. Poster presented at the Society for Research in Child Development Conference. Tampa, FL, 2003.
43. Milich R, Dodge KA. Social information processing in child psychiatric populations. J Abnorm Child Psychol 1984;12:471–490.
44. Murphy DA, Pelham WR, Lang AR. Aggression in boys with attention deficit hyperactivity disorder: methylphenidate effects on naturalistically observed aggression, response to provocation, and social information processing. J Abnorm Child Psychol 1992;20:451–465.
45. Bloomquist ML, August GJ, Cohen C, Doyle A, Everhart K. Socialproblem solving in hyperactive-aggressive children: how and what they think in conditions of automatic and controlled processing. J Clin Child Psychol 1997; 26: 172–180.
46. Melnick SM, Hinshaw SP. What they want and what they get: the social goals of boys with ADHD and comparison boys. J Abnorm Child Psychol 1996;24:169–185.

47. Thurber JR, Heller TL, Hinshaw SP. The social behaviors and peer expectation of girls with attention deficit hyperactivity disorder and comparison girls. J Clin Child Adolesc Psychol 2002;31:443–452.
48. Thomeer ML. The social knowledge and peer relationships of girls with ADHD in comparison to boys with ADHD and non-disordered children. Diss Abstr Int 1996; 57(06):4061.
49. Gresham FM, MacMillan DL. Social competence and affective characteristics of students with mild disabilities. Rev Educ Res 1997;67:377–415.
50. Gaub M, Carlson CL. Behavioral characteristics of DSM-IV ADHD subtypes in a school-based population. J Abnorm Child Psychol 1997;25:103–111.
51. Gaub M, Carlson CL. Gender differences in ADHD: a meta-analysis and critical review. J Am Acad Child Adolesc Psychiatry 1997;36:1036–1045.
52. Hartung CM, Willcutt EG, Lahey BB, Pelham WE, Loney J, Stein MA, Keenan K. Sex differences in young children who met criteria for attention deficit hyperactivity disorder. J Clin Child Adolesc Psychol 2002;31:453–464.

15
Reading Disabilities in Children With Attention Deficit Hyperactivity Disorder

Juliana S. Bloom, Carlin J. Miller, Mauricio A. Garcia, and George W. Hynd

1. INTRODUCTION

The term learning disabilities (LD) describes a broad category of developmental disorders and refers to a deficit in learning in one or more domains, which can include reading, mathematics, and writing *(1)*. Diagnosis is based on behavioral information and assumes adequate intelligence, intact sensory systems, and the absence of a handicapping condition or environment that would cause a person to have significant difficulty learning *(2)*. Although intervention can be effective, these difficulties in learning are persistent throughout the life-span *(3)*.

Subsumed under the broad category of LD, reading disability (RD), also known as dyslexia, has been most widely researched and is the best understood disorder at this time, and will thus be the focus of this chapter. In the past decade, a consensus has been reached among researchers that, for the majority of children with RD, the core deficit is difficulty with phonological processing *(3,4)*, although research continues to support an orthographic or visual deficit *(5)* and a rapid naming speed deficit *(6)*. The underlying cognitive deficits in RD are presumed to be related to neurobiological abnormalities, which will be discussed in detail later in this chapter.

A plethora of research has supported the idea that RD tends to run in families *(7)* and, in fact, research suggests that 50% of the variance in reading problems can be explained by genetic influences *(8)*. Several studies have specifically implicated chromosomes 6 and 15 *(9)*. Traditionally, RD was thought to affect more boys than girls *(10)* but some research has suggested that the increased prevalence in boys is a result of selection bias and that, in fact, girls and boys are equally affected by the disorder *(11)*.

LD often co-occur with attention deficit hyperactivity disorder (ADHD), a disorder of inattention and behavioral disinhibition affecting between 3 and 5% of children *(2)*. Although it is difficult to determine the concordance rate between ADHD and LD because of the different diagnostic definitions of both disorders used by researchers, it is clear that children with ADHD are more likely to have a LD than typically developing children *(12)*. Whereas 3–6% of the childhood population is estimated to have a LD *(13)*, the percentage of children with ADHD who have a co-occurring LD is significantly higher. Between 8 and 39% of children with ADHD meet criteria for RD, 12–27% have a spelling disability, and 12–30% have a

From: *Attention Deficit Hyperactivity Disorder: From Genes to Patients*
Edited by: D. Gozal and D. L. Molfese © Humana Press Inc., Totowa, NJ

math disability *(12)*. The high concordance rate of these two disorders has led to speculation surrounding the nature of the relationship between the two disorders. Is ADHD a consequence of LD, are learning problems a consequence of ADHD, or are the two disorders separate in etiology but frequently comorbid? These, and other questions, deserve attention.

2. COMMONALITIES BETWEEN ADHD AND RD

2.1. Cognitive Deficits

The cognitive deficits found in ADHD and RD have been the focus of much research, with the focus on inattention, language problems, and memory deficits. In the following sections, the research on the common and differentiating cognitive deficits found in ADHD and RD will be reviewed, with a summary of the literature contained in Table 1.

2.1.1. Inattention

The main commonality between individuals with ADHD and RD is the presence of difficulties with attention present in each group *(14,15)*. Attention is a multidimensional construct that can refer to "alertness, arousal, selectivity, sustained attention, distractibility, or span of apprehension" *(12)*. Individuals with ADHD have, by the definition of the disorder, age-inappropriate difficulties with attention and tend to have most difficulty with sustained attention, particularly during uninteresting or dull tasks, such as homework or independent classwork *(12)*. Thus, children with ADHD tend to avoid difficult or unappealing schoolwork or have difficulty concentrating on such schoolwork. Children with RD also tend to avoid schoolwork, particularly language-based tasks like reading and writing, because they can be too difficult or overwhelming. Thus, behaviorally, school-aged children with ADHD and RD tend to look alike when engaged in schoolwork. In fact, some researchers have found that inattention is present in both disorders *(16)* and many children with learning disabilities without ADHD have significant attention problems *(15)*. The overlap in dysfunctions of attention and the high concordance rate between the two disorders have caused researchers to question the nature of the relationship between the two disorders and the role of attention dysfunction in both disorders *(16–18)*.

August and Garfinkel presented three possible explanations for the presence of inattention in individuals with RD *(16)*. First, inattention is a nonspecific behavior that increases as a consequence of the child's reaction to reading difficulty; second, inattention precedes reading difficulty and affects the child's academic performance; and, as a third possibility, inattention is unrelated to RDs but the two conditions are frequently comorbid. Pennington, et al. introduced a "phenocopy" hypothesis of ADHD in the presence of RD *(19)*. According to Pennington et al.'s hypothesis, when comparing RD, ADHD, and RD/ADHD groups, the RD/ADHD or comorbid group shows cognitive deficits similar to those found in the pure RD children, and show only behavioral characteristics of children with ADHD—among them, the inattention symptom. Thus, the inattention found in RD is an associated cognitive problem of RD but does not represent the disorder ADHD.

There are several studies that have analyzed and contrasted cognitive skills among groups of children with pure ADHD, pure RD, and comorbid ADHD/RD. These studies vary widely in their methodology, but have allowed researchers to test the hypotheses regarding the overlap of ADHD and RD with regard to attention.

Kupietz used the continuous performance test (CPT) to evaluate similarities and differences in performances by children with developmental reading disabilities (DRD) and those

Table 1
Cognitive Deficits in ADHD and Reading Disabilities

Authors	Participants	Diagnostic criteria	Findings
August and Garfinkel, 1990	From 115 ADHD boys, an RD subgroup was subdivided. • 7–17 yr of age • No diagnosed neurological or pervasive disorder • IQ ≥ 80 in the Peabody Picture Vocabulary Test-Revised (PPVT-R) 70 children diagnosed with ADHD 45 children diagnosed with comorbid ADHD/RD 50 normal boys (control group)	ADHD: diagnoses based on a semistructured interview administered to the parents and a comprehensive diagnostic evaluation To classify an ADHD child as ADHD/RD: Either the Reading or Spelling subtest of the Wide Range Achievement Test-Revised had to be 85 or less, and at least 15 points below his PPVT-R IQ	1. The results on the Corners hyperactivity index showed attentional and behavioral problems on both groups 2. Some of the ADHD patients presented attention deficit plus RD whereas others only attentional difficulties 3. The measures of attention from the cognitive battery failed on distinguishing members from the pure ADHD and the ADHD/RD groups, possibly becaused a lack of clear differentiation between groups
Hynd et al., 1995	Two studies The first compared children with RD to those with RD plus comorbid psychopathology, primarily ADHD (RD+) • 6–15 yr of age • 27 males, 7 females • 17 diagnosed with RD, 17 diagnosed with RD+ The second compared children with RD to children with ADHD on neurolinguistic measures • 8–11 yr of age with parents • 27 males, 7 females • 16 diagnosed with RD, 18 diagnosed with ADHD	RD: ≥ 20-point discrepancy between IQ and reading achievement RD+: Meet DSM-IV criteria for diagnosis of ADHD, depression, or dysthymia, rating scales from parents and teachers, structured interview with parents ADHD: Meet DSM-IV criteria for diagnosis of ADHD, rating scales from parents and teachers, structured interview with parents	Study 1: 1. There were no significant differences between RD and RD+ on neurolinguistic measures Study 2: 2. The RD group had relative deficits in phonological processes and language 3. Neurolinguistic deficits are specific to RD even when comorbid psychopathology exists

(Continued)

Table 1
(Continued)

Authors	Participants	Diagnostic criteria	Findings
Johnson et al., 1999	• 80 children • 7–13 yr of age 40 children with ADHD and 40 with UADD (DSM-III-R) were matched on FSIQ, grade, and gender Both groups with ADHD were subdivided into with and without RD, leaving four groups: ADHD+LD, ADHD-LD, UADD+LD, and UADD-LD	ADHD/UADD: Clinical sample from an ADHD-LD clinic at a university teaching hospital, with FSIQ ≥ 85 and no comorbid disorders. RD: ≥ 15-point discrepancy between IQ and reading achievement or reading achievement at least one gradex at least their current placement	1. Children with ADHD + LD and UADD + LD had greater memory deficits 2. Children with ADHD had significantly more memory deficits than children with UADD
Korkman and Pesonen, 1994	Sixty children with ADHD, LD, and the comorbid condition. Average verbal or verbal IQ No significant emotional or conduct problems • 8 yr old children • 45 boys, 15 girls • ADHD ($n = 21$), LD ($n = 12$), and ADHD/LD ($n = 27$)	ADHD: Meet DSM-III criteria for diagnosis of ADHD LD: < 6th percentile on a spelling achievement test	1. All groups had difficulties with visual-motor precision and name retrieval 2. Children with ADHD showed deficits in impulse control 3. Children with LD were impaired in phonological awareness, verbal memory, and verbal IQ 4. Children with ADHD/LD showed deficiencies from both groups and had more pervasive attention and visual-motor programs
Kupietz, 1990	Three groups: Developmental Reading Disabled (DRD), DRD + ADHD, and normal controls (NC) • 7–12 yr of age • FSIQ ≥ 80 11 children with DRD (9 boys, 2 girls)	DRD: Met DSM-IIIR criteria; in addition, they achieved an estimated reading level 75% or less of expected for their grade placement. DRD/ADHD: Met DSM-III criteria; and also, they had to receive a mean teacher rating of at least 1.5 on	1. All three groups showed a decrement in sustained attention indicated by a decline in correct detections from the first to the second half of the CPT 2. DRD and DRD/ADHD were clearly differentiated from NC by the CPT 3. An age compensation effect was found in the DRD group, but was not observed in the

(Continued)

Table 1
(Continued)

Authors	Participants	Diagnostic criteria	Findings
	13 children with comorbid DRD/ ADHD (11 boys, 2 girls) 11 controls (8 boys, 3 girls)	the hyperactivity factor of the Conners Teacher Rating Scale. NC: no IQ scores were available, but they had no history of classroom behavioral problems. Conners and reading measures were normal	DRD/ADHD group
Mayes et al.,1994	• 119 children referred to a diagnostic clinic for attention, learning, and mood problems • 8–16 yr old • FSIQ ≥ 85	ADHD: DSM-IV diagnosis agreed upon by two professionals; only ADHD-CT used in this study LD: Achievement score significantly lower ($p < .05$) than predicted based on FSIQ	1. LD was present in 70% of children with ADHD LD written expression two times more common than reading, math, or spelling 2. Children with ADHD/LD had more severe learning and attention problems than those with LD and ADHD alone 3. Children with LD had attention problems and children with ADHD had learning problems, suggesting a continuum of disorders
Närhi and Ahonen, 1995	• 8–12 yr old • 73 males • VIQ/PIQ ≥ 80 21 males diagnosed with pure RD 25 males diagnosed with comorbid ADHD/RD 17 males diagnosed with pure ADHD 10 NCS	ADHD: Score of 18 or more on the Attention Scale of the Child Behavior Checklist-Teacher Report Form RD: Based on an aged-normed text reading test, time, speed, accuracy, and number of correct read words were measured. They calculated a quotient of correct read words per time unit and the children were classified as RD or non-RD using a cutoff point of a T-score of 30	1. Naming speed is a marker deficit of RD, regardless of the presence or absence of attentional problems 2. The poor reading performance of the comorbid group is not becaused poor attentional skills but it is the result of deficient reading acquisition 3. No specific executive dysfunctions in the pure ADHD group as was hypothesized were found

(Continued)

Table 1
(Continued)

Authors	Participants	Diagnostic criteria	Findings
Pennington et al., 1993	• 70 boys • 7–10 yr old • FSIQ ≥ 80 • RD (n = 15), ADHD (n = 16), ADHD/RD (n = 23), and control (n = 16) groups	ADHD: ≥SD above the mean in hyperactivity and pervasivesness, with an age of onset before the age of 6 RD: Significant discrepancy between observed and expected reading levels, based on intelligence, age, and educational experience	1. Children with RD were significantly impaired on phonological processes but had normal performance on executive functioning measures 2. Children with ADHD were significantly impaired on executive functioning but normal performance had on phonological processesing measures 3. The comorbid group resembled the RD-only group, suggesting that ADHD is secondary to RD in this group
Shaywitz et al., 1995	• 186 children • 7.5–9.5 yr old • English as primary language 43 children diagnosed with RD 59 children diagnosed with comorbid RD/ADHD 34 children diagnosed with ADHD 50 no impairment	RD: defined by using both discrepancy and low-achievement definitions. ADHD: met at least eight items of the DSM-III-R criteria for ADHD diagnosis by parents' endorsement; and/or scores 1.5 SD above the mean on the Attention, Activity, and Impulsivity scales of the Yale Children's Inventory.	1. The ADHD group performed lower on the measure of attentional skills (visual attention) 2. On individual testing, pure ADHD patients performed well on those linguistic measures that was very difficult for those with pure RD and RD/ADHD, but performed less well on a measure of selective attention 3. This study evidences that RD and ADHD are two distinct disorders that can co-occur frequently, where RD core symptom is an impaired phonological processing, inattention can be found in both but it is considered core symptom on ADHD, and where children with only RD have similar behavioral and cognitive profile to those with comorbidity RD/ADHD

DSM-IV, *The Diagnostic and Statistical Manual of Mental Disorders*, 4th edition; RD, reading disabilities; UADD, undifferentiated attention deficit disorder; LD, learning disabilities; PIQ, Picture IQ; VIQ verbal IQ; FSIQ, full-scale IQ; CPT, continuous performance Test; SD, standard deviation.

with ADHD *(17)*. In both groups, a sustained attention decrement from the first half to the second half of the task was found. The DRD group showed a larger decrement; however, they also showed improvement with age, which was not found in the ADHD group. August and Garfinkel found similar results for attentional and behavioral problems on the Revised Conners Teacher Questionnaire *(16)*. However, on the cognitive battery the measures of attention did not distinguish members of the pure ADHD and the ADHD/RD groups. In contrast to the behavioral scales, the authors found that some of the ADHD patients presented with attention deficit in addition to RDs, although others presented only with attentional difficulties *(16)*.

Other studies have shown conflicting results with regard to the presence or absence of inattention among children with RD and ADHD. For example, Närhi and Ahonen *(20)* compared four groups—pure RD, pure ADHD, comorbid RD/ADHD, and clinical controls—on measures of executive functions and rapid naming. Rapid automatized naming speed had been found to be predictive of reading skills before reading acquisition, in children from grades 1 and 2 *(20)*. In their conclusions, the authors reported that naming speed is a marker deficit of RD, regardless of the presence or absence of attentional problems. They also found that the poor reading performance of the comorbid group was owing not to poor attentional skills but to deficient reading acquisition. In addition, the hypothesized specific executive dysfunction was not found in the pure ADHD group. Specifically, they concluded, "The problems in reading acquisition of children in the comorbid group are due to factors that are also found in the purely reading-disabled group and are not explainable by attentional deficits" *(20)*. Those results are consistent with a later study developed by Nigg et al. *(21)*, in which the naming task performance provided evidence to distinguish, in an ADHD group, a cognitive subgroup with comorbid RD. Attention was not analyzed in this study.

Shaywitz et al. *(18)* also studied the relationship between ADHD and RD. As in the previous examples, they found differences in the attentional skills among children with ADHD, ADHD/RD, and RD. Behavioral characteristics and cognitive skills were assessed in this study. Children with RD showed poor performance on the phonological awareness, rapid naming, and speech production measures. On the other hand, children with ADHD and ADHD/RD demonstrated deficits in behavior and attention that were not found in children with RD alone. The comorbid group showed characteristics of both disorders: cognitive/linguistic deficits like those found in RD alone, and behavioral/attentional problems as found in ADHD alone. It is important to note that these deficits were additive, not synergistic, in the comorbid group.

Evidence suggests that RD and ADHD are two distinct disorders that can co-occur frequently. In RD the core symptom is an impaired phonological processing, while in ADHD the core symptoms are behavioral problems and executive functions, including inattention. Thus, the majority of studies to date support August and Garfinkel's *(16)* third explanation for the presence of inattention in RD and ADHD children, namely that RD and ADHD are separate disorders that frequently co-occur. Furthermore, studies suggest that the cognitive deficits in comorbid ADHD/LD are additive, not synergistic *(22–24)*.

2.1.2. Language

Although language problems in children with RD have been well documented, it appears that language dysfunction of a different nature also occurs in children with ADHD. Children with ADHD tend to talk excessively and in a disorganized fashion *(12)*. Previous research has shown that children with ADHD have difficulty on tasks of verbal fluency and are more likely to have an expressive rather than a receptive language disorder. These findings suggest that language problems in a child with ADHD are related to an inability to organize, monitor, and produce language, or the executive processes in language *(12)*.

Purvis and Tannock examined the language abilities of children with ADHD, RD, ADHD/RD, and controls *(23)*. Results indicated the presence of receptive and expressive language problems in children with RD. For children with ADHD, deficits were characterized by difficulties organizing and monitoring language. Children with comorbid ADHD and RD experienced both sets of deficits. Thus, this study suggests that children with ADHD and RD have a dysfunction of language, which is related to the semantics of language processing in children with RD and related to executive functions in children with ADHD.

2.1.3. Memory

Memory deficits have been associated with RD and ADHD in the literature for many years. Findings generally have suggested that children with RD have memory deficits that are limited to the verbal domain *(22,25,26)*, whereas memory deficits in ADHD are found across domains in working memory *(12)*. However, working memory deficits have also been found by some researchers in children with RD *(27)*, although, consistent with the theory of domain specificity, they are limited to phonological information *(28)*. When RD and ADHD are comorbid, memory deficits were more severe than in children with pure RD or pure ADHD *(22)*.

2.2. Internalizing and Externalizing Problems in ADHD and RD

2.2.1. Internalizing Disorders in LD and RD

Research suggests that individuals with LDs may be at risk for internalizing disorders *(26,29,30)*. Theory has held that individuals with LD experience psychological maladjustment owing to repeated academic failures, which predispose the individual to internalization *(29)*. Research supports the idea that LDs are associated with elevated levels of internalizing behavior, such as anxiety, withdrawal, depression, and low self-esteem *(26)*. However, the internalization does not reach clinically significant levels in individuals with LD *(29,30)*. These findings may be because of the fact that research in this area has been conducted on individuals with all subtypes of LD, which is a very heterogenous group *(29)*. In fact, there is a growing body of research that suggests that individuals with nonverbal LDs are much more likely to have psychosocial disturbance and behavioral problems than individuals with language-based LD, such as RD *(1,29)*. This idea is supported by the fact that, in a study of internalizing behavior in a group of parents of children with reading problems, no relationship was found between parent reading fluency and internalizing behavior *(30)*. Further research is needed to determine the prevalence of internalizing disorders in individuals with nonverbal or language-based LD.

2.2.2. Internalizing Disorders in ADHD

Children with ADHD are significantly more likely than controls to meet criteria for an internalizing disorder, with approx 25% of children with ADHD meeting criteria for a comorbid anxiety or mood disorder *(12)*. Rates of comorbid internalizing disorders are higher for individuals with cormorbid ADHD and LD than in children with LD who do not have ADHD *(12)*, suggesting that the presence of ADHD increases the risk of an anxiety or mood disorder. Although many have theorized that this concordance rate stems from failure in school and with peers, there is also evidence that some individuals with ADHD may be genetically predisposed for internalization. Research suggests that although anxiety disorders are transmitted independently from ADHD in families with comorbid children, there is evidence of a genetic linkage between depression and ADHD *(12)*. Thus, strong evidence exists to support the idea that internalizing disorders occur frequently in individuals with ADHD.

2.2.3. *Externalizing Disorders in LD and RD*

There is evidence for an elevated level of externalizing disorders in individuals with LD—particularly in hyperactivity, delinquency, and aggression—but, as with internalizing disorders, the elevations are not clinically significant and can again be attributed to those individuals with nonverbal LD *(29)*. In addition, studies are often confounded by the presence of ADHD in samples of children with LD *(1,30)*. Further research is necessary to determine the nature of the relationship between RD and externalizing disorders.

2.2.4. *Externalizing Disorders in ADHD*

Externalizing disorders, such as oppositional defiant disorder (ODD) and conduct disorder (CD), are found frequently in individuals with ADHD *(12)*. Prevalence rates range from 54 to 67% for individuals with ADHD who meet criteria for ODD, and 20–56% for individuals with ADHD who meet criteria for CD. These extremely high rates of prevalence have led some researcher to question whether these disorders were distinct, but research has shown that these disorders do exist independently of one another and have different developmental trajectories *(12)*. It is likely that the impulsivity and difficulty following rule-governed behavior found in ADHD contributes to the development of externalizing disorders in individuals with ADHD.

2.3. *Social Problems*

Research has found that social skills deficits have been found in individuals with both ADHD and LD *(12,26)*. Research on social skills deficits in individuals with LD, however, have used groups of individuals with all subtypes of LD *(26)*. It has been well documented that individuals with nonverbal LD tend to demonstrate social impairments *(31)*, and it is possible that this group has influenced the results of previous studies *(26)*. Further research is needed to determine the presence of social impairments in individuals with language-based LDs.

Theory has held that children with ADHD are rejected from peer groups owing to their communication problems, aggression, and disruptive behavior. In fact, research has shown that this social rejection by peers often occurs within 20–30 min of entering a social situation *(12)*. Social isolation and rejection lead to a deficit in social skills and, possibly, an increase in hostile attribution biases, which will further the cycle. It has been estimated that more than half of children with ADHD have social skills deficits.

2.4. *Underachievement/School Problems*

LDs—in particular, RDs—often lead to special-education placements for children who are struggling in school. The presence of ADHD symptoms, whether or not a formal diagnosis is made, compounds these struggles for the child, his or her teacher, and the family. According to Pfiffner and Barkley, ADHD often leads to significant problems at school, including but not limited to disruptive classroom behavior, academic under-performance, need for tutoring, grade retention, special education placement, school suspension and expulsion, and school dropout *(32)*. Research suggests that children with comorbid ADHD and RD have significantly more learning difficulties than children with either single disorder *(15)*.

Much of the symptom overlap between ADHD and RD is related to the previously described attention problems and difficulties with other comorbid disorders. These attention problems may lead to learning problems and vice versa *(33)*, although many children with LDs without ADHD also have significant attention problems *(15)*. The child with comorbid ADHD and RD has difficulty learning because of both the attention problems and the underlying reading problems. It may become a situation in which the child has difficulty paying attention, is not successful at learning to read, and his or her motivation drops. As the child falls further behind, he or she develops avoidance strategies and behavior problems that are more common in the classroom, but may also be present in other environments. In some cases, as attention improves, academic difficulties may also improve *(34)*. There is also evidence to suggest that as symptom severity increases, academic impairment also increases *(35)*.

3. NEUROBIOLOGICAL COMMONALITIES IN ADHD AND RD

Many commonalties are to be found in the neurobiological basis of ADHD and RD. What follows are brief descriptions of the neurobiology of ADHD and RD, as well as common findings. For more information on the neurobiology of ADHD, please *see* Chapter 9.

3.1. Neurobiology of ADHD

Generally, two kinds of methods are used in research to study the relationships between brain morphology/functioning and ADHD: brain imaging and neuropsychological correlations. ADHD has traditionally been associated with dysfunction in the frontal lobes, because of the association between the behavioral characteristics of ADHD and frontal-lobe functions. Some studies have differentiated normal controls from children with ADHD by using neuropsychological measures for the frontal lobe systems, but others failed in differentiating between individuals with ADHD and other clinical groups *(36–38)*.

Since the widespread use of imaging techniques for research purposes began in the 1990s, magnetic resonance imaging (MRI) studies have supported the idea that a distributed circuit underlies ADHD. This circuit includes right prefrontal brain regions, the caudate nucleus, globus pallidus, and a subregion of the cerebellar vermis. In recent research, three different circuits have been defined *(39)*. First, is a dorsolateral circuit, which would subserve executive function and include the dorsolateral cortex, dorsal caudate nucleus head, internal globus pallidus, mediodorsal nucleus of the thalamus, and the dorsal cortex of areas 9 and 10 of the frontal lobes. The second proposed circuit is the orbitofrontal circuit, which is formed by two parallel subcircuits: the lateral orbitofrontal circuits send projections to the ventromedial caudate nucleus, and the medial orbitofrontal circuits send projections to the ventral putamen and nucleus accumbens. Both circuits have been associated with the control of behaviors and emotions. The third circuit is the anterior cingulate circuit, which is related to motivational and inhibitory control *(39)*.

A major area of interest in the neurobiology of ADHD relates to frontal lobe size, asymmetry, and volume. Work by Hynd and colleagues demonstrated that although normal children evidence bigger left than right anterior-width measurements of the frontal lobes, this normal anterior asymmetry is not found in children with ADHD *(40)*. According to Hynd et al.'s study, children with ADHD have often shown significantly smaller right anterior width measurements than normal *(40)*. Pueyo et al. also found a reversed pattern of asymmetry for the frontal lobe; specifically, they found a reduction of the right frontal lobe size in the ADHD group *(41)*.

Another brain region frequently examined by researchers is the caudate nucleus. Pueyo et al. found a reverse pattern of asymmetry for the caudate nucleus in ADHD vs controls, with the right being larger *(41)*. Pineda and colleagues analyzed the alterations of the asymmetry and size of the caudate nucleus in two groups of ADHD children—combined type and inattentive type—and one control group *(39)*. In contrast with previous studies *(41–45)*, the authors did not find significant differences among measurements of the caudate in ADHD children when compared with normal controls or between ADHD subgroups. They concluded that their results did not support the hypothesis of the reversal asymmetry of the caudate nucleus discussed in previous studies *(39)*.

Another line of research on the neurobiological basis of ADHD is focused on cellular development and is based on a qualitative inspection of brain imaging. One study found gray-matter heterotopias and enlarged posterior fossa abnormalities in patients with ADHD *(46)*. These neurobiological aberrations occur during the second trimester of gestation, and likely play an important role in ADHD psychopathology *(46)*. However, these neurodevelopmental anomalies alone are not considered sufficient to explain the psychopathology of ADHD.

The normal brain mechanism of attention has been extensively studied *(47–49)*. The involvement of atypical levels of neurotransmitters has also been researched, supported by neurophysiological and neurochemical studies *(50–52)*. According to these theories, some neurotransmitters, specifically the catecholamines, dopamine and norepinephrine, have been implicated in ADHD. These neurotransmitters are thought to affect attention, inhibition, response of the motor system, and motivation. An imbalance in the formation of one of these neurotransmitters results in decreased stimulation of certain brain stem regions, such as the locus coeruleus, affecting arousal level and frontal lobe functioning. The efficacy on ADHD of treatment with psychostimulants has provided support for these ideas by showing that altering neurotransmitter activity alleviates ADHD symptomatology *(53,54)*.

3.2. *Neurobiology of RDs*

As early as the turn of the last century, researchers had begun to believe that reading deficits were the result of underlying differences in brain development. Hinshelwood correctly hypothesized that these neurodevelopmental differences were primarily in the angular and supramarginal gyri of the left hemisphere *(55)*. Although research has subsequently documented neurobiological differences in individuals with dyslexia throughout the brain, Hinshelwood's early hypothesis centered on those areas that have continued to be the focus of dyslexia research.

According to Riccio and Hynd, empirical studies have provided supporting evidence for the "widespread reorganization of the neurological system in individuals with dyslexia" *(56)*. Areas involved in the processing of language and visual information have received much of the research focus. Areas involved in language processing and implicated in dyslexia research include the planum temporale, Broca's areas, the angular gyrus, and the perisylvian region *(40,56–60)*. The magnocellular pathway, particularly the lateral geniculate nucleus of the thalamus, and the occipital cortex have also been reported to be linked to the visual processes involved in reading *(61)*. Additionally, dyslexia research has also highlighted the role of the corpus callosum in neurolinguistic deficits *(62)*.

The perisylvian region, particularly the planum temporale, has received most of the research attention in dyslexia studies. An early study of postmortem brains demonstrated that leftward asymmetry of the planum temporale is typical, with 65% of brains showing leftward asymmetry *(63)*. That study also reported that 11% of individuals had rightward asymmetry and 24% had symmetrical plana. Although premortem reading ability or reading history was not reported in the study, the leftward asymmetry of the planum temporale was clearly more typical in a postmortem population. A later study reported postmortem results from a young man who had been diagnosed with dyslexia during childhood *(64)*. According to that study, postmortem examination of the brain revealed symmetrical plana and polymicrogyri in the perisylvian region. Numerous other studies have also demonstrated that rightward asymmetry or symmetrical plana are more common in individuals with dyslexia than in the general population *(40,65–69)*.

In addition to documented rightward asymmetry or symmetry of the plana frequently present with dyslexia, cortical abnormalities in the temporoparietal region have also received some research attention. According to several studies, neuronal migration errors, also known as focal dysplasias or heterotopias, are also more common in individuals with dyslexia than the general population *(66)*. These migration errors are most commonly in the temporoparietal region with dyslexia *(70)*. Additionally, polymicrogyri, or an usually large number of atypically small folds in the surface of the brain *(71)*, are also more frequent in individuals with dyslexia than in the general population, particularly in the perisylvian region *(64, 66)*.

The gyral and sulcal morphology of the perisylvian region, which includes the planum temporale, has also been described as being frequently atypical in individuals with dyslexia. Steinmetz and colleagues developed a subtyping system to describe the gyral morphology of the region, which includes the shape and position of the posterior ascending ramus of the Sylvian fissure and the inferior postcentral sulcus *(72)*. Using both postmortem measurements and MRI images of live individuals, the system includes four subtypes. According to the initial studies reported by Steinmetz and colleagues, 65–67% of individuals have the most common subtype (Type I) in the left hemisphere and 82–85% in the right hemisphere, without regard to reading ability *(72)*. In contrast, 12–36% of individuals had the less-typical subtypes (Types II–IV) in the left hemisphere and 15–18% in the right hemisphere. When the same subtyping system was applied to individuals with neurolinguistic deficits and their biological relatives, studies have demonstrated that there was an increased incidence of atypical morphology and a decreased incidence of typical morphology when compared with the initial population *(59,73)*.

3.3. *Neurobiological Commonalities Across ADHD and RD*

In addition to the research on ADHD and RD summarized in previous sections, there is a growing body of literature addressing the commonalities across RD and ADHD from the neurobiological perspective. Although these disorders appear to be independent of each other *(24)*, there is significant evidence to suggest that the frequent co-occurrence of ADHD and RD might be expected based on similarities found in volumetric, biochemical, psychophysiological, and genetic studies. In the following sections, this research on the neurobiological commonalities across ADHD and RD will be reviewed, with a summary of the literature contained in Table 2.

3.3.1. Volumetric Evidence

The regions of interest in the volumetric studies of the comorbidity of ADHD and RD are very similar to those regions targeted in the previously reviewed literature, namely the

Table 2
Common Neurobiological Bases of ADHD and Reading Disabilities

Authors	Participants	Diagnostic criteria	Findings
Clarke et al., 2002	• 8–12 yr of age • 18 males in each group • FSIQ ≥ 85 20 children with ADHD 20 children with comorbid ADHD/RD 20 controls	ADHD: agreement on clinical assessment by pediatrician and psychologist with regard to DSM-IV diagnostic criteria; average reading ability ADHD/RD: agreement on clinical assessment by pediatrician and psychologist with regard to DSM-IV diagnostic criteria; reading performance ≥2 yr below chronological age	1. ADHD/RD group had relatively more τ activity, less α activity, and higher τ/α ratio than the ADHD group 2. EEG differences between ADHD/RD and ADHD groups were likely the result of RD independent of ADHD influences on EEG
Doyle et al., 2001	• 6–18 yr of age • FSIQ ≥ 80 • Middle-class SES and higher • All female 140 ADHD probands with 417 first-degree relatives 122 comparison probands (without ADHD) with 369 first-degree relatives	ADHD: DSM-III-R criteria unequivocally met based on K-SADS-E and SCID LD: used estimated FSIQ and academic achievement scores to compute a regression equation	1. Presence of LD did not change risk for ADHD 2. When LD and ADHD were both present in a family, risk for comorbidity was higher among family members 3. No evidence for nonassortative mating for ADHD and LD
Foster et al., 2002	• 8–12 yr of age • FSIQ ≥ 75 12 clinical controls 9 children with dyslexia (RD) 23 children with ADHD 10 children with comorbid ADHD/RD	Clinical controls: children were referred for neuropsychological evaluation but did not meet diagnostic criteria for any disorder Dyslexia: ≥20-point discrepancy between FSIQ and reading achievement ADHD: diagnostic criteria not stated	1. No significant differences between children with ADHD and children with RD on dichotic listening task 2. Rightward asymmetry of planum temporale was associated with atypical left ear advantage, regardless of diagnostic category

(Continued)

Table 2
(Continued)

Authors	Participants	Diagnostic criteria	Findings
Halperin et al., 1997	• 7–11 yr of age • 22 males 8 children diagnosed with comorbid ADHD/RD 14 children diagnosed with ADHD	ADHD: met DSM-III-R criteria for ADHD diagnosis on structured interview with parent with corroborating elevated teacher and parent report scores on behavior rating scales; ≥85 on reading achievement measure ADHD/RD: met DSM-III-R criteria for ADHD diagnosis on structured interview with parent; ≤80 on reading achievement measure	1. ADHD/RD group had significantly higher level of norepinephrine metabolite (MHPG) 2. MHPG levels were not associated with hyperactivity or impulsivity levels
Halperin et al., 1993	• 7–11 yr of age • Medication free > 4 weeks prior to study • FSIQ > 80 11 males diagnosed with comorbid ADHD/RD 13 males diagnosed with ADHD	ADHD: met DSM-III-R criteria for ADHD diagnosis on structured interview with parent; ≥85 on reading achievement measure ADHD/RD: met DSM-III-R criteria for ADHD diagnosis on structured interview with parent; ≤80 on reading achievement measure	1. ADHD/RD group had significantly higher level of norepinephrine metabolite (MHPG) 2. Groups did not differ on dopamine metabolite (HVA) levels
Hynd et al., 1990	• Caucasian • 24 males (8 per group) • FSIQ ≥ 85 10 normal controls 10 children diagnosed with ADD/H 10 children diagnosed with dyslexia (RD)	Normal controls: no history of learning or behavior problems; no significant medical, social, or emotional problems ADD/H: no family history of learning problems; Meet DSM-III criteria for ADD/H; history of favorable response to stimulant medication Dyslexia: average IQ; history of difficulty learning to read; ≥20-point discrepancy between IQ and reading achievement	1. Rightward asymmetry was more common in children with dyslexia than children with ADHD or normal controls 2. 70% of children with ADD/H had leftward (typical) asymmetry 3. Both children with dyslexia and children with ADD/H had significantly smaller right anterior width measurements

(Continued)

Table 2
(Continued)

Authors	Participants	Diagnostic criteria	Findings
Light et al., 1995	• 104 twin pairs from the Colorado Reading Project • 76 males • 8–20 yr of age • English-speaking homes 61 identical twin pairs with of age at least one member diagnosed with RD and both members have ADHD 43 same-sex fraternal twin pairs with at least one member diagnosed with reading disability and both members diagnosed with ADHD	RD: history of school reading problems; classified by discriminant reading score; FSIQ ≥ 90 ADHD: DICA composite ≥6; behavior problems present since at least 7 yr of age	1. 45% of the proband deficit in reading was owing to genetic factors that also influenced hyperactivity 2. Heritable variation accounted for 70% of the observed covariance between reading and hyperactivity measures 3. Heritable influences partly explained the comorbidity of RD and ADHD
Mangina, et al., 2000	• Preadolescents • Right-handed 10 children with ADHD/LD 10 normal controls	ADHD/LD: met DSM-IV criteria for learning disorders, ADHD, and behavior disorders; Achenbach T-scores ≥70; school grades ≤ 51%; FSIQ ≥ 85	1. Preadolescents with ADHD/LD were clearly differentiated from normal controls by EEG activity (bilateral underactivation) over the prefrontal and frontal regions 2. Cingulate gyri also appeared to be involved in regulating cognition and behavioral adjustment in normal controls
Semrud-Clikeman et al., 1996	• 6–16 yr old • Caucasian • FSIQ: 87–149 • 24 males 10 normal controls 10 children diagnosed with ADHD: combined type	Normal controls: no history of learning or behavior problems; no significant medical, social, or emotional problems ADHD: no history of significant learning problems; meet DSM-IV criteria for diagnosis (reporter/s not stated)	1. Neuroanatomical measures (right frontal region width and right insula length) differentiate between normal controls and those with developmental disorders 2. Length of left plana, left insula, and right plana did not differentiate between groups

(Continued)

Table 2
(Continued)

Authors	Participants	Diagnostic criteria	Findings
	10 children diagnosed with dyslexia (RD)	Dyslexia: history of difficulty learning to read; ≥20-point discrepancy between IQ and reading achievement	3. Width of left frontal region did not differentiate between groups
Willcutt, et al., 2000	• 823 same-sex twin pairs • 8–16 yr old 313 pairs with at least one member with RD 510 twin pairs with no member with RD	RD: used 2 discrepancy criteria (age achievement and IQ achievement) with 1.65 SD below mean as cutoff ADHD: DICA score ≥ 8 on maternal report	1. 95% of the phenotypic covariance between RD and inattention was the result common genetic influences 2. 21% of phenotypic covariance between RD and hyperactivity/ impulsivity was because of common genetic influences

FSIQ, full-scale IQ; EEG, electroencephalogram; k-SADS-E, SCID, MHPG, 3-metnoxy-4-hydroxy phenylglycol; HVA, homovanillic acid; DICA, Diagnostic Interview for Children and Adolescents; ADD/H.

structures of the perisylvian region including the planum temporale. These studies generally use data from MRI to measure specific structures in the brain. The number of studies comparing children with ADHD to children with RD is limited to three studies.

In an early study, Hynd and colleagues found that children with RD and those with ADHD had significantly smaller anterior width in the right cerebral hemisphere than the left *(40)*. The study also reported that children with ADHD were more likely to have the typical pattern of leftward asymmetry of the plana length than children with RD. In contrast, children with RD were more likely to have rightward asymmetry.

In a follow-up study, Semrud-Clikeman and colleagues used a more powerful statistical procedure and expanded the measurements to include other structures using the same subjects *(74)*. Their study reported that multiple structures, including bilateral plana lengths, left insula length, and width of the left frontal region did not differentiate among children with RD, children with ADHD, and normal controls. In contrast, other neuroanatomical measurements differentiated normal controls from children with RD or ADHD, but did not differentiate between the two clinical groups. Specifically, children with RD and children with ADHD, using strictly defined diagnostic criteria, were clearly different from children without ADHD or RD in terms of the width of their right frontal region and the length of their right insula.

In another follow-up to the 1990 Hynd et al. study, Foster and colleagues recently reported that children with ADHD could not be differentiated from children with RD by their performance on a dichotic listening task *(65)*. Rightward asymmetry of the planum temporale, regardless of diagnostic category, was clearly associated with an atypical left ear advantage for listening tasks. Overall, these studies suggest that although there may be subtle differences in brain development associated with each of the disorders independently, there may be significant overlap in performance by individuals with ADHD and RD.

3.3.2. *Biochemical Abnormalities*

The reports of biochemical differences in children with ADHD and RD are limited to two related studies. In both studies, Halperin and colleagues compared norepinephrine and dopamine metabolite levels of children with ADHD to children with comorbid ADHD and RD *(75,76)*. In both studies, children with the comorbid diagnoses had significantly higher levels of the norepinephrine metabolite 3-methoxy-4-hydroxy phenylglycol (MHPG), than children with a diagnosis of ADHD. Furthermore, the earlier study reported that the groups could not be differentiated by dopamine metabolite levels (homovanillic acid; 76). The authors hypothesized that because MHPG levels were not associated with hyperactivity or impulsivity levels on behavior rating scales, these higher levels were likely related to the additive attention problems that were the result of the comorbid diagnoses *(75)*.

3.3.3. *Abnormalities in Level of Neural Activation*

As the use of functional magnetic resonance imaging (fMRI) becomes more widespread, studies comparing neural activation levels in children with RD and ADHD should become more common. Up to this point, two studies have used electroencephalogram (EEG) results to report on activation differences and similarities in children with ADHD and RD. One study examined differences in activation levels between normal controls and preadolescents diagnosed with comorbid LD and ADHD *(77)*. According to their results, preadolescents who were diagnosed with ADHD/LD had significant underactivation in the prefrontal and frontal regions bilaterally when compared with controls. The authors also posited, based on results, that the cingulated gyri appeared to be involved in cognition and behavior in the control participants but not the children diagnosed with ADHD/LD.

In a more recent study, Clarke and colleagues compared children with ADHD, children with comorbid ADHD and RD (ADHD/RD), and control children *(78)*. Their results suggested significant differences in general patterns of activation between children with ADHD and children with comorbid ADHD/RD. These differences included higher levels of τ activity, lower levels of α activity, and a higher τ/α ratio in the ADHD/RD group compared with the ADHD group. The authors hypothesized that the EEG results by group were the result of associated effects of RD alone, and were independent of those effects associated with ADHD alone.

3.3.4. *Evidence From Genetic Studies*

As interest in genetic research continues to increase following the completion of the human genome sequencing, it is anticipated that this will be a growing line of research. Thus far, studies comparing children with ADHD to children with RD have been limited in scope. A study by Light and colleagues, using data from the Colorado Reading Project, reported that some of the same genetic factors that influenced reading performance also influenced levels of hyperactivity *(79)*. In other words, there are heritable factors that partly explain the high rate of comorbidity of ADHD and RD. Gillis and colleagues reported similar results *(80)*.

In a more recent study, Doyle and colleagues reported that the presence of a learning disability does not directly influence the risk for ADHD from the genetic perspective *(81)*. The study also reported that the presence of LD and ADHD in a family member increased the risk for comorbidity in other family members. There was also no evidence for nonassortative mating, or nonrandom pairing of individuals with ADHD and RD, in their sample, which removed a potential confound in their results.

4. SUMMARY OF CONSISTENT FINDINGS

4.1. *Common Cognitive Features of RD and ADHD*

Research suggests that ADHD and RD are, in fact, separate and distinct disorders that frequently co-occur *(18,19, 40)*. Although symptoms of inattention are present in both disorders *(14,15)* and reading performance may be impaired in both groups, the disorders can be differentiated by their respective cognitive deficits *(18)*: children with ADHD show impairments in attention, behavioral disinhibition, and/or hyperactivity *(14)*, whereas children with RD show impairments in phonological processing. Furthermore, although both groups demonstrate language impairments, in children with ADHD those impairments are related to executive functioning while in children with RD the deficits are in the verbal/phonological realm *(23)*. Memory deficits have been found in working memory in both groups, although in children with RD the working memory deficits are limited to the verbal domain *(28)*. Thus, ADHD and RD can be differentiated by the different cognitive deficits found in each.

4.2. *Common Social/Emotional Features of RD and ADHD*

The evidence supporting increased prevalence rates of internalizing disorders, externalizing disorders, and social skill deficits in ADHD is much stronger than evidence connecting those disorders and RD. Further research focusing on the subtypes of LD is needed to elucidate the relationship between internalizing disorders and RD.

4.3. *Common Neurobiological Features of RD and ADHD*

RD and ADHD share some of the same underlying neurobiological basis. The width of the right frontal region *(74)*, the length of the right insula *(74)*, underactivation of the prefrontal and frontal regions *(77)*, and abnormal levels of the norepinephrine metabolite MHPG *(52)* have all been found in groups of children with ADHD and LD. These areas correspond to those that have been implicated in ADHD alone but not in RD alone. This may suggest that, in individuals with the comorbid condition, the neurobiological basis of the disorder is confined to the frontal lobes and thus, in that subgroup of individuals, reading problems result from attention problems. However, more research on comorbid groups is needed to test this hypothesis.

5. THEORETICAL IMPLICATIONS AND FUTURE DIRECTIONS

There are three subtypes of ADHD: the primarily inattentive type, characterized by a sole significant dysfunction of attention; the hyperactive–impulsive type, characterized by deficits in behavioral inhibition; and the combined type, which meets criteria for both the hyperactive–impulsive and primarily inattentive subtypes *(82)*. There has been some controversy over the inclusion of the primarily inattentive subtype as Barkley *(12,14)* and other researchers contend that this subtype is a distinct disorder from ADHD, one that is not related to behavioral regulation or filtering/selection problems, but rather a group of individuals whose poor attention stems from deficits in working memory and a slow cognitive style *(14)*. Barkley also contends that this subtype has more benign outcomes throughout development, because of lower levels of impulsiveness and comorbidity with externalizing disorders, such as CD and ODD *(14)*.

The proposed shift in conceptualization of ADHD will be extremely important to the understanding of the relationship between ADHD and RD and the relationship between ADHD and other forms of LD. If ADHD is reconceptualized as two disorders—one of attention, sluggish cognitive tempo, and working memory deficits, and the other of behavioral disinhibition—it is possible that the first disorder will have a very high concordance rate with language-based LD, as those two disorders appear to share many features. Although many studies have found that RD and ADHD are etiologically distinct disorders, research will be necessary to determine if this is so for RD when compared with both subtypes of ADHD. In addition, research comparing ADHD and LD needs to focus on creating homogenous groups of individuals with LD, as evidence has shown that subtypes of LD may have very different etiologies, symptoms, associated features, and developmental course *(29)*. Finally, future research will need to focus on the subtypes of ADHD and LD, the cognitive deficits, social–emotional difficulties, and associated features of each, and how they may be interrelated and differentially treated.

ACKNOWLEDGMENTS

Preparation of this chapter was supported in part by a grant to the fourth author (GWH) from the National Institute for Child Health and Human Developmental, National Institutes of Health (#26890–07).

REFERENCES

1. Lyon GR, Fletcher JM, Barnes MC. Learning disabilities. In: Mash EJ, Barkley RA, eds. Child psychopathology, 2nd ed. New York: Guilford Press, 2003;520–588.
2. American Psychiatric Association. Diagnostic and statistical manual of Mental disorders, 4th ed., text revision. Washington: American Psychiatric Association 2000.
3. Shaywitz SE, Shaywitz BA. Cognitive and neurobiologic influences in reading and in dyslexia. Dev Neuropsych 1999;16:383–384.
4. Siegel LS. Phonological processing deficits as the basis of a reading disability. Dev Rev 1993;13:246–257.
5. Eden GF, VanMeter JW, Rumsey JM, Zeffiro TA. The visual deficit theory of developmental dyslexia. Neuroimage 1996;4:S108–S117.
6. Wolf M, Bower PG. The double-deficit hypothesis for developmental dyslexia. J Ed Psych 1999;91:415–438.
7. Miller CJ, Sanchez J, Hynd GW. Neurological correlates of reading disabilities. In: Swanson L, Graham S. eds. Handbook of research on learning disabilities. New York: Guilford Press, 2003:242–255.
8. Wadsworth SJ, Olson RK, Pennington BF, DeFries JC. Differential genetic etiology of reading disability as a function of IQ. J Learn Dis 1992;33:192–199.
9. Grigorenko EL, Wood FB, Meyer MS, Hart LA, Speed WC, Shuster A, Pauls DL. Susceptibility loci for distinct components of developmental dyslexia on chromosomes 6 and 15. Am J Gen 1997;60:27–39.
10. Geschwind N, Galaburda A. Cerebral lateralization: biological mechanisms, associations, and pathology: a hypothesis and program for research. Arch Neurol 1985;42:428–459.
11. Shaywitz SE, Shaywitz BA, Fletcher JM, Escobar MD. Prevalence of reading disability in boys and girls: results of the Connecticut Longitudinal Study. JAMA 1990;264:998–1002.
12. Barkley, RA. Attention-deficit hyperactivity disorder: a handbook for diagnosis and treatment, 2nd ed. New York: Guilford Press, 1998.
13. Kibby MY, Hynd GW. Neurobiological basis of learning disabilities. In: Hallahan DP, Keogh BK, eds. Research and global perspectives in learning disabilities: essays in honor of William M. Cruickshank. Mahwah: Lawrence Erlbaum, 2001;25–42.

14. Barkley RA. Attention-deficit hyperactivity disorder. In: Mash EJ, Barkley RA, eds. Child psychopathology, 2nd ed. New York: Guilford Press, 2003;75–143.
15. Mayes SD, Calhoun SL, Crowell EW. Learning Disabilities and ADHD: Overlapping spectrum disorders. J Learn Dis 2000;33:417–424.
16. August GJ, Garfinkel BD. Comorbidity of ADHD and reading disability among clinic-referred children. J Abnorm Child Psych 1990;18,1:29–45.
17. Kupietz, SS. Sustained attention in normal and in reading disabled youngsters with and without ADDH. J Abnorm Child Psych 1990;18,4:357–372.
18. Shaywitz BA, Fletcher JM, Holahan JM, KK et al. Child Neuropsych 1995;1,3:170–186.
19. Pennington BF, Groisser D, Welsh MC. Contrasting cognitive deficits in attention deficit hyperactivity disorder versus reading disabilities. Dev Psych 1993;29:511–523.
20. Närhi V, Ahonen T. Reading disability with or without attention deficit hyperactivity disorder: do attentional problems make a difference? Dev Neuropsych 1995;11:337–349.
21. Nigg JT, Carte ET, Hinshaw SP, Treuting JJ. Neuropsychological correlates of childhood attention-deficit/hyperactivity disorder: explainable by comorbid disruptive behavior or reading problems. J Abnorm Psych 1998;107:468–480.
22. Johnson BD, Altmaier EM, Richman LC. Attention deficits and reading disabilities: are immediate memory deficits additive? Dev Neuropsych 1999;15:213–226.
23. Purvis KL, Tannock R. Language abilities in children with attention-deficit hyperactivity disorder, reading disabilities, and normal controls. J Abnorm Child Psych 1997;25:133–144.
24. Shaywitz BA, Fletcher JM, Holahan JM, et al. Interrelationships between reading disability and attention-deficit/hyperactvity disorder. Child Neuropsych 1995;1:170–186.
25. Korkman M, Pesonen A. A comparison of neuropsychological test profiles of children with attention deficit hyperactivity disorder and/or learning disorder. J Learn Dis 1994;27:383–392.
26. Lyon GR. Learning disabilities. In: Mash EJ, Barkley RA, eds. Child Psychopathology. New York: Guilford Press, 1996;390–435.
27. Siegel LS. Basic cognitive processes and reading disabilities. In: Swanson L, Graham S, eds. Handbook of research on learning disabilities. New York: Guilford Press, 2003;158–181.
28. Swanson HL, Saez L. Memory difficulties in children and adults with learning disabilities. Basic cognitive processes and reading disabilities. In: Swanson L, Graham S, eds. Handbook of research on learning disabilities. New York: Guilford Press, 2003;182–198.
29. Greenham SL.Learning Disabilities and psychosocial adjustment: a critical review. Child Neuropsych 1999;5:171–196.
30. Miller CJ, Hynd GW. Parent contributions to child reading achievement, phonological processing skills, rapid naming ability, and internalizing disorder. In preparation.
31. Semrud-Clikeman M, Hynd GW. Right hemispheric dysfunction in nonverbal Learning disabilities: social, academic, and adaptive functioning in adults and children. Psych Bull 1990,107:196–209.
32. Pfiffner LJ, Barkley RA. Treatment of ADHD in school settings. In: Barkley RA, ed. Attention-deficit hyperactivity disorder: a handbook for diagnosis and treatment. New York: Guilford Press, 1998:458–490.
33. Marshall RM, Hynd GW, Handwerk MJ, Hall J. Academic underachievement in ADHD subtypes. J Learn Dis 1997;30:635–642.
34. Auro T, Ahonen T, Tolvanen A, Lyytinen H, de Barra HT. Contribution of ADHD characteristics to the academic treatment outcome of children with learning difficulties. Dev Neuropsych 1999;15:291–305.
35. Barry TD, Lyman RD, Klinger LG. Academic underachievement and attention-deficit/hyperactivity disorder. J Sch Psych 2002;40:259–283.
36. Barkley RA. The ecological validity of laboratory and analogue assessment methods of ADHD symptoms. J Abnorm Child Psych 1991;19:149–177.
37. Matier-Sharma K, Perachio N, Newcorn JH. Differential diagnosis of ADHD: are objective measures of attention, impulsivity and activity level helpful? Child Neuropsych 1995;1:118–127.
38. Lazar JW, Frank Y. Frontal systems dysfunction in children with attention-deficit hyperactivity disorder and learning disabilities. J Neuropsychiatry Clin Neurosci 1998;10:160–167.

39. Pineda DA, Restrepo MA, Sarmiento RJ. et al. Statistical analyses of structural magnetic resonance imaging of the head of the caudate nucleus in Colombian children with attention-deficit hyperactivity disorder. J Child Neurol 2002;17:97–105.
40. Hynd GW, Semrud-Clikeman M, Lorys AR, Novey ES, Eliopulos D. Brain morphology in developmental dyslexia and attention deficit disorder/hyperactivity. Arch Neurol 1990;47:919–926.
41. Pueyo R, Mañeru C, Vendrell P, Mataró M, Estévez-González, A García-Sánchez C, Junqué C. Trastorno por déficit de atención con hiperactividad. Asímetrias cerebrales observadas en resonancia magnética [Attention deficit hyperactivity disorder. Cerebral asymmetries observed on magnetic resonance]. Revista de Neurologia 2000;30:920–925.
42. Hynd GW, Hern KL, Novey ES. Attention-deficit hyperactivity disorder (ADHD) and asymmetry of the caudate nucleus. J Child Neurol 1993;8:339–347.
43. Castellanos FX, Giedd JN, Eckburg P, et al. Quantitative morphology of caudate nucleus in attention deficit hyperactivity disorder. Am J Psychiatry 1994;151:1791–1796.
44. Castellanos FX, Giedd JN, Marsh WL, et al. Quantitative brain magnetic resonance imaging in attention-deficit hyperactivity disorder. Arch Gen Psychiatry 1996;53:607–616.
45. Mataró M, García-Sánchez C, Junqué C, Estévez-González A, Pujol J. Magnetic resonance imaging measurement of the caudate nucleus in adolescents with attention-deficit hyperactivity disorder and its relationship with neuropsychological and behavioral measures. Arch Neurol 1997;54:963–968.
46. Nopoulos P, Berg S, Castellanos FX, Delgado A, Andreasen NC, Rapoport J. Developmental brain anomalies in children with attention-deficit hyperactivity disorder. J Child Neurol 2000;15:102–108.
47. Posner MI, Petersen SE. The attention system of the human brain. Ann Rev Neurosci 1990;13:25–42.
48. Clark CR, Geffen GM, Geffen LB. Catecholamines and attention: 1. Animal and clinical studies. Neurosci Behav Res 1987a;11:341–352.
49. Clark CR, Geffen GM, Geffen LB. Catecholamines and attention: 2. Pharmacological studies in normal humans. Neurosci Behav Res 1987b;11:353–364.
50. Zametkin AJ, Rapoport JL. Neurobiology of attention deficit disorder with hyperactivity: Where have we come in 50 years? J Am Acad Child and Adolesc Psychiatry 1987;26:676–686.
51. Halperin JM, Newcorn JH, Schwartz ST, McKay KE, Bedi G, Sharma V. Plasma catecholamine metabolite levels in ADHD boys with and without reading disabilities. J Clin Child Psychol 1993;22:219–225.
52. Halperin JM, Newcorn JH, Koda VH, Pick L, McKay KE, Knott P. Noradrenergic mechanisms in ADHD children with and without reading disabilities: A replication and extension. J Am Acad Child and Adolesc Psychiatry 1997;36:1688–1697.
53. Pelham WE, Greenslade KE, Vodde-Hamilton M, et al., Relative efficacy of long acting stimulants on children with attention deficit-hyperactivity disorder: A comparison of standard methylphenidate, sustained release methylphenidate, sustained release dextroamphetamine, and pemoline. Pediatrics 1990;86,226–237.
54. Riccio CA, Hynd GW, Cohen MJ. Etiology and neurobiology of ADHD. In: Bender WM, ed. Understanding ADHD. Upper Saddle River, NY: Merrill Publishers, 1996.
55. Hinshelwood J. Congenital word-blindness. Lancet 1900;1:1506–1508.
56. Riccio CA, Hynd GW. Neuroanatomical and neurophysiological aspects of dyslexia. Topics Lang Dis 1996;16:1–13.
57. Galaburda AM. The planum temporale. Arch Neurol 1993;50:457.
58. Hynd GW, Semrud-Clikeman M. Dyslexia and brain morphology. Psychol Bull 1989;106:447–482.
59. Leonard C, Voeller KK, Lombardino L, et al. Anomalous cerebral structure in dyslexia revealed with magnetic resonance imaging. Arch Neurol 1993;50:461–469.
60. Temple CM. Reading disorders. In: Temple CM, ed. Developmental cognitive neuropsychology. East Sussex, UK: Psychology Press, 1997;163–223.
61. Zeffiro T, Eden G. The cerebellum and dyslexia. Perpetrator or innocent bystander?: comment from Thomas Zeffiro and Guinevere Eden to Nicholson et al. Trends Neurosci 2001;24:512–513.

62. Hynd GW, Morgan AE, Edmons JE, Black K, Riccio CA, Lombardino L. Reading disabilities, comorbid psychopathology and the specificity of neurolinguistic deficits. Dev Neuropsychol 1995;11:311–322.
63. Geschwind N, Levitsky W. Human brain: left-right asymmetricies in temporal speech region. Science 1968;161:186–187.
64. Galaburda AM, Kemper TL. Cytoarchitectonic abnormalities in developmental dyslexia. Ann Neurol 1979;6:94–100.
65. Foster LM, Hynd GW, Morgan AE, Hugdahl K. Planum temporale asymmetry and ear advantage in developmental dyslexia and attention-deficit/hyperactivity disorder (ADHD). J Intl Neuropsychol Soc 2002;8:22–36.
66. Galaburda AM, Sherman G, Rosen GD, Aboitiz F, Geschwind N. Developmental dyslexia: Four consecutive patients with cortical abnormalities. Ann Neurol 1985;18:222–233.
67. Humphreys P, Kaufman WE, Galaburda A. Developmental dyslexia in women: Evidence for a subgroup with reversal of cerebral asymmetry. Ann Neurol 1990;28:727–738.
68. Larsen JP, Hoien T, Lundberg I, Odegaard H. MRI evaluation of the size and symmetry of the planum temporale in adolescents with developmental dyslexia. Brain and Lang 1990;39:289–301.
69. Semrud-Clikeman M, Hynd GW, Novey ES, Eliopulos D. Dyslexia and brain morphology: relationships between neuroanatomical variation and neurolinguistic tasks. Learn Ind Diff 1991;3:225–242.65
70. Palamini A, Andermann F, deGrissac H, et al. Stages and patterns of centrifugal arrest of diffuse neuronal migration disorders. Dev Med Child Neurol 1991;35:331–339.
71. Aicardi J. Diseases of the nervous system in childhood. New York: MacKeith Press, 1992.
72. Steinmetz H, Ebeling U, Huang Y, Kahn T. Sulcus topography in the parietal opercular region. Brain and Lang 1990;38:515–533.
73. Hiemenz JR, Hynd GW. Sulcal/gyral pattern morphology of the perisylvian language region in developmental dyslexia. Brain and Lang 2000;74:113–133.
74. Semrud-Clikeman M, Hooper SR, Hynd GW, Hern K, Presley R, Watson T. Prediction of group membership in developmental dyslexia, attention deficit hyperactivity disorder, and normal controls using brain morphometric analysis of magnetic resonance imaging. Arch Clin Neuropsychol 1996;11:521–528.
75. Halperin JM, Newcorn JH, Koda VH, Pick L, McKay KE, Knott P. Noradrenergic mechanisms in ADHD children with and without reading disabilities: A replication and extension. J Am Acad Child Adolec Psychiatry 1997;36:1688–1697.
76. Halperin JM, Newcorn JH, Schwartz ST, McKay KE, Bedi G, Sharma V. Plasma catecholamine metabolite levels in ADHD boys with and without reading disabilities. J Clin Child Psych 1993;22:219–225.
77. Mangina CA, Beuzeron-Mangina JH, Grizenko N. Event-related brain potentials, bilateral electrodermal activity and Mangina-Test performance in learning disabled/ADHD pre-adolescents as compared to age-matched normal controls. Intl J Psychophys 2000;37:71–85.
78. Clarke AR, Barry RJ, McCarthy R, Selikowitz M. EEG analysis of children with attention-deficit/hyperactivity and comorbid reading disabilities. J Learn Dis 2002;35:276–285.
79. Light JG, Pennington BF, Gilger JW, DeFries JC. Reading disability and hyperactivity disorder: evidence for a genetic etiology. Dev Neuropsychol 1995;11:323–335.
80. Gillis JJ, Gilger JW, Pennington BF, DeFries JC. Attention deficit disorder in reading-disabled twins: Evidence for a genetic etiology. J Abnorm Child Psychol 1992;20:303–315.
81. Doyle AE, Faraone SV, DuPre EP, Biederman J. Separating attention deficit hyperactivity disorder and Learning disabilities in girls: a familial risk analysis. Am J Psychiatry 2001;158:1666–1672.
82. American Psychiatric Association. Diagnostic and statistical manual of mental disorders, 4th ed. Washington, DC: American Psychiatric Association, 1994.

16

Attention Deficit Hyperactivity Disorder and the Brain

Evidence From Electrophysiological Studies

Alexandra P. Fonaryova Key, Melissa Ferguson, and Dennis L. Molfese

1. INTRODUCTION

This chapter examines the electrophysiological correlates of attention deficit hyperactivity disorder (ADHD) in children. As a growing number of children are diagnosed with this disorder, researchers are increasingly interested in ADHD and the cognitive processes of affected children. According to Schroeder and Gordon *(1)*, ADHD is the most frequently diagnosed childhood disorder, with a prevalence of 3–7% among school-aged children *(2)*. Although ADHD affects adults as well, this chapter focuses on the occurrence of this disorder in children. The sections below present brief diagnostic criteria of ADHD, according to the *Diagnostic and Statistical Manual of Mental Disorders*, 4th Edition (DSM-IV) *(2)*, provide an explanation of the diagnostic subtypes of the disorder, highlight comorbidity and subtype issues relating to event-related potentials (ERPs), examine electrophysiological findings regarding attention in children with the disorder, and investigate electrophysiological correlates of the disorder in relation to drug interventions. (For additional in-depth reviews of ADHD and ERPs, *see* refs. *3* and *4*).

2. DIAGNOSIS

According to the DSM-IV *(2)*, ADHD is characterized by the existence of inattention and/or hyperactivity–impulsivity. Inattention is characterized by carelessness, inattention to detail, distractibility, failure to listen, problems with organization, forgetfulness, and inability to follow directions. The behaviors that characterize hyperactivity are fidgeting; failure to remain seated in situations in which it is expected; inappropriate movement, such as running or climbing; difficulty staying quiet when it is expected; and excessive talking. Impulsivity is characterized by difficulty in being patient and frequently interrupting others during conversations or activities. Such patterns of behavior must occur at a level that is maladaptive for at least 6 mo and the individual must exhibit at least one of the distinguishing categories of behavior: inattention or hyperactivity–impulsivity. To be diagnosed with ADHD, the child must display at least six of the nine specified symptoms of inattention or hyperactivity–impulsivity. The symptoms of ADHD must begin before 7 yr of age and interfere in at least two settings, such as school and home. In addition, for a diagnosis of ADHD, the presenting symptoms cannot be explained by

From: *Attention Deficit Hyperactivity Disorder: From Genes to Patients*
Edited by: D. Gozal and D. L. Molfese © Humana Press Inc., Totowa, NJ

the existence of schizophrenia, pervasive developmental disorder, psychotic disorder, or any other mental disorder *(2)*.

3. SUBTYPES OF ADHD

When diagnosing ADHD, there are three subtypes that can be specified based on the main symptoms that the child has displayed over the previous 6-mo period. Although some children may exhibit indicators of all the characteristic behaviors (inattentiveness, hyperactivity, and impulsivity), the subtypes allow for the designation of the principal behaviors that cause impairment in the child's life *(2)*. The subtypes are: combined type, predominantly inattentive type, and predominantly hyperactive–impulsive type. When designating a predominant subtype, it is important to consider the symptom presentation and the number of symptoms present for the previous 6 mo. For example, if six or more symptoms of inattention have been present along with fewer than six symptoms of hyperactivity–impulsivity, ADHD predominantly inattentive type is diagnosed, and vice versa for ADHD, predominantly hyperactive–impulsive type. In the case of ADHD, combined type, the most commonly diagnosed subtype in children and adolescent populations, more than six symptoms of inattention and hyperactivity–impulsivity must have occurred over the prior 6-mo period for this characterization to apply *(2)*.

4. USE OF ERPs IN STUDY OF ADHD

ADHD is a disorder that may cause significant impairment in a child's life, resulting in academic, social, and interpersonal difficulties. Previous research has focused on the performance of children diagnosed with ADHD on behavioral tasks assessing attention regulation, memory, and inhibition that are thought to relate to these difficulties. As a result, researchers are increasingly interested in the corresponding brain responses that accompany such behaviors. One procedure used to determine the brain mechanisms utilized by children with ADHD is the use of the ERP. The ERP recorded from the scalp is a synchronized portion of the ongoing electroencephalographic pattern. It is usually represented as a complex waveform made of positive- and negative-going peaks. Such waveforms are thought to indicate changes in brain electrical activity overtime as reflected by changes in the amplitude or height of the wave as well as the latency or timing of the peaks *(5)*. What distinguishes the evoked potential from the more traditional electroencephalogram (EEG) measure is that the ERP is time-locked to the onset of some event in the person's environment. The ongoing EEG activity reflects a wide range of neural activity related to a plethora of neural and body self-regulating systems, as well as various sensory and cognitive functions ongoing in the brain at that time. The ERP, on the other hand, because of this time-locked feature, has been shown more likely to reflect both general and specific aspects of the evoking stimulus and the individual's perceptions and decisions regarding that stimulus. It is this time-locking feature that enables researchers to pinpoint, with some degree of certainty, portions of the electrical response that occurred while a person's attention was focused on a discrete event.

The ERP is not an exact and completely stable pattern reflecting only those discrete neural events directly related to the evoking stimulus, the task, or the response to such an event, which begins at levels well below that of the cortex as the stimulus information is transformed by the sensory systems and progresses through the brainstem, into the midbrain, and on upward into the higher brain centers. Such signals that originate within the brain must travel through a variety of tissues of different densities, conductivity, and composition (e.g., neurons, glial cells, fiber tracts, cerebrospinal fluid, bone, muscle) before they reach the recording electrodes placed on the scalp. Consequently, the final version of the ERP recorded at the scalp is a composite of a variety of complex factors, some of which relate directly to the stimulus situation and some of which do not. Moreover, as changes occur moment by moment in these factors, changes will occur at the same time in the amplitude of the ERP waveform, reflecting both these non-task-related changes, as well as changes in a variety of task-related cognitive factors. Because of this moment-by-moment variability in the ERP, which results in part from continuous changes in the physiology of the participant, many researchers collect several ERPs to a stimulus within a single recording session, sum these responses, and then calculate an average evoked response. It is reasoned that this averaged response is more likely to have buried within it the repetitive activity that reflects the processing of the stimulus from one time to the next. The non-stimulus-related activity that is not time-locked to the onset of the stimulus would be expected to average out or be minimized in the averaged waveform of the ERP. Subsequently, additional analyses are conducted on the averaged waveforms. These analysis approaches offer a range of options including amplitude and latency measures performed on various peaks of the averaged ERP, area measures, discriminant-function procedures, and other multivariate approaches such as principal components analysis.

The ERP procedure has several strengths, among them its ability to employ identical procedures with all participants, regardless of age or species. Consequently, direct comparisons can be made between various participant groups in terms of discrimination abilities. Although the ERP wave shapes change from infancy to adulthood and differ across different species, one can assess whether the brain responses recorded from these different populations reliably discriminate among different stimuli, participant groups, and task characteristics. These methods also provide information concerning both between-hemisphere, within-hemisphere, and front–back brain differences. The procedure provides time-related data that identify the different points in time when such information is detected and processed. Finally, under certain conditions, ERPs can be used to identify brain structures that generate these responses. Because of these advantages, the ERP procedure is valuable in the investigation of brain activity differences in ADHD children, as compared with other groups of children who have not been diagnosed with the disorder.

5. ERPs AND ADHD

ERPs provide additional information that complements and supplements behavioral data regarding the cognitive processes of children diagnosed with ADHD. Because the occurrence of ADHD is hypothesized to have a biological basis, it is important to determine the underlying brain activity that is involved in cognitive processing that distinguishes individuals with ADHD from those without the disorder. ERPs offer valuable insight into information processing, because this method facilitates the examination of cognition while children are engaged in various tasks, allowing the detection of underlying neural processing from different brain areas. Changes in neural activity, as evidenced by the ERP waveforms, reflect cognitive differences related to task demands. This technique extends the limitations of behavioral data in assessing children with ADHD, allowing cognitive processing to become apparent, which may not otherwise be observable with behavioral tasks alone

Through the combination of ERP and behavioral tasks, researchers have examined the ERP waveforms of children diagnosed with ADHD, as compared with those of normal control children. Results established the existence of differences in brain activity between such groups indicative of variations in the processing of information. Observed discrepancies in brain responses imply different underlying cognitive processes in response to specific stimuli.

Many studies using ERP procedures to measure the impact of ADHD on children's performance largely focus their investigations on a single portion of the ERP, the component known as the P3, or the third positive peak after stimulus onset. In fact, investigations of the P3 characteristics across developmental and cognitive studies with normal and atypical populations make it the most extensively researched ERP component.

The P3 is a pronounced positive peak in the ERP waveform that occurs in response to an unexpected stimulus (also called a target) approx 300 ms following stimulus onset. Currently, the most typical paradigm for eliciting this P3 component, also known as P3b, is the oddball paradigm where a target stimulus is presented infrequently (10–30% of trials) among more frequently occurring distracter stimuli (nontargets). For a P3 to be elicited, the subject must pay attention and respond to the stimuli and the ratio of target to distracter stimuli must be low (the fewer targets, the larger the peak). P3 amplitude is affected by attention *(6,7)*, stimulus probability, and stimulus relevance as well as by the amount of processing resources available, such as in single vs dual tasks *(8)*, the quality of selection *(9)*, and attention allocation *(10)*. P3 latency was reported to vary with stimulus complexity *(11)*, effectiveness of selection *(12,13)*, and sustained attention *(6)*. Further, P3 latency was reported to be related to cognitive abilities, with shorter latencies associated with better performance *(14,15)*.

The functional interpretation of the classic P3 is diverse—some view it as an indicator of memory updating *(16)* whereas others believe that it reflects a combination of processes that vary by task and situation, including more elaborate active stimulus discrimination and response preparation *(17)*. P3 latency is assumed to reflect the duration of stimulus evaluation *(16)*.

Sources of the P3 are not clearly identified but at least some are expected to be in the medial temporal lobe *(18)*, including the hippocampal region related to memory *(19,20)*, parahippocampal gyrus, amygdala, or thalamus *(21)*. Lesion data suggest that there may be multiple generators, including the temporoparietal junction *(22)*. Tarkka et al. *(23)* investigated the possible sources and reported that selecting only one region (e.g., hippocampus or thalamus) resulted in poor model fit, but combining the different locations produced a better model. Their findings are consistent with earlier observations using magnetoencephalography analyses that located sources in the floor of sylvian fissure (superior temporal gyrus), as well as deeper sources in the thalamus and/or hippocampus *(24,25)*.

However, no single ERP peak corresponds to a single cognitive function; instead, multiple components may be associated with any given cognitive process. The following sections outline a series of studies investigating ERP correlates of ADHD.

6. ADHD AND ATTENTIONAL PROCESSES

ADHD is commonly thought of as increased distractability, or difficulty sustaining attention during a specific task. However, the reasons for these frequently observed difficulties are less clear. Investigating various forms of attentional processes in children with ADHD, such as orientation, selection, and allocation, can shed more light on the disorder.

6.1. Orientation

Perchet et al. *(26)* investigated different stages of attention such as anticipatory processing, priming, target detection, and response selection in 24 children with ADHD, aged 6–10.5 yr (mean = 8.5 ± 1.4 yr) and 13 controls, aged 6–9 yr (mean = 7.4 ± 0.8 yr) using a Posner's attention-orienting paradigm with valid (60%), invalid (20%), and no-cue (20%) conditions. ERPs were recorded from 19 electrodes but only three sites were analyzed (Cz, Pz, Oc interpolated from O1 and O2). The researchers reported no group differences in ERP responses to cues. For target stimuli, controls produced a larger P1 component to valid vs invalid or no-cue trials, whereas the ADHD group showed no differences. On the other hand, children with ADHD had shorter N2–RT intervals than controls, with the shortest interval occurring for valid trials and longest interval for no-cue trials. Finally, the ADHD group had a substantially smaller contigent negative variation (CNV)/readiness potential (RP) than controls. The authors concluded that ADHD participants benefited less from trial cues, but target detection was intact as evidenced by the lack of N2–P3 differences. Motor response selection was abnormally accelerated and finished prior to complete stimulus processing. Finally, ADHD children showed no anticipation for targets in no-cue trials, attributed to an overall deficit in executive functions.

6.2. Selection

Robaey et al. *(12)* studied 12 boys with ADHD (n = 6, age <7.6 yr; n = 6, age >7.6 yr) and an equal number of controls. ERPs were recorded from 14 electrodes in a series of visual oddball tasks. Standard stimuli probability was 70%, whereas targets occurred 30% of the time. The tasks involved responding to words or pictures that did not belong to the "fruit" category. The other two tasks involved geometric shapes of various sizes or number sequences. Targets were stimuli where the shapes were arranged out of order for their size or when the number sequences changed. ADHD children generated larger P250 (frontocentral) increases to targets for both classification and seriation tasks, whereas larger N250 (parieto-occipital) and smaller P500 (parieto-occipital) occurred on the seriation task. The classification task generated shorter P350 latencies. A discriminant analysis indicated that P350 latency correctly classified 79.2% of the subjects. The authors concluded that ADHD increased change-orienting reactions to targets, but that there was a lack of automatic processing of saliency.

Karayandis et al. *(27)* recorded visual EPRs in 17 males with ADHD, aged 6–9 yr (mean = 7.17 ± 0.82 yr) and the same number of controls (mean = 7.66 ± 1.11 yr) during a visual choice task. The children had to respond differently to standard (75%) and deviant (25%) stimuli (pictures of animals). ERPs were obtained from 30 electrodes (20 electrodes in Electrocap plus 10 additional leads positioned at half-distance between them). The results indicated no group differences in early components over the occipital regions. However, latency of N1, P2, and N2 (left hemisphere) over frontal areas was delayed in ADHD. Further, N2 amplitude was smaller in ADHD over right frontal areas. For the later components, controls showed greater discrimination between frequent and rare stimuli as evidenced by greater P450 amplitude differences over left parietal leads. Finally, the ADHD group was characterized by an additional frontal N530 component, largest after the rare stimuli, while this component was absent in the controls who showed positivity in that range. Similarly, the negative slow wave was larger for rare stimuli in ADHD, whereas the differences were smaller in controls.

Lazzaro et al. *(28)* examined selection processes in 54 males with ADHD, aged 11–17 yr (mean = 13.7 ± 1.4 yr) and sex- and age-matched controls (mean = 13.4 ± 1.5 yr). Twenty of the ADHD group were on medication but withheld it for two or more weeks prior to testing. ERPs were recorded from 19 sites during an auditory oddball where a 1000-Hz tone served as the standard stimulus and a 1500-Hz tone was the deviant (probability = 15%). For group comparisons the researchers chose only three midline sites (Fz, Cz, Pz). Overall, the ADHD group had larger P2 and smaller N2 amplitudes. Latencies for N2 and P3 were significantly delayed. However, using a similar paradigm, Johnstone and Barry *(9)* did not note any latency differences but observed comparable amplitude effects. They examined 10 children with ADHD, aged 74–164 mo (mean age = 124.5 ± 25.5 mo) and age-, sex-, and IQ-matched controls (mean age = 128.2 ± 22.26 mo). ERPs were obtained from 17 electrodes (Electrocap) during an auditory oddball task (target probability = 15%). Targets were 1500-Hz tones and standards were 1000-Hz tones, presented in pseudorandom order with fixed interstimulus interval. The researchers reported that compared with controls, ADHD children had smaller N2 over frontal regions and larger N2 over the posterior areas in response to nontarget stimuli. Further, the ADHD group exhibited larger P3b for target stimuli over frontal regions and smaller p3b over posterior regions. The differences in findings may be attributed to a smaller number of participants and a wider age range used in the study.

Satterfield et al. *(29)* used a multimodal selective attention task with 15 ADHD and 15 control children, tested at age 6 yr and again at age 8 yr. One of the modalities was to be attended and responded to, whereas the other was to be ignored. In the auditory modality, stimuli were 1000-Hz clicks 10 ms long with targets (25%) being louder (83 dB) than standards (75%; 75 dB). In the visual modality, the targets were brighter checkerboard flashes (5.4 lux) among dimmer standard flashes (1.6 lux). Visual feedback was provided for correct and incorrect responses and children earned or lost a nickel for each correct or incorrect response, respectively. ERPs were obtained from 19 electrodes. The researchers indicated that the N2 amplitude was smaller in ADHD boys at age 6 yr but not different from controls at age 8 yr. For P3b, P350, and SP1, considered to be indicators of attention tuning (attended minus unattended) amplitudes were consistently higher in controls at age 8 yr owing to larger responses to attended auditory targets. Further, P350, SP1, and SP2 were sensitive to group differences in responses to attended targets but not to unattended targets. Processing negativity (NdL) differences were present at 6 yr of age but not at 8 yr at Fz. At Cz only controls had an NdL component at age 8 yr. Finally, no peak latency group differences were significant. The authors concluded that with age, control subjects demonstrated improvements in attentional tuning (between modality channels) and attention to stimulus types (target vs standard), whereas ADHD children showed no such change; instead, their ERPs indicated greater processing of attended stimuli.

Jonkman et al. *(30)* tested 18 ADHD children (mean age = 10.6 ± 2 yr) and 18 controls (mean age = 10 ± 1.2 yr) using a slightly different paradigm with attended and unattended channels being of the same modality. For auditory task, stimuli (1000-Hz and 1100-Hz tones) were presented separately but equiprobably to the left and right ear with probability of standard stimuli 80% and deviants 20%. For the visual task, the stimuli were presented in different colors and the orientation of diagonal gratings differed between standard and deviant stimuli. Subjects were instructed to attend to one channel (ear or color) only and to respond to target stimuli only. ERPs were recorded from four midline locations. The results indicated that for auditory tasks, frontal N1 amplitude to unattended channel stimuli was greater in controls. N2 amplitude was higher to unattended rather than attended deviant stimuli in controls, and ADHD children showed no effect. P3b amplitude was reduced in ADHD. Finally, controls had larger frontal and central NdL to standards over central region. For deviants, controls showed greater frontal early positivity and lesser negativity for attended deviants than ADHD children. For visual task, ADHD children had larger P1 to deviant over standard stimuli. Frontal P3 was significantly larger for deviant stimuli in controls for both attended and unattended channels. P3b was larger in controls over Pz and Oz. Further, the authors examined the relationship between performance and ERP measures and noted a correlation between P3b amplitude to targets and number of hits ($r = 0.80$, $p < 0.001$ for auditory and $r = 0.51$, $p < 0.03$ for visual tasks).

Taylor et al. *(13)* studied visual search ability in 11 ADHD children aged 7–8 yr (mean = 8.04 yr) and 10 children aged 9–10 yr (mean = 10.01 yr), as well as the same numbers of controls. ERPs were recorded using 19 electrodes. One set of tasks assessed parallel processing using change in size or color to identify targets (20% of trials), although other equally salient non-target items could also be present (17% of target trials). The other set was focused on serial processing where targets were characterized by conjunction of features (35% of trials). The researchers reported no group effects on P3 latency for ADHD children except for the serial task where controls had longer latencies. There were no group effects for P3 amplitude. The results were interpreted to indicate no group differences in overall processing strategies across tasks, but the ADHD group performed search in serial tasks as if they were parallel, i.e., in many cases completing the selection based on an automatic pop-out of a single feature rather than a conjunction of the target features.

Van der Stelt et al. *(31)* examined 24 boys with ADHD (aged 7–12 yr, mean = 9.1 ± 1.3 yr) and age-matched controls (mean = 9.3 ± 1.4 yr) using a more complicated visual search task where targets were characterized by a different spatial arrangement of the components (no gap), as well as color (task-relevant vs irrelevant). All stimulus types were presented with equal probability (25%). ERPs were recorded using 29 electrodes. When focusing on color, controls demonstrated frontal selection positivity at 190–290 ms over frontopolar and frontal sites, whereas this effect was absent in ADHD children who showed larger late processing negativity LPN over frontopolar sites because of larger late positivity to irrelevant nontarget stimuli. For the target stimuli, ADHD children had smaller P3b over T7 and P7 sites to relevant target and nontarget stimuli and demonstrated greater hemisphere differences at these sites compared to controls. The authors suggested that ADHD may impair selection based on color or more complex features but not the discriminative processes.

6.3. *Sustained Attention*

Strandburg et al. *(6)* investigated differences in sustained attention using two versions of Continuous Performance Task (CPT) with 16 ADHD children (mean age = 12.2 ± 2.4 yr) and 16 controls (mean age = 12.9 ± 1.8 yr). In single CPT, children had to respond to the target digit "8" (probability = 20%), whereas the same digit could appear among the distracters (probability = 36%). In the dual CPT, any digit repeated twice in a row was the target, whereas a nontarget digit could appear as a distracter on 41% of the trials. ERPs were obtained from three midline leads (Fz, Cz, Pz) and from electrodes over the temporal, parietal, and occipital regions in each hemisphere. There were no significant group differences for CNV or P1/N1 components. Processing negativity showed right laterality for the ADHD children only, but there were no group differences in amplitude or latency. P3 amplitude was reduced in ADHD for target stimuli in the single CPT but not in the dual CPT. P3 latencies were longer in ADHD for nontarget items. In the late portion of the wave (peaks at 580 ms and 760 ms), controls were characterized by increased frontal negativity to target stimuli. Further, at 580 ms, greater group differences were present for the single CPT compared with dual CPT. The authors concluded that there were no observable ADHD effects on early stages of attentional preparation or the amount of resources needed for task performance; however, ADHD did result in the reduced ability to detect targets and process response-relevant information. Using a traditional CPT-AX, Overtoom et al. *(7)* attempted to differentiate inattention and impulsivity in 16 boys with ADHD (mean age = 10.4 ± 1.4 yr) and 16 control children (14 boys; mean age = 10.3 ± 1.5 yr). ERPs were obtained from four midline leads. Hit P3 amplitude was smaller in ADHD than in controls over Pz. There were no differences in N2 responses to inhibition stimuli (AnoX) over Fz. For additional analyses, the researchers compared data from six children with oppositional defiant disorder (ODD) with controls and noted smaller N2, whereas the remaining 10 ADHD children were not different from the controls. The results indicated that ADHD children had more problems with inattention rather than with impulsivity and only ODD children showed deficits in the latter.

6.4. *Allocation*

Jonkman et al. *(10)* examined the attentional capacity of 14 children with ADHD, aged 7–13 yr (mean = 9.6 ± 2.2 yr) and matched controls using a probe paradigm where task-irrelevant stimuli were inserted among the task stimuli in easy and hard tasks (identification of specific color or sequence of colors, target probability 50%). The probes varied in appearance (60% standard, 20% deviant in orientation, and 20% novel) and did not require any response. ERPs were obtained from four midline leads. For the task stimuli, the results indicated that the ADHD group showed no increase in P3 amplitude with the increase in task difficulty. Further, ERPs of ADHD participants were characterized by smaller N1. Controls displayed larger negative central component (NC) in easy vs hard task while ADHD children showed no load effect. With regard to the probe stimuli, only P1 discriminated control and ADHD children with the control children showing larger amplitudes for deviant probes in the easy task. The authors concluded that ADHD children showed deficits not in attentional capacity but in allocation of attention.

6.5. *Inhibition*

Pliszka et al. *(32)* used a visual stop-signal task requiring children to withhold a response on 25% of the trials to investigate inhibitory control in 10 ADHD children (mean age = 11 ± 1.2 yr) and 10 controls (mean age = 11.3 ± 0.9 yr). Stop signals occurred with a random delay of 200–600 ms. ERPs were recorded with a 64-channel high-density electrode cap. Brain activity of the control group was characterized by a large N2 over right anterior inferior region elicited by the stop signal, although this component was significantly smaller in the ADHD ERPs. Additionally, scalp topography of the slow positive wave on the "go" trials differed between the two groups. For the controls, SPW was larger for failed than for successful inhibition trials over the right frontal region. The ADHD group had smaller slow positive wave (SPW) to failed inhibitions as compared with controls and showed no difference between successful and failed inhibitions within the group.

Overtoom et al. *(33)* studied 16 ADHD boys, aged 7–12 (mean age = 10.4 ± 1.4 yr) and 16 controls (14 boys) of the same age (mean age = 10.3 ± 1.5 yr) using a variation of the "stop task" where the task stimuli were visual and the stop signal was auditory (40% of trials). Additionally, the stop signal was presented with two different delays (125 vs 200 ms) after the trial stimulus. ERPs were obtained from four midline locations. Successful inhibition effect was identified as a greater positivity within a 100–400 ms range. Using a shorter delay, only controls showed differences in ERPs to successful vs failed inhibitions in 100–200 ms range, while the ADHD group showed smaller differences beginning at a later point (150–200 ms). Further, only the control group showed a significant inhibition effect over Fz and Cz in the 250–400ms window, although ADHD children had an inhibition effect present only at Cz and only at 250–300 ms. In the later portion of the wave (500–700 ms), failed inhibitions were characterized by larger amplitudes in control than in ADHD children. The authors concluded that ADHD children exhibited a specific impairment in reaction to the stop signal. They noted that their observations of inhibition-related positivity differences are not consistent with findings of other researchers but attributed that to the differences in the modality of the stop signal.

In further support of processing differences among children with ADHD, Yong-Liang et al. *(34)* examined inhibitory processes and behavioral measures in 21 boys with ADHD and 21 control boys (age 6–9 yr). A go/no-go task (no-go: 33%) was completed either before or after the stimulus-response compatibility task. Recordings were made from 30 electrode sites. Results showed no differences in reaction time between the groups, but demonstrated that control children made significantly more correct responses to the "go" condition, than children with ADHD, who made more unnecessary responses to the "no-go" stimuli. Children with ADHD, who completed go/no-go as the second task, had decreased frontal N2 amplitude. In contrast, right anterior frontal N2 amplitude was larger in control children when they were presented with the go/no-go task as the second task, and it was larger when the go/no-go task was presented first to the children in the ADHD group. In addition, the P650 amplitude was smaller for all groups for the no-go condition, and this decrease in amplitude was more prominent in the children with ADHD. The authors suggest the existence of difficulties with inhibition regulation in children diagnosed with ADHD, as a result of the differences of N2 based on task order and the discrimination of go and no-go conditions, as evidenced by the P3b.

6.6. Response Selection

Yong-Liang et al. *(35)* investigated the existence of a "response choice deficit" in children with ADHD, using a stimulus–response compatibility paradigm and a go/no-go task. It was hypothesized that a response choice deficit would result in extended reaction times, fewer correct responses, and larger ERPs in response to the incompatible stimuli in the task, in children with ADHD. ERPs were recorded from 30 electrodes, in 21 boys with ADHD and 21 control boys (age 6–9 yr). The behavioral results indicated no reaction-time differences between the groups. ERP analyses revealed longer frontal N100 and occipital P100 latencies in the children with ADHD. Larger frontal negativity (N360) was observed in the children with ADHD, to the stimuli that were incompatible, in comparison with the normal control children. Results indicated a difference in P3 for the children with ADHD, because of the order of the presentation of the tasks. More specifically, when the children in the ADHD group were presented with the stimulus–response compatibility task first, this group exhibited larger P330 amplitudes to the incompatible stimuli. In contrast, when the children with ADHD completed another task (go/no-go) prior to the stimulus-response compatibility task, the resulting P330 amplitude was smaller. Both groups exhibited larger parietocentral P650 amplitudes to the incompatible stimuli when the stimulus–response compatibility task was presented first. Further, central P650 amplitude increases were observed in the ADHD group when the stimulus–response compatibility task was completed following the go/no-go task, whereas central P650 amplitude decreased in the control group. The authors concluded that the behavioral data did not support a response choice deficit among children with ADHD, due to the fact that children in this group did not exhibit slower or more inaccurate responses than the children in the control group. The condition effect of task order suggests that children with ADHD initially employ more means of processing stimuli in the stimulus–response compatibility task, but when it was completed following the go/no-go task, the children relied on different processing strategies of the task and the response. In this situation, the children are more familiar with the experimental conditions, suggesting that they are more readily able to assess the situation and their responses to the presented stimuli.

6.7. *Summary: Attention Processes*

Examination of various attention processes in children with ADHD resulted in the conclusion that basic orienting processes may not be impaired in children with ADHD and that the modality of the stimulus (e.g., visual, auditory) generally does not have a significant effect. Most of the deficits are attributed to later stages of information processing. Based on the electrophysiological data, children with ADHD were characterized by greater processing of attended stimuli and increased sensitivity to changes in the stimuli. However, they relied on simpler selection strategies, especially when the task involved comparing multiple features of complex stimuli, and often did not benefit from pretrial cues or the salient features of the stimuli. In regard to inhibition and response selection, children with ADHD demonstrated no differences in brain activity associated with successful and failed inhibitions. ERPs of the ADHD group were characterized by reduced amplitudes and delayed latencies to failed inhibitions compared with the controls. Further, inhibition effects were sensitive to the experimental procedures and varied based on the order of the inhibition task among other tasks in the testing sessions. The above studies provide evidence that task order may be a key consideration in the assessment of ERPs of children with ADHD. Performance on certain tasks may be hindered or assisted dependent on the order in which a child with ADHD completes each task.

Across the tasks involving various attention processes, N2 and P3 components were most frequently identified as sensitive to group differences. Both were typically characterized by reduced amplitudes and delayed latencies (with exception of *12,13*) compared with control children. Attempt to relate ERP data to behavioral results indicated that P350 latency could be used to discriminate children with ADHD from the controls. Further, ADHD-related effects were also sometimes noted for amplitudes and latencies of other components, such as P1, N1, SPW, and (L)PN, but the findings were less consistent (*see* Table 1 for an overview).

7. ERPs AND SUBTYPES OF ADHD

Because diagnosis of ADHD involves the differentiation of clinical subtypes dependent on the predominant symptom presentation, researchers have become interested in investigating ERP differences between such diagnostic groups.

DeFrance et al. *(36)* conducted a study to investigate ERP differences between 34 children with ADHD, predominantly hyperactive/impulsive (ADHD-IM, mean age = 9.8 yr), 17 children with ADHD, predominantly inattentive (ADHD-IA, mean age = 9.7 yr), and 20 normal control children (mean age = 9.9 yr). The researchers used a go-go task consisting of a "passive" task, in which the children were instructed to visually observe the stimuli that were presented, and an "active" task, during which the children were instructed to press the right mouse button when a "0" appeared on the screen, and to press the left mouse button for any other number. The task was designed to differentiate between ERP activity that was a result of effortful processing *(37)* and that which was owing to attention *(38)*. ERPs were recorded from 28 electrode sites. Results demonstrated larger P250 amplitudes in children in the ADHD groups in the effortful phase of the task. In order to examine processing differences between the passive and effortful phases of the experiment, the researchers used the difference waveform, which was determined by subtracting the passive wave from the effortful wave. The authors used this procedure to identify differences in processing that were associated with effortful cognition. The difference waveform reflected variations in processing between the three experimental participant groups. The ADHD-IM (impulsive type) group had larger P250 amplitude and smaller P3b (P500) amplitude than the control group. In contrast, children with ADHD-IA (inattentive type) exhibited smaller P500 amplitude, and more left hemisphere processing of the P250 and P350 than the other two groups. According to this study, the aspect that discriminated the ADHD-IM children from the ADHD-IA group was the left hemisphere distribution for the ADHD-IA children for the P250 and P350. According to the authors, the results of this study support the existence of distinct attentional disorder subtypes; the subtypes were accurately classified by ERP data, in concordance with diagnostic criteria.

Group differences have also been demonstrated in auditory tasks using an oddball paradigm. Kuperman et al. *(39)* conducted a study with elementary-school children, investigating ERP differences in 12 children with ADHD, 16 children with undifferentiated ADD (UADD) (children without hyperactivity), and 12 control children. ERPs were recorded from 18 electrode sites using an auditory oddball paradigm, in which the children were instructed to attend to the number of rare auditory tones that were presented during the experimental session. The results demonstrated group differences, with ADHD children displaying longer N100 latencies to the common tone, and control children exhibiting greater P3 amplitudes to the rare tone than the other two groups. P3 amplitude did not differ significantly between the ADHD and UADD groups. Group hemisphere differences were also found. Children with ADHD and UADD had smaller P3 left-hemisphere amplitude to the common tone; the ADHD group had larger left-hemisphere N1 amplitudes to the common tone, and decreased left hemisphere P3 latency to the rare tone. The researchers concluded that there are variations in ERPs among ADHD, UADD, and controls, and that the children with ADHD and UADD may have difficulties in the judgment of stimuli and may employ fewer attentional mechanisms than children from the other two groups.

8. ERPs AND COMORBIDITY

ADHD is a disorder that is often comorbid with other psychological disorders. Children diagnosed with ADHD often have co-occurring learning and behavioral disorders. A number of studies have attempted to determine whether the differences that are expressed by such children are the result of ADHD or could be attributed to the existence of other psychological problems (*see* Table 2 for an overview).

8.1. ADHD and LD

Many researchers have focused on learning disabilities and ADHD, and have investigated both the comorbidity of the two disorders, and the existence of each disorder alone, with no second comorbid disorder. Frank et al. *(40)* assessed differences in ERPs between 18 children with learning disabilities (LD) (mean age = 10.6 yr), 36 children with both LD and ADHD (mean age = 11.9 yr), and 27 normal control children (mean age = 11.9 yr), using an oddball auditory task, in which the children were instructed to count the rare tones. ERPs were recorded from the Cz. The authors reported smaller P3 amplitudes to the rare, target stimuli in the task in children with ADHD/LD, compared with normal children. There were no significant differences found between the LD and ADHD/LD groups in P3 amplitude, implying that ADHD did not largely contribute to the differences observed. The researchers concluded that the results imply that the smaller P3 amplitude that was observed in the children with LD and ADHD/LD is indicative of information processing differences and is not exclusively associated with the attentional, impulsive or hyperactive characteristics of ADHD.

In a later study, Frank et al. *(41)* examined electrophysiological differences associated with age and diagnosis. The study used an auditory oddball paradigm and included six participant groups, with 29 adults without a diagnosis (mean age = 24.5 yr), 43 normal control children (mean age = 11.8 yr), 12 children with ADHD (mean age = 9.5 yr), 33 children with LD (mean age = 10.5 yr), 63 children with ADHD/LD (mean age = 9.1 yr), and 11 children with conduct disorder (mean age = 10.5 yr). ERPs were recorded with electrodes placed on the scalp at Cz. The results demonstrated longer P3 latencies and smaller P3 amplitude in children diagnosed with ADHD/LD, as compared with normal children and children with conduct disorders. Normal control children had larger P3 amplitudes than ADHD/LD children. Age differences were significant for amplitudes of N1 and N2, as well as for N4 latency in children 8–12 yr and 12–18 yr of age. In the LD group, N2 amplitude was positively correlated with age. In the ADHD/LD group, there were also significant correlations for ERPs and age: latencies of N1 and N4 were negatively correlated with age, whereas P3 amplitude and amplitude difference between rare and frequent responses were positively correlated with age. The authors suggested that the results of this study imply that the variation in P3 amplitude and latency in the groups of children diagnosed with LD and ADHD/LD is due to differences in processing, and is not directly related to attentional difficulties. Because there were no significant differences in the P3 between normal children and those diagnosed with ADHD only, this suggests that the differences exist because of information processing dissimilarity, not problems with attention regulation. In addition, because there were no significant interactions between the diagnostic and age groups, the authors concluded that "electrophysiological abnormalities in LD and ADHD do not significantly change with age during childhood."

Overall, none of the reported studies were able to discriminate between children with ADHD only and those with ADHD/LD. Both groups were characterized by smaller P3 amplitude, suggesting processing differences in children with ADHD and LD, as compared to normal children. These findings imply that observed processing differences in children with ADHD and comorbid LD may not be exclusively related to attentional problems but to a larger common difference in information processing.

8.2. ADHD and Behavior Disorders

Not only is ADHD comorbid with learning disabilities, but studies have also been conducted investigating the brain responses of children with ADHD and behavioral disorders. Linden et al.

(42,43) investigated ERPs and reaction time in children with ADHD, children with ADHD and ODD, and control children, 5–12 yr of age, using an oddball paradigm. The results showed that children with ADHD and ADHD/ODD had longer N2 and P3 latencies, P3 amplitude differences, and slower reaction times in comparison to the control group. Results also yielded an N1 amplitude group difference for the ADHD group and the children with ADHD/ODD.

In addition, the researchers examined age effects on the ERPs of the children that participated in the study. Age differences were found for N1 and P2 latency of the children with ADHD and the children with ADD/ODD. Such variations in the ERPs were no longer apparent with increasing age. More specifically, the young children with ADHD only (aged 5–9 yr) had longer N1 and P2 latencies, but in 12-yr-old children such differences were no longer observed. There was a significant interaction of age and group, with the older children (10–12 yr of age) with ADHD exhibiting smaller N1 amplitudes and the younger children with ADHD showing larger N1 amplitudes than the other groups that were included in the study. The 10–12-yr-old children with ADHD/ODD and the 5–9-yr-old children with ADHD had greater P2 latencies. This study also demonstrated an age effect that was not specific to subgroup. P2 amplitudes were greater for the children in the older group than for the children in the younger group. The researchers concluded that early components of the ERP waveform (N1, P2) distinguish the clinical groups from normal control children.

8.3. Summary: Comorbidity

Overall, ERP studies investigating comorbidity between ADHD and other learning and behavioral disorders demonstrate that at the moment there are no clear indicators that would allow to discriminate pure ADHD group from children with other concurrent disabilities. These findings further suggest that observed ERP differences (e.g., reduced P3 amplitude) between the ADHD and control groups may not be attributed solely to attention difficulties and may indicate other deficiencies or contributions of other disorders.

9. ERPs AND IQ

Researchers have also been interested in the correspondence between the ERP waveforms and the cognitive intelligence measures. Robaey et al. *(44)* investigated the relation of ERPs to verbal and visuospatial intelligence measures on the Wechsler Intelligence Scale for Children-Revised (WISC-R), and Piagetian intelligence measures in 19 children with ADHD (mean age = 7 yr 5 mo) and 30 control children (mean age = 7 yr 7 mo), using classification and seriation tasks. Fourteen electrodes were used to record ERPs. Results demonstrated significant correlations between verbal skills, visuospatial performance and conservation abilities, and ERP amplitudes of the waveforms. For the control group, results showed a negative correlation between verbal scores and ERPs, as demonstrated in decreased parieto-occipital P350 and parieto-occipital P500 amplitude with increasing verbal IQ. A negative correlation was also found for performance measures and frontal P250 and parieto-occipital N250 amplitudes, with decreased P250 and N250 amplitudes related to higher visuospatial performance scores. Furthermore, for the Piagetian intelligence measures a significant negative correlation was found for frontal P250 amplitude, whereas significant positive correlations were obtained for P500 amplitudes. Finally, amplitude of the parieto-occipital P350 was also correlated with these measures, but the direction of the relationship varied based on stimulus (target or distractor) and score type (raw vs scaled).

Some of the findings in this study for children with ADHD are similar to the findings for normal control children, whereas others are inconsistent. In children with ADHD, a negative correlation was obtained between verbal skills and frontal P250 amplitude. Likewise, a negative correlation was found between verbal abilities and parieto-occipital P500 amplitude. The correlations that were observed in the study for ADHD children on verbal skills were greater for nontarget waveforms and significant over the right hemisphere. The correlations between visuospatial performance and ERP amplitudes for the ADHD group were significant on the right hemisphere for N250 to target stimuli and the right hemisphere for P500 to nontarget stimuli. More specifically, P250 and N250 waves were negatively correlated with scores on picture arrangement, positively correlated with block design scores. In contrast to the control group, the only significant correlation for the Piagetian measures in the ADHD group was a negative correlation for N250 amplitude. As a result, the authors suggested that distinct ERP patterns are apparent for different types and levels of intelligence. They concluded that ERPs could be useful tools for evaluating the elements of intelligence. Robaey and his colleagues proposed that different forms of intelligence utilize different processing components of the brain, as evidenced by ERP waveforms.

More broadly, ERPs may be indicative of verbal and visuo spatial performance, as suggested by the correlational findings. Because ERPs are reflective of underlying neural processing, they may provide valuable information regarding complex cognitive processes, as revealed by intellectual abilities and intelligence test performance.

10. SCALP TOPOGRAPHY STUDIES

Oades et al. *(45)* recorded auditory ERP and mismatch negativity (MMN) responses to three tones from 19 scalp locations from 12 controls, 12 ADHD children, and 10 children with Tourette's syndrome (8–15 yr of age) during the standard oddball task. ADHD children generated faster latency N1 components, suggesting that they process perceptual information faster at an earlier stage of development. The scalp location for the largest P2 component was shifted toward anterior electrode sites compared with controls (similarly reported by ref. *46*; but qualified by ref. *47*). ADHD children also did not show the usual right-biased P3 asymmetry or the frontal vs parietal P3 latency difference. This absence of P3-based hemisphere differences has been noted in other studies for ADHD children *(48)*.

Steger et al. *(48)* investigated bilateral neural processing in 15 ADHD and 16 age-matched control boys (mean age for each group = 10.8 yr). Unlike a number of studies reviewed, mean IQ was lower for ADHD (98.43) than control children (107.15). ERPs were recorded from 32 scalp locations. Overall, P3 amplitude to targets was smaller in ADHD children, a finding consistent with other studies. Such a decrease could reflect reduced resource allocation to targets (*see also* ref. *10*). The attenuation of the lateralized readiness potential for left-hand responses of ADHD children supports a specific motor preparation deficit in ADHD. Additionally, the decline in responding controlled by the right hemisphere resembles that noted earlier by Oades et al. *(45)*.

11. INFORMATION-PROCESSING STRATEGY

Frank et al. *(49)* assessed differences in short-term memory between normal developing children and adults and ADHD children. Visual ERPs were recorded from 30 normal adults (17–34 yr), 17 normal children (8–16 yr), and 14 children with ADHD (8–14 yr) during a Sternberg memory search paradigm. Visual ERPs were recorded from electrodes at Cz, Pz, and Oz sites in response to nonmeaningful visual geometric shapes followed by a fixation point and then a test stimulus. On half the trials a test stimulus matched one item in the set. Analyses that focused only on Cz noted that when the number of items increased from two to four, the number of errors and RT increased, although P3 amplitude decreased, suggesting a self-terminating strategy. That is, the ADHD children made their decision to respond before reviewing the entire stimulus. The authors concluded that ADHD children demonstrate a different pattern of information processing in comparison with normal children and adults.

12. ATTENDING TO TARGETS TRIAL BY TRIAL

Lazzaro et al. *(47)* investigated P300 single trial-by-trial variability in 17 unmedicated adolescents with attention deficit hyperactivity disorder. Using averaged ERPs, as well as the response variance curve (RVC) to measure single-trial ERP variability relative to their average, Lazzaro et al. recorded ERPs during an auditory oddball task. No differences in P300 amplitude or latency were found between controls and the ADHD group. However, when patients were initially placed on dextroamphetamine (mean daily dose = 0.5 mg/kg) and 10 patients switched to methylphenidate (MPH) (mean daily dose = 0.75 mg/kg) because they exhibited aggressive behavior, they showed a significant reduction in maximum RVC variability compared to their unmedicated state. No other differences were found for overall P300 amplitude.

In a related study of time-on-task, Heinrich et al. *(46)* investigated both performance measures and endogenous ERP components in ADHD and healthy children during an auditory selective attention task. Investigators examined changes in brain responses on each successive trial. Participants included 24 normal developing boys (mean age = 10 yr, 7 mo) and 24 boys who met DSM-III-R criteria (mean age = 10 yr, 5 mo). Children responded to the higher of two tones presented to the ear by pressing a button. ADHD children detected fewer targets than did healthy children although both groups performed equally well in the beginning (less than 1 min).

Subsequent analyses of the ERP data were conducted on a trial-by-trial basis. To obtain a reliable estimate of the single trial ERP, a recursive wavelet node single-sweep training algorithm was used. Thus, wavelet nodes with comparable time-frequency characteristics like the nodes of the averaged ERP were obtained for each single trial response. No overall effects were found between healthy and ADHD children for frontal negativity and parietal positivity. However, healthy and ADHD children did differ in time-on-task dynamics for frontal negativity. The increase in frontal negativity observed in both groups to target-attended stimuli might indicate that more attention resources had to be allocated for ADHD children to reach adequate performance and this increase in resources required that the child spend more time on task. In ADHD children, this process started earlier compared to healthy children. Moreover, ADHD children did not appear to mobilize more resources during this task in contrast to healthy children who reached their maximum value around the 30th target-attended trial. In contrast to the distinct quadratic course of frontal negativity in the control group, smaller higher-order fluctuations were present in the ADHD group. This could be related to shorter attention spans and generally fluctuating cognitive behavior. The lack of group differences in parietal positivity was interpreted to indicate that the underlying neurophysiological processes (e.g., stimulus evaluation processes) were not impaired in the ADHD children and that these processes did not contribute to their poorer performance.

13. DRUG EFFECTS

A review of many of these studies noted a focus on the use of MPH and its impact on attention as indexed by both behavioral measures (reaction time [RT], number of correct responses, error rates, etc.) and ERP measures, mainly the P3a and P3b ERP components. For the most part, treatment studies that compare ADHD children treated with MPH with nontreated ADHD children and normal controls report variations in peak amplitudes and latencies related to drug interventions (*see* Table 3 for an overview).

In a relatively early ERP study investigating the effects of MPH on brain and behavior responses, Miller et al. *(50)* recorded changes in the ERP when 19 boys with ADHD were administered MPH and compared with 13 normal controls (8–10 yr). These ADHD children comprised a special population that was described as free from any other identified handicapping conditions including LDS. Although no differences were found on a selective attention Stroop task, ERP components did differ between groups. Specifically in response to targets (infrequent stimuli), ADHD boys produced larger P3b amplitude and shorter mean latencies compared with controls. In contrast, controls generated shorter P3a peaks than ADHD boys to nontargets (*see also* ref. *51*).

With medication, however, effects changed. In general, for target stimuli, controls and treatment groups produced shorter N1 latencies (i.e., responded faster) than the placebo group in the retest condition compared to the baseline condition. In addition, N1 amplitude was smaller for treated children than for controls. In contrast, treated children generated larger N2 amplitudes than controls. Peak amplitudes were also larger for the treatment group for P1, P3a, and P3b, a finding consistent with many of the MPH treatment studies.

The authors argued that the shorter target N1 latencies in ADHD boys suggested that they are unable to selectively attend to the target events in the same manner as normals. However, given the nature of the task, it is possible (as suggested by ref. *10*) that the ADHD children engaged a default strategy that precluded much of the encoding of the stimuli.

Given the behavior performance improvements (correct responses, RT) noted for both target and nontarget stimuli, it appears that MPH enhances early selective attention and stimulus recognition.

Jonkman et al. *(52)* assessed the impact of MPH on attention using a probe ERP study to investigate differences between children with and without ADHD. Visual ERPs and behavior measures were obtained from 28 children (7–13 yr) from electrodes placed over Fz, Cz, Pz, and Oz scalp locations. In the first experiment, during the easy task, participants pressed a button whenever a blue rectangle was detected and another button to all rectangles of another color. In the hard task, participants compared each rectangle with the preceding rectangle. Although controls were more accurate across tasks, no differences were noted in RT between the ADHD children and controls. However, although the P3 amplitudes for both groups were comparable for the easy task, only controls showed a marked amplitude increase in the hard task. The authors interpreted these findings to indicate that the ADHD were not able to assign more attention capacity to the more demanding task. Thus they argued that ADHD children experience a deficiency in capacity allocation and not simply capacity shortage.

The second experiment tested whether MPH would affect later performance for the ADHD children and increase the amplitude of the P3 during the hard task. Overall, correct responses increased but RT did not differ between the placebo and MPH conditions. In contrast P3 amplitude was larger for the MPH than the placebo condition. It did not differ, though, between conditions. The authors continued to conclude that individuals with ADHD experience a deficiency in capacity allocation.

In a series of well-designed and controlled studies, Sunohara and colleagues *(53,54)* investigated the effects of MPH on attention in children with ADHD. In the first study, Sunohara et al. *(53)* compared ERPs recorded from 13 medication responders, 13 nonresponders, and 13 control children in a double-blind study. Both ADHD groups were tested on four separate occasions during a 4-wk double-blind, placebo-controlled assessment of MPH effectiveness. Each child was tested on baseline, placebo, and lower and higher doses of MPH in random order. Psychoeducational and cognitive tasks were administered each week to assess child's response to medication. ERPs were recorded 1.5–3 h after midday administration of MPH or placebo from a set of 13 electrodes during two oddball tasks: a visual feature detection task and a semantic classification task. Mean age for all children was 11.47 yr. When off medication, no differences were noted between the two ADHD groups. However, when on MPH, longer latency N2 and P3b responses were noted for the nonresponders than for responders. This finding paralleled cognitive performance differences between the two ADHD groups while on medication, with higher error rates occurring for the nonresponders.

Sunohara et al. *(54)* studied MPH effects in ADHD by recording ERPs during attention task performance in 20 normal controls (mean age = 10.5 yr) and 20 children with ADHD under different dose conditions (mean age = 10.8 yr). Using a double-blind, placebo-controlled crossover trial design across a consecutive 2-d period, the ADHD group was assessed off drug (baseline) and on placebo, low (0.28 mg/kg), and high (0.56 mg/kg) dose levels of MPH. At baseline, the ADHD children were more impulsive and inattentive than controls and had shorter P2 and N2 latencies and longer P3 latencies. Low-dose MPH was associated with reduced impulsivity (fewer false alarms) and decreased P3 latencies, whereas the higher dose level was associated with reduced impulsivity and less inattention (more hits), as well as increased P2 and N2 latencies and decreased P3 latencies. No peak amplitude changes were noted. No adverse effects of the higher dose were noted, for any of the children. These results suggest differential dosage effects and a dissociation between dose levels and aspects of processing.

In a related study, Winsberg et al. *(55)* also recorded ERP differences in 14 hyperkinetic MPH responders (mean age = 126.7 mo) and 14 control children (mean age = 126.7 mo). Control IQs were higher than those of the hyperkinetic children. Responses on the Conners Abbreviated rating scale and Conners Teacher's rating scale were recorded twice per week. EEG was then recorded beginning 1 h prior to administration of medication or a placebo and finished within 18–24 h of administration of the last dose. Controls received no medication or placebo treatments. Participants were involved in active and passive oddball tasks.

ERP peak amplitudes and latencies were measured for five separate peaks: for MMN, N1 at 50–150 ms, P2 at 150–250 ms, N2 at 150–250 ms, and P3 at 250–550 ms. Behavioral differences were found between the two groups when the hyperkinetic children were not receiving MPH but disappeared following drug administration to the target group. Placebo-treated ADHD children had significantly lower percent correct detections and slower RT to correct detections than MPH-treated ADHD children.

As in the case of Sunohara et al. *(54)*, Winsberg et al. also found an increase in P3 amplitude. Following administration of MPH, a significantly earlier and larger peak was generated in response to deviant stimuli in both the active and passive response conditions when compared with the controls and placebo treatment conditions. The MPH group generated significantly larger P3 amplitudes in response to standards in the active condition compared with the placebo and control groups. Additionally, a series of negative correlations occurred between RT to correct detections and P3 amplitude for the ADHD–MPH group, but not for placebo group.

Zillessen et al. *(56)* also assessed changes in the P300 component. They further replicated the effects reported by Sunohara et al. *(54)* and Winsberg et al. *(55)*. In a test of 17 right-handed boys (mean age = 9.5 yr), children were tested twice while unmedicated during a CPT and twice in a medicated CPT condition. Children pressed a mouse button if the letter "*O*" (80 times = 20%) occurred immediately before the letter "*X*". They noted that while receiving MPH, a larger P3a component occurred. No effects were seen in later processes.

Not all studies report increased P3 amplitude effects with medication in ADHD children. Taylor et al. *(13)* tested 21 ADHD children (16 males, 7–10 yr of age) and 21 control children (14 males, 8–10 yr of age) in a series of serial and parallel processing tasks. Although no P3 latency or amplitude effects were noted between groups, the current task did not require sustained attention, thereby explaining the lack of significant P3 changes owing to medication.

Across studies it appears that the lack of significant differences between MPH-treated and normal control groups for the N1 and P2 components suggests that the basic physiological components of the nervous system remain intact for the ADHD population. Under correctly medicated conditions these children appear to encode and process sensory aspects of incoming stimuli in a normal fashion. Likewise, the consistent finding of increased P3 amplitudes and faster RT in MPH treated groups suggests that ADHD children are more physiologically alert and accurate when receiving the medication. In fact, given larger P3 peak amplitudes resulting from MPH treatment it appears that the child becomes physiologically hypervigilant. These conclusions are tempered by some findings suggesting that not all children with ADHD-like symptoms respond behaviorally or electrophysiologically in a manner that indicates hightened vigilance as indexed by performance increases or increased P3 amplitudes *(57)*.

14. SUMMARY

In general, across studies, control children typically produce larger ERP components (P1, P3) than ADHD children who are not medicated. With medication, however, such peak amplitude differences often disappear. A number of investigators conclude that overall perceptual processes are intact in ADHD children and that these processes do not contribute to their poorer performance. Furthermore, basic orienting processes, regardless of modality, do not appear to be impaired in children with ADHD.

Most ADHD-related deficits are attributed to later stages of information processing. In general, ADHD children rely on simpler selection strategies, especially when the task involves comparing multiple features of complex stimuli. It appears that such children seldom benefit from pretrial cues or increasing the salient features of stimuli. Concerning inhibition and response selection, children with ADHD exhibited few differences in ERP brain activity associated with successful or failed inhibitions. Later-occurring components, such as N2 and P3 components, were most frequently identified as sensitive to differences between ADHD children and controls. Both were typically characterized by reduced amplitudes and delayed latencies (with the exception of 12,13) compared with control children. In this connection, given the relation between ERPs and behavioral results it has been suggested that P350 latency could be used to discriminate children with ADHD from controls in some tasks.

Table 1
ADHD and Basic Attentional Processes

Authors	Year	Hypotheses	Subjects ADHD	Subjects Control	Electrodes (analyzed)	Design	Results
				Orientation			
Perchet et al.	2001	ERP indicators of anticipatory processes, attentional priming, target detection, and response selection/ reprogramming	28 (25 males), age 6.5–11 yr (mean = 8.4 ± 1.5 yr *ERP data*: 24 (21 males), age 6–10.5 yr (mean = 8.5 ± 1.4 yr)	22 (13 males) age 5.5–9 yr (mean = 7.2 ± 1.3 yr) *ERP data*: 13 (10 males), age 6–9 yr (mean = 7.4 ± 0.8 yr)	Cz, Pz, Oc = (O1+O2)/2 Ref: nose Filters: 0.1–30 Hz	Posner's orienting paradigm (60% valid, 20% invalid, 20% uncued trials)	P1: no differences across target conditions for ADHD; Shorter N2–RT interval in ADHD CNV/RP area smaller in ADHD
				Selection/Search/Detection			
Satterfiled et al.	1990	Examine longitudinal effects on auditory attention tuning, abnormal development in ADHD, development of P3b differences with age, reduction of Nd differences	15 (all males, 10 with conduct 5 with oppostional–defiant disorder [ODD] test 1: age 5.8–7.1 yr (mean = 6.3 ± 0.4 yr); test 2: 8 yr (mean = 8.9 ± 0.4 yr);	15 (all males) test 1: age 5.8–7.1 yr (mean = 6.3 ± 0.4 yr); test 2: 8 yr (mean = 8.9 ± 0.3 yr)	19 (Electrode cap) Ref: linked ears Filters: 0.1–50 Hz (1–50 Hz for Fp1/2)	Auditory/visual selective task (stimulus intensity reduced at 8-yr retest)	Auditory target : analysis P2–N2 smaller in ADHD at 6 yr, no difference at 8 yr. Controls > ADHD for P350, P3b, SP1, greater increase to target in controls
Robaey et al.	1992	Orienting to rare targets (P2) and controlled processes (N2c, P3b) will be different across groups	12 (all males without comorbid disorders) age = 6–8 yr (6: age < 7.6 yr, 6: age > 7.6 yr)	12 (all males) age = 6–8 yr (6: age < 7.6 yr, 6: age > 7.6 yr)	14 (single electrodes) Ref: linked ears Filters: 0.08–40 Hz *Analyzed*: number of electrodes	Four visual tasks (categorization and seriation: words, pictures, numbers), 30% targets (15 trials)/block,2	P250, N250 greater in ADHD; P500 smaller; shorter latencies P350 Discriminant analysis: latency P350

(Continued)

Table 1 (*Continued*)

Authors	Year	Hypotheses	Subjects		Electrodes	Design	Results
			ADHD	Control	(analyzed)		
					varied by peak 200 ms/750 ms	blocks	
Johnstone et al.	1996	AERPs to target/nontarget	10 (8 males) age = 6.2–13.7 yr (mean =1 0.4 ± 2.1yr)	10 (8 males) age = 6.2–13.7 yr (mean = 10.7 ± 1.9 yr)	17 (Electrocap) linked ears Ref: Filters: 0.1–25Hz *Analyzed:* 9 regions (overlapping)	Auditory task 15% targets (1500 Hz tone), 85% standards (1000 Hz tone)	No latency effects; N2 smaller in ADHD over forntal areas and larger over posterior regions; P3b to nontargets larger in ADHD
Taylor, et al.	1997	Differences in serial vs parallel processing	21 total 11 (8 males) age = 7–8 yr, (mean = 8.04 yr); 10 (8 males) age = 9–10 yr, (mean = 10.01 yr)	21 total 11 (8 males) age = 7–8 yr, 8.03 yr); 10 (6 males) age 9–10 yr, (mean = 9.10 yr)	19 Ref: spinal Filters: 0.1–30 Hz	Parallel task: search by color or shape Serial task: search by color and shape	P3 latencies longer in controls in serial task
Jonkman et al.	1997	Assess ADHD-related differences in early selection in visual and auditory tasks	18 (16 males) age = 7–13 yr (mean = 10.6 ± 2 yr)	18 (all males) age = 7–13 yr (mean = 10 ± 1.2 yr)	Fz, Cz, Pz, Oz, Ref: linked earlobes Filters: 0.15–30 Hz	Auditory and visual selective attention (20% targets, half in the relevant channel)	Auditory: N1 and N2 larger in controls to stimuli in nonattended channel; no such differences for ADHD P3b and PN smaller in ADHD
Karayandis et al.	2000	Assess differences in early visual processing/stimulus discrimination and evaluation	17 (all males, 6 with ODD) age = 6.4–9.8 yr (mean = 7.17 ± 0.82 yr)	17 (all males) age = 7.05–10 yr (mean = 7.66 ± 1.11 yr)	30 (20 Electrocap + 10 extra) Ref: linked earlobes Filters: 0.1–30 Hz *Analyzed*: number of	Visual task (25% target), respond to both	N1, P2 delayed in ADHD; greater discrimination of St in controls (N2 amplitude), N2 earlier in controls over left front; opposite trend on latency

					electrodes varied by peak.		(increase in ADHD). P450 rare–frequent differences larger in controls N530 larger in ADHD (especially for rare St). NSW has larger St effects in ADHD
Lazzaro et al.	2001	Relation of τ activity to ERPs	54 (all males: 47combined type, 7 hyperactive–impulsive) age = 11–17 yr (mean = 13.7 ± 1.4 yr)	54 (all males) age = 11–17 yr (mean = 13.4 ± 1.5 yr)	19 (electrocap), Ref: linked earlobes Filters: low-pass 50 Hz *Analyzed*: for group comparisons, used Fz, Cz, Pz only	Auditory task (tones), 15% targets	P200 larger in ADHD, smaller N200, N200, and P300 delayed.
van der Stelt et al.	2001	Identify functional loci of visual selection and assess developmental effects	24 (all males, 23 combined type, without comorbid disorders) age = 7–12 yr (mean = 9.1 ± 1.3 yr)	24 (all males) age = 7–12 yr (mean = 9.3 ± 1.4 yr)	29 (cap) Ref: right mastoid Filters: 0.16–40 (20.7) Hz	Visual selective attention (color or semantic selection)	ADHD: smaller frontal slow positivity and P3b; No latency differences
				Inhibition			
Pliszka et al.	2000	Examine functional organization of inhibition	10 (all males; combined type) mean age = 11 ± 1.2 yr	10 (all males) mean age = 11.3 ± 0.9 yr	64 (Electrocap) Ref: right mastoid Filters: 0.01–100 Hz *Analyzed*: grand averages, scalp topography, and 24 electrodes averaged into 8 regions	Stop task	N2 amplitude smaller in ADHD over right frontal inferior region; SPW more positive in controls

(Continued)

Table 1 (*Continued*)

Authors	Year	Hypotheses	Subjects: ADHD	Subjects: Control	Electrodes (analyzed)	Design	Results
Yong-Liang et al.	2000	Inhibitory processes and behavioral measures of ADHD and control children	21 boys with ADHD (age = 6–9 yr)	21 boys (age = 6–9 yr)	Fz, Cz, Pz, Oz, Fp1/Fp2, Af3/Af4, F3/F4, F7/F8, Fc3/Fc4, T7/T8, C3/C4, C1/C2, Cp3/Cp4, Tp7/Tp8, P3/P4, P7/P8, O1/O2 Ref: linked earlobes Filters: 0.1–30 Hz	Mixed go/no-go paradigm (30% no-go) Stimulus Response Compatibility Task	ADHD: N2 and P650 amplitude differences as a function of task order
Overtoom et al.	2002	Is poor inhibition caused by poor stop signal processing?	16 (all males, 6 comorbid ODD, 1 anxiety, 3 developmental disorders) age = 7–12 yr (mean = 10.4 ± 1.4 yr)	16 (14 males) age = 7–12 yr (mean = 10.3 ± 1.5 yr)	Oz, Pz, Cz, Fz Ref: linked mastoids Filters: 0.15–200 (40) Hz	Stop task	Controls show greater difference in success/fail to inhibit in early and late stages. Inhibition effect in ADHD significant over Cz, additional Fz involvement for controls
				Sustained Attention			
Strandburg et al.	1996	Unclear	16 (13 males) mean age = 12.2 ± 2.4 yr	16 (9 males) mean age = 12.9 ± 1.8 yr	9 (Fz, Cz, Pz, T5, T6, P3, P4, O1, O2), Ref: linked earlobes Filters: 0.1–30 Hz	Single CPT, dual CPT	ADHD have smaller P3 (when controlled for age) and longer latencies; smaller frontal negativity
Overtoom et al.	1998	ADHD shows more inattention and	16 (all males, 6 comorbid ODD,	16 (14 males) age = 6–14 yr	Fz, Cz, Pz, Oz Ref: linked	Continuous performance	P3 hit amplitude smaller in ADHD

		impulsivity ADHD differ in patterns of brain activity	1 anxiety, 3 developmental disorders) age = 6–14 yr (mean = 10.4 ± 1.4 yr)	(mean = 10.3 ± 1.5 yr)	mastoids Filters: 0.15–200 (40) Hz	task	N2 amplitude smaller in ODD only
				Allocation			
Jonkman et al.	2000	Examine attentional capacity and/or *allocation* problems	14 (13 males; 6 scored lower than 15 on Conners; 5 below clinical level on CBCL) age = 7–13 yr (mean = 9.6 ±- 2.2 yr)	14 (12 males) age = 7–13 yr (mean = 10.1 ± 1.5 yr)	Fz, Cz, Pz, Oz Ref: linked earlobes Filters: 0.15–40 Hz	Eriksen "Flanker," easy and hard decision tasks	No P3 amplitude increase to targets from easy to hard condition in ADHD (present in controls) Controls > ADHD for N1
Yong-Liang et al.	2000	Assessed "response choice deficit" in children with ADHD and control children	21 boys with ADHD (age = 6–9 yr)	21 boys (age = 6–9 yr)	Fz, Cz, Pz, Oz, Fp1/Fp2, Af3/Af4, F3/F4; F7/F8, Fc3/Fc4, T7/T8, C3/C4, C1/C2, Cp3/Cp4, Tp7/Tp8, P3/P4, P7/P8, O1/O2 Ref: linked earlobes Filters: 0.1–30 Hz	Mixed stimulus response compatibility paradigm, go/no-go task (30% no-go)	ADHD: longer frontal N100 and occipital P100 latencies, larger frontal negativity (N360) to incompatible stimuli, and occipital P330 and parietocentral P650 differences as a function of task order

ERP, event-related potential; ADHD, attention deficit hyperactivity disorder; AERP, auditory event-related potential; CPT, continuous performance test.

Table 2
ADHD and Related Issues

Authors	Year	Hypotheses	Subjects: ADHD	Subjects: Control	Electrodes (analyzed)	Design	Results
				ADHD subtypes			
DeFrance et al.	1996	Investigate ERP differences between the hyperactive–impulsive and inattentive subtypes of ADHD and normal controls	34 children with ADHD-IM (25 males, 9 females; mean age = 9.8 yr) 17 children with ADHD-IA (8 males, 9 females; mean age = 9.7 yr)	20 control children (10 males and 10 females; mean age = 9.9 yr)	28 electrode sites Ref: linked earlobes Filters: 0.1–40 Hz	Go-go Task, consisting of a "passive" and "effortful" condition	ADHD: larger P250 amplitude in effortful task. ADHD-IM: larger P250 amplitude and smaller P3b (P500) amplitude. ADHD-IA: smaller P500 amplitude and more left hemisphere distribution of P250 and P350.
Johnstone et al.	2001		50 children with ADHD-Comb 50 children with ADHD-IA type age = 8–17 yr 11 mo (2-yr age groups: 8–10, 10–12, 12–14, 14–16, and 16–18 yr) 10 children in each group	100 children (2-yr age groups: 8–10, 10–12, 12–14, 14–16, and 16–18 yr) 10 children in each group	17 sites (Electrocap) Ref: linked ears Filters: 0.01–35 Hz	Auditory oddball paradigm (15%: 1500 Hz, 85%: 1000 Hz)	Compared with controls, ADHD groups had smaller P3b ADHD-IA: altered N1 topography, larger P2, smaller N2, altered P3b topography. ADHD-Comb: smaller N1; altered P2, N2, and P3b topography. ADHD-IA vs Comb: No amplitude differences for any peaks; opposite N1 and P2 topography, altered N2 and P3 distributions

			Comorbid disorders				
Frank et al.	1994	ERP differences between children with LD and LD/ADHD	18 children with LD (mean age = 10.6 yr); 36 children with LD/ADHD (mean age = 11.9 yr);	27 controls (mean age = 11.9 yr)	Cz Ref: left ear Filters: 1–100 Hz	Two tone oddball discrimination auditory task (80%: 1000 Hz, 20%: 2000 Hz)	LD and ADHD/LD: reduced P3 amplitude to rare stimuli. No signifi cant differences between LD and ADHD/LD in P3 amplitude
Linden et al.	1996	Differences between ADHD, ADHD/ODD, and normal children and determine developmental age impact on ADD subgroups	45 children (5–12 yr)	14 normal children (5–12 yr)	One active scalp electrode and one EOG channel	Auditory oddball task (75%: 526 Hz, 25%: 885 Hz)	ADHD/LD: longer N2 and P3 latencies and P3 amplitude differences ADHD and ADHD/ODD: age differences in N1 and P2 ERPs, differences no longer apparent with increasing age.
Frank et al.	1998	ERP age differences in children with ADHD, LD, ADHD-LD, conduct disorder (CD), and normal control children and adults	12 children with ADHD (mean age = 9.5 yr); 33 children with LD (mean age = 10.5 yr); 63 children with ADHD/LD (mean age = 9.1 yr); 11 children with CD (mean age = 10.5 yr)	29 normal adults (mean age = 24.5 yr); 43 normal children (mean age = 9.5 yr)	Cz Ref: left ear Filters: 1–100 Hz	Two tone oddball discrimination auditory task (80%: 1000 Hz, 20%: 2000 Hz)	ADHD/LD: longer P3 latencies and smaller P3 amplitude Significant age differences for children 8–12 yr and 12–18 yr for N2 amplitude, N4 latency, and N1 amplitude.LD: N2 amplitude positively correlated with age ADHD/LD: N1 latency negatively correlated, N4 latency negatively correlated, P3 amplitude positively correlated, with age

(Continued)

Table 2 (*Continued*)

Authors	Year	Hypotheses	Subjects: ADHD	Subjects: Control	Electrodes (analyzed)	Design	Results
Mangina et al.	2000	Differences in ERPs and Mangina Test performance in ADHD/LD, behaviorally disordered children from normal control children	10 LD/ADHD, behaviorally disordered children (8 males, 2 females; mean age = 10.9 yr)	10 normal control children (7 males, 3 females; mean age = 10.6 yr)	Fp1, Fp2, F3, F4, F7, F8, T3, T4, T5, T6, C3, C4, P3, P4, O1, O2, Fpz, Fz, Cz, Pz, Oz Ref: linked mastoids Filters: low-pass 30 Hz	Memory Workload Task Mangina Test	Control: larger anterior N450 amplitude, P450 latency increased as a function of increasing memory load, P450 amplitude showed a quadratic trend
Banaschewski et al.	2003	Investigated comorbidity of ADHD and ODD	15 children with hyperkinetic disorder (mean age = 9.9 yr); 16 children with hyperkinetic CD (mean age = 9.8 yr); 15 children with ODD/CD (mean age = 10.7 yr)	18 controls (mean age = 10.1 yr)	19 electrodes Ref: FCz Filters: 0.1–30 Hz)	Continuous Performance Task	ODD/CD: smaller P3a amplitudes than controls ODD/CD and HCD: smaller P3b amplitude
			Cognitive abilities other than attention				
Robaey et al.	1995	ERP correlates of WISC-R and Piagetian intelligence measures in ADHD and normal control children	19 children (17 males, 2 females; mean age = 7 yr 5 mo)	30 children (15 males, 15 females; mean age = 7 yr 7 mo)	F4, C4, P4, O2, F3, C3, p3, O1, Fc4, Cp4, Po2, Fc3, Cp3, Po1 Ref: linked ears Filters: 0.08–40 Hz	Two classification tasks Two seriation tasks	*Control:* Negative correlations for: 1. Verbal scores and parieto-occipital P350 and P500 amplitude. 2. Performance scores and frontal P250 and parieto-occipital N250 amplitudes.

						3. Negative correlation for Piagetian intelligence measure and frontal P250 amplitude. 4. Significant correlations between parieto-occipital P350 and P500 amplitudes and Piagetian intelligence measures. ADHD: negative correlations between: 1. Frontal P250 and parieto-occipital P500 amplitude and verbal skills. 2. P250 and N250 waves and Picture Arrangement scores. 3. N250 amplitude and Piagetian measures. 4. Positive correlation between P250 and N250 waves and Block Design scores.
Oades et al.	1996	12 (11 males) 7.5–13.5 yr No medication	12 controls (7 males) 8.2–12.9 yr 10 (9 males) Tourette's (TS) 8.2–15.2 yr	32 electrode cap Ref: linked ears Filters: 0.3–70 Hz	Oddball task to elicit MMN to three tones varying in pitch and frequency of presentation	*ADHD* exhibited shorter latencies. Both ADHD and TS generated very large P2 amplitudes at more anterior sites.

(Continued)

Table 2 (*Continued*)

Authors	Year	Hypotheses	Subjects: ADHD	Subjects: Control	Electrodes (analyzed)	Design	Results
Frank et al.	1996	Memory differences	14 children with ADHD/LD (mean age = 1 1.1 yr)	30 adults (mean age = 23.4 yr);17 children (mean age = 12 yr)	Cz, Pz, and Oz Ref: left ear Filters: 1–100 Hz	Visual Memory Search paradigm	ADHD/LD: decreased P3 latency, and smaller P3 amplitude for mismatch condition
Lazzaro et al.	1997	Differences in variability of processing between ADHD and controls	17 (12–16 yr) males No medication	17 (12–16 yr) males	Fz, Cz, Pz Ref: linked earlobes Filters: 0.5–70 Hz	Analyzed response variance curve during oddball auditory task	Greater single trial variability in ADHD males for P300
Steger et al.	2000	Possible deficits at visual and premotor areas	15 males 8.2–12.6 yr No medication	16 males 8.2–12.6 yr No medication	32 electrode cap Ref: FPz Filters: 0.1–70 Hz	Recorded force between thumb and index finger during bilateral responding task	Small, specific visuoattention, central and motor processing deficits noted in ADHD males but not controls
Heinrich et al.	2001	Examine on-line time task analysis	24 unmedicated males (9–15 yr)	24 males (9–15 yr)	F3, Fz, F4, C3, Cz, C4, P3, P4 Ref: mastoid Filters: .03-120 Hz	Selective attention task	ADHD: smaller frontal negativity, earlier increase in omission errors. No reaction time differences between ADHD and controls

ERP, event-related potential; ADHD, attention deficit hyperactivity disorder; IA, inattentive; Comb, combined; IM, impulsive; LD, learning disabilities; ODD, oppositional–defiant disorder; EOG, electro-oculogram; HCD; hyperkinetic conduct disorder; WISC-R, Wechsler Intelligence Scale for Children, Revised; MMN, mismatch negativity.

Table 3
ADHD and Effects of Medication

Authors	Year	Hypotheses	Subjects: ADHD	Subjects: Control	Electrodes (analyzed)	Design	Results
Young et al.	1995	Pre- and postdrug P3b amplitude changes, predict children who) respond to MPH	35 children (21 males, mean age = 12.3 yr)	None	19 electrodes (Electrocap) Filters: 1–30 Hz	Auditory oddball P300 paradigm before and after single-dose trial of MPH	Of 15 predicted responders, 12 were actual responders, 3 actual nonresponders. Of 11 predicted nonresponders, 2 actual responders, 9 actual nonresponders
Miller et al.	1996	Evaluate impact of MPH	19 males (9, MPH group; 10, placebo group) age = 8–10 yr	13 (males) 8–10 yr	19 electrode cap Ref: linked earlobes Filters: 1–30 Hz	Stroop task	MPH resulted in shorter N1 latencies, increased P1, N2, P3a, P3b. Differential effect on ERPs to targets/nontargets
Sunohara et al.	1997	Compare two ADHD groups (nonresponders and responders to MPH) and normal controls	13 non-responders to MPH (mean age = 11.47 ± 1.20 yr) 13 responders to MPH (mean age = 11.43 ± 0.98 yr) WISC-R verbal or performance IQ > 85	13 normally developing children (mean age = 11.43 ± 1.18 yr) WISC-R verbal or performance IQ > 85	Fpz, Fz, Cz, Oz, C3, C4, Pz, P3, P4, T3, T4, T5, T6 Ref: spine/clavicle pair. Filters: 0.1–30 Hz	Orthographic and semantic classification task	Both ADHD groups had longer P3b latencies on baseline than controls. P3b latencies: Controls < high MPH responders < low MPH responders Shorter latencies in orthographic task compared with semantic task

(Continued)

Table 3 (*Continued*)

Authors	Year	Hypotheses	Subjects: ADHD	Subjects: Control	Electrodes (analyzed)	Design	Results
Taylor et al.	1997	Effects of MPH	21 total 11 (8 males) age = 7–8 yr (mean = 8.04 yr); 10 (8 males) age = 9–10 yr, (mean age = 10.01 yr)	21 total 11 (8 males) age = 7–8 yr (mean = 8.03 yr); 10 (6 males) age = 9–10 yr (mean age = 9.10 yr)	19 (Neuroscan), Ref: spinal Filters: 0.1–30 Hz	Parallel task: search by color or shape Serial task: search by color and shape	No P3 amplitude changes attributed to medication
Winsberg et al.	1997	Investigated neurophysiological action of MPH	14 hyperactive children mean age = 111.36 mo	14 children mean age = 126.71 mo	Fpz, Fz, Cz and Pz and at left and right mastoids Ref: nose Filters: 0.3–35 Hz	Passive auditory paradigm and an active auditory attention task	No differences between groups in N1, P2, MMN, N2 latency or amplitude. MPH group: shorter latency P3 to deviant stimuli in active condition
Smithee et al.	1998	Does MPH affect children's responses to response frequency (ratio of targets/non targets) and stimulus sequence (alternation vs repetition)	26 children	No controls	Fz, Cz, Pz Ref: linked earlobes Filters: 0.5–30 Hz	Double-blind trial for two consecutive weeks each of placebo and MPH	MPH treatment increased accuracy and speed among younger children, reduced reaction-time variability No effect on ERPs
Sunohara et al.	1999	Investigate impact of MPH on specific aspects of attention at different dose levels	20 children 10–12 yr (16 males, 4 females, mean age = 10.5 yr) with primary diagnosis	20 age-matched controls without ADHD (16 males, 4 females, mean age = 10.8 yr)	Electro-Cap 27 active electrodes Ref: spinal Filters: 0.1–30 Hz	Continuous Performance Test (CPT) double paradigm: children respond	Low MPH: reduced impulsivity (fewer false alarms); shorter P3 latency High MPH: reduced impulsivity and inattention

			of ADHD			after seeing a repeated letter during observation of a long string of visual stimuli	(more hits); increased P2 and N2 latencies, decreased P3 latency No effect on amplitudes.
Jonkman et al.	2000	Assess impact of MPH on performance	14 (7–13 yr)	14 (7–13 yr)	Fz, Cz, Pz, Oz Ref: linked mastoids Filters: 0.15–40 Hz	Visual probe task	MPH increased P3 amplitudes in easy and hard tasks but did not impact probe ERP amplitudes
Zillessen et al.	2001	Investigate changes in topographic P300-features to MPH and to different attention processes in primer and distractor conditions	17 right-handed males (7.2–11.7 yr, mean age = 9.5 yr) Mean IQ 106 (range 83–121)	None	21 gold electrodes Ref: reference-independent analysis Filters: 0.3–70 Hz	CPT Children tested twice in unmedicated condition (CPT1, CPT2) and twice in medicated condition (CPT3, CPT4).	Significantly higher amplitudes for primer than for distracters, Significantly higher P3a amplitudes for the medicated than for the unmedicated children

ADHD, attention deficit hyperactivity disorder; MPH, methylphenidate; WISC-R, Wechsler Intelligence Scale for Children, Revised; IQ, intelligence quotient; ERPs, event-related potentials

REFERENCES

1. Schroeder C, Gordon B. Assessment and treatment of childhood problems: a clinician's guide (2nd ed.). New York: Guilford Press, 2002.
2. American Psychiatric Association. Diagnostic and statistical manual of mental disorders 4th ed. Washington, DC: American Psychiatric Association, 1994.
3. Barry R, Clarke A, Johnstone S. A review of electrophysiology in attention-deficit/hyperactivity disorder: I. Qualitative and quantitative electroencephalography. Clin Neurophysiol 2003;114; 171–183.
4. Barry RJ, Johnstone SJ, Clarke A. A review of electrophysiology in attention-deficit/hyperactivity disorder: II. Event-related potentials. Clin Neurophysiol, 2003:114;184–198.
5. Calloway E, Gruae S, Shatton M. Brain electrical potentials and individuals' psychological differences. New York: Grune & Stratton, 1975.
6. Strandburg, RJ, Marsh JT, Brown W, Arsanow R, Higa J, Harper R, Guthrie D. Continuous-processing-related event-related potentials in children with attention deficit hyperactivity disorder. Biol Psychiatry 1996;40:964–980.
7. Overtoom, CC, Verbaten MN, Kemner C, et al. Associations between event-related potentials and measures of attention and inhibition in the Continuous Performance Task in children with ADHD and normal controls. Am Acad Child Adolesc Psychiatry 1998;37:977–985.
8. Donchin E, Miller GA, Farwell LA. The endogenous components of the event-related potential—a diagnostic tool? Prog Brain Res 1986;70: 87–102.
9. Johnstone SJ, RJ Barry Auditory event-related potentials to a two-tone discrimination paradigm in attention deficit hyperactivity disorder. Psychiatry Res 1996;64:179–192.
10. Jonkman LM, Kemner C, Verbaten MN, Van Engeland H, Camfferman G, Buitelaar JK, et al. Attentional capacity, a probe ERP study: differences between children with attention-deficit hyperactivity disorder and normal control children and effects of methylphenidate. Psychophysiology 2000;37:334–346.
11. McCarthy G, Donchin E. A metric for thought: a comparison of P300 latency and reaction time. Science 1981:211:77–80.
12. Robaey P, Breton F, Dugas M, Renault B. An event-related potential study of controlled and automatic processes in 6–8-year-old boys with attention deficit hyperactivity disorder. Electroencephalogr Clin Neurophysiol 1992;82:330–340.
13. Taylor MJ, Sunohara GA, Khan SC, Malone MA. Parallel and serial attentional processes in ADHD: ERP evidence. Dev Neuropsychol 1997;13:531–540.
14. Emmerson R, Dustman R, Shearer D, Turner C. P3 latency and symbol digit performance correlations in aging. Exper Aging Res 1990;15:151–159.
15. Polich J, Martin S. P300, cognitive capability, and personality: a correlational study of university undergraduates. Pers Indiv Differences 1992;13:533–543.
16. Donchin E, Coles M. Is the P300 component a manifestation of context updating? Behav Brain Sci, 1988;11:357–427.
17. Verleger R. Event-related potentials and memory: A critique of the context updating hypothesis and an alternative interpretation of P3. Behav Brain Sci, 1988;11:343–356.
18. O'Donnel B, Cohen R, Hokama H, Cuffin B, Lippa C, Shelton M, Drachman D. Electrical source analysis of auditory ERPs in medial temporal lobe amnestic syndrome. Electroencephalogr Clin Neurophysiol 1993;87:394–402.
19. Donchin E. Surprise! . . . Surprise? Psychophysiology 1981;18, 493–513.
20. Paller KA, McCarthy G, Roessler E, Alllison T, Wood C. Potentials evoked in human and monkey medial temporal lobe during auditory and visual oddball paradigms. Electroencephalogr Clin Neurophysiol, 1992;84:269–279.
21. Katayama Y, Tsukiyama T, Tsubokawa T. Thalamic negativity associated with the endogenous late positivity component of cerebral evoked potential (P300): recordings using discriminative aversive conditioning in humans and cats. Brain Res Bull, 1985;14:223–226.
22. Knight RT, Scabini D, Woods DL, Clayworth CC. Contributions of temporal-parietal junction to the human auditory P3. Brain Res 1989;502:109–116.

23. Tarkka I, Stokic D, Basil L, Papanicolaou A. Electric source localization of the auditory P300 agrees with magnetic source localization. Electroencephalogr Clin Neurophysiol 1995;96:538–545.
24. Papanicolaou A, Baumann S, Rogers R. Source estimation of late components of emitted tone evoked magnetic fields. In: Hoke M, Erne S, et al., eds., Biomagnetism: clinical aspects. Amsterdam: Elsevier, 1992:177–180.
25. Rogers R, Papanicolaou A, Baumann S, Bourbon W, Alagarsamy S, Eisenberg H. Localization of P3 sources using magnetoencephalography and magnetic resonance imaging. Electroencephalogr and clin Neurophysiol, 1991;79:308–321.
26. Perchet C, Revol O, Fourneret P, Mauguierre F, Garcia-Larrea L. Attention shifts and anticipatory mechanisms in hyperactive children: an ERP study using the Posner paradigm. Biol Psychiatry 2001;50:44–57.
27. Karayanidis F, Robaey P, Bourassa M, DeKoning D, Geoffroy G, Pelletier G. ERP differences in visual attention processing between attention-deficit hyperactivity disorder and control boys in the absence of performance differences. Psychophysiology 2000;37:319–333.
28. Whitmont S, Meares R, Clarke S. The modulation of late component event related potentials by pre-stimulus EEG theta activity in ADHD. Int J Neurosci 2001;107:247–264.
29. Satterfield JH, Schell AM, Nicholas T, Satterfield B, Freese T. Ontogeny of selective attention effects on event-related potentials in attention-deficit hyperactivity disorder and normal boys. Biol Psychiatry 1990;28:879–903.
30. Jonkman LM, Kemner C, Verbaten M, et al. Event-related potentials and performance of attention-deficit hyperactivity disorder: children and normal controls in auditory and visual selective attention tasks. Biol Psychiatry 1997;41:595–611.
31. van der Stelt O, van der Molen M, Boudewijn-Gunning W, Kok A. Neuroelectrical signs of selective attention to color in boys with attention-deficit hyperactivity disorder. Cogn Brain Res, 2001;12:245–264.
32. Pliszka SR, Liotti M, Woldorff M. Inhibitory control in ch0ildren with attention-deficit/hyperactivity disorder: event-related potentials identify the processing component and timing of an impaired right-frontal response-inhibition mechanism. Biol Psychiatry 2000;48:238–246.
33. Overtoom CC, Kenemans JL, Verbaten M, et al. Inhibition in children with attention-deficit/hyperactivity disorder: a psychophysiological study of the stop task. Biol Psychiatry 2002; 51, 668–676.
34. Yong-Liang G, Robaey P, Karayanidis F, Bourassa M, Pelletier G, Geoffroy G. ERPs and behavioral inhibition in a go/no-go task in children with attention-deficit hyperactivity disorder. Brain Cogn 2000;43:215–220.
35. Yong-Liang G, Robaey P, Karayanidis F, Bourassa M, Pelletier G, Geoffroy G. Stimulus-response incompatibility effects on event-related potentials in children with attention-deficit hyperactivity disorder. Brain Cogn 2000;43:211–215.
36. DeFrance JF, Smith S, Schweitzer F, Ginsberg L, Sands S. Topographical analyses of attention disorders of childhood. Int J Neurosci 1996;87:41–61.
37. Goodin DS, Squires KC, Henderson BH, Starr A. Age-related variations in evoked potentials to auditory stimuli in normal human subjects. Electroencephalogr Clin Neurophysiol 1978;44:447–458.
38. Schneider W, Shiffrin R. Controlled and automatic human information processing: I. Detection, search, and attention. Psychol Rev 1977;84:1–66.
39. Kuperman SB, Johnson B, Arndt S, Lindgren S, Wolraich M. Quantitative EEG differences in a nonclinical sample of children with ADHD and undifferentiated ADD [comment]. J Am Acad Child Adolesc Psychiatry 1996;35:1009–1017.
40. Frank Y, Seiden JA, Napolitano B. Event-related potentials to an oddball auditory paradigm in children with learning disabilities with or without attention deficit hyperactivity disorder. Clin Electroencephalogr 1994;25:136–141.
41. Frank Y, Seiden JA, Napolitano B. Electrophysiological changes in children with learning and attentional abnormalities as a function of age: event-related potentials to an oddball paradigm. Clin Electroencephalogr 1998;29:188–193.
42. Linden M, Gevirtz R, Isenhart R, Fisher T. Event related potentials of subgroups of children with attention deficit hyperactivity disorder and the implications for EEG biofeedback. J Neurother Winter 1996;40–49.

43. Linden M, Gevirtz R, Isenhart R, Fisher T. Event related potentials of subgroups of children with attention deficit hyperactivity disorder and the implications for EEG biofeedback. J Neurother Spring/Summers 1996;1–11.
44. Robaey PS, Cansino, Dugas M, Renault B. A comparative study of ERP correlates of psychometric and Piagetian intelligence measures in normal and hyperactive children. Electroencephalogr & Clin Neurophysiol 1995;96:56–75.
45. Oades RD, Dittmann-Balcar A, Schepker R, Eggers C, Zerbin D. Auditory event-related potentials (ERPs) and mismatch negativity (MMN) in healthy children and those with attention-deficit or tourette/tic symptoms. Biol Psychol 1996;43:163–185.
46. Heinrich H, Moll GH, Dickhaus H, Kolev V, Yordanova J, Rothenberger A. Time-on-task analysis using wavelet networks in an event-related potential study on attention-deficit hyperactivity disorder. Clin Neurophysiol 2001;112:1280–1287.
47. Lazzaro I, Anderson J, Gordon E, Clarke S, Leong J, Meares R. Single trial variability within the P300 (250–500 ms) processing window in adolescents with attention deficit hyperactivity disorder. Psychiatry Res 1997;73:91–101.
48. Steger J, Imhof K, Steinhausen H, Brandeis D. Brain mapping of bilateral interactions in attention deficit hyperactivity disorder and control boys. Clin Neurophysiol 2000;111:1141–1156.
49. Frank Y, Seiden J, Napolitano B. Visual event related potentials and reaction time in normal adults, normal children, and children with attention deficit hyperactivity disorder: Differences in short-term memory processing. Int J Neurosci 1996;88:109–124.
50. Miller DC, Kavcic V, Leslie JE. ERP changes induced by methylphenidate in boys with Attention Deficit Hyperactivity Disorder. J Attention Dis 1996;1:95–113.
51. Smithee JA, Klorman R, Brumaghim JT, Borgstedt AD. Methylphenidate does not modify the impact of response frequency or stimulus sequence on performance and event-related potentials of children with attention deficit hyperactivity disorder. J Abnorm Child Psychol 1998;26:233–245.
52. Jonkman LM, Kemner C, Verbaten M, et al. Effects of methylphendidate on event-related potentials and performance of attention-deficit hyperactivity disorder children in auditory and visual selective attention tasks. Biol Psychiatry 1997;41:690–702.
53. Sunohara GA, Voros JG, Malone MA, Taylor MJ. Effects of methylphenidate in children with attention deficit hyperactivity disorder: a comparison of event-related potentials between medication responders and non-responders. Int J Psychophysiol 1997;27:9–14.
54. Sunohara GA, Malone MA, Rovet J, Humphries T, Roberts W, Taylor MJ. Effect of methylphenidate on attention in children with attention deficit hyperactivity disorder (ADHD), ERP evidence. Neuropsychopharmacology 1999;21:218–228.
55. Winsberg BG, Javitt DC, Silipo GS. Electrophysiological indices of information processing in methylphenidate responders. Biol Psychiatry 1997;42;434–445.
56. Zillessen KE, Scheuerpflug P, Fallgatter AJ, Strik WK, Warnke A. Changes of the brain electrical fields during the continuous performance test in attention-deficit hyperactivity disorder-boys depending on methylphenidate medication. Clin Neurophysiol 2001;112:1166–1173.
57. Young ES, Perros P, Price GW, Sadler T. Acute challenge ERP as a prognostic of stimulant therapy outcome in attention-deficit hyperactivity disorder. Biol Psychiatry 1995;37:25–33.

17

Anatomical and Functional Neuroimaging Studies of Children and Adolescents With Attention Deficit Hyperactivity Disorder

Jonathan C. Pfeifer, Melissa DelBello, Scott Holland

1. INTRODUCTION

Attention deficit hyperactivity disorder (ADHD) is one of the most prevalent behavioral disorders in pediatric populations *(1,2)*. Researchers have hypothesized that ADHD has a biological etiology *(3)*. Indeed, twin studies have provided evidence to suggest that ADHD is an inherited disorder *(4)* and a variety of genes have been identified, which have been associated with an increased susceptibility to developing ADHD *(5)*. The core characteristics of ADHD, which include inattentiveness, impulsivity, and hyperactivity, are thought to be the result of dysfunctional noradrenergic and dopaminergic pathways residing in discrete brain regions *(6,7)*. As a result of recent advances in neuroimaging technologies, there has been an increasing number of neuroimaging studies investigating the neurophysiological basis of ADHD *(3)*. Some studies have concentrated on anatomical pathology, probing for variations in the neuroanatomical structures of ADHD patients, such as differences in volumes of distinct brain regions. In contrast, other studies have focused on physiological functions of the central nervous system, such as regulation of blood flow, which may be responsible for the behavioral manifestations of the disorder. The following chapter will begin with a brief review of neuroimaging techniques that have been utilized to investigate the neurobiological basis of ADHD. Next, we will review the findings of structural and functional neuroimaging studies involving children and adolescents with ADHD. We will also discuss recent findings from functional neuroimaging studies that have begun to investigate the mechanisms of action of pharmacological treatments for ADHD. Finally, we will examine some of the limitations of existing studies and propose neuroimaging investigation that might help further clarify the neurophysiology of ADHD.

2. NEUROIMAGING TECHNIQUES

2.1. Structural Neuroimaging

2.1.1. Computed Tomography

Computed tomography (CT), one of the first cross-sectional neuroimaging modalities, has been utilized for more than 30 yr to examine the central nervous system (CNS). CT produces two-dimensional views of multiple axial brain slices from numerous one-dimensional

From: *Attention Deficit Hyperactivity Disorder: From Genes to Patients*
Edited by: D. Gozal and D. L. Molfese © Humana Press Inc., Totowa, NJ

projections captured from varying angles *(8)*. The attenuation of the X-rays on various paths through the CNS causes contrast. This contrast creates lighter or darker areas seen on the image, allowing one to discriminate between various anatomical sites. In medicine, CT has traditionally been used to evaluate CNS lesions, such as tumors, infarction, or gross structural changes, as well as define areas of blood–brain barrier breakdown when used with intravenous contrast *(8)*. Although less expensive than magnetic resonance imaging (MRI), CT is limited for several reasons *(8)*. First, it exposes subjects to ionizing radiation, creating ethical concerns when used for solely for research purposes. Second, visualization of the basotemporal cortex and posterior fossa may be obscured owing to artifacts in structures near bone. Third, visualization of white-matter disease is poor, as is contrast resolution between grey and white matter. Finally, there is risk of an allergic reaction to the iodine-based contrast that is commonly used. In addition to these restrictions, other confounding factors, such as the diagnostic heterogeneity of the ADHD patients, has limited the interpretability of early CT studies *(9–12)*. However, these investigations helped define the framework of methodologies that followed in later neuroimaging studies of ADHD patients.

2.1.2. *Magnetic Resonance Imaging*

MRI has been used for the majority of studies investigating anatomical differences between youth with ADHD and healthy controls. MRI provides images with high resolution, without subjecting the patient to ionizing radiation *(11)*. In addition, any plane of view may be visualized, the most common being the sagittal, axial, and coronal. Because of its safety profile, subjects can be scanned multiple times, allowing for longitudinal studies to be performed in which the time-dependent effects of such parameters as medical treatment and development can be assessed. Furthermore, the low biological risk of MRI is also justification for including healthy subjects in investigations that include pediatric samples. In addition, MRI is superior for detecting white-matter lesions and avoiding bony artifacts that may be associated with CT *(8)*. Images are produced primarily using the magnetization of hydrogen nuclei in water molecules. Atomic nuclei with an odd number of protons or neutrons have an innate spin, creating a magnetic dipole moment. When the atoms comprising a subject's brain tissue are placed within a strong magnetic field, the nuclei attain their lowest energy state, so that their magnetic dipole moments are aligned in a parallel fashion with respect to the magnetic field. The nuclei within the magnetic field spin around the axis of the field (precession), which causes a release of energy. This energy is localized and detected by the scanner in the form of radiofrequency electromagnetic waves. An external radiofrequency pulse is then added to perturb the resonance of the nuclei, displacing the dipoles from the plane parallel to the magnetic field. Upon removing the external radiofrequency magnetic field pulse, the nuclei return to their lowest energy state (relaxation), again becoming parallel to the magnetic field. Using magnetic field gradients and Fourier transformation, the detected signals are converted into an image. The resolution of some of the newer high-field MR scanners can reach approx 300 μM, increasing the validity of studies quantifying brain regions as their borders become more distinct. Although traditionally utilized to evaluate brain structures clinically, MRI has evolved. Newer applications of MR technology, including magnetic resonance spectroscopy (MRS), functional magnetic resonance imaging (fMRI), and diffusion imaging, have allowed investigators to probe into the biochemical and physiological (functional) basis of ADHD neuropathology.

2.2. Functional Neuroimaging

2.2.1. Single-Photon Emission Computed Tomography

One of the most widely used functional neuroimaging techniques for studying ADHD has been single-photon emission computed tomography (SPECT). SPECT has the capacity to measure regional cerebral blood flow (rCBF), as well as localize and determine the densities of various receptors in vivo *(8)*. rCBF is considered to be an indirect measure of neural activity and glucose metabolism in corresponding brain areas. Subjects participating in SPECT studies are injected intravenously with a flow tracer conjugated to a radionuclide (^{99m}Tc is a common example). The flow tracer may then localize to a receptor or where there is increased blood perfusion. The concentration of the bound radionuclide is imaged by detecting fleeting γ-rays, or photons, which are emitted as the radioisotope decays. The uptake of the tracer can also be quantified accurately. Various molecules have been used to localize specific receptor sites, such as TRODAT for the dopamine transporter (DAT-1). In addition to providing specific receptor information, SPECT is relatively affordable because of the fact that a cyclotron is not required for SPECT radioisotope production. The radioactive decay half-life of most SPECT isotopes is relatively long, so the compounds may be manufactured in one location and shipped for use in another.

Although SPECT has yet to be used in the diagnosis of patients with psychiatric disorders, it is utilized clinically in the assessment of developmental anomalies, seizures, and tumors *(13)*. SPECT is not typically used for research purposes in pediatric populations, because it utilizes ionizing γ-radiation.

2.2.2. Positron Emission Tomography

Positron emission tomography (PET) is an imaging technique that can measure rCBF, oxygen and glucose metabolism, cerebral blood volume, and the extraction of water across the blood–brain barrier *(8)*. Neurological receptor binding may also be examined, with specific radiotracers designed for such targets as the D2 dopamine, 5-HT2 serotonin, glutamate-*N*-methyl-D-aspartate, histamine, and opiate receptors. Images are based on the tracer's ability to emit a short-lived particle known as a positron. In order to manufacture positron-emitting radioisotopes, a cyclotron is necessary to generate isotopes of carbon (^{11}C), nitrogen (^{13}N), oxygen (^{15}O), or fluorine (^{18}F). During the process of imaging, positrons collide with nearby electrons, and end up producing two photons that travel in the exact opposite direction. The image is created by the detector, using a "coincidence circuit," which recognizes the simultaneous ionization. The spatial resolution of PET is between 5 and 6 mm. Because the energy of the γ-photons detected in PETs raises energy higher than those used in SPECT, its sensitivity is somewhat higher. Additionally, because of the coincidence detection, PET produces cross-sectional images inherently. Although a powerful and promising technique with a higher sensitivity than SPECT, PET is expensive, and therefore, its availability is limited. The typical positron-emitting isotopes are short-lived (several hours) and must be manufactured near the site of usage.

2.2.3. Functional Magnetic Resonance Imaging

fMRI is a relatively new neuroimaging technique that permits investigators to simultaneously produce high-resolution anatomical images as well as information regarding changes in blood flow between an active and resting state. The advantages of fMRI compared with SPECT or PET include that it is noninvasive and the subject is not exposed to ionizing radiation.

Images of blood flow are based on the varying magnetic properties between oxyhemoglobin and deoxyhemoglobin. When brain activity is increased beyond a certain threshold, the amount of oxygen in the blood supply to that brain region surpasses the amount of oxygen being utilized. The ratio of oxyhemoglobin to deoxyhemoglobin increases, which is the parameter detected by the scanner. This method has commonly been referred to as the blood-oxygen-level-dependent, or BOLD, technique. A variation of fMRI, T2 relaxometry, has been utilized to evaluate steady-state perfusions of various brain regions over time *(14)*.

2.2.4. Magnetic Resonance Spectroscopy

MRI is a neuroimaging technique that enables investigators to quantify chemical species in the CNS in vivo. In contrast to SPECT, MRS directly measures the concentration of certain metabolites in the brain. This technique can be used to investigate the relative concentrations of common biological isotopes, such as hydrogen (^{1}H), lithium (^{7}Li), carbon (^{14}C), fluorine (^{19}F), sodium (^{23}Na), and phosphorus (^{31}P). To be observable by MRS, a nucleus must have a nonzero spin property and be present in a sufficient concentration ($\geq$ 100 nmol typically). MRS can measure specific neurochemical compositions and concentrations within a brain region. For example, chemicals noted in the proton spectrum, including choline, *N*-acetylaspartate (NAA), creatine, glutamate/glutamine/γ-aminobutyric acid, and myoinositol can be quantified in this fashion *(15)*.

Using the aforementioned techniques, specific neuroanatomical and neurophysiological abnormalities have been identified in children and adolescents with ADHD. There are several diagnostic and rating instruments that have been used to evaluate pediatric patients with ADHD, including the Diagnostic Interview for Children and Adolescents *(16)* and the Child Behavior Checklist *(17)*. Additionally, since group differences in IQ scores confound findings from neuroimaging studies of ADHD youth, some investigators have used the Wechsler Intelligence Scale for Children *(18)* to evaluate IQ scores in order to adjust for group differences. In addition, other investigators have correlated regional brain structure and/or function with performance on neurocognitive tests, including those measuring attention and inhibition, to examine specific regional brain abnormalities in ADHD youth *(19)*.

3. STRUCTURAL NEUROIMAGING OF ADHD YOUTH

3.1. Cerebrum and Frontal Cortex

MRI studies evaluating the neuroanatomical substrates of ADHD have revealed involvement of the entire cerebrum, as well as several specific brain regions. Castellanos et al. have reported reductions of almost 5% in total cerebral volume, as well as a variance of lateral ventricular asymmetry in ADHD subjects vs controls matched for age and sex *(20–22)*. Other groups report 8.3% reductions in total cerebral volume in boys with ADHD compared with controls *(23)*.

One of the most consistent finding in ADHD youth has been abnormalities in frontostriatal brain regions *(11,24)*. Additionally, right-sided abnormalities are reported more commonly than left-sided abnormalities *(25)*. Indeed, one of the first MRI studies of ADHD youth reported smaller right "anterior" width measurement as compared to age- and sex-matched healthy controls *(26)*. Also consistent with this theory, Filipek et al. reported smaller right frontal regions in ADHD boys compared with healthy controls *(27)*. Moreover, Casey et al. reported significant correlations between performance on response inhibition tasks and anatomical measures of the prefrontal cortex and caudate nuclei that were predominantly in the right hemisphere, supporting a role of right frontostriatal circuitry in response inhibition and ADHD *(19)*. In a study with similar findings, decreased right hemispheric white matter was associated with poor performance on tasks requiring prolonged attention *(28)*.

Recently, studies have examined histologically and functionally distinct subregions of the frontal cortex. For example, Mostofsky et al. reported reduction in frontal white-matter volume that was specific to the left hemisphere and bilateral reduction in frontal gray-matter volume that was more specific to the right hemisphere. Subparcellation of the frontal lobe revealed smaller prefrontal, premotor, and deep white-matter volumes, suggesting that ADHD encompasses dysfunctions attributable to abnormal development of more than one frontal cortical region. Kates et al. reported smaller *prefrontal* cortical gray- and white-matter volumes in ADHD patients as compared with healthy controls *(29)*. In contrast to the right-sided dysfunction theory of ADHD, one study reported smaller left orbitofrontal cortical volumes in adults with ADHD *(30)*.

3.2. Subcortical Brain Regions

The basal ganglia, containing components, such as the caudate, putamen, and globus pallidus, is intimately connected to various circuitries responsible for control of a wide range of activities, including, motor and executive functioning. Several studies report decreased size of the globus pallidus in ADHD youth *(20,31)*. However, these reports vary as to whether the findings are right- or left-sided. In general, reports have not found putamen volumes to differ between ADHD youth and healthy controls *(20,31)*, although posterior ventral putamen lesions have been associated with an increased risk of ADHD symptomology in children *(32)*.

Studies examining caudate structure in ADHD youth have produced conflicting results *(3,24)*. The caudate modulates input from frontal brain areas, such as the orbitofrontal and dorsolateral cortices *(33)*. Therefore, it has been viewed to play a role in regulation of attention and inhibition *(28)*. Castellanos et al. reported a lack of normal caudate asymmetry, as well as smaller right caudate volumes in ADHD boys compared with healthy controls *(34)*. Other studies have reported normal asymmetry to be left greater than right caudate volume *(11,24,27,28,35,36)* and that this pattern was reversed in ADHD subjects *(27,35)*. Semrud-Clikeman et al. reported that left caudate head size was associated with higher scores on the externalizing scale of the Child Behavior Checklist; subjects with ADHD demonstrated elevated scores and smaller left caudate heads *(28)*. Furthermore, reversed asymmetry (right [R] > left [L]) of the caudate was associated with poorer performance on the Stroop test, which measures the capacity for response inhibition. The majority of subjects with reversed asymmetry were ADHD patients. Pineda et al. assessed caudate volume differences among healthy controls, inattentive ADHD patients, and combined ADHD patients, and found that subjects in all three groups demonstrated left > right caudate volumes, and no differences in volumes were found among groups *(37)*. In contrast, Schrimsher et al. found that ADHD symptomology is predicted by the degree of right > left caudate asymmetry *(38)*. Decreased caudate size in ADHD patients has been reported to diminish with age, suggesting that perhaps delayed development of the caudate may cause an increased risk of exhibiting ADHD symptoms *(21)*. However, this finding may be the result of trends for caudate volume to decrease with age being more apparent in controls than in ADHD subjects *(34,39)*. Smaller caudate has also been seen in patients with a monozygotic twin not diagnosed with this disorder, indicating that environmental factors may play a large role in one's neuroanatomical make up *(40)*. Further investigation is required to correctly define "normal" asymmetry, as well as to determine the role of the caudate in the pathophysiology of ADHD *(27)*.

The corpus callosum, the "connector" of the two hemispheres of the cortex, has been speculated to be involved in ADHD. This structure is one of the most recognizable brain structures in MR images, and is usually identified in midsagittal sections *(11)*. One study reported a smaller midsagittal cross-sectional area of two anterior regions of the corpus callosum, the rostrum and the rostral body, which correlated with teacher and parent ratings of ADHD symptoms *(41)*. A second study reported that children with Tourette's syndrome had increased area of the corpus callosum as compared with controls; however, the rostral body was again found to be smaller in ADHD children *(42)*. The rostral body has interconnections with the premotor cortex, caudate, and orbital prefrontal region, all of which are thought to be involved in regulation of inhibition *(41)*. Other areas of the corpus callosum have been shown to be smaller in children with ADHD, including the genu, isthmus, and the splenium *(43–45)*. Together, these studies indicated that corpus callosal abnormalities are associated with ADHD.

It is increasingly recognized that in addition to its role of coordinating motor activities, the cerebellum is also involved in regulating cognitive functions. The cerebellum has neural projections to other brain areas that are involved in regulation of emotion and attention *(46)*. Castellanos et al. have reported decreased cerebellar volumes in ADHD patients *(20–21)*. Specifically, two studies have reported decreased size of the inferior posterior lobe (lobules VIII-X) of the posterior vermis *(22,46)*. Decreased size of the posterior inferior lobe has also been reported by Berquin et al. *(47)*. Evidence of cerebellar morphological deviation, in conjunction with such findings as decreased white matter in the parietal-occipital regions of ADHD patients *(27)*, suggests that pathologies of posterior brain regions are involved in the neuropathophysiology of ADHD *(46)*.

4. FUNCTIONAL NEUROIMAGING OF ADHD YOUTH

Typically, functional neuroimaging studies in ADHD patients have been performed in conjunction with a cognitive task. During functional imaging studies it is important that cognitive stimuli activate brain regions thought to be deficient in a specific disorder *(48)*. The neuroanatomical studies described in the previous section provide a guide to appropriate designs for functional imaging studies targeted to be involved in ADHD. Paradigms commonly used in subjects with ADHD include go/no-go tasks, continuous performance tasks, and the Stroop test, which are designed to measure attention and inhibition by factoring parameters such as response time or correct motor responses. Therefore, investigators using functional imaging techniques have attempted to measure differences in task performance and regional brain activation between patients with ADHD and healthy controls.

Some of the initial functional neuroimaging studies of ADHD youth used 18 [F] fluor-2-deoxy-D-glucose PET to determine cerebral blood flow and found an 8% decrease in global metabolism in adult patients with childhood-onset ADHD as compared with healthy controls. Specifically, they identified decreased rates of metabolism in several prefrontal and premotor areas *(49)*. However, the authors were unable to replicate these results in a sample of adolescents with ADHD *(50)*. Using a go/no-go task, Durston et al. demonstrated that subjects with ADHD had a more profuse pattern of activation as compared with controls *(51)*. Controls showed greater activation in the area of the left caudate; however, in several other brain regions, such as the superior frontal gyrus, the precuneus, and the inferior parietal lobe, ADHD subjects had increased activation.

A SPECT study reported by Amen and Carmichael observed that 65% of ADHD patients had decreased perfusion to the prefrontal cortex during task performance, whereas only 5%

of controls demonstrated this pattern of response *(52)*. The majority of ADHD patients whose perfusion did not decrease in this study exhibited decreased prefrontal perfusion at rest. Likewise, Kim et al. reported decreased perfusion of prefrontal and temporal regions of the right cerebral hemisphere during rest *(53)*. Consistent with the hypothesis of decreased function of right prefrontal regions in patients with ADHD, Rubia et al. documented decreased function of the right mesial prefrontal cortex in ADHD boys during stop and delay tasks, suggesting that this area may regulate motor output that is not task-specific *(54)*. In this study, brain regions that were hypofunctional during the stop task only included the right inferior prefrontal cortex and left caudate, indicating that abnormalities in the right prefrontal cortex and its connections to the basal ganglia underlie the neurophysiology of ADHD. Abnormal asymmetry of blood perfusions (left > right) in the prefrontal regions of ADHD subjects during response-inhibition tasks has been reported, suggesting that deficits in the right frontal lobes of ADHD patients may be secondary to increased blood flow to the left hemisphere *(55)*. Finally, decreased activation of the anterior cingulate cortex, thought to be associated with stimulus and response selection, has been reported in ADHD patients during tasks of attention *(56)*.

Alterations in blood flow of the striatum have also been observed in patients with ADHD. For example, decreased blood flow to the putamen was observed in ADHD subjects as compared with healthy controls using T2 relaxometry *(14)*. Decreased blood flow to the striatum may also cause disturbances in attention towards verbal stimuli *(57–58)*. Perhaps the striatal deficits are responsible for the clinical manifestation of "not listening."

Although abnormalities in the caudate and prefrontal regions are most consistently implicated in the neurophysiology of ADHD, other brain regions have also been identified to have abnormal perfusion patterns in ADHD patients. For example, Kaya et al. reported that decreased perfusion of the right medial and lateral temporal cortices in ADHD children was present during resting conditions and was associated with higher ratings on both the DuPaul teachers' questionnaire and Conners' ratings for hyperactivity and restlessness *(59)*. Kim et al. have shown decreased cerebellar perfusion at rest in ADHD patients, again indicating its likely involvement in the pathology of ADHD *(53)*. Increased perfusion of the posterior occipital and parietal lobes has also been documented in ADHD patients during rest *(53)*. Interestingly, left > right asymmetrical perfusion has been observed in these regions in ADHD patients with severe symptoms while performing tasks of inhibition *(55)*.

Endophenotypes associated with ADHD are now being realized to perhaps have an etiology defined at the receptor level. Dougherty et al. stated a 70% increase in density of DAT in adult patients with ADHD relative to 30 controls, suggesting that varying levels of DAT are involved in the molecular pathology of ADHD *(60)*. Increased binding of TRODAT-1 to DAT has also been demonstrated in adult populations with ADHD controls *(61,62)*. However, another study using $[^{123}I]2\beta$-CIT has shown no differences in DAT levels between ADHD patients and controls *(63)*. It is theorized that such examples of increased DAT levels could either be an accommodation to long-term excess dopamine levels, or the result of a constitutively overactive expression of DAT causing there to be lower levels of synaptic dopamine *(6)*. Although these studies have managed to find differing patterns of activation and protein expression among various phenotypes, the majority have neglected investigation into the genotype of this disorder. To better assess the contribution of inheritance and genetics to the molecular pathology of ADHD, future investigators should consider the genotype of the patients in imaging studies. Preliminary findings indicate that ADHD patients homozygous for

Table 1
Functional Neuroimaging Studies of ADHD Youth

Author (year)	Subjects' mean age (yr ± SD)	Imaging modality	Probes	Control task	Results
Durston et al. (2003)	7 ADHD (8.6 ± 1.6) 7 healthy controls (8.7 ± 1.5)	fMRI	Go/no-go task (Pokemon characters)	2 or 4 go trials preceding no-go trials (foil task)	Frontostriatal regions activated differently in ADHD vs controls. ADHD. Controls with increased activity in the left caudate nucleus.
Rohde et al. (2003)	8 ADHD; 4 homozygous for the 10-repeat allele at the *DAT1* gene, 4 without the repeat	^{99m}Tc-ECD SPECT	Resting	Resting	Higher rCBF in medial frontal and left basal ganglia regions in ADHD patients with the 10-allele repeat at the *DAT1* gene.
Vles et al. (2003)	6 ADHD boys (age range 6–10 yr)	^{123}I-Ioflupane SPECT and ^{123}I-benzamide SPECT	MPH treatment (3–4 mo at 0.25–0.6 mg/kg/d)	Resting	Downregulation of DAT and D2 receptor expression s/p 3–4 mo of MPH treatment. R > L asymmetry of DAT expression dissipated s/p MPH treatment.
Kaya et al. (2002)	13 ADHD (9.5 ± 1.6) 7 healthy controls (8.8 ± 1.9)	^{99m}Tc-HMPAO SPECT	Resting		Decreased perfusions of the right medial and lateral temporal cortices in ADHD children, corresponding to higher ratings on both the DuPaul Teachers Questionnaire and Conners' ratings for hyperactivity and restlessness.
Anderson et al. (2002)	10 ADHD (9.3 ±1.6) 6 healthy controls (10.2 ± 1.5)	T2 Relaxometry	0.0, 0.5, 0.8, or 1.5 mg/kg/d MPH divided bid x 1 wk	CPT	Increased T2 a relaxation time (decreased perfusion) in the cerebellar vermis in ADHD patients with a higher degree of motor hyperactivity, and reduced T2 relaxation time (increased perfusion) in ADHD patients without hyperactivity after being administered moderate/high doses of methylphenidate.

Langleben et al. (2002)	22 ADHD treated with MPH for average of 12 wk (10), 7 controlss *(10)*	^{99m}Tc-ECD SPECT probe	Go/no-go task	Six alternating go/no-go blocks(25s). Task performed 2.5 min before 99m Tc-ECD injection	Increased rCBF in the premotor, motor, and anterior cingulated cortices in patients 36 h status post their last dose of MPH compared to perfusion when taking their normally prescribed MPH regimen.
Kim et al. (2002)	40 ADHD (9.7 ± 2.1) 17 healthy controls (10.4 ± 2.2)	^{99m}Tc-HMPAO SPECT	At rest		In resting conditions, ADHD subjects had decreased perfusion in the right middle frontal gyrus, right medial orbitofrontal gyrus, right middle temporal gyrus, and the medial cerebellar cortex bilaterally compared to controls ADHD subjects also had increased perfusion in the left postcentral angular gyrus, the right postcentral and angular gyri, left inferior and superior occipital gyri, and right precentral gyrus.
Kim et al. (2001)	32 right-handed, ADHD boys (10.6 ± 5.6)	^{99m}Tc-HMPAO SPECT probe	MPH treatment (8 weeks, mean dose 0.7 mg/kg)	Resting	Increased blood perfusion of the thalami, caudate, and frontal lobes after 8 wk of MPH treatment, with concordant improvement in behavior rating scales.
Langleben et al. (2001)	20 ADHD boys (10.2) 4 healthy controls (10.9)	^{99m}Tc-ECD (ethylcysteinate) SPECT probe	Go/no-go task	Six alternating go/no-go blocks (25s). Task performed 2.5 min before ^{99m}Tc-ECD injection	L > R prefrontal and asymmetry of rCBF in severe and moderate groups. L > R occipitoparietal asymmetry of rCBF in severe group during the tasks of response inhibition.

(Continued)

Table 1
(Continued)

Author (year)	Subjects' mean age (yr ± SD)	Imaging modality	Probes	Control task	Results
Langleben et al. (2001)	20 ADHD boys (10.2) 4 healthy controls (10.9)	^{99m}Tc-ECD (ethylcysteinate) SPECT probe	Go/no-go task	Six alternating go/no-go blocks (25s). Task performed 2.5 min before ^{99m}Tc-ECD injection	L > R prefrontal and asymmetry of rCBF in severe and moderate groups. L > R occipitoparietal asymmetry of rCBF in severe group during the tasks of response inhibition.
Ilgin et al. (2001)	6 males and 3 females with ADHD (9.8 ± 2.3)	^{123}1 IBZM SPECT	MPH treatment (3 months), dose of 0.5–1.5 mg/kg/day (initial dose of 0.2–0.5 mg/kg/day)	Resting	Downregulation of D2 receptor expression s/p 3 months of MPH treatment. Therapeutic response greater in those with higher base line D2 receptor levels.
Teicher et al. (2000)	11 ADHD boys (9.3 ± 1.6) 11 healthy controls (10.2 ± 1.5)	T2 relaxometry	Go/no-go task		Less perfusion (as measured by T2 relaxometry) in the putamen (bilaterally) in ADHD patients vs controls. Decrease in T2 relaxometry time for putamen in hyperactive subjects (moreperfusion) and an increased T2 relaxometry for putamen time in "less-active" subjects after treatment with MPH.
Rubia et al. (1999)	7 ADHD boys (15.7) 9 healthy controls (15.0)	fMRI	Stop task and delay task	Airplane	ADHD subjects demonstrated decreased function of the right inferior prefrontal cortex and left caudate during the stop task, and decreased function of the right mesial prefrontal cortex in both tasks.

Vaidya et al. (1998)	10 ADHD boys (10.5 ± 1.4) 6 healthy controls (9.3 ± 1.5)	fMRI	Go/no-go task	Stimulus and response-controlled, each 5 min with go and no-go blocks with or without MPH	ADHD boys off MPH had reduced striatal activation on stimulus controlled-task, and higher frontal activation in response inhibition tasks vs controls. MPH was shown to increase frontal activation in patients and controls, but increased striatal activation only in ADHD patients and decrease it in controls.
Lou et al. (1998)	12 ADHD boys (9.6), 6 healthy controls (8)	Xenon^{133} SPECT probe	Sequence of animal names utilized as auditory stimuli	1. White noise (500–1000-Hz) 2. Passive listening 3. Selecting name of a "dangerous animal" from sequence given (target detection)	Decreased perfusion of blood to the right striatum during target selection (a measure of attention to verbal stimuli) anterior gyrus cinguli was activated during the control of passive listening and the striatal and inferofrontal areas were activated during target detection, inferring these are involved in semantic processing of verbal stimuli and attention, respectively.
Amen and Carmichael (1997)	54 medication-free ADHD patients (11) 18 medication-free psychiatric outpatients (11)	^{99m}TC hexamethylpropylene amine oxide SPECT	Conners Continuous Performance Test	Resting	65% of ADHD subjects had decreased perfusion to the prefrontal cortex during the performance task vs 5% of controls.
Ernst et al. (1994)	20 ADHD (6 females, 14.7 ± 1.6) 19 healthy controls (5 females, 14.3 ± 1.4)	[^{18}F]fluorodeoxy-glucose PET	Auditory CPT	Resting	No differences in global metabolism in ADHD subjects. vs. controls. Female ADHD pts had a 19.6% decreased level of cerebral metabolism vs ADHD boys, and a 15.0% decreased in metabolism vs control females.

(Continued)

Table 1
(Continued)

Author (year)	Subjects' mean age (yr ± SD)	Imaging modality	Probes	Control task	Results
Zametkin et al. (1990)	10 ADHD (14.5 ± 1.5) 10 HV (14.3 ± 1.4)	[^{18}F]fluor-2-deoxy-D-glucose PET	Auditory CPT	Resting	Authors found no differences in global glucose metabolism, nor found any differences in absolute metabolism in 60 areas analyzed in ADHD vs controls. When values were normalized, decreased metabolism was found in the left anterior frontal, right posterior temporal area, and a portion of the left posterior frontal area. Increased metabolism was found in a more inferior region of the left posterior frontal region in ADHD subjects, when rates were normalized.
Lou et al. (1989)	6 ADHD (8.2) 13 ADHD "with other neurological symptoms" (9.5) 9 controls (range = 7–15 yr)	Xenon^{133} SPECT probe	At rest/ 4 "pure" patients and 9 ADHD patients "with other neurological symptoms" given 10–30 mg MPH before a second scan	Resting	Decreased perfusion in the right striatum of pure ADHD patients, and decreased perfusion of the striatum (bilaterally) in ADHD patients "with other neurological symptoms" compared to controls. Increased perfusion of primary sensory and sensory motor regions in both ADHD groups vs controls. ADHD patients. MPH increased perfusion in striatal and periventricular regions, with a trend for decreased blood flow to primary sensory regions.

MHP, methylphenydate; PET, positron emission tomography; SPECT, single-photon emission computed tomography; fMRI, functional magnetic resonance imaging; ECD, ethyleysteinate; HMPAO; CPT, continous performance test; L, left; R, right.

the 10-repeat allele at the *DAT1* gene to have increased perfusion in the left basal ganglia and medial frontal areas as compared with ADHD patients without this repeat *(64)*. Other studies have reported no significant difference in brain morphometry between ADHD subjects with and without the dopamine 4 receptor *(DRD 4*7)* repeat allele *(65)*.

5. MRS STUDIES IN ADHD YOUTH

There have been relatively few MRS studies of ADHD youth. McMaster et al. reported that ADHD youth have increase in frontostriatal glutamatergic tone as compared with healthy volunteers *(66)*. In a follow-up study, the same group studied ADHD children medication-naïve and after treatment and reported that the glutamate/glutamine/γ-aminobutyric-acid to creatine/phosphocreatine ratio significantly decreased in the striatum *(67)*. Consistent with these findings, Courvoisie et al. recently reported increased glutamate/glutamine in frontal regions bilaterally and increased NAA and choline in the right frontal area of ADHD children compared with healthy controls *(68)*. Other MRS studies have reported decreased NAA, a putative marker of neuronal function, in the striatum of ADHD boys, which was not altered following one dose of methylphenidate (MPH) *(69)*. In contrast, another study reported NAA decrease in the dorsolateral prefrontal cortex that was specific to girls with ADHD *(70)*. In a study of adults, decreased NAA in the dorsolateral prefrontal cortex was reported in the ADHD group as compared with healthy controls *(71)*. To date, MRS studies in ADHD youth have been limited by their small sample size and primarily examining only frontostriatal regions of interest. Future investigations using MRS and examining other regions of interest and medication effects in larger samples are necessary.

6. FUNCTIONAL NEUROIMAGING AND PSYCHOPHARMACOLOGY IN ADHD YOUTH

Medications are the mainstay of treatment for ADHD *(72)*. Specifically, psychostimulants such as MPH are effective for the treatment of ADHD. MPH is hypothesized to exert its effects by modifying neuronal activity of dopaminergic and noradrenergic pathways *(73)*. Recent imaging studies are beginning to demonstrate *how* and *where* MPH work within the CNS. Moreover, not only is MPH a very efficacious treatment for ADHD, but evidence also exists that medications may lead to normalization of structural abnormalities. For example, unmedicated patients have been shown to have smaller total white-matter volumes vs medicated ADHD patients and controls *(21)*.

Blood perfusion patterns within the CNS are also modified by stimulants, often in conjunction with improvement in psychological assessments. One of the first imaging studies to evaluate the effects of stimulants on glucose metabolism revealed no change in ADHD patients taking MPH or D-amphetamine on a *long-term* basis, even though clinical ratings illustrated symptom improvement *(75)*. In the same study, 60 specific brain regions were analyzed and there were no significant changes in patients taking D-amphetamine. However, patients taking MPH exhibited decreased metabolism in the right anterior putamen and increased metabolism right posterior frontal region. In a previous study carried out by the same group, global glucose metabolism was not observed after *short-term* administration of stimulants *(75)*. However, several brain regions had increased or decreased blood flow in comparison with the later study, which demonstrates the importance of evaluating the temporal effects of stimulants on neurofunction in patients with ADHD. A study utilizing SPECT evaluated rCBF in boys with ADHD pre- and post-8 wk of MPH treatment and found greater blood supply in the caudate, frontal lobes, and thalami following treatment, which was associated with significant improvement on behavior rating scales *(76)*, suggesting that MPH improves blood flow *specifically* in frontostriatal-thalamic circuits *(76)*. In contrast, Langleben et al. reported that MPH *decreases* blood perfusion in brain areas implicated in ADHD *(77)*. In this study, ADHD patients 36 h following discontinuation of MPH had increased rCBF in the premotor, motor, and anterior cingulate cortices, although they were taking their prescribed dosage of MPH, suggesting that MPH might inhibit these regions, which may correspond to its therapeutic effects of inhibiting motor hyperactivity. However, it is unknown whether the findings of this study the result of the therapeutic effects of MPH, or simply a withdrawal phenomenon *(39,77)*. MPH may also regulate motor hyperactivity in some patients with ADHD by altering perfusion to the cerebellar vermis, which receives dopaminergic projections from the ventral tegmental area. One study reported that high doses of methylphenidate increase T2 relaxation time in the vermis in hyperactive ADHD patients, and conversely, reduce T2 relaxation time in patients without hyperactivity *(78)*.

Other studies that have assessed the effects of MPH in non-ADHD controls demonstrate that the effects of MPH may be both similar and different in controls than in ADHD patients. For example, fMRI studies have revealed that MPH increases activation in frontal regions and decreases activation in striatal regions in patients with ADHD and controls *(79)*, consistent with the hypothesis that the motor and cognitive symptoms of ADHD may be explained as the consequences of excess dopamine activity in subcortical structures and a deficiency of dopamine in the cortex, respectively *(80)*.

Neuroimaging methodologies also have the potential to show the manner in which the expression of certain proteins involved in the pathogenesis of ADHD may be downregulated in response to pharmacological interventions. For example, Dressel et al. found that untreated adult ADHD patients had an increased striatal binding of ^{99m}Tc TRODAT-1 to the DAT in comparison to age-matched controls *(61)*. After methylphenidate treatment, specific binding decreased, complementing clinical improvement in these same patients. The authors speculated that the downregulation of DAT in response to MPH would increase dopamine in the synaptic gap, and possibly lead to improvement in clinical symptoms. Similarly, Krause et al. have shown that 4 wk of MPH treatment can significantly decrease density of DAT by almost 30% *(62)*. D2 dopamine receptors may also be downregulated in response to MPH, and it has been reported that patients with higher baseline levels of D2 receptors respond more favorably to MPH treatment *(81)*. Vles et al. have also reported decreased expression of the D2 receptor and DAT in response to MPH treatment, and postulate that decreased expression of D2 receptors may be the result of decreased DAT expression, and the resulting increase of dopamine in the synaptic cleft *(82)*.

7. CONSIDERATIONS FOR FUTURE NEUROIMAGING STUDIES OF ADHD YOUTH

In summary, neuroimaging studies have yielded differences primarily in three brain regions: the frontal lobe, the basal ganglia, and the cerebellum. Furthermore, there are a number of studies reporting abnormal asymmetry and differences in global brain volume. However, localized frontal and striatal abnormalities have been consistently detected in childhood ADHD, leading investigators to hypothesize that an abnormal frontostriatal network is involved in the pathophysiology of ADHD.

There are several limitations of prior neuroimaging studies of ADHD youth that may guide the design of future investigations. For example, the small sample size of most studies has resulted in reduced statistical power, limiting the interpretation of the results. Studies with small sample sizes of children and adolescents, which present during various developmental stages will likely result in high variability in structural and functional studies. Because the effects of ADHD on brain size and function are apparently subtle, these abnormalities might not be identified in small studies. Future multisite studies may be helpful to obtain data on larger samples in order to make adjustments for clinical and demographic variables in small sample sizes.

Additionally, many studies have included only males. Although the prevalence of ADHD is greater in males, future studies evaluating the neurostructural and neurofunctional abnormalities in ADHD girls are necessary. Indeed, prior investigations have reported gender differences in cerebral function of ADHD subjects. For example, Ernst et al. reported that girls with ADHD had a 19.6% decrease in cerebral metabolism as compared to boys with ADHD, and a 15% decrease in metabolism as compared to healthy control girls *(83)*. Another study by the same group evaluated the effect of aging on cerebral glucose metabolism in ADHD subjects and reported that older age was associated with decreased cerebral metabolism in women with ADHD, but not in men with ADHD or controls of ether sex *(84)*, suggesting that this trend may be secondary to sex hormone differences between males and females that are associated with development. In a more recent study, Castellanos et al. evaluated a group of 50 female ADHD patients and 50 female controls and found smaller total cerebral volumes and posterior-inferior cerebellar vermal volumes in ADHD females *(22)*. In contrast, some of the findings of previous studies of male ADHD subjects, such as caudate asymmetry, were not identified, suggesting that there may be sex differences in the neuroanatomy of ADHD.

Another limitation of studies has been the variability among investigations in controlling for motion artifact, especially considering that there is an increased risk of subject restlessness when studying ADHD populations. Bite-bars *(79)* have been used in the past, but more effective methods to decrease movement are needed. Future studies must also consider age of onset of ADHD and address abnormalities in developmental trajectories. For example, levels of dopamine containing neurons, dopamine metabolites, and DAT all reportedly decrease with age of ADHD patients.

The effects of medications should also be considered when designing future neuroimaging studies *(27)*. Specifically, MRS may be useful to identify neurochemical predictors of treatment response and neurochemical effects of treatments.

Finally, few studies have examined the differential neurobiology of the patients with the different subtypes of ADHD. Future functional and structural neuroimaging studies may be helpful to determine the differential neurobiology between subtypes of ADHD. In order to establish a more biologically based classification scheme, further studies should try to demonstrate whether the clinical subtypes of ADHD show distinct structural or functional differences. Moreover, neuroimaging studies may be useful is establishing the differential neurobiology of pediatric ADHD and bipolar disorder, which may lead to more accurate diagnoses and, therefore, more effective interventions *(85)*.

Although there are many neuroimaging investigations in subjects with ADHD, there are numerous inconsistencies in the results of these studies *(3)*. Thus specific biological markers of ADHD have yet to be defined and the clinical applications of such findings are not yet regimented. It is unlikely that neuroimaging will be the diagnostic standard for ADHD in the near future. Nonetheless, future prospective longitudinal neuroimaging studies, using newer technologies such as diffusion tensor imaging, may allow us to identify the neurostructural, neurofunctional, and neurochemical abnormalities, as well as abnormal neuronal pathways, that occur in children and adolescents with ADHD. Large sample sizes are likely to be necessary to unequivocally identify candidate brain regions that are involved in ADHD. Additionally, these investigations will allow us to begin to understand how the neurodevelopmental trajectories of ADHD youth differ from normal.

REFERENCES

1. Tayler E, Chadwick O, Heptinstall E, Danckaerts M. Hyperactivity and conduct problems as risk factors for adolescent development. J Acad Child Adolesc Psychiatry 1996;35:1213–1226.
2. Barkley RA, ed. Attention deficit hyperactivity disorder: a handbook for diagnosis and treatment. New York: Guilford Press, 1990.
3. Baumeister AA, Hawkins MF. Incoherence of neuroimaging studies of attention deficit/hyperactivity disorder. Clin Neuropharmacol 2001;24:2–10.
4. Thapar A, Holmes J, Poulton K, Harrington, R. Genetic basis of attention deficit and hyperactivity. Brit J Psychiatry 1999;174:105–111.
5. Comings DE, Gade-Andavalou R, Gonzalez N, et al. Multivariate analysis of associations of 42 genes in ADHD, ODD, and conduct disorder. Clin Genet 2000;58:31–40.
6. Solanto MV. Dopamine dysfunction in AD/HD: integrating clinical and basic science research. Brain Behav Res 2002;130:64–71.
7. Biederman J, Spencer T. Attention-deficit/hyperactivity disorder (ADHD) as a noradrenergic disorder. Biol Psychiatry 1999;46:1234–1242.
8. DelBello MP, Kowatch RA. Neuroimaging in pediatric bipolar disorder. In: Geller B and DelBello MP, eds. Bipolar Disorder in Childhood and Early Adolescence. New York: Guilford Press, 2003:158–174.
9. Nasrallah HA, Loney J, Olson SC, McCalley-Whitters M, Kramer J, Jacoby B. Cortical atrophy in young adults with a history of hyperactivity in childhood. Psychiatry Res 1986;17:241–246.
10. Shaywitz BA, Shaywitz SE, Byrne T, Cohen DJ, Rothman S. Attention deficit disorder: quantitative analysis of CT. Neurology 1983; 33:1500–1503.
11. Giedd JN, Blumenthal J, Molloy E, Castellanos FX. Brain imaging of attention deficit/hyperactivity disorder. Ann NY Acad Sci 2001;931:33–49.
12. Zametkin AJ, Liotta W. The neurobiology of attention-deficit/hyperactivity disorder. J Clin Psychiatry 1998;59:17–23.
13. O'Tauma LA, Treves ST. Brain single-photon emission computed tomography for behavior disorders in children. Semin Nucl Med 1993; 23:255–264.
14. Teicher MH, Anderson CM, Polcari A, Maas LC, Renshaw PF. Functional deficits in basal ganglia of children with attention-deficit/hyperactivity disorder shown with functional magnetic resonance imaging relaxometry. Nat Med 2000;6:470–473.
15. Strakowski SM, DelBello MP, Adler C, Cecil CM, Sax KM. Neuroimaging in bipolar disorders. Bipolar Disord 2000;2:148–164.
16. Welner JS, Reich W, Herjanic B, Jung K, Amado H. Reliability, validity, and child agreement studies of the Diagnostic Interview of Children and Adolescents (DICA). J Am Acad Child Adolesc Psychiatry 1987;26:649–653.
17. Achenbach TM, Edelbbrock C. Manual for the child behavior checklist and revised child behavior profile. Burlington: University of Vermont Department of Psychiatry, 1983.
18. Wechsler D. Manual for the Weschler Intelligence Scale for Children-Revised. New York: Psychological Corporation, 1974.
19. Casey BJ, Castellanos FX, Giedd JN, et al. Implication of right frontostriatal circuitry in response inhibition and attention-deficit/hyperactivity disorder. J Am Acad Child Adolesc Psychiatry 1997;36:374–383.

20. Castellanos FX, Giedd JN, Marsh WL, et al. Quantitative brain magnetic resonance imaging in attention-deficit hyperactivity disorder. Arch Gen Psychiatry 1996;53:607–616.
21. Castellanos FX, Lee PP, Sharp W, et al. Developmental trajectories of brain volume abnormalities in children with attention-deficit/hyperactivity disorder. JAMA 2002;288:1740–1748.
22. Castellanos FX, Giedd JN, Berquin PC, et al. Quantitative brain magnetic resonance imaging in girls with attention deficit/hyperactivity disorder. Arch Gen Psychiatry 2001;58:289–295.
23. Mostofsky SH, Cooper KL, Kates WR, Denckla MB, Kaufman WE. Smaller prefrontal and premotor volumes in boys with attention-deficit/hyperactivity disorder. Biol Psychiatry 2002;52:785–794.
24. Hendren RL, DeBacker I, Pandina GJ. Review of neuroimaging studies of child and adolescent disorders from the past 10 years. J Acad Child Adolesc Psychiatry 2000;39:815–828.
25. Heilman KM, Voeller KKS, Nadeau SE. A possible pathophysiologic substrate of attention deficit hyperactivity disorder. J Child Neurol 1991; 6 Suppl:S76–81.
26. Hynd GW, Semrud-Clikeman M, Lorys AR, Novey ES, Eliopulos D. Brain morphology in developmental dyslexia and attention deficit disorder/hyperactivity. Arch Neurol 1990;47: 919–926.
27. Filipek PA, Semrud-Clikeman M, Steingard RJ, Renshaw PF, Kennedy DN, Biederman J. Volumetric MRI analysis comparing subjects having attention-deficit hyperactivity disorder with normal controls. Neurology 1997;48:589–601.
28. Semrud-Clikeman M, Steingard RJ, Filipek, P, Biederman J, Bekken K, Renshaw PF. Using MRI to examine brain-behavior relationships in males with attention deficit disorder with hyperactivity. J Am Acad Child Adolesc Psychiatry 2000;39:477–484.
29. Kates WR, Frederiske M, Motofsky SH, et al. MRI parcellation of the frontal lobe in boys with attention deficit hyperactivity disorder or Tourette syndrome. Psychiatry Res 2002;116:63–81.
30. Hesslinger B, Tebartz van Elst L, Thiel T, Haegele K, Henning J, Ebert D. Frontorbital volume reductions in adult patients with attention deficit hyperactivity disorder. Neurosci Lett 2002;328:319–321.
31. Aylward EH, Reiss AL, Reader MJ, Singer HS, Brown JE, Denckla MB. Basal ganglia volumes in children with attention-deficit hyperactivity disorder. J Child Neurol 1996;11:112–115.
32. Max JE, Fox PT, Lancaster JL, et al. Putamen lesions and the development of attention-deficit/hyperactivity disorder. J Am Acad Adolesc Psychiatry 2002;41:563–571.
33. Alexander GE, DeLong MR, Strick PL. Parallel organization of functionally segregated circuits linking basal ganglia and cortex. Ann Rev Neurosci 1986;9:357–381.
34. Castellanos FX, Giedd JN, Eckburg P, et al. Quantitative morphology of the caudate nucleus in attention deficit disorder. Am J Psychiatry 1994;151:1791–1796.
35. Hynd GW, Hern KL, Novey ES, et al. Attention deficit-hyperactivity disorder and asymmetry of the caudate nucleus. J Child Neurol 1993;8:339–347.
36. Mataro M, Garcia-Sanchez C, Junque C, Estevez-Gonzalez A, Pujol J. Magnetic resonance imaging measurement of the caudate nucleus in adolescents with attention-deficit hyperactivity disorder and its relationship with neuropsychological and behavioral measures. Arch Neurol 1997;54:963–968.
37. Pineda DA, Restrepo MA, Sarmiento RJ, et al. Statistical analyses of structural magnetic resonance imaging of the head of the caudate nucleus in Colombian children with attention-deficit hyperactivity disorder. J Child Neurol 2002;17:97–105.
38. Schrimsher GW, Billingsley RL, Jackson EF, Moore BD. Caudate nucleus volume asymmetry predicts attention-deficit hyperactivity disorder (ADHD) symptomatology in children. J Child Neurol 2002;17:877–884.
39. Castellanos FX. Proceed, with caution: SPECT cerebral blood flow studies of children and adolescents with attention deficit hyperactivity disorder. J Nucl Med 2002;43:1630–1633.
40. Castellanos FX, Sharp WS, Gottesmann RF, Greenstein DK, Giedd JN, Rapoport JL. Anatomic brain abnormalities in monozygotic twins discordant for attention deficit hyperactivity disorder. Am J Psychiatry 2003;160:1693–1696.

41. Giedd JN, Castellanos FX, Casey BJ, et al. Quantitative morphology of the corpus collosum in attention deficit hyperactivity disorder. Am J Psychiatry 1994;151:665–669.
42. Baumgardner TL, Singer HS, Denckla MB, et al. Corpus callosum morphology in children with Tourette syndrome and attention deficit hyperactivity disorder. Neurology 1996;47:477–482.
43. Semrud-Clikeman M, Filipek PA, Biederman J, et al. Attention deficit hyperactivity disorder: magnetic resonance imaging morphometric analysis of the corpus collosum. J Am Acad Child Adolesc Psychiatry 1994;33:875–881.
44. Hynd GW, Semrud-Clikeman M, Lorys AR, Novey ES, Eliopulos D, Lyytinen H. Corpus callosum morphology in attention-deficit hyperactivity disorder: morphometric analysis of MRI. J Learn Disabil 1991;24:141–146.
45. Lyoo IK, Noam GG, Lee CK, Lee HK, Kennedy BP, Renshaw PF. The corpus callosum and lateral ventricles in children with attention-deficit hyperactivity disorder: a brain magnetic resonance imaging study. Biol Psychiatry 1996;40:1060–1063.
46. Mostofsky SH, Reiss AL, Lockhart P, Denckla MB. Evaluation of cerebellar size in attention-deficit hyperactivity disorder. J Child Neurol 1998;13:434–439.
47. Berquin PC, Giedd JN, Jacobson LK, et al. Cerebellum in attention-deficit hyperactivity disorder: a morphometric MRI study. Neurology 1998;50:1087–1093.
48. Rubia K. The dynamic approach to neurodevelopmental psychiatric disorders: use of fMRI combined with neuropsychology to elucidate the dynamics of psychiatric disorders, exemplified in ADHD and schizophrenia. Behav Brain Res 2002;130:47–56.
49. Zametkin AJ, Nordahl TE, Gross M, et al. Cerebral glucose metabolism in adults with hyperactivity of childhood onset. New Eng J Med 1990;323:1361–1366.
50. Zametkin AJ, Liebenauer LL, Fitzgerald GA, et al. Brain metabolism in teenagers with attention-deficit hyperactivity disorder. Arch Gen Psychiatry 1993;50:333–340.
51. Durston S, Tottenham NT, Thomas KM, et al. Differential patterns of striatal activation in young children with and without ADHD. Biol Psychiatry 2003;53:871–878.
52. Amen DG, Carmichael BD. High-resolution brain SPECT imaging in ADHD. Ann Clin Psychiatry 1997;9: 81–86.
53. Kim NN, Lee JS, Shin MS, Cho SC, Lee DS. Regional cerebral perfusion abnormalities in attention deficit/hyperactivity disorder: statistical parametric mapping analysis. Eur Arch Psychiatry Clin Neurosci 2002;252:219–225.
54. Rubia K, Overmeyer S, Taylor E, et al. Hypofrontality in attention deficit hyperactivity disorder during higher-order motor control: a study with functional MRI. Am J Psychiatry 1999;156:891–896.
55. Langleben DD, Austin G, Krikorian G, Ridlehuber HW, Goris ML, Strauss HW. Interhemispheric asymmetry of regional cerebral blood flow in prepubescent boys with attention deficit hyperactivity disorder. Nuclear Med Comm 2001;22:1333–1340.
56. Bush G, Frazier JA, Rauch SL, et al. Anterior cingulate cortex dysfunction in attention-deficit/hyperactivity disorder revealed by fMRI and the counting Stroop. Biol Psychiatry 1999;45:1542–1552.
57. Lou HC, Andresen J, Steinberg B, McLaughlin T, Friberg L. The striatum in a putative network activated by verbal awareness in normals and in ADHD children. Euro J Neurol 1998;5:67–74.
58. Lou HC, Henriksen L, Bruhn P, Borner H, Nielson JB. Striatal dysfunction in attention deficit and hyperkinetic disorder. Arch Neurol 1989;46: 48–52.
59. Kaya GC, Pekcanlar A, Bekis R, et al. Technetium-99m HMPAO brain SPECT in children with attention deficit hyperactivity disorder. Ann Nuclear Med 2002;16:527–531.
60. Dougherty DD, Bonab AA, Spencer TJ, Rauch SL, Madras BK, Fischman AJ. Dopamine transporter density in patients with attention deficit hyperactivity disorder. Lancet 1999;354:2132–2133.
61. Dressel S, Krause J, Krause K-H, et al. Attention deficit hyperactivity disorder: binding of [^{99m}Tc]TRODAT-1 to the dopamine transporter before and after methylphenidate treatment. Euro J Nuc Med 2000;27:1518–1524.
62. Krause K-H, Dresel SH, Krause J, Kung HF, Tatsch, K. Increased striatal dopamine transporter in adult patients with attention deficit hyperactivity disorder: effects of methylphenidate as measured by single photon emission computed tomography. Neuro Letter 2000;285:107–110.

63. van Dyck CH, Quinlan DM, Cretella LM, et al. Unaltered dopamine transporter availability in adult attention deficit hyperactivity disorder. Am J Psychiatry 2002;159:309–312.
64. Rohde LA, Roman T, Szobot C, Cunha RD, Hutz MH, Biederman J. Dopamine transporter gene, response to methylphenidate and cerebral blood flow in attention-deficit/hyperactivity disorder: a pilot study. Synapse 2003;48: 87–89.
65. Castellanos FX, Lau E, Taybei N, et al. Lack of an association between a dopamine-4 receptor polymorphism and attention-deficit/hyperactivity disorder: genetic and brain morphometric analysis. Mol Psychiatry 1998;3:431–434.
66. MacMaster F, Carrey N, Sparkes S, Kusumakar V. Proton spectroscopy in medication-free pediatric attention-deficit/hyperactivity disorder. Biol Psychiatry 2003;53:184–187.
67. Carrey N, MacMaster F, Fogel J, et al. Metabolite changes resulting from treatment in children with ADHD: a 1H-MRS study. Clin Neuropharmacol 2003;26:218–221.
68. Courvoisie H, Hooper S, Fine C, Kwock L, Castillo M. Neurometabolic functioning and neuropsychological correlates in children with ADHD-H: preliminary findings. J Neuropsychiatry Clin Neurosci 2004;16:63–69.
69. Jin Z, Zang Y, Zeng Y, Zhang L, Wang Y. Striatal neuronal loss or dysfunction and choline rise in children with attention-deficit hyperactivity disorder: a 1H-magnetic resonance spectroscopy study. Neurosci Lett 2001;315:45–48.
70. Yeo R, Hill D, Campbell RA, et al. Proton magnetic resonance spectroscopy investigation of the right frontal lobe in children with attention-deficit/hyperactivity disorder. J Am Acad Child Adolesc Psychiatry 2003;42:303–310.
71. Hesslinger B, Thiel T, Tebartz van Elst L, Hennig J, Ebert D. Attention-deficit disorder in adults with or without hyperactivity: where is the difference? A study in humans using short echo (1)H-magnetic resonance spectroscopy. Neurosci Lett 2001;304:117–119.
72. Olfson M, Gameroff MJ, Marcus SC, Jenson PS. National trends in the treatment of attention deficit hyperactivity disorder. Am J Psychiatry 2003;160:1071–1077.
73. Volkow ND, Wang G, Fowler JS, et al. Relationship between blockade of dopamine receptors by oral methylphenidate and the increases in extracellular dopamine: therapeutic implications. Synapse 2002;43:181–187.
74. Matochik JA, Liebenauer LL, King AC, Szymanski HV, Cohen RM, Zametkin AJ. Cerebral glucose metabolism in adults with attention deficit hyperactivity disorder after chronic stimulant treatment. Am J Psychiatry 1994;151:658–664.
75. Matochik JA, Nordahl TE, Gross M, et al. Effects of acute stimulant medication on cerebral metabolism in adults with hyperactivity. Neuropsychopharm 1993;8:377–386.
76. Kim BN, Lee JS, Cho SC, Lee DS. Methylphenidate increased regional cerebral blood flow in subjects with attention deficit/hyperactivity disorder. Yonsei Med J 2001;42:19–29.
77. Langleben DD, Acton PD, Austin G, et al. Effects of methylphenidate discontinuation on cerebral blood flow in prepubescent boys with attention deficit hyperactivity disorder. J Nucl Med 2002;43:1624–1629.
78. Anderson CM, Polcari A, Lowen SB, Renshaw PF, Teicher, MH. Effects of methylphenidate on functional resonance relaxometry of the cerebellar vermis. Am J Psychiatry 2002;159:1322–1328.
79. Vaidya CJ, Austin G, Kirkorian G, et al. Selective effects of methylphenidate in attention deficit hyperactivity disorder: a functional magnetic resonance study. Proc Natl Acad Sci 1998;95:14,494–14,499.
80. Castellanos FX. Toward a pathophysiology of attention-deficit/hyperactivity disorder. Clin Pediatr 1997;36:381–393.
81. Ilgin N, Senol S, Gucuyener K, Gokcora N, Atavci S, Senor S. Is increased availability associated with response to stimulant medication in ADHD? Develop Med Child Neurology 2001;43: 755–760.
82. Vles JS, Feron FJ, Hendriksen JG, Jolles J, van Kroonenburgh MJ, Weber WE. Methylphenidate down-regulates the dopamine receptor and transport system in children with attention deficit hyperkinetic disorder (ADHD). Neuropediatrics 2003;34: 77–80.

83. Enrst M, Liebenauer MA, King C, Fitzgerald GA, Cohen RM, Zametkin AJ. Reduced brain metabolism in hyperactive girls. J Am Acad Child Adolesc Psychiatry 1994;33:858–868.
84. Ernst M, Zametkin AJ, Phillips RL, Cohen RM. Age-related changes in brain metabolism in adults with attention deficit/hyperactivity disorder and control subjects. J Neuropsychiatry 1998;10:168–177.
85. Biederman J, Farone SV, Mick E, et al. Attention-deficit hyperactivity disorder and juvenile mania: an overlooked comorbidity? J Am Acad Child Adolesc Psychiatry 1996;35:997–1008.

18

State Regulation and Attention Deficit Hyperactivity Disorder

Jaap van der Meere

1. INTRODUCTION

Parents, teachers, and clinicians continue saying that the behavior of children with attention deficit hyperactivity disorder (ADHD) can be extremely variable. For activities that are of interest (i.e., watching television), the children can sit still and maintain attention for hours. Their performance accuracy declines rapidly, however, if the task at hand is not appealing, which may happen during (neuro) psychological testing. Here, the clinician needs all his or her experience to keep the child on track in order to estimate the child's true potential. Once the requirements for testing are finally met (i.e., the child sits still, listens carefully, and is motivated), the clinician is exhausted, and the child shows "no deficits." This huge variability of behavior may lead to confusing interpretations in our research field. For instance, on the one hand, many researchers consider the classroom to be an optimal condition to study the effects of methylphenidate (MPH) on impulsive and overactive behavior, whereas on the other hand, children with ADHD have more daytime sleep episodes than the norm *(1)*. The role of behavioral variability in ADHD is also emphasized by genetic studies, showing that variable responding during reaction-time (RT) tests mediates the genetic effects, not ability factors *per se*, including delay aversion *(2)* or stopping an intended response *(3)*.

In sum, there are reasons to claim that insight into the source of behavioral variability provides an essential key to the understanding of ADHD. However, having arrived at this point, the question emerges as to which cognitive model research has to be carried out when the intimate relationship between behavior and its biological/motivational context is not a favorable subject in the field of neurocognitive science.

2. WHICH MODEL TO CHOOSE TO STUDY ADHD

For decades behavior scientists have been interested in phenomena, such as overt and covert attention, filtering relevant from irrelevant information, memory, motor-presetting, inhibition, and so on. In line with this, the development of information-processing models has been impressive, becoming increasingly precise and well-specified, especially with regard to models linking psychophysiological indices (i.e., evoked potentials and neuroimaging data) with overt behavior, which provide promising data on what takes place in the brain

From: *Attention Deficit Hyperactivity Disorder: From Genes to Patients*
Edited by: D. Gozal and D. L. Molfese © Humana Press Inc., Totowa, NJ

between perception and action. However, although no one would deny that factors, such as sleep loss, stress, fatigue, noise, incentives, punishment, time on task, time of day, knowledge of results, supervision, presentation rate of stimuli, temperature, and alcohol, affect the quality of information processing, the influence of these so-called energetic factors has rarely been considered in the current cognitive theories. On the contrary, these factors are generally seen as confounding factors. At best they are considered modulatory. This could well be the result of the modern *Zeitgeist*: the dominance of the metaphor of the computer, in which computational mechanisms are emphasized and motivation and energetics ignored *(4)*. Nevertheless, it is obvious that in order to model real-life cognitive performance any comprehensive account of cognition would ultimately have to incorporate the effects of energetic factors.

In this spirit, leading researchers in the field of experimental psychology met in Les Arcs, France, from August 23 through 28, 1985. The meeting was sponsored by the North Atlantic Treaty Organization Scientific Affairs Division and provided a perfect forum to discuss the possibilities of a marriage between the 20th century computer metaphor and the 19th century energy metaphor (e.g., energy mobilization; ref. *5*), or to use their own words, to restate one of the classic problems of psychology—that of accounting for motivational or intensive aspects of behavior *(6–10)*—as opposed to structural or directional aspects. The results were put together in a *pièce de resistance* titled *Energetics and Human Information Processing*, edited by Hockey, Coles, and Gaillard *(11)*. An important conclusion made by the forum was that the original assumption of a unitary, nonspecific process based on activation of the brain stem reticular formation was too simple, given that work in the field of neurobiology had demonstrated evidence of discrete neurotransmitter systems with quite specific information-processing functions and central roles in regulation of behavior. In contrast, there were strong arguments to differentiate between different types of energetic supply. A key model discussed in Les Arcs was the cognitive energetic model by Sanders *(4,12–14)*, together with its counterpart: the neurophysiological oriented model by Pribram and McGuinness *(15)*; *see* Fig. 1.

In this model, task efficiency is considered as a product of elementary cognitive stages (level 1) and their energy distribution (levels 2 and 3). The elementary stages at level 1 are stimulus encoding, memory search, binary decision, and motor preparation. These stages may be seen as structural processes, i.e., processes that mediate between stimulus and response. They are assumed to function serially and discretely, meaning that contingent stages operate in strict succession, with each stage finishing before the next can begin. The stages are involved in executive functioning, such as divided and focused attention *(16,17)* and (motor) set shifting *(18)*. The availability of the elementary (computational) stages at level 1 is related to the arousal and activation levels of the subject (level 2).

Arousal is defined as a time-locked phasic physiological response to input *(15)*. McGuinness and Pribram *(19)* related the arousal system to the amount of information in the stimulus and to surprise, novelty, or complexity levels in selective attention tasks. In short, the arousal system refers to the "what is it?" reaction. In addition, they speculated that the arousal system is related to emotional reactivity. The core brain system associated with arousal extends from the spinal cord through the brainstem reticular formation including the hypothalamic sites. The amygdala and related frontal cortical structures are involved in the control of the core brain arousal system. The dominant neurotransmitters in the arousal system are serotonin and noradrenaline *(20,21)*.

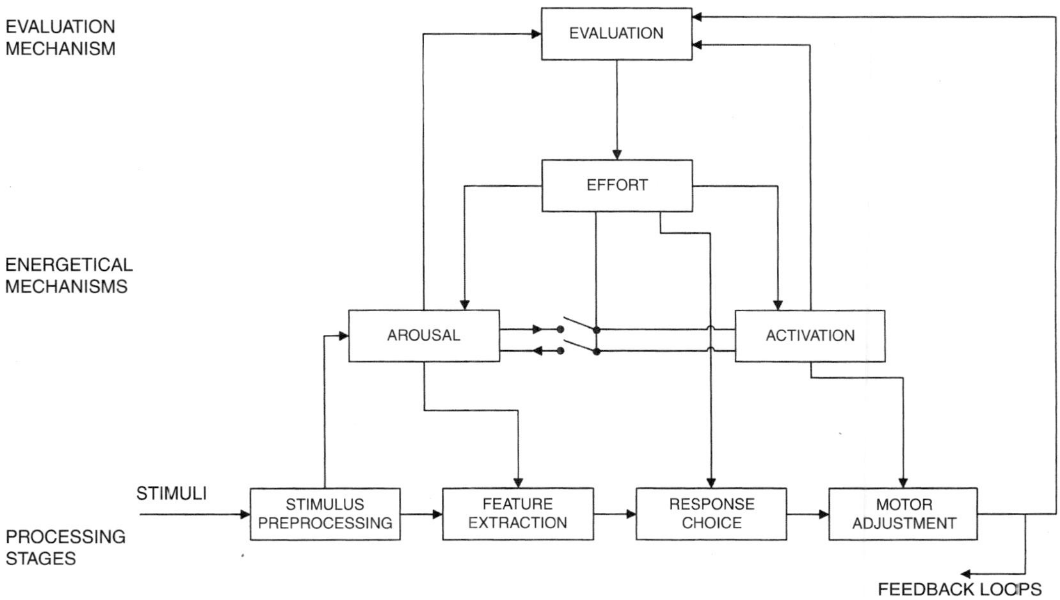

Fig. 1. The cognitive energetic model.

The activation system refers to a tonic long-lasting voluntary readiness for action: the "what is to be done?" reaction. Structures involved in the activation system are the dorsal thalamus and the basal ganglia with, in particular, the corpus striatum of the forebrain *(15,19)*. Dopamine is the most important neurotransmitter *(22)*.

The effort system (level 3) is under control of an evaluation mechanism, which scans the momentary state of the arousal and activation levels. A suboptimal state of arousal and/or activation is compensated through the effort mechanism by either activating or inhibiting the arousal and/or activation pool/resources. Thus, unlike the traditional activation theory, in which the energetical processes are essentially stimulus-driven *(10,23)*, in the view of Pribram and McGuiness the energetic resources may be controlled through strategic resource-management decisions. Therefore, in essence the Pribram and McGuiness model builds on the work of Broadbent *(24)* and Kahneman *(25)*, wherein motivation is not only a driving or energizing force but also a key factor involved in the initiation, maintenance, and regulation of action.

In sum, state monitoring means checking for discrepancies between an individual's actual state and his required (target) state. If there is a discrepancy, it is evaluated and action is taken to restore equilibrium. Within this perspective, Hockey *(26)* formulated the following four different types of actions:

1. Active regulation of the individual's actual state, which is influenced by stressors, such as time-on-task.
2. Change of the criteria for optimal performance, so that the individual's required state is closer to his or her actual state (and, as a result, accepting errors).
3. Action oriented toward direct control of the environmental influences on the individual's actual state (for instance, closing windows to shut out the noise of traffic).
4. No action.

Only the first type of action may attract costs to physiological subsystems: primarily the limbic system in a circuit involving the cingulate cortex, hippocampus, septal nuclei, and the anterior hypothalamus, with the hippocampus playing the major role in this circuit *(15)*.

It is to be noted here that the earlier-discussed marriage between the 20th century computer metaphor and the 19th century energy metaphor is reflected in Sanders' model *(4)* by the linkage of level 1 with levels 2 and 3, wherein the quality of elementary cognitive steps is dependent upon the energetic (arousal and activation) state of the subject.

Using Sternberg's additive factor method *(18)*, Sanders showed that the processing stages at level 1, as well as the energetic levels 2 and 3, could be separately influenced by so-called task manipulations. For instance, when the task duration is short and when subjects are motivated, stimulus degradation, set size, and response compatibility manipulations affect the stages of, respectively, stimulus encoding, central processes, and motor preparation. Arousal is influenced by noise (overarousal) and stimulus repetition (underarousal). Motor activation is influenced by stimulus uncertainty (i.e., varying the presentation rate of stimuli) and amphetamine. Effort, in turn, is affected by factors, such as knowledge of results and time-on-task. Sleep loss affects both arousal and activation.

In summary, based on the outcome of reaction-time studies, Sanders created an impressive body of knowledge on the effects of energetic state on the quality of input and output stages of the information-processing chain. Given the theme of the current chapter, the first question is how direct effects on computational stages (level 1) can be distinguished from indirect effects, which depend on variations in energetic supply (levels 2 and 3). The rule of thumb is that direct computational factors usually have their effects on all the individual trials during reaction-time tests, and, hence, shift the whole distribution of reaction times. Characteristic for energetic factors, on the other hand, is that their effect varies strongly between individual trials. Therefore, their effect will be most pronounced at the higher end of the distribution and may indeed be absent in the lower end *(27)*. Within this context, Leth-Steensen et al. *(28)* performed a detailed statistical analysis of the response times of children with ADHD vs control children, fitting the ex-Gaussian distributional model to the individual response time data. The children with ADHD showed a large amount of abnormally slow responses. This was considered as a typical feature of a deficient allocation of energetic resources (the effortful maintenance of optimal activation levels needed for maintaining a consistent state of motor preparation). However, before discussing in detail research findings in terms of the Sanders' model, time is ripe to compare the model with the attention framework of Posner and colleagues, which is currently among the most influential models in the United States.

Posner and colleagues *(29–32)* have postulated three distinct but interconnected neuroanatomical networks. The posterior attention system (PAS) is particularly involved in selective attention, i.e., shifting attention to a target in space. The posterior parietal lobe has been shown to play an active role in disengaging attention. Also part of this system are the superior colliculus of the midbrain, involved in moving attention to another location, and the pulvinar nucleus of the thalamus, associated with engaging attention at a new location. The PAS receives noradrenergic input from arousal modulating structures in the medulla, among which the locus coeruleus (LC) is the most important *(33)*.

The anterior attention system is involved in detecting and comparing events and selecting appropriate responses. Broadly speaking, it is considered to exercising executive control and bringing an object into conscious awareness *(31)*. The network is involved in effortful attention processing of stimuli and training. The gyrus cingulate is associated with these functions.

The third system is the vigilance or alertness system, which refers to maintaining a sustained state of alertness. The right frontal and right parietal areas are part of this network. The LC is also part of this network, as the structure strongly controls right frontal areas.

It is unfortunate that it is as yet unclear whether generalization from the cognitive-energetic framework to the concepts of Posner's theory is actually justified. Neither has there been a proper analysis of Pribram's predominantly limbic structures as compared to Posner's cortical structures. Yet it is interesting that evidence for a functional distinction between an input system (Posner's posterior structure), an output system (Posner's frontal lobe structure), and a central control system (Posner's anterior structure) emerge in all current descriptions of attention mechanisms *(4)*. For example, we may consider the alertness network, which has the function of maintaining an alert state to correspond with the noradrenergic arousal system as described by Pribram and McGuinness *(15)*. Another correspondence could be the fact that the vigilance network, defined as levels 2 and 3 in Sanders' model, influences both the posterior and anterior network involved in executive functioning.

Reviews written from the energetic perspective *(34–39)* have underlined that there is little, if any, evidence that pure ADHD is associated with a divided or focused attention disturbance, with a response inhibition deficit, or with an inability to shift from controlled processing into automatic processing. However, children are delayed in their motor preparation and inhibition processes especially when the presentation rate of the stimuli is slow. In terms of the Sanders model this could indicate poor state regulation: i.e., underactivation and poor effort allocation. The findings make Posner's PAS and anterior attention system networks unlikely candidates to be associated with ADHD; this could be different with regard to Posner's vigilance network as a difficulty in remaining in an alert state. In Section 3, a series of RT studies will be discussed suggesting that children with ADHD have difficulties remaining in an alert state, particularly in conditions with a slow presentation rate of stimuli.

3. EVENT RATE FINDINGS

According to Sanders' theory, the signal rate of the go/no-go signals may alter the state of the subject, a fast condition may induce "overactivation," resulting in fast-inaccurate responding, whereas the slow condition may induce "underactivation," resulting in slow-inaccurate responding. Therefore, to counteract a decrement in task efficiency, subjects have to correct their state in the fast and slow conditions. With this in mind, the working hypothesis in our research was, "If children with ADHD do not effectively change (adapt) their state then task inefficiency will be most pronounced in the fast and slow conditions, wherein state regulation is assumed to be essential, whereas the effect of signal rate on task performance will be less pronounced in control children who effectively correct their state."

It appeared that the effect of signal rate on the test performance in the ADHD group was most pronounced in the slow condition. Children with ADHD were slow and variable responders to go signals and at the same time showed poor impulse control toward no-go trials. The findings were interpreted that children with ADHD are easily underactivated. In other words, when the test is boring (as is evidently the case when stimuli are slowly presented) they are the first to show poor task efficiency. When the test is activating (which is the case with a fast presentation rate) the children with ADHD are (almost) indistinguishable from controls *(40)*. A developmental study indicated that the ability of state control is at least 2 yr delayed in children with ADHD *(41)*. Potgieter et al. *(42)* have replicated these findings. They compared a control group with prematurely born children with and without ADHD using the same go/no-go instrument. It appeared that the prematurely born children had no problems with response inhibition compared to the control group. However, prematurely born children with ADHD showed slow and variable responses to go signals and had a problem inhibiting their responses to no-go signals in the slow condition, not in the fast condition.

With respect to the discriminant validity problem it is of importance to emphasize that performance is disproportionately impaired by a fast event rate condition in adults with high-functioning autism (HFA), whereas no differences in RT performance are observed between these individuals and the control group in the slow event rate condition. This finding is explained in terms of overactivation in HFA, which normalizes under a slow event rate *(43)*, whereas poor RT performance (including poor response inhibition) occurred independently of task event rate in children with combined ADHD and comorbid tic disorder *(40)*, in children with early and continuously treated phenylketonuria *(44)*, in learning-disabled children without ADHD *(45)*, and in children with mild mental retardation plus conduct disorder *(46)*. Thus, poor response inhibition in such populations is not associated with a state regulation deficit. It is most likely that a cognitive deficit located at the first level of the information processing chain of Sanders' model provides a better explanation for the decreased task performance in these populations.

The finding that the task performance improves in conditions with a fast presentation rate and declines in conditions with a slow presentation rate has also been reported in studies in which other paradigms were used. Sheres et al. *(47)* administered the stop paradigm using similar event rate conditions as used in the go/no-go studies by van der Meere and colleagues. They too found a significant relationship between slow event rate and poor task performance (i.e., slow RT, not poor response inhibition) in children with ADHD with or without, oppositional defiant disorder. Similarly, Purvis and Tannock *(48)*, using the Conners Continuous Performance Test in which letters were presented with interstimulus intervals of either 1, 2, or 4 s, showed that children with ADHD were similar to children without ADHD at 1-s intervals but were slower than children without ADHD at the other intervals. Walker and colleagues *(49)* studied adults with ADHD. They demonstrated that although the predictive power of a diversity of impulsivity tests was poor in discriminating ADHD from other psychiatric disorders, the ADHD group displayed a slower and more variable RT performance especially in slow event rate conditions. Finally, Sonuga-Barke *(50)* found that the task performance of children with ADHD on a computerized version of the Matching Familiar Figure Test was lower than the controls on the trial conditions of 5 and 15 s, but similar to the controls on the 10-s trials.

Clearly the aforementioned studies used different tasks and different stimulus presentation rates. This may have produced slightly different results—i.e., some studies reported decreased RT efficiency in children with ADHD in a condition with a presentation rate of 4 s, and others during a presentation rate of 8 s. However, in spite of the fact that the effect of presentation rate on RT performance is probably highly idiosyncratic, it seems reasonable to suppose that children with ADHD are poor performers (i.e., slow and variable responses with many errors) when the presentation rate is low. They perform much better when the presentation rate is high, because a high presentation rate compensates their under activated motor state. In this context, van der Meere et al. *(51)* investigated response inhibition during a self-paced condition in children with ADHD. In this condition a go or no-go signal appeared on the display as soon as the child had pressed the response button. It appeared that the ADHD and the normal control group speeded up their responses producing an interstimulus interval of about 600 ms. This speeding up led to an increase in errors to the same extent in both groups.

The robustness of the event rate effect remains also under sustained attention conditions of more than 30 min. Here, children with ADHD were found to have a rapid decline in task efficiency over time with a slow presentation rate, but not with a fast presentation rate *(34)*. This finding is also explainable in terms of the activating effect of the high event rate. Behavioral observations during sustained attention demands suggested that the excessive motor activity in children with ADHD *(52,53)*, including visual behavior *(54,55)* could be a strategy used to stay awake and alert.

4. STATE REGULATION AND ITS PSYCHOPHYSIOLOGICAL COSTS

The reaction time findings showed that the task performance of the normal control group remained remarkably stable as a function of event rate manipulation, and the earlier discussed energetic control framework argues that the maintenance of performance stability is an active process under control of the individual, requiring the management of cognitive resources through the mobilization of mental effort. In the last decades, several psychophysiological indices of effort allocation have been formulated, such as amplitudes of evoked potentials, heart rate variability, respiration, electrodermal activity, pupil diameter, rate and amplitude of eye blinks, endocrine responses (catecholamines and cortisol), and muscle activity. The reader is referred to Mulder *(56)* for an extensive review on these indices in relation to the cognitive-energetic model of Sanders. The following subheadings will be confined to heart rate variability issues and event-related potentials.

4.1. Heart Rate Variability

Spectral analysis of the heart rate time series allows us to examine the sympathetic and parasympathetic neural modulation of the heart. Modulation at frequencies from 0.03 to 0.15 Hz (the so-called midfrequency band) corresponds primarily to baroreceptor-mediated regulation of blood pressure. This frequency band involves modulation by both sympathetic and parasympathetic (vagal) influences. Modulation at frequencies greater than 0.15 Hz are respiration-modulated, and are defined as the high-frequency component. A plethora of research has shown that the more effective the compensatory state regulation is in the protection of performance, the more decreased the amplitude of the frequencies from 0.03 to 0.15 (the midband) *(56–60)*.

In view of the earlier discussed event rate findings, the compensatory control model predicts that the midband will be higher in children with ADHD and HFA relative to the normal control group. This is indeed what empirical research has found. Borger and van der Meere *(55)* evaluated the midfrequency band during fast and slow presentation rates. As expected, with fast stimulus presentations the speed and variability of responding by the children with ADHD was similar to the controls. However, with slow stimulus presentations, reactions of the ADHD group became slower and more variable than the control children. Further analysis showed that the ADHD group had a higher amplitude in the midfrequency band than the control group in the slow condition, whereas no between-group differences were found in the fast condition. It was concluded that children with ADHD allocated less effort in the slow condition. With respect to time-on-task effects, two studies *(61,62)* reported that children with ADHD and children diagnosed with pervasive developmental disorder not otherwise specified both had problems remaining motivated in order to maintain a stable performance throughout a memory recognition task. Both groups expressed a performance decline over time and higher amplitudes in the midfrequency band relative to a normal control population. Consequently, reduced vagal modulation, reflecting poor state regulation, was suggested in both children with ADHD and children falling into the autism spectrum. However, in view of the behavioral data discussed earlier, it is assumed that the ADHD group has problems in enhancing their underactivated state during a boring condition, whereas the pervasive developmental disorder not otherwise specified group may have problems in decreasing an elevated activation level during a state-enhancing condition.

4.2. *Evoked Response Potentials*

It has been argued that more effort allocation is related to a larger parietal P300 amplitude *(56)*. So, the general finding of psychophysiological research focused on ADHD, reviewed by van der Meere *(34)*, that the amplitude of this component is reduced in such children indicates that they allocate less effort to remain in an optimal state. Recent evoked-potential research carried out on the lines of the cognitive energetic model *(63)* demonstrated that children with ADHD responded slower in a go/no-go condition with a slow presentation, which was accompanied by a diminished P300 amplitude, suggesting less effort allocation. No differences in speed of responding and P300 amplitudes were found between children with ADHD and a peer control group. In the fast condition, the children with ADHD made more errors of commission, which was associated with an enlarged P200 amplitude, suggesting overarousal *(56)*. In sum, the results are compatible with the state regulation deficit hypothesis showing that children with ADHD have a small optimal state window: they are easily underactivated and overactivated. A developmental study indicated that the ability to regulate state, expressed in amplitudes of evoked potentals, increased as function of age *(64)*.

5. NEUROANATOMICAL STRUCTURES AND THE CARDIOVASCULAR SYSTEM

This section describes the neuroanatomical structures and physiological mechanisms involved in the interaction between the brain and the cardiovascular system in order to maintain an optimal blood flow, and, as a consequence, an optimal supply of energy and oxygen to all the components of the body. A key mechanism in this domain is the baro reflex. Figures 2 and 3 are schematic presentations of the direct (dotted) and indirect (dashed) afferent connections of the anterior cingulate cortex and the insular cortex to the important structures in the baroreflex.

The parasympathetic (or vagal) system controls about 75% of the fastest effector (i.e., heart rate) in the baro reflex. The sympathetic system controls the remaining 25% of this effector and further controls the maximum elastance of the heart, the venous volume, and the systemic resistance. The larger parts of the vagal projections to the heart originate in the nucleus ambiguous (NA), which is located in the medullary part of the reticular formation. The NA begins posterior of the facial nucleus and extends caudally to the first cervical level of the spinal cord, from the perspective of the afferents from the nervus tractus solitarius, which functions as a control center. The figures show that the LC and the NA are important structures with respect to cardiac reactivity. The former structure is closely linked to vigilance performance *(65,66)*, and the latter has a major role in the polyvagal theory of Porges *(67)* and is, because of its interaction with the facial nerve, believed to mediate complex behaviors such as attention, motion, emotion, and communication.

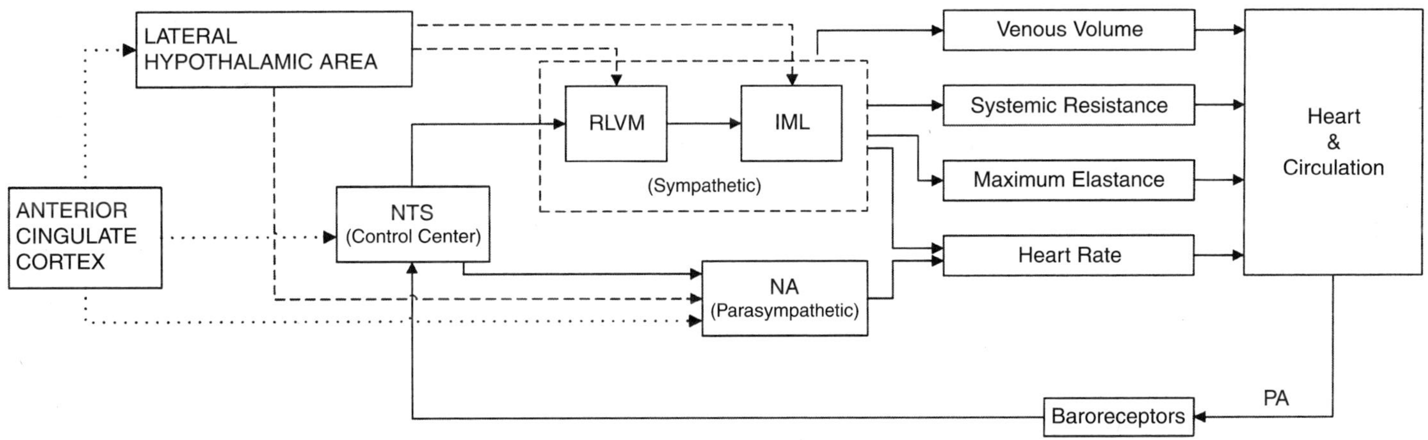

Fig. 2. The connection between brain structures and the baro reflex. RVLM, rostral ventrolateral medulla; IML, intermediolateral cell column; NTS, nucleus tractus solitarius.

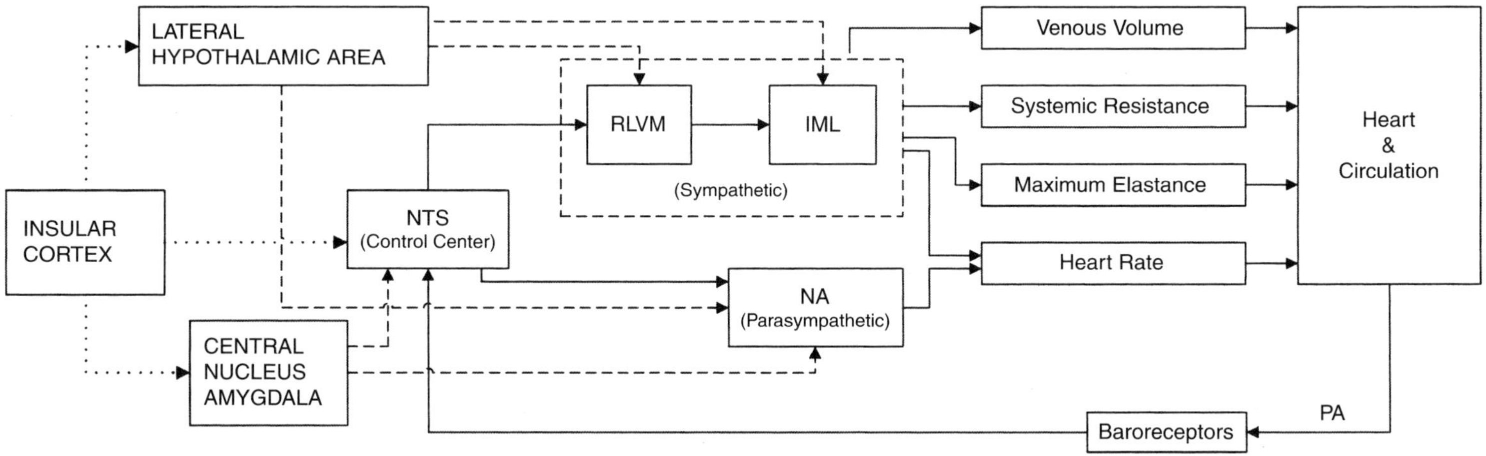

Fig. 3. The connection between brain structures and the baro reflex. RVLM, rostral ventrolateral medulla; IML, intermediolateral cell column; NTS, nucleus tractus solitarius.

That the NA plays an essential role in ADHD was recently suggested by van der Meere and Borger *(68)*. They evaluated children's midfrequency band in association with their facial movements, measured using the Facial Action Coding System *(69)*, during sustained attention demands. Movements of eyebrow, eyes, lips, tongue, and so on are innervated by the facial nerve. The source nucleus of the facial nerve is the border of the NA, which as discussed earlier, together with the nucleus tractus solitarius forms the rostral ventrolateral medulla and the vagal dorsal motor nucleus, the cardiac control center of the brain. In view of this, the study's main prediction was that facial expressions were coupled to the visceromotor regulation of the cardiac function by through the NA vagal efferents. This was indeed the case in the control group. The correlation between facial expressions and the midband amplitude was 0.60. This suggested that the more effort allocated to regulate state, the lower the amplitude in the mid frequency band and the more facial expressions. In the ADHD group, however, such correlations were absent. It was concluded that more research is needed to examine the role of the NA in the field of ADHD.

6. INTERIM CONCLUSION

Research findings based on Sanders' cognitive energetic model of information processing leads to the conclusion that ADHD is associated with brainstem injury, probably located at the LC and NA. It is to be noted that these structures play a central role in the alertness and vigilance network, as defined by Posner. However, it is important to emphasize at this point that many of the associations between structure and function discussed above are often based on indirect evidence and are always biased by the relatively artificial definitions of the suggested psychological processes. Whether or not the model of poor state regulation in ADHD turns out to be completely correct, it undoubtedly could play a major role in coordinating research efforts in our field and in serving as a foundation for future, more accurate, theory building.

With this in mind, one of the problems that has to be resolved in future research is that a variety of disorders other than ADHD has been repeatedly suggested to be accompanied by deficient parasympathetic (vagal) modulation processes, such as anxiety-related disorders *(70,71)*, major depression *(72)*, and schizophrenia *(73,74)*. On the one hand, one may argue that this overlap is not surprising, given that ADHD is considered as a precursor for maladaptive behavior at a later age. On the other hand, most of the studies just mentioned have evaluated cardiac control during steady-state conditions, which makes them difficult to interpret in terms of cardiac adaptivity. Thus, experimental designs contrasting such disorders and tapping cardiac reactivity are strongly recommended.

The suggestion that HFA might also be associated with brainstem injury fits well with the ideas of Rodier *(75)*, who claimed, on the basis of research findings in adults exposed to thalidomide while still in the womb, that autism may originate in the early weeks of pregnancy. Others have also emphasized in the past that a defective motivational framework may explain the attentional deficits in children with autism *(76)*. This being said, the dissociation between ADHD and HFA as presented in Fig. 3 calls for a direct comparison, given the many failures to differentiate both disorders at a cognitive level *(77)*.

In the following final headings of this chapter, factors will be discussed that may enhance the underactivated state in children with ADHD, i.e, methylphenidate, reward, and monitoring.

7. MPH AND STATE REGULATION

The effect of MPH on the behavior of children with ADHD is generally evaluated by questionnaires. As stated by Rapport et al. *(78)*, one of the most serious difficulties with the use of rating scales to assess the effects of medication is that they fail to provide information on associated changes in adaptive functioning. From this perspective, our research group has carried out several continuous performance tests, showing that MPH enhances task performance in children with ADHD *(79)* and in children with epilepsy and ADHD *(80)*. Findings were interpreted as follows: time-on-task triggers underactivation in subjects and MPH is lifting the activation state, which in turn results in enhanced task performance. Thus, MPH improves the task performance when conditions are boring (slow event rate). But what happens when children on MPH are executing a test with a high presentation rate of stimuli, which leads to overactivation? Our research group carried out two studies to answer this question. In the first study we used a double-blind crossover design in which 109 children with ADHD were randomly assigned without replacement to placebo, MPH, and clonidine. The primary dependent variables were reaction time and errors on the earlier discussed go/no-go test with interstimulus intervals of 1, 4, and 8 s. As expected, performance of the ADHD children was worst in the condition with a slow event rate. But surprisingly, no difference in task efficiency was found between the three groups in either the fast or slow condition. So we had to conclude that the state regulation deficit in ADHD is resistant to MPH and clonidine *(81)*. The MPH dosage was 0.6 mg/kg in a twice-a-day schedule with a dosage at breakfast of 0.3 mg/kg. In our second study *(82)*, we investigated the effects of MPH using the same go/no-go test but in contrast to the former experiment, the MPH dosage was not similar for each child but titrated on the basis of parent interviews. Findings indicated that MPH improved the reaction time profile during the condition with a slow event rate. However, errors increased dramatically in the condition with a fast presentation rate. Thus, the two energizers together, MPH plus a fast presentation rate, induced a reduction in the children's task efficiency. Findings are easily understood in terms of the stimulus shift hypothesis of Kinsbourne *(83)*, i.e., MPH raises the baseline activation level producing a decline in task performance because the fast condition is the most activating condition. Overall, findings may be compatible with Bergman et al. *(84)*, who claimed that MPH has its maximal impact on cognitive areas that are least impaired, and minimal impact on cognitive areas that are most impaired, i.e., poor state regulation in the opinion of the author of the current chapter.

8. REWARD AND STATE REGULATION

The question whether reward lifts the underactivated state toward a more optimal state has yet to be settled. The empirical results are equivocal. First, we have the important work by Sonuga-Barke and colleagues who postulated that children with ADHD are delay-aversive, rather than reward maximizers *(85,86)*. Similarly, Solanto *(87)* reported that reward is not a crucial factor in ADHD. She showed that the number of anticipatory responses during delayed response learning in children with ADHD and in control children is equally affected by reinforcement and response costs. Using the stop task, Oosterlaan and Sergant *(88)* also found that the impact of reward and response costs on response inhibition is the same in children with ADHD and control children. However, Slusarek and colleagues *(89)*, in contrast, found that reward interfered with the ability to withhold responding during the stop test in children with ADHD. Two studies of our research group suggest that task efficiency of

ADHD children with comorbid oppositional defiant disorder and children with conduct disorder (delinquent type) is sensitive for reward, but that the task efficiency of children with pure ADHD is not *(51,90)*. The findings underline the need to differentiate between ADHD and disruptive behavior *(91)* and await further research.

9. MONITORING AND STATE REGULATION

Van der Meere et al. *(79)* determined whether supervision would have a positive influence on the sustained attention abilities in children with ADHD. They found that the drop in performance efficiency over time was prominent in children with ADHD especially when working in the absence of the experimenter. When the experimenter was silently sitting behind the child who executed the continuous performance test, the decline in task efficiency over time was less pronounced, suggesting that even passive monitoring affects reallocation of effort during task performance.

This said, it is to be emphasized that in our field surprisingly little research has looked at the influence of the presence of other people on the task efficiency of children with ADHD. This is the more surprising given that historically the study of social facilitation and inhibition belongs to classic topics of experimental social psychology. The work of Zajonc *(92)* in particular teaches us about the potential arousal value others may have. He suggested a theoretical framework to account for the observation that the presence of others leads to an increment of general drive. However, as is the case with every theory, Zajonc's drive-theoretical explanation was substantially criticized. As a cognitive alternative to the drive-theoretical explanation, Duval and Wicklund *(93)* and Wicklund *(94)* proposed a theory of objective awareness. Here, specific stimuli such as mirrors, cameras, and the presence of another person are believed to focus the subject's attention inward (upon oneself) as the subject gets aware of his or her status. This inward focusing would give rise to an evaluation of possible discrepancies between the subject's intrinsic level of aspiration (the ideal self) and the subject's actual level of performance (the actual self), in terms of salient performance criteria. The eventually noted discrepancy between the ideal self and the actual self leads to an increasing motivation to reduce this discrepancy. For the careful reader it is obvious that these concepts come close to the earlier discussed actual and required state proposed by Hockey *(26)*. At this point, it is worthwhile to mention that the mere presence of others has a lowering effect on the midfrequency band *(95)*.

A merger of knowledge derived from both social psychology and our field would possibly facilitate more precise questions concerning the social conditions triggering the symptoms of ADHD. It is speculated here that the study of the effects of different modes of supervision executed by different persons (e.g., caretakers, peers) on state regulation in children with ADHD may offer promising intervention alternatives in the near future.

10. ETIOLOGY OF POOR STATE REGULATION

Family, adoption, and twin studies all have provided important insights into the etiology of ADHD. Similarly, the role of early caregiving in the development of ADHD is likely to be more significant than was previously assumed. Therefore, it seems safe to conclude that there are multiple pathways to ADHD *(96)*. In this perspective, longitudinal research focusing on state regulation is needed to get more insight into the developmental pathway of ADHD.

State control in neonates and infants has a large tradition in the field of ethology and neurobiology. For instance, Wolff *(97)* formulated different behavioral states in infants on the basis of prolonged observations using indices such as respiration, body movements, gaze behavior, and eyes open/closed. The behavioral states, in turn, were associated with different levels of responsiveness of the infant. Prechtl *(98)* elaborated on the issue of behavioral states and developed a diagnostic tool for assessing the quality of the nervous system of newborn, preschool, and school-aged children. More recently, Porges *(99)* argued that baseline vagal tone, derived from the respiratory component of heart rate variability, constitutes an important index of self-regulatory autonomic and behavioral responsiveness of the neonate, and that the measure is associated with dimensions of temperament: reactivity, self-regulation and expressivity *(100)*.

Given the topic of the current chapter, the study of Izard et al. *(100)* is important because they found that heart rate variability was higher in insecurely attached infants than in securely attached infants. Although it would be premature to suggest that insecure attachment is a precursor of ADHD *(101)*, the similarities in cardiovascular findings suggest that the midfrequency band may be seen as a promising measure in longitudinal research. The measure really awaits application in longitudinal research on well-known risk factors involving caretakers, such as alcoholism and depression, but also on less-recognized factors, such as maternal rigidity. For instance, Butcher et al. *(102)* showed that maternal rigidity, measured in the first year of preterm children, was strongly associated with children's mental performance at 7.5 yr of age. It was concluded that rigidity limits the mother's ability to adapt her parenting behavior to her child's needs. It is well-recognized that children born preterm, like children with ADHD, are less predictable and less readable than their full-term age mates.

11. STATE REGULATION AND THE CHILD'S ENVIRONMENT

It is well-recognized that the behavior of children with ADHD may drive parents, teachers, and peers into despair. What is particularly puzzling for the child's environment is the variability of behavior: some situations elicit normal behavior, whereas others don't. What might be even more irritating is the fact that a particular situation has never been a problem for the child in the past, but now it suddenly is. The concept of (poor) state regulation might provide caretakers a framework for understanding these sudden changes in behavior.

For parents it would be important to know that ethological observations of children with ADHD during social interaction with a nonfamiliar adult (e.g., a student) indicated that these children act on their environment in order to trigger verbal and nonverbal temporal stimulation, i.e., structure providing behavior to enhance their nonoptimal state *(103)*. What makes these findings so interesting is that it took the children only a few minutes to trigger these structure-providing behaviors in the student who had no established emotional relationship with the child. In fact, the student was unaware of the purpose of the study. In view of this, it is easy to imagine that the task of parenting a child with ADHD is much more demanding and time-intensive than parenting a child without the disorder. In the context of stimulation-seeking behavior the studies of Antrop et al. *(104, 105)* are of importance. Here children with ADHD and a control group were observed during a waiting period of 15 min. The results indicated that children with ADHD showed a greater decline in behavior in the presence of stimulation of touching objects and movement of trunk, and that those who underestimated the time of the waiting period were more apt to seek additional stimulation than those who overestimated the waiting period.

For teachers it may be instructive to know that ethological studies of gaze behavior during a reaction-time test indicated that children with ADHD were looking away from the stimulus source (i.e., a TV screen) about 60 times every 4 min. However, a microanalysis of their visual behavior indicated that they timed their looking-away behavior strategically—that is, they looked away from the monitor only in the interval between two successive trials *(106,107)*. It was concluded that children's gazing behavior, rather than constituting inattentive and inappropriate behavior, was an attempt to increase their activation state in order to fulfill the test requirements. This conclusion comes close to claims made by Palm et al. *(52)* and Weinberg and Harper *(53)*, who suggested that the excessive motor activity of children with ADHD could be a strategy to stay awake and alert. In fact, in terms of Hockey's model of state control these behaviors may be seen an example of actions oriented toward direct control of the environmental influences on the individual's actual state.

12. CONCLUSION

The idea that motivation is an important mediator in the behavioral problems in many children with ADHD is not new *(108–111)*. The same holds for the nonoptimal arousal concept in ADHD *(112,113)*. However, much of the research so far has been primarily task-driven rather than theory-driven, and the concepts of motivation and arousal were loosely defined and used interchangeably. In order to overcome these shortcomings, the aim of this chapter was to redefine the concepts along the lines of Sanders' and Hockey's model of state regulation. We concluded that ADHD is associated with poor state regulation with the LC and especially the NA as important structures. The tonic firing rate of the cardiac vagal motor neurons located at the NA is described by Porges *(67,114)* as the smart vagus because of its association with attention, motion, emotion, and communication.

The author is aware that there are many competing hypotheses on the brain areas involved in ADHD. One is the frontal lobe hypothesis, suggesting that ADHD is the result of a general disorganization in behavior linked to problems of inhibition that are mediated by a genetically based abnormality in the functioning of the frontal structures responsible for so-called executive functions *(115)*. And indeed, there are well-documented changes in the structure and function of the right frontal cortex in ADHD *(116)*. However, multiple studies did not unequivocally support such dysfunctions, neither behaviorally nor electrophysiologically *(117)*.

The hypothesis that ADHD is associated with brainstem injury has rarely been considered because the brain stem (on a simplistic level) is associated by many neurobiologists with basic functions, such as breathing, eating, balance, motor coordination, and so forth, whereas many of the characteristics of ADHD, such as poor attention and poor impulse control, are believed to be controlled by higher-level regions of the brain. Because empirical evidence is emerging that attention and impulse control abilities in children with ADHD are closely related to their activation state, we hope that future neurobiological research will concentrate more on basic functions than is the case today. Such research may drastically change the way the disorder is conceptualized. We must not forget that the postulated brain stem involvement is far from incompatible with the postulated dopaminergic hypothesis in ADHD *(117)*, given that the LC is one of the most important noradrenergic structures of the brain *(33)*. In addition, in the Sander's model of state regulation and energy allocation, the term "energy" was merely used as a metaphor and was not intended to refer to physical energy. However, evidence is growing that on a local level, the regional blood flow and glucose consumption of the brain appear to depend on neuronal structures involved in mental activities related to the earlier discussed cognitive paradigms of Sternberg, Shiffrin and Schneider, and Sanders

(118). From this perspective, it is hypothesized that at least some form of ADHD may be viewed as cortical, energy-deficit syndromes secondary to catecholamine-mediated hypofunctionality of astrocyte glucose and glycogen metabolism, which provides activity-dependent energy to cortical neurons *(119)*.

Besides evaluating the psychophysiological and neural circuitry, an attempt has been made to place the concept of poor state control in a social context. We would like to emphasize that the study of the midfrequency band has demonstrated that it constitutes a useful parameter for studying emotional processes and temperament *(120)*. As such the midfrequency band may hopefully also provide an essential tool for studying another hallmark characteristic of the disorder, i.e., the social skill deficits observed in many of these children, most dramatically expressed by their disturbed peer relations. Reasoning along these lines, we must never forget the outcome of the classic follow-up study of Cowen et al. *(121)* showing that negative nominations by third-grade classmates was, relative to teacher ratings and psychometric results, by far the best predictor of later psychiatric problems.

REFERENCES

1. Lecendreux M, Konofal E, Bouvard M, Falissard B, Mouren-Simeoni M.Ch. Sleep and alertness in children with ADHD. J Child Psychol Psychiatry 2000;41:803–812.
2. Kuntsi J, Stevenson J. Psychological mechanisms in hyperactivity: II. Mediators of genetic effects. J Child Psychol Psychiatry 2001;42:211–219.
3. Swanson J, Oosterlaan J, Murias M, Schuck S, Flodman P, Spence A, et al. Attention deficit/hyperactivity disorder children with a 7-repeat allele of the dopamine receptor D4 gene have extreme behavior but normal performance on critical neuropsychological tests of attention. Proc Nat Acad Sci 2000;9:4754–4759.
4. Sanders AF. Elements of human performance: reaction processes and attention in human skills. London: Lawrence Erlbaum, 1998.
5. Cannon. Bodily changes in pain, hunger, fear and rage. New York; Appleton-Century-Crofts, 1986 (originally published in 1915).
6. Freeman GL. The energetics of human behavior. Ithaca, NY: Cornell University Press, 1948.
7. Duffy E. Emotions: an example of the need for reorientation in psychology. Psychol Rev, 1934; 41:184–198.
8. Duffy E. An explanation of 'emotional' phenomena without the use of the concept 'emotion.' J Gen Psychol, 1941;25:283–293.
9. Duffy E. The concept of energy mobilization. Psychol Rev, 1951;58:30–40.
10. Duffy EA. Activation and behavior. New York: Wiley, 1962;3–29.
11. Hockey GRJ, Coles MGH, Gaillard AWK. Energetical issues in research on human information processing. In: Hockey GRJ, Gaillard AWK, Coles MGH eds. Energetics and human information processing. Dordrecht, The Netherlands: Martinus Nijhoff, 1986.
12. Sanders AF. Towards a model of stress and human performance. Acta Psychologica 1983;53:61–97.
13. Gopher D, Sanders AF. S-Oh-R: Oh stages! Oh resources! In: Prinz W, Sanders AF eds. Cognition and motor behavior, Heidelberg: Springer Verlag, 1984;231–253.
14. Gopher D. In defence of resources: on structure, energies, pools and the allocation of attention. In: Hockey GRJ, Gaillard AWK, Coles MGH eds. Energetics and human information processing. Dordrecht: The Netherlands, 1986;353–372.
15. Pribram KH, McGuinness D. Arousal, activation and effort in the control of attention. Psychol Rev 1975;82:116–149.
16. Shiffrin RM, Schneider W. Controlled and automatic human information processing: Perceptual learning, automatic attending, and a general theory. Psychol Rev 1977;84:127–190.

17. Schneider W, Shiffrin, RM. Controlled and automatic human information processing: Detection, search and attention. Psychol Rev 1977;84:1–66.
18. Sternberg S. Discovery of processing stages; extensions of Donders' method. In: WG. Koster ed. Attention and performance, Amsterdam; North Holland 1969:2:276–315.
19. McGuinness D, Pribram K. The neuropsychology of attention: emotional and motivational controls. In: Wittrock MC ed. The brain and psychology. New York: Academic Press, 1980;95–140.
20. Damasio AR. Decartes error. emotion, reason, and the human brain. New York: Avon Books, 1994.
21. LeDoux JE. The emotional brain: the mysterious underpinnings of emotional life. New York: Simon & Schuster, 1996.
22. Robbins TW. Arousal and attention: psychopharmacological and neuropsychological studies in experimental animals. In: Parasuraman R ed. The attentive brain. Cambridge MA: MIT Press, 1998;189–219.
23. Malmo RB. Activation : a neurophysiological dimension. Psychol Rev 1959;66:367–386.
24. Broadbent DR. Decision and stress. London: Academic Press, 1971.
25. Kahneman D. Attention and effort. Englewood Cliffs, NJ: Prentice-Hall, 1973.
26. Hockey GR. Compensatory control in the regulation of human performance under stress and high workload: a cognitive energetical framework. Biol Psychol, 1997;45:73–93.
27. Sanders FA, Hoogeboom W. On the effects of continuous active work on performance. Acta Psychologica 1970;33:414–431.
28. Leth-Steensen C, King Elbaz Z, Douglas VI. Mean reaction times, variability, and skew in the responding of ADHD children: a response time distributional approach. Acta Psychologica 2000;104:167–190.
29. Posner MJ. Chronometric explorations of mind: the third Paul M. Fitts lectures. Hillsdale, NJ: Lawrence Erlbaum, 1978.
30. Posner MJ, Peterson SE. The attention system and the human brain. Ann Rev Neurosci 1991;13:25–42.
31. Posner MJ, Raichle ME. Networks of attention. In: Posner M, Raichle M, eds. Images of the mind. New York: Scientific American Library, 1994;153–179.
32. Posner MJ, Rothbart MK. Attentional mechanisms and conscious experience. In: Milner AD, Rugg MD eds. The neuropsychology of consciousness, London: Academic Press, 1991;91–112.
33. Posner MJ. Interaction of arousal and selection in the posterior attentional network. In: Baddely A, Weiskrantz L, eds. Attention, awareness and control. A tribute to Donald Broadbent. New York; Oxford University Press, 1993;390–405.
34. Van der Meere JJ. The role of attention. In: Sandberg S, ed. Monographs on child and adolescent psychiatry. Hyperactivity disorders. Second edition. Cambridge: Cambridge University Press. 2002;162–213.
35. Sergeant JA, van der Meere JJ. The diagnostic significance for ADD(H) classification, a future DSM. In: Sagvolden T, Borggrevink HM, Archer T. eds. Attention deficit disorder and hyperkinetic syndrome. New York: Lawrence Erlbaum, 1989;149–163.
36. Sergeant JA, van der Meere JJ. Convergence of approaches in localizing the hyperactivity deficit. In Lahey BB, Kazdin AE, eds. Advances in clinical child psychology. New York: Plenum Press, 1990a;207–246.
37. Sergeant JA, van der Meere JJ. Additive factor method applied to psychopathology with special reference to childhood hyperactivity. Acta Psychologica 1990;74:277–296.
38. Sergeant JA, van der Meere JJ. Towards an empirical child psychopathology. In: Routh DK ed. Disruptive behaviour disorders in childhood, New York: Plenum Press, 1994;59–78.
39. Sergeant JA, van der Meere JJ. Ritalin: an energetical factor? In: Greenhill LL, Osman BB eds, Ritalin. Theory and practice, New York: Mary Ann Liebert, 1999;321–340.
40. Van der Meere JJ, Gunning B, Stemerdink N. The effect of presentation rate on task performance in ADHD children with and without tics. J Percept Motor Skills, 1995;81:259–262.

41. Van der Meere JJ, Stemerdink BA. The development of state regulation in normal children: an indirect comparison with ADHD. Dev Neuropsychol 1999;16:213–225.
42. Potgieter S, Borger N, van der Meere JJ, de Cock P. Motor inhibition in very low birth weight children associated with ADHD. Dev Med Child Neurol 2000;42:17–18.
43. Raymaekers R, van der Meere J, Roeyers H. Event rate manipulation and its effect on arousal modulation and response inhibition in adults with high functioning autism. J Clin Exp Neuropsychol 2004;26:74–82.
44. Stemerdink BA, van der Meere JJ, van der Molen MW, Kalverboer AF, Hendrikx MMH, Huisman J, et al. Information processing in patients with early and continuously-treated phenylketonuria. Eur J Pedia 1995;154:739–746.
45. Van der Meere JJ, Vreeling HJ, Sergeant JA. A motor presetting experiment in hyperactive, learning disabled and control children. J Child Psychol Psychiatry 1992;33:1347–1354.
46. Van der Meer D-J, van der Meere JJ. Response inhibition in children with conduct disorder and borderline intellectual functioning. Child Neuropsychol (in press).
47. Sheres, Oosterlaan Sergeant. Response execution and inhibition in children with AD/HD and other disruptive disorders: The role of behavioural activation. J Child Psychol Psychiatry, 2001;42:347–357.
48. Purvis KL, Tannock R. Phonological processing, not inhibitory control differentiates ADHD and reading disability. J Am Acad Child Adolesc Psychiatry 2000;4:485–494.
49. Walker AJ, Shores EA, Trollor JN, Lee T, Sachdev PS. Neuropsychological functioning of adults with attention deficit hyperactivity disorder. Clin Neuropsychol 2000;22:115–24.
50. Sonuga-Barke EJS. Interval length and time-use by children with ADHD: a comparison of four models. J Abnorm Child Psychol 2003;44:257–264.
51. Van der Meere JJ, Marzocchi GM, de Meo T. Response inhibition and attention deficit hyperactivity disorder with and without oppositional defiant disorder screened from a community sample. Dev Neuropsychol (submitted).
52. Palm L, Persson E, Bjerre I, Elmqvist D. Sleep and wakefulness in preadolescent children with deficits in attention, motor control and perception. Acta Paediatrica 1992;81:618–624.
53. Weinberg WA, Harper CR. Vigilance and its disorders. Neurol Clin 1993;11:59–78.
54. Alberts E. Facial behavior in children: tension and attention during the performance of a task. In: Kalverboer AF, ed. Developmental biopsychology: experimental and observational studies in groups "at risk". Ann Arbor: University of Michigan Press, 1990;69–93.
55. Borger NA, van der Meere JJ. Motor control and state regulation in children with ADHD: a cardiac response study. Special issue: Biol Psychol 2000;51:247–267.
56. Mulder G. The concept and measurement of mental effort. In: Hockey GRJ, Gaillard AK, Coles MGH, eds. Energetics and human information processing. Martinus Nijhoff Publishers. NATO ASI Series 1986;175–198.
57. Mulder LJM, Veldman JBP, Elgersma AF, Mulder G, van Roon A. Respiratory pattern, invested effort, and variability in heart rate and blood pressure during the performance of mental tasks. In: Di Rienzo M, Mancia G, Parati G, Pedotti A, Zanchetti A, eds. Computer analysis of cardiovascular signals, Amsterdam: IOS Press, 1995;219–33.
58. Veldman JBP, Gaillard AWK. Physiological workload reactions to increasing levels of task difficulty. Ergonomics 1998;41:656–669.
59. Althaus M, Mulder LJM, Mulder G, van Roon AM, Mindraa RB. Influence of respiratory activity on the cardiac response pattern to mental effort. Psychophysiol 1998;35:420–430.
60. Borger NA, Wiersma RJ, van der Meere JJ. 0.10 hz heart rate variability component and sustained attention (Abstract). J Psychophysiol 2000;14:260–261.
61. Borger N, van der Meere JJ, Ronner A, Alberts E, Geuze R, Bogte H. Heart rate variability and sustained attention in ADHD children. J Abnorm Child Psychol 1999;27:25–33.
62. Althaus M, Mulder LJM, Mulder G, Aarnoudse CC, Mindraa RB. Cardiac adaptivity to attention-demanding tasks in children with a pervasive developmental disorder not otherwise specified (PDD-NOS). Biol Psychiatry 1999;46:799–809.

63. Wiersema RJ, Van der Meere JJ, Roeyers H, Van Coster R, Bayens D. State regulation, error processing and event-related potentials in ADHD. (submitted).
64. Wiersema RJ, Van der Meere JJ, & Roeyers H. Development of state regulation and error processing: an ERP study. (submitted).
65. Aston-Jones G, Rajkowski J, Cohen J. Role of locus coeruleus in attention and behavioral flexibility. Biol Psychiatry 1999;46:1309–1320.
66. Berridge CW. Arousal and attention related actions of the locus coeruleus-noradenergic system: potential target in the therapeutic actions of amphetamine-like stimulants. In: Solanto MV, Arnsten AFT, Castellanos FX, eds. Stimulant drugs and ADHD: basic and clinical neuroscience. New York: Oxford University Press 2000;158–184.
67. Porges SW. Orienting in a defensive world: Mammalian modifications of our evolutionary heritage: a polyvagal theory. Psychophysiol 1995;32:301–318.
68. Van der Meere JJ, Borger NA. Sustained attention, heart rate variability and facial expressions in children with ADHD. (submitted).
69. Ekman P, Friesen WV. Manual for the Facial Action Coding System. Palo Alto, CA: Consulting Psychologists Press, 1978.
70. Rechlin T. Decreased parameters of heart rate variability in amitriptyline treated patients: Lower parameters in melancholic depression than in neurotic depression—a biological marker? Biol Psychiatry 1994;36:705–707.
71. Friedman BH, Thayer JF. Autonomic balance revisited: panic anxiety and heart rate variability. J Psychosomatic Res 1998;44:133–151.
72. Mezzacappa E, Steingard R, Kindlon D, Saul JP, Earls F. Tricyclic antidepressants and cardiac autonomic control in children and adolescents. J Am Child Adoles Acad Psychiatry 1998;37:52–59.
73. Malaspina D, Bruder G, Dalack GW, Storer S, van Kammen M, Amador X, et al. Diminished cardiac vagal tone in schizophrenia: associations to brain laterality and age of onset. Biol Psychiatry 1997;42:612–617.
74. Angelink MW, Malessa R, Kamcili W, Zeit T, Lemmer W, Bertling R, Lieser E. Cardiovascular autonomic reactivity in schizophrenics under neuroleptic treatment: A potential predictor of short-term outcome? Neuropsychobiology 1998;38:19–24.
75. Rodier PM. Converging evidence for brain injury in autism. Dev Psychopathol 2002;14:537–557.
76. Garretson HB, Fein D, Waterhouse L. Sustained attention in children with autism. J Autism Dev Disord 1990;20:101–114.
77. Sergeant JA, Geurts H, Oosterlaan J. How specific is a deficit of executive functioning for attention deficit hyperactivity disorder? Behav Brain Res 2002;130:3–28.
78. Rapport MD, Loo S, Denney C. The paired associate learning task: is it an externally valid instrument for assessing methylphenidate response in children with attention deficit disorder. J Psychopathol Behav Assess 1995;17:125–144.
79. Van der Meere JJ, Shalev RS, Borger NA, Gross-Tsur V. Sustained attention, activation and MPH in ADHD. A research note. J Child Psychol Psychiatry 1995;36:697–703.
80. Gross-Tsur V, Manor O, Van der Meere JJ, Joseph A, Shalev R. Epilepsy and ADHD: is methylphenidate safe and effective? J Pediatr 1997;130:40–44.
81. Van der Meere JJ, Gunning B, Stemerdink BA. The effect of methylphenidate and clonidine on state regulation in ADHD children. J Abnorm Child Psychol 1999;40:291–298.
82. Van der Meere JJ, Shalev R. MPH, state regulation and the cardiac response. (submitted).
83. Kinsbourne M. Testing models for attention deficit hyperactivity disorder in the behavioral laboratory. In: Conners K, Kinsbourne M, eds. Attention deficit hyperactivity disorder. Medizin Verlag GmbH, Munchen, 1990;51–69.
84. Bergman A,Winters L, Cornblatt B. Methylphenidate: effects on sustained attention. In: Greenhill LL, Osman BB, eds. Ritalin, theory and patient management. New York: Mary Ann Liebert Publishers, 1991;223–232.

85. Sonuga-Barke EJS, Taylor E, Sembi S, Smith J. The effects of delay of choice. J Child Psychol Psychiatry 1992;33:387–398.
86. Sonuga-Barke EJS, Houlberg K, Hall M. When is impulsiveness not impulsive: the case of hyperactive children's cognitive style. J Child Psychol Psychiatry 1994;35:1247–53.
87. Solanto MV. The effects of reinforcement and response-cost on a delayed response task in children with attention deficit hyperactivity disorder: a research note. J Child Psychol Psychiatry, 1990;31:803–808.
88. Oosterlaan J, Sergeant J. Effects of reward and response cost on response inhibition in ADHD, disruptive, anxious, and normal children. J Abnorm Child Psychol 1998;26:161–174.
89. Slusarek M, Velling S, Bunk D, Eggers C. Motivational effects on inhibitory control in children with ADHD. J Am Acad Child Adolesc Psychiatry 2001;40:355–363.
90. Van der Meere JJ, Hughes KA, Borger NA, Sallee FR. The effect of reward on sustained attention in ADHD children with and without CD. In: Sergeant JA, ed. Eunethydis. Trumpi Partner, Zurich, Switzerland: 1995;241–253.
91. Lahey BB, Loeber R. Framework for a developmental model of oppositional defiant disorder and conduct disorder. In: Routh DK, ed. Disruptive behavior disorders in childhood. New York: Plenum Press, 1994;139–180.
92. Zajonc RB. Social facilitation. Science 1965;149:269–274.
93. Duval S, Wicklund RA. A theory of objective self-awareness. New York: Academic Press, 1972.
94. Wicklund RA. Objective self-awareness. In: Berkowitz L, ed. Advances in experimental social psychology, New York: Academic Press, 1975;8:233–277.
95. Pruyn ATH, Aasman J, Wijers B. Social influences on mental processes and cardiovascular activity. In: Orlebeke JF, Mulder G, van Doornen LJP, eds. The psychophysiology of cardiovascular Control. New York: Plenum Press, 1985;365–377.
96. Sandberg S. Pscyhosocial contributions. In: Sandberg S, ed. Hyperactivity and attention disorders of childhood. Cambridge: Cambridge University Press, 2002:367–416.
97. Wolff PH. The causes, controls and organization of behavior in neonates. Psychological Issues, 5, (No. 1, Monograph 17), 1966.
98. Prechtl HFR. The optimality concept. Early Hum Dev 1980;4:201–203.
99. Porges SW. Vagal tone: an autonomic mediator of affect. In: Garber J, Dodge A, eds. The development of emotion regulation and dysregulation. Cambridge: Cambridge University Press, 1991;111–128.
100. Izard CE, Porges SW, Simons RF, Haynes OM, Hyde C, Parisi M, Cohen B. Infant cardiac activity: Developmental changes and relations with attachment. Dev Psychol 1991;27:432–439.
101. Glazer D. Child abuse and neglect and the brain: a review. J Child Psychol Psychiatry 2000;41: 97–116.
102. Butcher PhR, Wijnberg-Williams BJ, Hegemann M, Stremmelaar EF, Schoemaker MM, van der Meere JJ, Bambang Oetomo S. Maternal rigidity is associated with level of intelligence in preterms at school age. Child Psychiatry Hum Dev (in press).
103. Stroes A, Alberts E, van der Meere JJ. Children with ADHD in social interaction with a non-familiar adult: and observational study. J Am Acad Child Adolesc Psychiatry 2003;42:295–302.
104. Antrop I, Roeyers H, van Oost P, Buysse A. Stimulus seeking and hyperactivity in children with ADHD. J Child Psychol Psychiatry 2000;41:225–231.
105. Antrop I, Buysse A, Roeyers H, van Oost P. Stimulus seeking and hyperactive behavior in children with ADHD: a reanalysis. Percept Motor Skills, 2002;95:71–90.
106. Alberts E, van der Meere, JJ. Observations of hyperactive behaviour during vigilance. J Child Psychol Psychiatry 1992;33:1355–1364.
107. Borger NA, van der Meere JJ. Visual behaviour of ADHD children during an attention test: An almost forgotten variable. J Child Psychol Psychiatry 2000;41:525–532.
108. Douglas VI, Peters KG. Toward a clear definition of the attentional deficit of hyperactive children. In: Hale GA, Lewis M, eds. Attention and the development of cognitive skills, New York: Plenum Press, 1979;173–248.

109. Rosenthal RH, Allen TW. An examination of attention, arousal, and learning dysfunction of hyperkinetic children. Psychol Bull 1978;85:689–715.
110. Routh DK. Hyperactivity. In: Magrab P, ed. Psychological management of pediatric problems, Baltimore, MD: University Park Press, 1978:3–48.
111. Sroufe LA. Drug treatment of children with behavioral problems. In Horowitz F, ed. Review of child developmental research, Chicago: University of Chicago Press, 1975;4:347–408.
112. Zenthall SS, Zenthall TR. Optimal stimulation: a model of disordered activity and performance in normal and deviant children. Psychol Bull 1983;94:446–471.
113. Douglas VI. Attentional and cognitive problems. In: Rutter M, ed. Developmental neuropsychiatry. New York; Guilford Press, 1983;280–328.
114. Porges SW. Orienting in a defense world. Mammalian modifications of an evolutionary heritage: a polyvagal theory. Psychophysiology, 1995;32:301–318.
115. Denckla MB. A theory and model of executive function. A neuropsychological perspective. In: Lyon GR, Krasnegor NA, eds. Attention, memory and executive function. Baltimore, MD: Brooks. 1996;263–178.
116. Oades RD. Frontal, temporal and lateralized brain function in childrern with attention defcit hyperactivity disorder (ADHD): a psychophysiological and neuropsychological viewpoint on development. Behav Brain Res 1998;94:83–95.
117. Sagvolden T, Sergeant JA. Special Issue. Attention deficit hyperactivity disorder. Behav Brain Research 1998;94:1–224.
118. Mulder G, Wijers AA, Lange JJ, Buijink BM, Mulder LJM, Willemsen ATM, Paans AMJ. The role of neuroimaging in the discovery of processing stages: a review. Acta Psychologica 1995;90:63–79.
119. Todd RT, Botteron KN. Is attention-deficit/hyperactivity disorder an energy deficiency syndrome? Biol Psychiatry 2001;50:151–158.
120. Thayer JF, Lane RD. A model of neurovisceral integration in emotion regulation and dysregulation. J Affective Dis 2002;61:201–216.
121. Cowen EL, Pederson A, Babigian H, Izzo LD, Trost MA. Long term follow-up of early detected vulnerable children. J Consult Clin Psychol 1973;41:438–446.

19

Sleep and Attention Deficit Hyperactivity Disorder

Louise M. O'Brien and David Gozal

1. INTRODUCTION

A growing number of studies have addressed the prevalence of sleep problems among children with attention deficit hyperactivity disorder (ADHD). As the major symptoms of ADHD (i.e., inattention, impulsiveness, and restlessness) are also characteristic of sleep deprivation, the role of sleep in ADHD is the focus of many investigations. Parental reports of sleep disturbances are common in children with ADHD *(1–8)*, and as such they were so widely presumed to be an intrinsic part of the clinical phenotype of ADHD that sleep problems were included as one of the previous *Diagnostic and Statistical Manual of Mental Disorders*, 3rd edition (DSM-III) diagnostic criteria for ADHD *(9)*. However, none of the more recent diagnostic manuals *(10,11)* have included sleep disturbance as a symptomatic criterion for ADHD. Therefore, because parental perception of sleep disturbance helped to define ADHD previously, it is not surprising that studies using earlier diagnostic criteria found a significant association between ADHD and sleep problems.

Sleep arousal disturbances include difficulties in falling asleep, in awakening, and in maintaining adequate alertness for daily activities; such disturbances are frequently reported in children with ADHD. Sleep difficulties have generally been attributed to core difficulties in regulation of arousal. Difficulty in staying alert when not engaged in stimulating activity is commonly reported by children with ADHD, particularly ADHD of the inattentive type. Alertness difficulties are reported even when sufficient sleep has been obtained the night before, and many individuals with ADHD become aware that they have to keep moving around or changing activities in order to maintain wakefulness. Conversely and as a frequently reported phenomenon, a sudden improvement in alertness will occur when children with ADHD start moving around. In such cases, the report is not that they do feel fatigued, as would be anticipated if they had not slept enough, but rather it is perceived as an inability to maintain a sufficient level of alertness or arousal unless engaged in stimulating activities. Such descriptions have occasionally led to the mislabeling of such individuals as having narcolepsy. Conversely, Navelet et al. *(12)* and Dahl et al. *(13)* have reported that some children with narcolepsy were misdiagnosed as having ADHD. Thus, there seems to be a logical association between the physiology of sleep and the presence of sleep disorders in ADHD, as sleep is an autonomically governed process reflecting cyclical changes in brain arousal *(14)*, while ADHD may result from irregular arousal functioning *(15)*. In 1996, Dahl inferred that the prefrontal cortex may have a critical role in integrative regulation of arousal, sleep,

From: *Attention Deficit Hyperactivity Disorder: From Genes to Patients*
Edited by: D. Gozal and D. L. Molfese © Humana Press Inc., Totowa, NJ

affect, and attention *(16)*. Indeed, previous neuroimaging studies of regional brain glucose consumption in adult subjects with childhood-onset ADHD documented relatively hypoactive cortical functioning in the frontal lobes concurrent with decreased alertness *(17)*. Similarly, positive associations between physiological indices of arousal obtained during the day and a history of sleep disturbance were reported in a study of children with ADHD *(18)*.

In addition to the potential implications of the putative mechanisms underlying wakefulness and alertness in the context of behavior, attention, and executive function, objective assessment of sleep problems in ADHD may be particularly important because objective disturbances of sleep, such as sleep disordered breathing (SDB) *(2,19–23)*, narcolepsy *(24)*, and periodic limb movement disorder of sleep (PLMS) *(25–29)* may all present daytime behavioral symptoms that resemble ADHD.

Therefore, in this chapter, we will review the literature pertaining to the subjectively reported and objectively documented sleep characteristics in children with ADHD and conversely examine the effects of specific sleep disorders on behavior and cognition.

2. SUBJECTIVE MEASURES OF SLEEP DISTURBANCE IN ADHD

The majority of studies investigating the relationships between sleep and ADHD are based on parental reports, and as such are not only markedly subjective, but also convey the inherent bias derived from the interpretation by the parent of their child's manifestations. Notwithstanding such major limitations in all these studies, the consistent conclusion from such studies indicates a high prevalence of sleep complaints among children with ADHD compared with control children *(1,3,5,7,8,30,31)*. Such sleep complaints are manifest as increased bedtime resistance *(7,8)*, difficulty in falling asleep *(1,5,7,8)*, more frequent nighttime awakenings *(1,7)*, and the presence of sleep-related anxiety *(3,7)*, and are commonly reported not only by the parents but also by the ADHD patients themselves. In fact, a relatively recent comprehensive review of the literature *(4)* revealed that parents of children with ADHD were five times as likely to report that their children have sleep problems compared with parents of healthy children. Often, the child is unwilling to go to bed at night but will also object to taking a nap even when clearly exhausted during daytime. Nonetheless, the inability of children with ADHD to fall asleep either during the day or during the evening hours may reflect a multitude of underlying issues. For example, the absence of a consistent bedtime routine is usually a frequent impediment to regular sleep latencies in healthy children, and the inability to implement this behavioral pattern before sleep may clearly and adversely affect the period between bedtime as imposed by the parents and the actual sleep onset. Another likely and frequent scenario is the occurrence of oppositional behaviors rather than a physiological alteration in the sleep-wake regulatory mechanisms during the evening hours. Intrinsic issues to the child that may generate difficulty in the onset of sleep include amplification of underlying processes, such as anxiety, which may be linked to fear of separation or of darkness. In addition, disruption of sleep itself through recurring nightmares may trigger an anticipatory objection to the bedtime routine. Therefore, all of these and many other confounding factors make it very difficult to determine the exact nature of the true relationships between ADHD and sleep initiation. A summary of subjective assessments of sleep disturbance in ADHD is shown in Table 1.

Using the revised DSM-III manual (DSM-III-R) *(10)* to minimize subject selection bias, Ball and colleagues *(3)* studied 102 children who met criteria for ADHD and 78 control children. The control group comprised children who had been referred to neuropsychology assessment

Table 1
Subjective Assessments of Relationship Between Sleep and ADHD

Ref.	Authors	Year	Subjects	Age	Diagnosis of ADHD	Control sample	Sleep assessment	Results
1	Kaplan et al.	1987	1. 40 ADHD (non-medicated)	3–6 yr	Pediatrician	1. 40 children from local day care centers	1. Two sleep questions	1. 60% ADHD reported inadequate amount of sleep compared to 25% controls
			2. 116 ADHD (non-medicated)	3–6 yr	Parent report plus DSM-III criteria	2. 88 males from local day care centers	2. Four sleep questions	2. Mean scores significantly higher in ADHD for all four questions
2	Trommer et al.	1988	36 ADHD; 12 ADD	9.3 ± 4 yr	Not reported	30 controls	Questionnaires	ADHD/ADD report more sleep disturbance
3	Ball et al.	1997	102 ADHD (28 with stimulant medication at time of test)	9 ± 3 yr	Parent report and formal psychological assessment	78 children referred for assessment; did not meet criteria for ADHD	Retrospective review of parent responses to sleep questions	ADHD more likely to report "problems with sleep;" "often up at night;" and "insists on night light"
32	Dagan et al.	1997	12 ADHD males	9.6 ± 1.6 yr	Psychiatric assessment	12 healthy males	Sleep–wake schedule, semi-structured interview, and sleep habits questionnaires	No differences observed between the two groups

(Continued)

Table 1
(Continued)

Ref.	Authors	Year	Subjects	Age	Diagnosis of ADHD	Control sample	Sleep assessment	Results
33	Marcotte et al.	1998	43 ADHD 11 learning disorder 25 ADHD/LD	6–12 yr	Neuropsychological and neurological assessment with DSM-III criteria	86 children from the local community	Sleep Screening Questionnaire for Parents	No differences between subgroups ADHD, LD, ADHD/LD. Total sample scored higher on Breathing Problems Scale, Sleepiness Scale, and Behavioral Scale than controls
5	Ring et al.	1998	13 ADHD; Methylphenidate for >4 wk	8 ± 3 yr	Interview by child psychiatrist	Healthy siblings of the children with ADHD	Structured sleep questionnaire	ADHD reported more difficulties with sleep initiation and maintenance
34	Corkum et al.	1999	79 unmedicated ADHD; 22 medicated ADHD	6–12 yr	Clinical diagnostic interviews	36 children from the community	Child Sleep Questionnaire—Parent Version; Child and Family Sleep History Questionnaire	Unmedicated ADHD had longer sleep duration than other groups; both ADHD groups had poorer sleep practices than controls; dyssomnias related to comorbid diagnoses and stimulant medication

7	Owens et al.	2000	46 ADHD (nonmedicated)	7.5 ± 1.5 yr	Formal psychological assessment	46 matched children from elementary school	Children's Sleep Habits Questionnaire and the Sleep Self-report questionnaire	ADHD reported higher scores on both questionnaires
8	Corkum et al.	2001	25 ADHD (medication naïve)	9.1 ± 1.4 yr	Formal psychological assessment	25 children from the community	Child Sleep Questionnaire	ADHD reported higher scores on five of six parameters
35	O'Brien et al.	2003	44 ADHD; 27 hyperactive	5–7 yr	Conners' Parent Rating Scale	39 controls	Sleep habits questionnaire	ADHD reported significantly more difficulty initiating sleep, restless sleep, awakenings, bruxism, enuresis, snoring, and daytime sleepiness than controls and were less willing to go to bed. Hyperactive children reported more difficulty initiating sleep and enuresis than controls

LD, learning disability.

center for evaluation but who did not fulfill criteria for ADHD. A retrospective review of sleep-related items from the Conners Parent Rating Scale *(36)* and the Personality Inventory for Children—Revised *(7)* was conducted. The authors found that significantly more parents of the children with ADHD answered positively to the general question from the Conners scale "problems with sleep," and also to the more specific question "often up at night" from the Personality Inventory. These results supported those of Kaplan et al. *(1)* who found that parents of children diagnosed with ADHD by their pediatricians were more likely to be perceived as obtaining an inadequate amount of sleep when compared to children without any reported behavior problems who were recruited from local day care centers. However, in the study by Kaplan et al., the authors acknowledged that the children with a diagnosis of ADHD may represent a unique subgroup of children who were taken to a physician for treatment. Therefore, these investigators conducted a second phase of this study, wherein they recruited children from local day care centers who were believed to be more active or more inattentive than normal and compared this group with a control group of children with no reported behavioral problems. All of the children with reported behavioral disturbances and none of the control children met DSM-III criteria for ADHD *(9)*. Parents answered the following four questions regarding their child's sleep:

1. Difficulty falling asleep.
2. Wakes during the night.
3. Wakes early.
4. Cries out during the night.

Highly significant differences were observed for each of the four questions between the children with ADHD and the controls. Nonetheless, Kaplan et al. suggested the possibility that parents of children who are unusually active may be more sensitive to their sleep problems. In a third and last phase of their study they attempted to address this issue by obtaining daily logs of sleep habits for three consecutive weeks. Information recorded included bedtime, sleep time, number of times the child got out of bed both before falling asleep and following any awakenings, enuresis, night sweats, sleep duration and time out of bed in the morning. This third phase showed that children with ADHD had significantly shorter nap durations, longer sleep time, more awakenings during the night, more bed-wetting episodes, and more night sweats than control children. Taken together, these data further support the relationship between ADHD and sleep disturbance, even when some objective measures are introduced. However, although one of the strengths of the study by Kaplan et al. was the attempt to record objective sleep measurements, sleep diaries are still highly prone to reporting biases because they are reliant on parental report. For example, if parents of children with ADHD are more sensitive and more acutely aware to their child's sleep disturbance, they may be less able to sleep at night, may be more likely to wake up during otherwise insignificant and physiological awakenings, and therefore will be more likely to be aware of their child's behaviors and to report them in the diaries.

3. OBJECTIVE ASSESSMENT OF SLEEP IN CHILDREN WITH ADHD

To prevent the potential problems imposed by parental reporting, objective measures of sleep disturbance were necessary. Several investigators have utilized actigraphs—i.e., small watchlike accelerometer recording devices that permit somewhat accurate derivation of sleep-wake state, latency to sleep onset, duration of sleep, and other sleep-related measures—to document sleep in children with ADHD. In addition, the gold-standard test, overnight polysomnography, was also used, and although labor-intensive and expensive, has provided valuable information and allow investigation of sleep architecture and sleep stage distribution in ADHD patients.

Despite the high frequency of sleep-related complaints, earlier objective assessments of sleep in children with ADHD have shown inconsistent findings, such that a very nebulous picture emerges from such studies. Furthermore, small sample sizes and inconsistent criteria in subject inclusion, as well as in the incorporation of control subjects, make comparisons of these studies difficult. The disparity between subjective and objective findings is best highlighted by Corkum et al. *(8)*, who compared 25 children with ADHD with 25 age-matched controls (mean age = 9 yr) utilizing parent and child reports of sleep quality and 7-d actigraphic recordings. Parents of children diagnosed with ADHD reported significantly more problems with sleep onset, morning awakenings, restless sleep, and bedtime resistance than children in the control group. However, when both actigraphy recordings and the children's reports of their own sleep were analyzed, the only variable that was significantly different between the two groups was bedtime resistance. Corkum and colleagues hypothesized that the significant difficulties that parents of children with ADHD report with their children's sleep may be related to the difficult and often oppositional behaviors manifesting as bedtime resistance rather than representing primary sleep disorders in ADHD. In addition, these objective-subjective incongruencies could also be related to differences introduced by retrospective and prospective collection of sleep measures.

In their review of the published literature on objective sleep characteristics in ADHD, Corkum et al. *(4)* inconsistent findings were the rule. Indeed, there was either an absence of any discernible differences in sleep variables among ADHD subjects and controls, or instead significant changes emerged in the sleep parameters. Contrary to information gained from studies utilizing subjective data, increased sleep onset latency is not commonly found. Although studies using sleep diaries *(1,8)* and actigraphy *(38)* reported longer sleep duration in children with ADHD, use of electroencephalogram (EEG) to determine sleep times yielded conflicting results. For example, Ramos Platon et al. *(39)* found prolonged sleep duration in ADHD, whereas Greenhill et al. *(40)* reported longer sleep duration in children who were medicated, but did not find any differences in nonmedicated children. Longer sleep onset latencies have been found in studies on both medicated *(40–42)* and nonmedicated children *(38)*; shorter sleep latencies have also been reported in two studies in nonmedicated children *(39,41)*. Despite the heterogeneous definitions of ADHD employed in these studies (ranging from formal psychological assessment to reports on a parent-based rating scales), and the medication status of the children, no consistent alterations in sleep onset latency have been found in the vast majority of the studies *(8,32,35,43–49)*. A summary of objectively assessed sleep disturbances are shown in Table 2.

Clinically, parents of children with ADHD complain of hyperactive and oppositional behaviors that occur throughout the day and into the evening. The extension of these behaviors to bedtime is the most likely explanation for the higher probability that parents of children with ADHD will report that their children have bedtime resistance and sleep-onset delay. Thus, children with ADHD may be displaying oppositional behaviors that prevent them from following rules and engaging in appropriate bedtime behaviors. On the basis of the aforementioned findings, the overall higher frequency of bedtimes and sleep-related problems appears to reflect more sleep limit-setting issues rather than representing sleep disorders *per se*.

Table 2
Objective Assessments of Relationship Between Sleep and ADHD

Ref.	Authors	Year	Subjects	Age	Diagnosis of ADHD	Control sample	Sleep assessment	Results
41	Small et al.	1971	Three hyperactive children; before and during medication	8.4 ± 0.6 yr	Psychiatric examination	Seven age-matched controls	Five nights of EEG (no medications); 1 mo on stimulants followed by three nights EEG then three nights of placebo	ADHD had shorter sleep latency and muscle activity during sleep in baseline condition. Medicated: ADHD had reduced number of sleep cycles, increased sleep latency, decreased awakenings, increased REM latency
44	Feinberg et al.	1974	Four male hyperkinetic children (no stimulants) and four hyperkinetic children on long-term stimulants	8.6 ± 1 yr	Physician-diagnosed	Six male age-matched controls	EEG recordings for one night	Medication associated with longer REM latency
42	Haig et al.	1974	Six hyperactive males (medicated); four children restudied postdrug.	8–14 yr	Inter-disciplinary clinic diagnosis	Six normal males	EEG recordings for five nights	Medicated hyperactive children had increased sleep latency and increased REM latency relative to controls. No differences found for on and off drug comparisons

50	Nahas and Krynicki	1977	Four hyperactive males (before and during medication)	7.3 ± 2.5 yr	Diagnosis of hyperactive impulse disorder	Published values	EEG recordings	Hyperactive group decreased REM and stage 4; increased stage 2 and state changes. No medication effects observed
43	Busby et al.	1981	11 non-medicated hyperkinetic males	10.6 ± 1.7 yr	Presence of core symptoms for DSM-III and elevated hyperactivity scores on Conners	11 males negative on Conners	EEG recordings for five nights	Hyperactive group had increased REM latency
51	Kahn	1982	16 hyper-kinetic males	6–12 yr	Neurological and psychological assessment	12 males	EEG recordings	Shortened REM latency in nine hyperkinetics
40	Greenhill et al.	1983	Nine ADHD males (before and during medication)	8.6 ± 1.4 yr	Psychological assessment; DSM-II criteria	11 children (four males) negative for mental disorder	EEG recordings for two nights pre-medication then two nights of EEG recording after 6 mo of drug therapy	Premedication; no differences. On medication, ADHD had longer sleep latency, and increased sleep time, with increased stage changes and increased REM cycles

(Continued)

Table 2
(Continued)

Ref.	Authors	Year	Subjects	Age	Diagnosis of ADHD	Control sample	Sleep assessment	Results
52	Porrino et al.	1983	12 hyperactive males (on and off medication)	6–12 yr	Psychological assessment; DSM-III criteria	12 age and classroom matched males	24-h motor activity monitor for 1 wk	Hyperactive group had higher level of movement during sleep
53	Busby and Pivik	1985	16 hyperactive males (eight medicated)	8–12 yr	DSM-III criteria and Conners' Parent and Teacher Rating scales	Eight controls from local schools	EEG and respiration for four nights (first two nights for adaptation)	Arousal responses to stimuli not different; however a lower threshold in nonmedicated children observed in stage 2
1	Kaplan et al.	1987	25 males with ADHD (medication free)	3–6 yr	Parent report plus DSM-III criteria	27 males from local day care centers	Sleep logs for 21 consecutive days	ADHD children more likely to have shorter naps, longer sleep at night, more awakenings, bedwetting, night sweats
39	Ramos Platon et al.	1990	13 ADD children (medication free)	9 ± 1.7 yr	Formal psychological assessment and DSM-III criteria	Published data on 43 children	EEG recordings with respiration and ECG for two nights	ADD had decreased sleep latency, increased sleep time and number of awakenings, and increased SWS. ADD had decreased REM and stage 1 sleep. Older ADD had longer REM latency

54	Palm et al.	1992	10 children with deficits in attention, motor control, and perception (medication free)	6–12 yr	Physician, psychologist and physio-therapist	18 controls	PSG, MSLT, and reaction times for two nights	Index children had a longer latency to sleep onset during night one. No other differences in sleep observed; index had children significantly longer reaction times
45	Tirosh et al.	1993	10 ADHD (before and during medication).	6–12 yr	Previous diagnosis of ADHD	10 matched controls	Actigraphy during baseline, placebo and methylphenidate for 8 d each	During medication there was a shorter sleep duration
32	Dagan et al.	1997	12 ADHD males (five medicated)	9.6 ± 1.6 yr	Psychiatric assessment	12 healthy males	Actigraphy for three nights	ADHD had poorer sleep efficiency, less quiet sleep, and increased activity
38	Gruber et al.	2000	38 ADHD males (medication naïve)	9.6 ± 2.7 yr	DSM-IV criteria based on teacher and parent ratings	64 males from a normative sample	Actigraphy for five nights and daily sleep logs.	ADHD had longer sleep onset latency, increased sleep duration and increase true sleep. No differences found in the sleep log data.

(Continued)

Table 2
(Continued)

Ref.	Authors	Year	Subjects	Age	Diagnosis of ADHD	Control sample	Sleep assessment	Results
46	Lecendreux et al.	2000	30 ADHD males; (psycho-stimulant naïve)	7.8 ± 1.6 yr	Psychiatric assessment using DSM-IV criteria	22 matched controls presenting with reading disorder	1 wk of hospitalization; EEG and ECG recordings overnight and during MSLT; computerized test of alertness	No differences in overnight study. MLST showed shorter sleep latency in ADHD; ADHD children had more daytime sleep episodes. ADHD performed worse on tests of reaction time
8	Corkum et al.	2001	25 ADHD (medication naïve)	9.1 ± 1.4 yr	Formal psychological assessment	25 children from the community	1. Actigraphy for 7 d 2. Sleep diary	1. No differences between groups 2. ADHD longer sleep time and more bedtime resistance
47	Konofal et al.	2001	30 male ADHD (medication-free)	5–10 yr	Psychiatric assessment with DSM-IV criteria	19 controls with learning disorders matched for age and sex	PSG and video performed on the 3rd night following adaptation	ADHD children had higher levels of nocturnal activity; sleep architecture otherwise not different
35	O'Brien et al.	2003	44 ADHD; 27 hyperactive	5–7 yr	Conners' Parent Rating Scale	39 controls from the community	PSG for one night	REM latency longer in ADHD than in hyper or controls; REM% shorter in ADHD than in hyper or controls

48	O'Brien et al.	2003	87 ADHD (53 medicated)	6.5 ± 1.4 yr	Report of confirmed diagnosis of ADHD	53 controls from the community	PSG for one night	Decreased REM% in ADHD; Medicated ADHD had trend toward longer REM latency
49	O'Brien et al	2003	47 ADHD from clinical sample 53 ADHD from community sample	8 ± 1.6 yr (clinical; sample) 6.6 ± 0.4 yr- (community sample)	Diagnosis by physician or psychologist for clinical sample; parental report of ADHD together with score >2SD on Conners for community samples	53 controls from the community	PSG for one night	ADHD had increased REM latency, decreased REM% than controls

MSLT, multiple sleep latency test; SWS, slow-wave sleep; ECG, echocardiogram; PSG, polysomnogram; SD, standard deviation.

4. SLEEP ARCHITECTURE IN ADHD

The proportion of time spent in different sleep stages in children with ADHD has been investigated in a number of studies dating back to the 1970s. Nahas and Krynicki *(50)* found a decreased percentage of rapid-eye-movement (REM) sleep and stage 4 sleep (Δ sleep) in nonmedicated hyperactive males when compared with published values in normal children. These changes were accompanied by a reciprocal elevation of stage 2 sleep. Conversely, increased Δ sleep was reported by Ramos Platon et al. *(39)* in a group of 13 medication-free attention deficit disorder children in comparison to published data. Clearly, the use of published normative values for comparison of findings in selected ADHD cohorts is not very valuable and does not allow for assessments of real differences that may exist in sleep architecture between the ADHD and control children. Notwithstanding these considerations, reported differences in REM sleep between ADHD and control children appear to be more reliably present. Indeed, Busby et al. *(43)* performed overnight polysomnography in a small number of children with ADHD (n = 11) and controls (n = 11) and found that REM sleep latency was significantly increased in the ADHD group, a finding that is in agreement with those of Haig et al. *(42)* and Feinberg et al. *(44)*. In contrast, Kahn *(51)* found decreased REM sleep latencies, and Ramos Platon et al. *(39)* found no significant differences in hyperactive and control children. Further, the studies by Haig et al. *(42)* and Feinberg et al. *(44)* found that the increase REM latency was present only in children who were medicated with stimulants. Despite such findings, it needs to be emphasized that a first-night effect could be one of the factors that may affect REM sleep latency, such that the putatively prolonged REM sleep latency among ADHD children could essentially reflect the fact that ADHD children are more sensitive to changes in the environment, and therefore more prone to develop a first-night effect in the sleep laboratory. However, when sleep EEG dynamics were followed in ADHD children for four consecutive nights, there was a tendency to maintain prolonged REM sleep latency across all nights *(43)*. In addition, the proportion of time spent in REM sleep has been found to decrease *(39,50)* in nonmedicated children with ADHD. More recently, in a series of more extensive studies from our laboratory, we confirmed that a prolonged REM latency is clearly present in children with significant symptoms suggestive of ADHD *(35)*, and that such delayed onset of REM findings were still present in children with reports of a diagnosis of ADHD obtained from both a clinical population and a community population *(49)*. Furthermore, O'Brien, et al. *(48)* also found a trend toward a longer REM latency in medicated children with ADHD compared with controls. Interestingly, we found on all three of these studies that the proportion of REM sleep as a function of total sleep duration was decreased in the ADHD groups. What are the implications of such findings? O'Brien et al. *(35)* found significant correlations between the magnitude of REM sleep disturbance and the degree of disturbance in neurocognitive measures, particularly in those associated with executive function. Such associations suggest that disruption of REM sleep may exert small effects on daytime functioning, a not-so-surprising finding, given that REM sleep plays important roles in memory consolidation of learned tasks *(55)*.

5. SDB AND ADHD: TRUE, FALSE OR UNRELATED?

A large body of evidence has now documented that children with either snoring or SDB often present with problems of attention and behavior that are remarkably similar to those observed in children with ADHD *(2,7,8,23,56–58)*. In addition, three separate population surveys encompassing almost 3300 children showed the presence of daytime sleepiness, hyperactivity, and aggressive behavior in children who snored *(2,59,60)*. It has been further suggested that up to one third of all children with frequent, loud snoring will display significant hyperactivity and inattention *(2)*. Based on the available literature, the relatively high prevalence of SDB (3% of children) and ADHD (5–6%) would predict that their coexistence may also be relatively frequent. However, the actual prevalence of SDB in children with ADHD far exceeded that predicted by the simple probability if these two disorders were mechanistically unrelated coexisting disorders. In fact, it has been suggested that up to 25% of children with a diagnosis of ADHD may actually have SDB *(23)*. Although such rather elevated figure estimates of the overlap between SDB and ADHD is probably less prominent if medication status and psychiatric comorbidity are accounted for in the analysis, the phenomenon still holds true but only for a subgroup of children with hyperactivity. In a recent study by our team *(35)*, we found that the prevalence of SDB in a cohort of children with ADHD does not appear to differ from the prevalence in the general population. However, an unusually high frequency of SDB was found among children with mild-to-moderate increases in hyperactivity, who did not meet the more stringent criteria necessary for the diagnosis of ADHD. This suggests that although SDB may induce significant behavioral effects manifesting as increased hyperactivity and inattention, it will not overlap with true clinical ADHD when the latter is assessed by more objective tools than just parental perception.

6. EFFECT OF STIMULANT MEDICATION ON SLEEP IN ADHD

Stimulant medications have long been the first line of treatment for children with ADHD, and routinely yield clear benefits in both behavioral patterns and attention deficits, independent of whether the assessments are part of laboratory research or field trials *(31)*. In addition to the improvements in the cardinal symptoms of inattention, impulsivity, and hyperactivity, substantial cognitive improvements have also been noted *(61)*. However, many of the putative sleep problems in children with ADHD have been attributed to the use of stimulants. Insomnia has long been reported to be a side effect of stimulant therapy despite the fact that the majority of studies have been based on parental report, rather than truly assess sleep latency and maintenance. Stein *(6)* found that almost one third of families with stimulant-treated children reported insomnia or increased sleep latency compared with 10% of untreated children with ADHD. Similarly, both Barkley *(31)* and Ahamenn et al. *(62)* found that stimulant medication was associated with insomnia. In contrast, Pataki et al. *(63)* did not find insomnia to be reported with significantly greater frequency in children medicated with methylphenidate compared to baseline or placebo periods.

There is some evidence that the medication schedule may influence sleep measures *(64–66)*. For example, delays in the first REM period and decreased proportion of REM sleep have been reported following nocturnal administration of stimulants *(64)*. Additionally, the type and dosage of the stimulant may affect sleep characteristics in children. Efron et al. *(67)* conducted a double-blind, crossover trial of methylphenidate and dexamphetamine, and reported that the latter caused more severe insomnia that methylphenidate. Tirosh et al. *(45)* reported that only sleep duration was affected (reduced) by methylphenidate hydrochloride compared with placebo, whereas others have reported prolongation of REM latency *(41,44)*, increases in the number of REM cycles *(40)*, or decreased proportion of REM *(64)*. We recently examined the potential effect of stimulants on objective sleep measures and found no differences in sleep parameters between children taking methylphenidate or dexamphetamine compared with nonmedicated children *(48)*. These results support earlier findings of Haig et al. *(42)* and Nahas and Krynicki *(50)*, who found no differences in sleep parameters in a small group of children before and during stimulant therapy. Thus, if stimulant medication is indeed associated with disrupted sleep, the disruptions are likely to be minimal and of little clinical consequence. Moreover, some of observed sleep disturbances could be related to drug rebound effects rather than medication effects *per se*.

The relationship(s) between ADHD, medication, and sleep is far from being a trivial one. However, small sample sizes, lack of control subjects, and skewed clinical populations drawn from tertiary referral centers potentially detract from the validity of any of the potential findings, and make it difficult if not impossible to compare across studies. Furthermore, these obstacles are further compounded by not knowing whether studies on nonmedicated children were conducted in children who never received psychostimulants vs children who had previously been on stimulant therapy, in whom sleep characteristics may have been influenced by residual medication effects. As a result of all these methodological issues, whether psychostimulant use is associated with sleep disturbance remains an unanswered question despite the widespread use of such medications for the treatment of ADHD symptoms.

7. SLEEP MOTOR HYPERACTIVITY AND ADHD

Studies using both actigraphy *(32,52)*, overnight polysomnography *(41,43)*, and more recently video analysis of nighttime motion *(47)* have reported that hyperactive children show an increased frequency of body movements during sleep. PLMS has been reported in greater frequency among children with ADHD compared to controls *(26,27)*, raising the speculation that PLMS and ADHD may share neurobiological mechanisms *(27,28)*. Indeed, children with PLMS are reported to have hyperactive behavior *(25)* and PLMS may be common among hyperactive children *(26–28,60)*. In one study by Picchietti et al. *(27)*, 15 out of 16 children with frequent PLMS (>25 per hour of sleep) had ADHD. Chervin and Archbold *(68)* further reported a dose-dependent association between hyperactivity, measured by the Conners Parent Rating Scale *(36)* and PLM index. Furthermore, treatment of PLMS will often lead to substantial behavioral improvements in hyperactivity *(69)*. However, most of these studies were conducted in tertiary-referral patient cohorts *(25–28,60,68)*. To further examine the possibility that skewed ADHD populations may lead to an overrepresentation of PLMS, O'Brien et al. *(49)* studied a community sample of children diagnosed with ADHD and compared it to both a group of control children and to a group of children referred for subspecialty evaluation at a tertiary medical center. Although this study did not find an increase in PLMS in the community sample of ADHD children, PLMS was found in 40% of children referred to the tertiary clinic. Of interest almost half of these children had arousals associated with PLMS events. These findings further raise the question of whether those children attending the clinical setting actually represent a subgroup of children with ADHD who are also more likely to have a nighttime disorder (i.e., PLMS). In other words, ADHD children referred to a tertiary specialty clinic may represent a subset of ADHD children who are at high risk for PLMS and associated sleep fragmentation, which in turn may exacerbate daytime behavior. This possibility is further substantiated by data from Crabtree et al. *(29)* who found that children with PLMS and ADHD had significantly more PLMS events associated with arousals than children without ADHD. As such, the number of arousals elicited by PLMS events during sleep may be more directly linked with hyperactivity rather than the overall number of PLMS *per se*. As such, children who exhibit an elevated PLMS index may have a reduced risk of presenting symptoms of ADHD if the PLMS events are not associated with arousals.

An alternative possibility may be that children presenting to sleep disorders centers are more likely to exhibit PLMS, whether or not they are diagnosed with ADHD. In this context, PLMS-associated arousals could be a result of the underlying pathophysiology of ADHD, rather than represent a pathophysiological mechanism facilitating the emergence of hyperactive behaviors and attention deficits. Chervin and Archbold *(68)* found that 26% of children presenting to their sleep disorders center who underwent polysomnography had a PLMS index greater than or equal to 5, and found no association between PLMS and inattention–hyperactivity in children. Conversely, Picchietti and Walters *(27)* found that 91% of children with PLMS in their clinic had a diagnosis of ADHD. The disparities among the various studies are therefore difficult to reconcile, and further support the need for additional research on the prevalence and significance of PLMS in children with ADHD.

8. ADHD, COMORBIDITY, AND SLEEP

In a setting of ADHD, comorbid psychiatric diagnoses, such as anxiety and behavioral disorders, may impose significant effects on the occurrence of sleep disturbances as reported by parents. However, the data are scanty on this issue, and the few studies available have not consistently included a clinical comparison group. Furthermore, the results of such studies are conflicting. Day and Abmayr *(70)* found that ADHD children with comorbid conditions were more likely to report problems with settling and going to sleep, as well as disruptions during sleep, whereas Marcotte et al. *(33)* found that the frequency of sleep-related problems did not differ between children with ADHD and those with a learning disorder. Corkum et al. *(34)* attempted to unravel the potentially complex relationships between ADHD comorbidities and medication status and sleep. These investigators reported that although children with ADHD were more likely to have more problematic sleep issues than their normally developing peers, they were not different from other children with psychiatric diagnoses (anxiety disorder, depression, conduct disorder, oppositional defiant disorder). The combined subtype of ADHD (presence of both hyperactive and inattentive behaviors) was associated with the presence of dyssomnias and sleep-related involuntary movements. However, *post hoc* analyses revealed that the dyssomnias were associated with stimulant medication and oppositional defiant disorder rather than ADHD *per se*, whereas sleep-related involuntary movements were highly associated with anxiety. More recently, Mick et al. *(71)* have provided additional data supportive of the findings by Corkum et al. *(34)*, and have suggested that the majority of sleep difficulties observed in ADHD children are accounted for by comorbid anxiety and pharmacotherapy with stimulants. Furthermore, comorbid anxiety was associated with a decreased likelihood of going to bed willingly, of falling asleep easily, and also with an increased likelihood of waking during the night. These findings suggest that bedtime struggles often reported in ADHD may be more closely related to the presence of comorbidities than ADHD *per se*. Thus, the relationship between ADHD and sleep disturbance is complex, and may depend on numerous factors that include the type of sleep problem, the presence of comorbidity, and the medication status. Further studies that include control groups recruited from psychiatric or neurologic subspecialty clinics may provide additional information on the sleep characteristics of these children, and help determine whether the differences observed are unique to ADHD or are shared by neuropsychiatric diseases in general.

9. SUMMARY

In conclusion, the associations between sleep disturbance and ADHD are complex and quite poorly defined at present. Parental report-based studies invariably yield findings of significantly more reported sleep disruptions in children with ADHD, whereas objective assessments have yet to uncover striking and consistent differences. Despite such considerations, it seems prudent to assess children with ADHD for the presence of sleep disturbances because identification of specific sleep disorders may facilitate improved control of ADHD-ascribed symptoms in these children. Future studies utilizing large sample sizes of rigorously diagnosed children and appropriately matched controls are required and need to include careful selection processes that incorporate information on comorbid disorders and medication history and schedules.

ACKNOWLEDGMENTS

The authors are supported by National Institutes of Health grant HL-65270, Department of Education Grant H324E011001, Centers for Disease Control grant E11/CCE 422081–01, and The Commonwealth of Kentucky Research Challenge Trust Fund.

REFERENCES

1. Kaplan BJ, McNichol J, Conte RA, Moghadam HK. Sleep disturbance in preschool-aged and hyperactive and nonhyperactive children. Pediatrics 1987;80:839–844.
2. Ali NJ, Pitson D, Stradling JR. Snoring, sleep disturbance and behaviour in 4–5 year olds. Arch Dis Child 1993;68:360–366.
3. Ball, JD, Tiernan M, Janusz J, Furr A. Sleep patterns among children with attention-deficit hyperactivity disorder: a re-examination of parental perceptions. J Pediatr Psychol 1997;22:389–398.
4. Corkum P, Tannock R, Moldofsky H. Sleep disturbance in children with attention-deficit hyperactivity disorder. J Am Acad Child Adolesc Psychiatry 1998;37:637–646.
5. Ring A, Stein D, Barak Y, et al. Sleep disturbances in children with attention-deficit/hyperactivity disorder: a comparative study with healthy siblings. J Learn Disabil 1998;31:572–578.
6. Stein MA. Unravelling sleep problems in treated and untreated children with ADHD. J Child Adolesc Psychopharmacol 1999;9:157–168.
7. Owens J, Maxim R, Nobile C, McGuinn M, Msall M. Parental and self-report of sleep in children with attention deficit/hyperactivity disorder. Arch Pediatr Adolesc Med 2000;154:549–555.
8. Corkum P, Tannock R, Moldofsky H, Hogg-Johnson S, Humphries T. Actigraphy and parental ratings of sleep in children with attention deficit/hyperactivity disorder (ADHD). Sleep 2001;24:303–312.
9. American Psychiatric Association. Diagnostic and statistical manual of mental disorders, 3rd ed. Washington, DC: American Psychiatric Association; 1980.
10. American Psychiatric Association. Diagnostic and statistical manual of mental disorders, 3rd ed. revised, Washington, DC: American Psychiatric Association, 1987.
11. American Psychiatric Association. Diagnostic and statistical manual of mental disorders, 4th ed. Washington, DC: American Psychiatric Association, 1994.
12. Navelet Y, Anders T, Guilleminault C. Narcolepsy in children. In: Narcolepsy: Proceedings of the First International Symposium on Narcolepsy. Advances in Sleep Research, vol. 3. Guilleminault C, Dement WC, Passouant P, eds. New York: Spectrum 1976:171–177.
13. Dahl RE, Holttum J, Ztrubnik L. A clinical picture of child and adolescent narcolepsy. J Am Acad Chil Adolesc Psychiatr 1994;33:834–841.
14. Ware JC, Orr WC. Sleep disorders in children. In: Handbook of clinical child psychology. Walker CM, Roberts MC, eds. New York: Wiley, 1983:381–405.

15. Laufer M, Denhoff E, Solomons G. Hyperkinetic impulse disorder in children's behavior problems. Psychosom Med 1957;19:38–49.
16. Dahl RE. Regulation of sleep and arousal: development and psychopathology. Dev Psychopathol 1996;8:3–27.
17. Zametkin AJ, Nodah TE, Gross M, et al. Cerebral glucose metabolism in adults with hyperactivity of childhood onset. New Engl J Med 1990;26:676–686.
18. Fisher BE, Rinehart S. Stress, arousal, psychopathology and temperament: a multi-dimensional approach to sleep disturbance in children. Personality indiv Diff 1990;11:431–438.
19. Guilleminault C, Eldridge F, Simmons FB, Dement WC. Sleep apnea in eight children. Pediatrics 1976;58:28–31.
20. Brouillette RT, Fernbach SK, Hunt CE. Obstructive sleep apnea in infants and children. J Pediatr 1982;100:31–40.
21. Stradling J R, Thomas G, Warley ARH, Williams P, Freeland A. Effect of adenotonsillectomy on nocturnal hypoxaemia, sleep disturbance, and symptoms in snoring children. Lancet 1990;335:249–253.
22. Ali NJ, Pitson D, Stradling JR. Sleep disordered breathing: effects of adenotonsillectomy on behaviour and psychological functioning. Eur J Pediatr 1996;155:56–62.
23. Chervin RD, Dillon JE, Bassetti C, Ganoczy DA, Pituch KJ. Symptoms of sleep disorders, inattention, and hyperactivity in children. Sleep 1997;20:1185–1192.
24. Guilleminault C, Pelayo R. Narcolepsy in prepubertal children. Ann Neurol 1998;43:135–142.
25. Picchietti DL, Walters AS. Restless legs syndrome and periodic limb movement disorder in children and adolescents: comorbidity with attention-deficit hyperactivity disorder. Child Adolesc Psychiatr Clin North Am 1996;5:729–740.
26. Picchietti DL, England SJ, Walters AS, Willis K, Verrico T. Periodic limb movement disorder and restless legs syndrome in children with attention-deficit-hyperactivity disorder. J Child Neurol 1998;13:588–594.
27. Picchietti DL, Walters AS. Moderate to severe periodic limb movement disorder in childhood and adolescence. Sleep 1999;22:297–300.
28. Picchietti DL, Underwood DJ, Farris WA, et al. Further studies on periodic limb movement disorder and restless legs syndrome in children with attention-deficit-hyperactivity disorder. Mov Disord 1999;14:1000–1007.
29. Crabtree VM, Ivanenko A, O'Brien LM, Gozal D. Periodic limb movement disorder of sleep in children. J Sleep Res 2003;12:73–81.
30. Trommer BL, Hoeppner JB, Rosenberg RS, Armstrong KJ, Rothstein JA. Sleep disturbance in children with attention deficit disorder. Ann Neurol (abstract) 1988;24:322.
31. Barkley RA. Attention deficit hyperactivity disorder: a handbook for diagnosis and treatment. New York: Guilford Press, 1990:76–77.
32. Dagan Y, Zeevi-Luria S, Sever Y, et al. Sleep quality in children with attention deficit hyperactivity disorder: an actigraphic study. Psychiatry Clin Neurosci 1997;51:383–386.
33. Marcotte AC, Thatcher PV, Butters M, Bortz J, Acebo C, Carskadon MA. Parental report of sleep problems in children with attentional and learning problems. Dev Behav Pediatr 1998;19:178–186.
34. Corkum P, Moldofsky H, Hogg-Johnson S, Humphries T, Tannock R. Sleep problems in children with attention-deficit/hyperactivity disorder: impact of subtype, comorbidity, and stimulant medication. J Am Acad Child Adolesc Psychiatry 1999;38:1285–1293.
35. O'Brien LM, Holbrook CR, Mervis CB, et al. Sleep and neurobehavioral characteristics in 5–7 year old children with parentally reported symptoms of ADHD. Pediatrics 2003;111:554–563.
36. Conners CK. Conners' Rating Scales-Revised. North Tonawanda, NY: Multi-Health Systems Publishing, 1997.
37. Wirt RD, Lachar D, Klinedinst JK, Seat PD. Multidimensional description of child personality: a manual for the Personality Inventory for Children. Los Angeles: Western Psychological Corp., 1982.

38. Gruber R, Sadeh A, Raviv A. Instability of sleep patterns in children with attention-deficit/hyperactivity disorder. J Am Acad Child Adolesc Psychiatry 2000;39:495–501.
39. Ramos Platon MJ, Vela Bueno A, Espinar Sierra J, Kales S. Hypnopolygraphic alterations in attention deficit disorder (ADD) children. Int J Neurosci 1990;53:87–101.
40. Greenhill L, Puig-Antich J, Goetz R, Hanlon C, Davies M. Sleep architecture and REM sleep measures in prepubertal children with attention deficit disorder with hyperactivity. Sleep 1983;6:91–101.
41. Small A, Hibi S, Feinberg I. Effects of dextroamphetamine sulphate on EEG sleep patterns of hyperactive children. Arch Gen Psychiatr 1971;25:369–380.
42. Haig JR, Schroeder CS, Schroeder SR. Effects of methylphenidate on hyperactive children's sleep. Psychopharmacologia 1974;37:185–188.
43. Busby K, Firestone P, Pivik RT. Sleep patterns in hyperkinetic and normal children. Sleep 1981;4:366–383.
44. Feinberg I, Hibi S, Braun M, Cavness C, Westerman G, Small A. Sleep amphetamine effects in MBDS and normal subjects. Arch Gen Psychiatry 1974;31:723–731.
45. Tirosh E, Sadeh A, Munvez R, Lavie P. Effects of methylphenidate on sleep in children with attention-deficit hyperactivity disorder. Am J Dis Child 1993;147:1313–1315.
46. Lecendreux M, Konofal E, Bouvard M, Falissard B, Mouren-Simeoni MC. Sleep and alertness in children with ADHD. J Child Psychol Psychiatry 2000;41:803–812.
47. Konofal E, Lecendreux M, Bouvard MP, Mouren-Simeoni MC. High levels of nocturnal activity in children with attention-deficit hyperactivity disorder: a video analysis. Psychiatry Clin Neurosci 2001;55:97–103.
48. O'Brien LM, Ivanenko A, Crabtree VM, et al. The effect of stimulants on sleep characteristics in children with attention deficit/hyperactive disorder. Sleep Med 2003;4:309–316.
49. O'Brien LM, Ivanenko A, Crabtree VM, et al. Sleep disturbances in children with ADHD. Ped Res 2003;54:237–243.
50. Nahas AD, Krynicki V. Effect of methylphenidate on sleep stages and ultradian rhythms in hyperactive children. J Nerv Met Dis 1977;164:66–69.
51. Kahn A. Sleep REM latency in hyperkinetic boys. Am J Psychiatry 1982;139:1358–1360.
52. Porrino LJ, Rapoport JL, Behar D, Sceery W, Ismond DR, Bunney WE Jr. A naturalistic assessment of the motor activity of hyperactive boys. I. Comparison with normal controls. Arch Gen Psychiatry 1983;40:681–687.
53. Busby K, Pivik RT. Auditory arousal thresholds during sleep in hyperkinetic children. Sleep 1985;8:332–341.
54. Palm L, Persson E, Bjerre I, Elmqvist D, Blennow G. Sleep and wakefulness in preadolescent children with deficits in attention, motor control and perception. Acta Paediatr 1992;81:618–624.
55. Karni A, Tanne D, Rubenstein BS, Askenasy JJ, Sagi D. Dependence on REM sleep of overnight improvement of a perceptual skill. Science 1994;265:679–682.
56. Guilleminault C, Korobkin R, Winkle R. A review of 50 children with obstructive sleep apnea syndrome. Lung 1981;159:275–287.
57. Guilleminault C, Winkle R, Korobkin R, Simmons B. Children and nocturnal snoring—evaluation of the effects of sleep related respiratory resistive load and daytime functioning. Eur J Pediatr 1982;139:165–171.
58. Owens J, Opipari L, Nobile C, Spirito A. Sleep and daytime behavior in children with obstructive sleep apnea and behavioral sleep disorders. Pediatrics 1998;102:1178–1184.
59. Ferreira AM, Clemente V, Gozal D, et al. Snoring in Portuguese primary school children. Pediatrics 2000;106:5:e64.
60. Chervin RD, Archbold KH, Dillon JE, et al. Inattention, hyperactivity, and symptoms of sleep disordered breathing. Pediatrics 2002;109:449–456.
61. Rapport MD, Kelly DL. Psychostimulant effects on learning and cognitive function: Findings and implications for children with attention deficit hyperactivity disorder. Clin Psychol Rev 1991;11:61–92.

62. Ahmann PA, Waltonen SJ, Olson KA, Theye FW, Van Erem AJ, LaPlant RJ. Placebo-controlled evaluation of Ritalin side effects. Pediatrics 1993;91:1101–1106.
63. Pataki CS, Carlson GA, Kelly KL, Rapport MD, Biancaniello TM. Side effects of methylphenidate and desipramine alone and in combination in children. J Am Acad Child Adolesc Psychiatry 1993;32:1065–1072.
64. Chatoor I, Wells KC, Conners CK, Seidel WT, Shaw D. The effects of nocturnally administered stimulant medication on EEG sleep and behavior in hyperactive children. J Am Acad Child Psychiatry 1983;22:337–342.
65. Stein MA, Blondis TA, Schnitzler ER, et al. Methylphenidate dosing: twice daily versus three times daily. Pediatrics 1996;98:748–756.
66. Kent JD, Blader JC, Koplewicz HS, Abikoff H, Foley CA. Effects of a late-afternoon methylphenidate administration on behavior and sleep in attention-deficit hyperactivity disorder. Pediatrics 1995;96:320–325.
67. Efron D, Jarman F, Barker M. Side effects of methylphenidate and dexamphetamine in children with attention deficit hyperactivity disorder: a double-blind, crossover trial. Pediatrics 1997;100:662–666.
68. Chervin RD, Archbold KH. Hyperactivity and polysomnographic findings in children evaluated for sleep-disordered breathing. Sleep 2001;24:313–320.
69. Walters S, Mandelbaum DE, Lewin DS, Kugler S, England SJ, Miller M. Dopaminergic therapy in children with restless legs/periodic limb movements in sleep and ADHD. Pediatr Neurol 2000;22:182–186.
70. Day HD, Abmayr SB. Parent reports of sleep disturbances in stimulant-medicated children with attention-deficit hyperactivity disorder. J Clin Psychol 1998;54:701–716.
71. Mick E, Biederman J, Jetton J, Faraone SV. Sleep disturbances associated with attention deficit hyperactivity disorder: The impact of psychiatric co-morbidity and pharmacotherapy. J Child Adolesc Psychopharmacol 2000;10:223–231.

20

Neuropsychological Performance in Adults With Attention Deficit Hyperactivity Disorder

Lisa Lee Weyandt

1. INTRODUCTION

Attention deficit hyperactivity disorder (ADHD) is characterized by developmentally inappropriate levels of attention, impulsivity, and overactivity; it is estimated to affect 5–10% of children and adolescents and 3–4% of adults *(1,2)*. ADHD was previously considered a disorder of childhood; however, follow-up studies suggest that the majority of individuals continue to exhibit ADHD symptoms throughout adolescence and adulthood. Longitudinal studies also indicate that these individuals are at greater risk for academic, social, and behavioral difficulties during childhood, adolescence, and adulthood, as well as psychiatric comorbidity (e.g., antisocial behavior, drug use, mood disorders) *(3–7)*. Relative to what is known about ADHD in children and adolescents, less empirical information is available concerning ADHD in adults. In fact, some researchers have questioned the validity of adult ADHD and have asserted that ADHD typically remits in adulthood *(8)*. Many others, however, disagree with this notion and attest to the persistence of ADHD throughout adolescence and adulthood *(9,10)*. Recently Faraone et al. *(11)* sought to determine whether ADHD is a valid disorder in adulthood, using the validity criteria of Robins and Guze *(12)*. Faraone et al. reviewed clinical, family, psychopharmacological, neurobiological, and adult ADHD outcome studies and concluded that adult ADHD is a valid disorder, although the authors emphasized that additional studies are needed to clarify the specific nature of ADHD in adulthood.

One factor that fuels the controversy surrounding ADHD in adulthood is that the precise etiology of ADHD is unknown. Findings from genetic, neurochemical, neuroimaging, and neuropsychological studies, however, collectively support a neurobiological basis for the disorder. For example, twin and adoption studies have demonstrated that genetic factors are etiologically important in the expression of ADHD *(13)*, and recently Willcutt, et al. *(14)* reported that monozygotic twins were significantly more likely than dizygotic twins to meet the criteria for ADHD (78% and 35%, respectively). Familial studies have found that individuals with ADHD are more likely to have siblings or parents with ADHD relative to families with no history of ADHD *(15)*. Genetic studies have found that despite shared environmental influences, ADHD is primarily influenced by genetic factors *(16)*. Neuroanatomical, neurochemical, and neuroimaging studies collectively have supported a physiological basis for ADHD, although some findings have been inconsistent. Several studies, for example, have reported differences in size and symmetry of anatomical brain structures (e.g., corpus callosum, cerebellum, striatum)

From: *Attention Deficit Hyperactivity Disorder: From Genes to Patients*
Edited by: D. Gozal and D. L. Molfese © Humana Press Inc., Totowa, NJ

when comparing individuals with and without ADHD, whereas other studies have not replicated these findings *(17–22)*. Numerous neurotransmitter, neurometabolite, cerebral blood flow, and glucose metabolism studies have also reported differences between those with and without ADHD, although the mechanism responsible for these differences remains elusive *(23–27)*.

2. NEUROBIOLOGICAL THEORIES AND EXECUTIVE FUNCTIONS

Several neurobiological theories have been advanced to explain the underlying pathophysiology of ADHD and most converge on abnormalities of frontal-subcortical networks and structures. As Teeter and Semrud-Clikeman suggested *(28)*, these theories can be classified into two groups: those that focus on abnormalities of subcortical structures and regions such as the basal ganglia, and those that focus on abnormalities of frontal and prefrontal cortices. Recent studies have also focused on the role of the right hemisphere in ADHD *(29)*, and others have found size differences in the cerebellum of children with and without ADHD *(17,30)*. The precise etiology of the structural and functional abnormalities implicated in ADHD is unknown but is likely resulting from interactions among genetic, physiological, and environmental factors that ultimately affect brain development and neuronal functioning. For example, evidence suggests that ADHD may be owing in part to polymorphisms in dopamine genes that modulate neurotransmission in subcortical and cortical regions *(31)*. It is also plausible that prenatal factors such as exposure to teratogens and other risk factors result in morphological abnormalities within the frontal-subcortical region *(32)*. These morphological abnormalities may contribute to the dysregulation of cognitive and behavioral systems that mediate the core behaviors deficient in ADHD, such as self-regulation, motor behavior, and higher-order neuropsychological processes known as *executive functions (33)*.

Executive functions are broadly defined as higher-order cognitive abilities that allow for strategic planning, cognitive flexibility, self-regulation, goal-directed behavior, and impulse control. Neuroanatomically, executive functions have been ascribed to the frontal lobes and, more specifically, the prefrontal cortex *(34)*. As noted by Fletcher, however, the physiological substrates that underlie executive functions are complex and likely involve intricate neural networks interconnected with numerous brain regions *(35)*. Supporting this notion is the fact that damage to brain regions other than the prefrontal lobes, such as the basal ganglia, can result in executive function deficits. Nevertheless, the prevailing neurobiological and neuropsychological theories of ADHD is focus on frontal-subcortical structures and circuitry *(36)*. These theories arose in part from the earlier "dysfunctional frontal lobe hypothesis" of ADHD.

Wender and colleagues *(37–38)* were among the first to suggest that ADHD symptoms were caused by dysfunction of the frontal-subcortical systems, and Mattes *(39)* specifically asserted that ADHD is the result of frontal lobe dysfunction. This theory was based on research with humans and experimental animals who had sustained frontal lobe damage, and subsequent to the damage exhibited symptoms analogous to ADHD: hyperactivity, distractibility, and problems with self-regulation and goal-directed behavior *(40–42)*. From this body of literature, it was deduced that the frontal lobes, in particular the prefrontal regions, play a primary role in executive functioning processes. More recent studies using Functional magnetic resonance imaging (fMRI) with normal subjects have revealed that the prefrontal cortex increases in activation during higher-order cognitive processing such as working memory, and the anterior cingulate cortex increases during neuropsychological task performance (Continuous Performance Test [CPT]) *(43,44)*. With regard to ADHD, neuroimaging research has found both structural and functional differences in individuals with ADHD relative to controls, such as decreased blood flow in the striatum and prefrontal regions *(25,45–47)*. fMRI studies have revealed that these brain regions increase in activity as a result of stimulant medication *(48)*. These findings, in conjunction with other neurobiological research and research with experimental animals, support a mediating role of the prefrontal cortex in executive functions.

With regard to the development of executive functions, research suggests that executive functions follow a multistage process of development, with older children performing better on executive function tasks than younger children *(49)*. Executive functions have also been studied in child clinical samples, such as children with early brain damage. Christ et al. for example, recently investigated the effect of early brain damage and compromised prefrontal brain development on executive function performance in children with bilateral spastic cerebral palsy (SCP) *(50)*. Their results indicated that children with SCP performed more poorly on neuropsychological tasks relative to controls. Executive function performance has also been investigated in children with phenyl ketonuria, Tourette's syndrome, autism, learning disabilities, and conduct disorder *(51–53)*. In adult samples, executive functioning has been studied in a variety of disorders such as Alzheimer's disease, multiple sclerosis, and schizophrenia *(54,55,56)*, to name a few. Results of these studies have been mixed in terms of the presence and extent of executive function deficits, as well as the type and severity of neuropsychological deficits characteristic of each sample. Relative to other clinical groups, executive functions have been studied most often in those with ADHD.

Given the similar pattern of behavioral and cognitive deficits observed in those with documented frontal lobe damage and those with ADHD, researchers have hypothesized that ADHD symptomology may be the result of frontal-subcortical dysfunction that ultimately causes impairment in neuropsychologicial functioning, i.e., deficits in executive functions. A large number of neuropsychological studies have been conducted comparing the performance of children with and without ADHD on a variety of neuropsychological measures. As noted by Weyandt *(56a)*, results from these studies are inconclusive but, relative to other child clinical samples, executive function deficits appear more consistently and the level of impairment tends to be more severe with children with ADHD, especially in the area of motor response inhibition *(51)*. Fewer studies have addressed neuropsychological functioning in adolescents with ADHD and among those that have, some studies have found group differences on neuropsychological executive function tasks, whereas others have not found these differences *(47,57–60)*. Barkley et al. reviewed 22 neuropsychological studies that investigated frontal lobe functioning in children and adolescents with ADHD and concluded that most of these instruments do not reliably discriminate between those with and without the disorder and hence have poor clinical utility *(61)*.

3. NEUROPSYCHOLOGICAL FUNCTIONING IN ADULTS WITH ADHD

Recently researchers have begun to explore neuropsychological functioning in adults with ADHD. Some have argued that neuropsychological tests are objective measures and consequently can provide further evidence of the validity of adult ADHD, and can be useful in the diagnosis of ADHD in adults *(63,64)*. From this perspective, if ADHD is a developmental disorder and symptoms persist into adulthood, the neuropsychological deficits, characteristic of children and adolescents with ADHD may be predictive of neuropsychological deficits in adulthood. Given that neuropsychological deficits, particularly executive function deficits, have been found (albeit inconsistently) in children with ADHD, researchers have hypothesized that parallel deficits would be present in adults with the disorder.

Similar to the child literature, studies investigating neuropsychological functioning in adults with ADHD have focused primarily on intelligence and executive function tasks. The purpose of the remainder of this chapter is to review select literature concerning neuropsychological performance in adults with ADHD. This chapter is not meant to be exhaustive but rather to summarize the general findings, methodological problems, and implications concerning neuropsychological studies with adults with ADHD.

For organizational purposes neuropsychological tasks have been categorized under subheadings that do not necessarily reflect the construct validity of the tasks (e.g., planning, inhibition). For simplicity and flow, ADHD is used throughout this chapter even when the diagnostic nomenclature may have been different at the time some of the studies were conducted. Table 1 summarizes the neuropsychological studies reviewed with respect to authors, measures, findings, and sample characteristics.

4. INTELLIGENCE MEASURES

Intelligence tests, or IQ screening measures, have been included in many adult ADHD studies for a variety of purposes: to investigate whether intelligence of adults with ADHD differs from controls, to determine whether certain subtests (e.g., freedom from distractibility index) can predict group memberships, or for covariate or matching purposes. The findings have been mixed but in general, consistent with the child literature, IQ tests do not appear to be a reliable tool for discriminating adults with and without ADHD.

Although some studies have reported differences in IQ *(65–67)* and Freedom from Distractibility *(66,68,69)* in adults with and without ADHD other studies have not found these differences *(63,70–76)*. Several studies have investigated subtest differences (e.g., digit span, digit symbol, arithmetic) and again, these findings have been inconsistent *(71,77–79)*. It is difficult to draw conclusions about these findings, as it is plausible that executive function deficits influence IQ test performance. It is equally plausible that intellectual capacity influences performance on executive function tasks. Denckla has suggested that there is a "complex overlap" between general intelligence and neuropsychological performance, specifically executive function performance *(80)*. She has also pointed out that despite high levels of intelligence, individuals may exhibit various types of executive function deficits. Murphy et al. have argued that that ADHD shares a portion (i.e., 10%) of the variance with IQ, that executive function performance is negatively correlated with ADHD symptom severity, and that executive function performance is positively correlated with IQ *(78)*. Indeed, Murphy et al. found that performance differences attenuated on several neuropsychological tasks when IQ was controlled for in subjects with and without ADHD. Given these findings, Murphy et al. suggested that future studies should report and control for IQ group differences. Weyandt et al. investigated the relationship between Wechster Adult Intelligence Scaled-Revised performance and an executive function task (CPT) and found that intelligence was not correlated with neuropsychological performance in a group of young adults with and without ADHD *(73)*.

Thus, several issues require further study and clarification with regard to intelligence and neuropsychological performance in adults with ADHD. Specifically, the relationship between intelligence and other measures of neuropsychological functioning needs to be better understood (e.g., do some measures correlate positively with intelligence while others have an inverse relationship?). The issue of whether intelligence test subtests can reliably discriminate between adults with and without ADHD, as well as whether certain subtests can reliably discriminate adult ADHD from other clinical disorders, needs to be elucidated. Of course,

Table 1
Summary of Neuropsychological Findings

Author	Measures	Findings	Sample size	Mean age
Hopkins, et al. 1979	1. MFFT			
	RT	Nonsignificant	ADHD = 70	19.5
	Errors	Significant ADHD>C	C = 42	19
	2. Embedded figures tests			
	Completion time	Significant ADHD>C		
	Number correct	Significant ADHD<C		
	Errors	Significant ADHD>C		
	3. Stroop			
	RT	Significant ADHD>C		
	Errors	Significant ADHD>C		
Gualtieri et al. 1985	1. Continuous performance task			
	Correct responses	Significant ADHD<C	ADHD = 22	
	Commission errors	Significant ADHD>C	C = 22	27.5
	2. Matching familiar figures test	Nonsignificant		
Klee et al. 1986	1. CPT			
	Omissions	Significant ADHD>C	ADHD = 12	20
	Commission errors	Nonsignificant	C = 12	28.8
	2. MFFT			
	Errors	Nonsignificant		
	RT	Nonsignificant		
	3. WAIS-R subtests			
	Arithmetic	Nonsignificant		
	Digit symbol	Significant ADHD<C		
Biederman et al. 1993	1. WAIS-R			
	FDIQ	Significant ADHD<C	ADHD = 284	38.9
	Full-scale IQ	Significant ADHD<C	C = 142	39

(Continued)

Table 1
(Continued)

Author	Measures	Findings	Sample size	Mean age
Arcia and Gualtieri 1994	1. Finger tapping	Significant ADHD<C	ADHD = 23	23.4
		Significant head injury<C	Head injury = 26	29.9
		Significant head injury<ADHD	Controls = 25	27.1
	2. CPT			
	Latency	Significant ADHD>C		
		Significant head injury>C		
	3. Symbol-digit substitution test	Nonsignificant		
	4. Pattern comparison	Nonsignificant		
	5. Pattern memory			
	RT	Significant head injury<ADHD		
	Correct	Significant ADHD<C		
	6. Serial digit learning			
	Error	Significant ADHD<C		
		Head injury<C		
Holdnack et al 1995	1. WAIS-R	Significant ADHD<C	ADHD = 25	30.6
			Control = 30	26.7
	2. Gordon diagnostic			
	Vigilance	Nonsignificant		
	Distractible	Significant ADHD>C		
	Impulse	Nonsignificant		
	3. Trails			
	A	Significant ADHD>C		
	B	Nonsignificant		
	4. WCST	Nonsignificant		
	5. CVLT	Significant ADHD<C		
Silverstein 1995	1. Shipley	Nonsignificant	ADHD = 17	36
			TS = 17	32
	2. Trails		C = 17	31
	A	Nonsignificant		
	B	Nonsignificant		

	3. Stroop	Nonsignificant		
	4. Perceptual Speed Test			
	Omission errors	Nonsignificant		
	Commission errors	Nonsignificant		
	Items completed	Significant ADHD<C		
	5. WAIS-R subtests			
	Digit symbol	Significant ADHD<C		
Horton 1996	1. WAIS-R	Nonimpaired	ADHD =11 Test norms	33.4
	2. Trails			
	A	Nonimpaired		
	B	Borderline impairment		
	3. Stroop	Nonimpaired		
	4. Rhythm Test	Nonimpaired		
	5. Speech sounds	Nonimpaired		
	6. Finger tapping	Nonimpaired		
	7. Spatial Relations	Borderline impairment		
	8. Wechsler Memory Scale	Impaired		
	9. Category test	Impaired		
Downey et al. 1997	1. TOVA		n = 41 ADHD n = 37 ADHD Comorbid norms	33.2 Not reported
	Omissions	Impaired		
	Commissions	Nonimpaired		
	Variability	Impaired		
	2. Stroop	Nonsignificant		
	3. Attentional capacity test	Significant ADHD<ADHD Comorbid		
	4. Bull category test	Significant ADHD>ADHD Comorbid		
	5. CVLT	Impaired		
	6. Finger tapping	Nonsignificant		

(Continued)

Table 1
(Continued)

Author	Measures	Findings	Sample size	Mean age
Roy-Byrne et al. 1997	1. CPT		Probable ADHD = 46	33.1
	RT for correct responses	Nonsignificant	C = 46	39.5
	RT SE block change	Nonsignificant		
	RT SE ISI change	Nonsignificant		
Taylor and Miller 1997	1. Trails		ADHD = 28	34.1
	A time	Significant ADHD<C (PLC)	Psychiatric = 231	34.1
	B time	Significant ADHD<C (PLC)	Control = 211	34.1
	2. Stroop			
	Color	Significant ADHD<C (PLC)		34.1
	Interference	Significant ADHD>C (PLC)		34.1
	Word	Nonsignificant		34.1
	3. WCST			
	Categories completed	Significant ADHD<C (PLC)		34.1
	Set	Significant ADHD<C (PLC)	ADHD<P	34.1
	4. WAIS-R			
	Est IQ	Significant ADHD<C (PLC)	ADHD>P	34.1
Epstein et al. 1998	1. CPT		ADHD = 60	35
	Commission errors	Significant ADHD>C	C = 72	25
	Omission errors	Significant ADHD>C		
	Hit reaction time	Nonsignificant		
	Hit reaction time SE	Nonsignificant		
Gansler et al. 1998	1. Visual CPTs		ADHD = 30	28.9
	Omissions	Significant ADHD>C	C = 10	
	Commissions	Significant ADHD>C		
	2. WCST	Nonsignificant		
	3. Progressive planning test	Nonsignificant		
	4. Trail making A	Significant ADHD<C		
	Trail making B	Nonsignificant		
	5. Logical memory	Nonsignificant		

	6. Visual reproduction	Nonsignificant		
	7. WAIS-R subtests	Nonsignificant		
Jenkins et al. 1998	1. WAIS-R IQ		ADHD = 22	33.6
	Full	Nonsignificant	C = 18	31.7
	Verbal	Nonsignificant		
	Performance	Nonsignificant		
	2. Paced auditory serial addition test	Significant ADHD<C		
	3. COWAT	Significant ADHD<C		
	4. WCST categories	Nonsignificant		
	5. CVLT			
	Learning	Significant ADHD<C		
	Long delay	Significant ADHD<C		
	6. Luria Motortask			
	errors	Significant ADHD>C		
	7. Digit Span	Nonsignificant		
Kovner et al. 1998	1. WAIS-R IQ	Nonsignificant	ADHD = 19	33.1
	Vocab	Nonsignificant	C = 10	29.3
	Block design	Nonsignificant		
	Digit span	Significant ADHD<C		
	2. Boston Naming Test	Nonsignificant		
	3. Benton test of facial recognition	Nonsignificant		
	4. Warrington Recognition Memory Test	Nonsignificant		
	5. CPT	Nonsignificant		
	6. Shifting sets test			
	RT	Significant ADHD>C		
Seidman et al. 1998	1. WAIS-R		ADHD = 64	36.3
	Full-scale IQ	Nonsignificant	C = 73	40.1
	FD-IQ	Nonsignificant		
	2. Rey-Osterrieth	Nonsignificant		

(Continued)

Table 1
(Continued)

Author	Measures	Findings	Sample size	Mean age
	3. Auditory CPT			
	Omissions	Significant ADHD>C		
	Commission	Nonsignificant		
	4. CVLT			
	Total words	Significant ADHD<C		
	Semantic	Significant ADHD<C		
	Recall	Significant ADHD<C		
	Forgetting	Nonsignificant		
	5. WCST	Nonsignificant		
	6. Stroop	Nonsignificant		
	7. Visual Cancellations Test	Nonsignificant		
Weyandt et al. 1998	1. TOVA	Nonsignificant	ADHD = 21	25.8
			C = 24	23.4
	2. Tower of Hanoi	Nonsignificant	ORD = 19	21.5
	3. WCST			
	Total errors	Significant ADHD>C (DRD>C)		
	Perseveration Errors	Significant ADHD>C (DRD>C)		
Corbett and Stanczak 1999	1. Stroop		ADHD = 27	37.1
	Color	Significant ADHD<C	C = 15	39.5
	Word	Nonsignificant		
	C/W	Nonsignificant		
	Interference	Nonsignificant		
	2. TOADN	Significant ADHD<C		
	TOADQ	Nonsignificant		
Lovejoy et al. 1999	1. Stroop color	Significant ADHD<C	ADHD = 26	41
			Controls = 26	
	2. Trails A Time	Significant ADHD>C		
	Trails B Time	Significant ADHD>C		

	3. CVLT	Nonsignificant		
	4. COWA	Significant ADHD<C		
	5. WAIS-R FFD	Significant ADHD<C		
	6. WAIS-R IQ	Nonsignificant		
Schreiber et al. 1999	1. Rey-Osterreith CP		ADHD = 18	30.3
	Cluster accuracy	Nonsignificant	C = 18	29.5
	Configural accuracy	Significant ADHD<C		
	Detail	Nonsignificant		
	Neatness	Significant ADHD<C		
	Planning	Significant ADHD<C		
	Fragmentation	Nonsignificant		
	Vertical expansion	Nonsignificant		
	Horizontal expansion	Nonsignificant		
	Perseveration	Nonsignificant		
	Total score	Nonsignificant		
Himelstein and Haperin 2000	1. Target Orientation Task		ADHD = 9	35.3
	RT	Significant ADHD>C	C = 23	22.9
	2. Competing Motor Programs Task	Nonsignificant		
	3. CPT			
	Correct response	Nonsignificant		
	RT	Nonsignificant		
Walker et al. 2000[a]	1. CPT		ADHD = 30	25.8
	Omission errors	Significant ADHD>C	Psych group = 30	35.1
	Commission errors	Significant ADHD>C	C = 30	25.8
	Hit RT	Nonsignificant		
	2. Stroop			
	Word	Significant ADHD<C		
	Color	Significant ADHD<C		

(Continued)

Table 1
(Continued)

Author	Measures	Findings	Sample size	Mean age
	Color/Word	Significant ADHD<C		
	Interference	Nonsignificant		
	3. COWAT	Significant ADHD<C		
	4. WAIS-R subtests			
	Arithmetic	Significant ADHD<C		
	D symbol	Significant ADHD<C		
	D forward	Nonsignificant		
	D back	Significant ADHD<C		
	5. Trails AB	Nonsignificant		
		Nonsignificant		
Dinn et al. 2001	1. Object alternation test	Significant ADHD-HI<C	ADHD = 25	35.6
			C=11	35.4
	2. Go/No-Go Task			
	RT	Significant ADHD-C>C		
	3. Stroop Errors			
		Significant ADHD-C>C		
	4. Controlled Word Fluency Test	Significant ADHD-C<C		
Epstein et al. 2001	1. CPT		ADHD = 25	33.6
	Commission errors	Significant ADHD>C		
	Omission errors	ADHD>Anxiety	Anxiety disorder = 15	37.7
		Nonsignificant	Controls = 30	33.4
	2. PVOT			
	Impulsive errors	Nonsignificant		
	3. Stop-Signal Task	Nonsignificant		
Johnson et al. 2001	1. Shipley	Nonsignificant	ADHD = 56	33.3
			C = 38	40.8
	2. Wechlser Memory			
	Logical Memory I	Significant ADHD<C		

	Logical Memory II	Significant ADHD<C		
	Visual Rep I	Nonsignificant		
	Visual Rep II	Significant ADHD<C		
	3. Trails AB	Nonsignificant		
		Significant ADHD>C		
	4. Stroop			
	Word	Significant ADHD<C		
	Color	Significant ADHD<C		
	Color/word	Nonsignificant		
	5. WCST			
	Cat Comp	Nonsignificant		
	Correct	Nonsignificant		
	6. CPT			
	Omission errors	Nonsignificant		
	Commission errors	Nonsignificant		
	RT Distraction	Significant ADHD>C		
	RT Vigilance	Nonsignificant		
	7. COWA	Nonsignificant		
Murphy et al. 2001	1. CPT		ADHD = 105	21.1
	Commission errors	Significant ADHD>C	ADHD = 64	21.2
	Omission errors	Nonsignificant		
	RT	Nonsignificant		
	Variability	Significant ADHD>C		
	2. Stroop			
	Interference	Significant ADHD<C		
	Number completed	Significant ADHD<C		
	Errors	Nonsignificant		
	3. WAIS-III			
	Digit Span	Significant ADHD<C		

(Continued)

Table 1
(Continued)

Author	Measures	Findings	Sample size	Mean age
	4. Simon game	Significant ADHD<C		
	5. COWAT	Significant ADHD<C		
Rapport et al. 2001	1. WAIS-R	Nonsignificant	ADHD = 35	32.9
	2. Stroop errors		Control = 32	33.2
	Color	Nonsignificant		
	Interference	Significant ADHD<C		
		Significant ADHD<C		
	3. WCST	Nonsignificant		
	4. Trails A	Nonsignificant		
	Trails B	Significant ADHD>C		
	5. COWAT	Nonsignificant		
	6. Letter number span	Nonsignificant		
	7. ROCF	Nonsignificant		
	8. Gordon Diagnostic			
	Distractibility	Nonsignificant		
	Vigilance	Nonsignificant		
	Impulse	Nonsignificant		
Murphy 2002	1. Stop-signal paradigm		ADHD = 18	27–58
	Latency no signal	Nonsignificant	C = 18	25–59
	Latency signal	Significant ADHD>C		
Murphy 2002	1. Tower of Hanoi		ADHD = 18	27–58
	Efficiency	Significant ADHD<C	C = 18	25–59
	Moves	Significant ADHD>C		
	Errors	Nonsignificant		
	Time	Nonsignificant		
	2. Trails			
	A time	Significant ADHD>C		
	B time	Significant ADHD>C		
	3. Benton Facial Recognition Test	Nonsignificant		

Nigg et al. 2002	1. Antisoccade Motor Inhibition Task Total Errors	Significant ADHD>C	ADHD = 22	23.1
			C = 21	21.6
	2. Negative Priming Cognitive Inhibition Task Overal-RT	Significant ADHD>C		
Weyandt, et al. 2002	1. WAIS-R FFD	Nonsignificant	ADHD = 17	25.5
	2. TOVA			
	Omission errors	Significant ADHD>C		
	Commission errors	Nonsignificant		
	Mean response time	Nonsignificant		
	Variability response time	Nonsignificant		
Woods et al. 2002	1. WAIS-R IQ		ADHD = 26	38.3
	Estimate	Nonsignificant	C = 26	39.2
	WAIS-R FDD	Significant ADHD>C		
	2. COWA	Significant ADHD>C		
	3. CULT	Significant ADHD>C		
	4. Stroop color/word	Significant ADHD<C		
	5. Trails A	Significant ADHD>C		
	Trail B	Significant ADHD>C		
	6. Object usage test	Nonsignificant		
	7. Smell identification test errors	Significant ADHD>C		

Note* no significant differences between ADHD and psychiatric group on any of the neuropsychological tasks.

RT, reaction time; WAIS-R, Wechsler Adult Intelligence Scale-Revised; TOVA, Test of Variables of Attention; ISI, interstimulus interval; COWAT, Controlled Oral Word Association Test; COWA, Contextualized Writing Assignment; ADHD-HI, ADHD-hyperactive/impulsive type; ADHD-C, ADHD-combined type; Est IQ, estimated full-scale IQ.

it is possible that the inconsistencies across studies reflect true sample differences; however, given the methodological confounds and differences across studies, it appears more likely that these factors are contributing to the disparate findings.

5. ATTENTION AND BEHAVIORAL INHIBITION MEASURES

A variety of neuropsychological tasks have been used as executive function, behavioral inhibition measures. Examples of these tasks include the Matching Familiar Figures Test (MFFT), Embedded Figures Test, Benton Facial Recognition Test, Posner Visual Orienting Task, stop-signal task, and CPTs. Gualtieri et al. *(81)* and Klee et al. *(77)*, for example, reported that adults with ADHD performed similar to controls on the MFFT, a test that purportedly measures impulsivity. Hopkins et al. *(117)*, however, found that adults with ADHD made significantly more errors than controls on the MFFT, but their reaction time did not differ from controls. Hopkins et al. also found that adults with ADHD took more time to complete the Embedded Figures Tests and made significantly more errors on the EFT than control subjects. The Benton Facial Recognition Test requires subjects to match unfamiliar faces, and Murphy et al. reported that adults with and without ADHD performed similarly on this task *(117)*.

With regard to response inhibition, Dinn, Robbins, and Harris found that adults with ADHD performed more poorly on the Object Alternation Test *(89)*. Epstein et al., however, did not find differences between subjects with and without ADHD on two impulsivity measures (Posner Visual Orienting Task; PVOT, stop-signal task) *(97)*. Murphy, however, found that adults with ADHD demonstrated deficits in inhibitory control using the stop-signal paradigm *(83)*.

5.1. Continuous Performance Tests

Several CPTs are available (e.g., Gordon Diagnostic System, tests of variables of attention, Conners Continuous Performance Test); in general they are designed to measure vigilance and behavioral inhibition using a series of visual and/or auditory stimuli. The findings have been inconsistent across studies, with some studies reporting significant differences between adults with and without ADHD with respect to commission *(70,78)* and omission errors, *(63,70,73,77)* vigilance, distractibility, and variability measures *(65,78)*, and reaction time *(76,84)*, whereas other studies have not found these differences *(65,74,85–87)*. Similarly, Silverstein et al. reported that adults with ADHD made more errors than controls on a perceptual speed test, but did not differ from controls with respect to omission or commission errors *(75)*. Even within a study, results have revealed significant differences on some aspects of the CPT (e.g., vigilance number correct, omission errors) but null findings on other CPT measures (e.g., commission errors, delay conditions) *(63,65,73,74,77,83)*. Furthermore, the clinical utility of CPTs is dubious as they have not been found to reliably discriminate among clinical groups *(88)*. Walker et al., for example, investigated the CPT performance of adults with ADHD relative to a psychiatric group and a control group and found that adults with ADHD made more errors of omission and commission compared with controls, but no significant differences were found between the clinical groups *(79)*. Similarly, Weyandt et al. did not find significant differences on commission errors between young adults with ADHD and developmental reading disorder *(85)*. Riccio et al. reviewed the diagnostic efficacy of CPTs for numerous disorders in adulthood and concluded that "the symptoms detected are components of many disorders and these processes are disturbed in many of the psychopathologies listed in the DSM-IV" *(88)*.

One approach to interpreting the discrepant findings across studies is to identify CPT measures that most often produce significant results. This approach is problematic, however, as the studies differ with respect to CPT measures employed, task parameters, and CPT-dependent variables. As noted by Riccio et al., "research findings may not be generalizable across even minor variations in tasks, and generalizability across these variations cannot be assumed but must first be proven" *(88)*. What can be concluded is that in some studies, adults with ADHD perform more poorly than controls, and that CPTs do not appear to reliably discriminate clinical groups. Additional research is needed, however, to investigate the relationship between various task parameters and CPT performance in adults with ADHD. Research is also needed to further investigate the CPT performance of various clinical groups and to determine whether a single CPT, or CPT variable(s) can differentiate clinical groups.

5.2. *Stroop Neuropsychological Screening Test*

The stroop neuropsychological screening test (SNST) is thought to measure selective attention, distractibility, and response inhibition and is commonly used as an executive function measure. Studies comparing adults with and without ADHD have produced conflicting results with some studies reporting differences on color, interference, or number completed measures *(67–69,74,78,79,82,89)*. but not on the word, number completed measures, interference or total errors *(67,74,78,79,90,91)*. Weyandt et al. investigated the SNST performance of college students who were classified as having significantly high or low ADHD symptoms, and found that these two groups did not differ significantly on the SNST *(92)*. Walker et al. recently investigated the performance of adults with ADHD relative to a psychiatric group and controls and reported that those with ADHD performed significantly worse on the SNST Color, Word, and Color/Word measures but not on the interference measure *(79)*. No differences were found between the ADHD and psychiatric groups which, consistent with other neuropsychological tasks, suggests that the SNST is useful in identifying normal from aberrant performance but may not be useful in differentiating clinical groups.

6. VERBAL FLUENCY TASKS

Various verbally mediated tasks appear in the literature. One that is used rather frequently is the Controlled Oral Word Association Test (COWAT). The COWAT purportedly measures set maintenance, interference, and word initiation. Some studies have found that adults with ADHD perform more poorly on this task relative to controls *(68,69,71,78,79)*. Dinn et al. for example, reported that adults with ADHD produced fewer words relative to control participants *(89)*. Other studies have not found differences on the COWAT *(74,76)*. Similar to the CPT literature, preliminary findings suggest that efficacy of verbal fluency tasks in discriminating clinical groups is questionable *(79)*.

7. COGNITIVE FLEXIBILITY AND PLANNING MEASURES

7.1. *Trail Making Tests*

Trail Making Tests Part A is thought to measure visual scanning and numerical sequencing abilities, as well as perceptual-motor speed, and Part B is designed to measure cognitive flexibility. The results have been mixed within and across studies. Some studies have reported that adults with ADHD performed more poorly on Part B *(68,74)* but similar to controls on Part A *(74,76)*. Other studies have found the opposite pattern of performance *(65,70)*, whereas other studies have found that adults with ADHD perform more poorly than controls on Parts A and B *(68,69,82)*. Still others have compared the performance of adults with ADHD to normative data and did not find they were significantly impaired on this task *(75,89)*. Recently, Walker et al. reported that adults with ADHD, a psychiatric group, and a control group performed similarly on Parts A and B *(79)*. Taylor and Miller also compared adults with ADHD to a psychiatric group and a control group and did find that the ADHD and psychiatric groups performed significantly worse than the control group on both trails. No difference was found between the ADHD and psychiatric groups *(67)*.

7.2. Wisconsin Card Sorting Test

The Wisconsin Card Sorting Test (WCST) is frequently included as a measure of cognitive flexibility. A number of measures can be examined, including categories completed, perseveration and nonperseveration errors, and failure to maintain set. One study reviewed reported WCST performance differences between adults with and without ADHD *(67)* and on a related task, the Category Test, Horton found that adults with ADHD demonstrated impaired performance *(90)*. Most studies have not found WCST performance differences in adults with ADHD relative to controls *(65,70,71,74,85)*. More robust differences are found with cases with documented frontal lobe damage according to a recent meta-analytic review by Demakis, who reported a WCST composite effect size of small to medium (–0.33) *(93)*. One interpretation of the lack of consistent deficits on the WCST among adults with ADHD is that the WCST is sensitive to more severe frontal dysfunction and less able to detect relatively milder impairments such as those that may characterize adults with ADHD.

Additional planning and motor tasks have been used in a few studies. For example, Gansler et al. included the Progressive Planning Test, but did not find differences between adults with and without ADHD *(70)*.

7.3. Rey-Osterreith Complex Figure

The Rey-Osterreith Complex Figure (ROCF) purportedly measures visuospatial and organizational abilities and has been used more frequently in the child literature than in the adult literature. Rapport et al. and Seidman et al. did not find differences in ROCF performance in adults with and without ADHD *(63,74)*. Schreiber et al. used the Boston Qualitative Scoring System to investigate whether adults with ADHD performed differently on the ROCF relative to controls *(94)*. Results revealed that groups did not differ on the overall 36-point score, however differences were found on three indices: configural accuracy, planning, and perseveration. Using a regression model, the sensitivity and specificity in discriminating ADHD from control subjects was 75 and 81%, respectively.

7.4. Tower of Hanoi

The Tower of Hanoi (TOH) is regarded as an executive function task that measures planning and problem-solving skills and has been used extensively in the child literature. Murphy found that adults with ADHD relative to controls were less efficient on the TOH and took significantly more moves to solve the puzzles *(82)*. The groups did not differ with respect to time required to complete the task or number of errors. Weyandt et al. did not find TOH performance differences in adults with ADHD relative to adults with developmental reading disorder or to control participants *(85)*.

8. MEMORY TASKS

Various memory tasks have been used to explore the performance of adults with and without ADHD and similar to other neuropsychological tasks, the findings have been mixed. For example, letter-number span is a task that purportedly measures working memory, which has been described as an important component of executive functioning *(95)*. Rapport et al. did not find differences between adults with ADHD relative to a control group on the letter-number span task *(74)*. Similarly, Gansler et al. compared the performance of adults with and without ADHD on logical memory and visual reproduction tasks and found no significant group differences in performance on these short-term memory tasks *(70)*. Horton, however, reported that adults with ADHD exhibited impaired memory skills on the Wechsler Memory Scale *(89)*. Additionally, Arcia and Gualtieri found that adults with ADHD performed more poorly than control subjects on visual and auditory memory tasks *(84)*.

The California Verbal Learning Test (CVLT) has also been included in several adult ADHD studies. The CVLT was designed to measure various aspects of memory and learning and is frequently described as an executive function task. Research by Holdnack et al. reported that adults with ADHD demonstrated acquisition deficits on the CVLT despite average to above-average IQ *(65)*. They interpreted their findings as adults with ADHD having search-and-retrieval difficulties as well as poor strategic planning. Seidman et al. found that adults with ADHD performed significantly more poorly than controls on total words learned, semantics, and recall measures of the CVLT and similar findings were reported by Woods et al. and Jenkins et al. *(63,69,71)*. In the study by Woods et al., no differences were found between groups on the rate of forgetting measure *(69)*. Lovejoy et al. did not find group differences in performance on this measure between adults with and without ADHD *(68)*.

9. ADDITIONAL NEUROPSYCHOLOGICAL TASKS

A number of neuropsychological tasks were used less frequently in the literature. For example, Gansler et al. used the Auditory Consonant Trigrams and did not find differences between adults with and without ADHD *(70)*. However, Jenkins et al. included the Paced Auditory Serial Addition Test in a battery on neuropsychological tests and found that adults with ADHD performed more poorly than controls *(71)*. Corbett and Stanczak, and Downey et al. reported that adults with ADHD performed more poorly on an auditory processing measure compared to controls *(91,96)*.

Murphy et al. included tasks, such as the Simon game (nonverbal working memory), digit span, and object use test (cognitive flexibility) and smell identification task *(78)*. Murphy et al. found that adults with ADHD performed more poorly than controls on the Simon game and digit span, but similar to controls on the object use test *(78)*. Himelstein and Halperin investigated the information processing performance of adults with and without ADHD using a target orientation task and a competing motor program task *(86)*. The results indicated that adults with ADHD had significant difficulty with motor output and response organization rather than sustained attention problems. Similar results were reported by Dinn et al. using a go/no-go task when examining the performance of adults with ADHD and by Jenkins et al. using the error measure of the Luria motor task *(71,89)*.

Horton used a battery of neuropsychological tasks and reported that adults with ADHD performed in the normal range on most of the tasks; rhythm test, speech sounds, and finger tapping *(90)*. Downey et al. and Arcia and Gualtieri also found that adults with ADHD did not differ from controls on a finger tapping test *(84,96)*. Arcia and Gualtieri did find, however, that adults with closed head injuries performed more poorly than controls on the finger-tapping test *(84)*. Last, odor identification has also been investigated with adults with ADHD. For example, Murphy et al. found that adults with ADHD made more errors on an odor identification task, and Gansler et al. reported that adults with ADHD predominantly inattentive type made more odor identification errors than adults with the hyperactive–impulsive subtype *(70,78)*. Errors in odor identification are of course not unique to ADHD and have been found in other clinical disorders with known frontal neuropathology, such as Alzheimer's disease *(54)*.

10. DISCUSSION

It is impossible to speculate on the meaning of the adult ADHD studies without first addressing the various methodological limitations that characterize many of the studies discussed in this chapter.

10.1. Subject Issues

First, the studies differ with respect to diagnostic methods and inclusionary criteria. For example, some studies relied primarily on clinical interviews, although others relied on self-report instruments to document the presence of adult ADHD. Studies also differed to the degree to which they assessed and examined comorbidity and ADHD subtypes. For example, many studies did not control for comorbidity or if comorbidity was addressed, small sample sizes limited the degree to which the effects of this factor could be assessed. Research consistently indicates a high level of psychiatric comorbidity in adults with ADHD, which can be a potential confound when interpreting abnormal neuropsychological task performance in adults with ADHD. Whether comorbidity contributes to executive function deficits is unclear. Several studies have suggested that comorbidity does contribute to neuropsychological deficits *(67,75)*; however, other studies suggest that executive function deficits may be independent of comorbidity. Specifically, Seidman et al. demonstrated that when comorbidity was controlled for, significant neuropsychological task performance differences remained between adults with and without ADHD on several, but not all, executive function tasks *(63)*. Murphy et al. also reported that comorbidity did not account for group differences in neuropsychological task performance *(78)*.

With respect to subtypes, Gansler et al. reported that adults with with ADHD performed differently on several neuropsychological tasks depending on their subtype *(70)*. Taylor and Miller, Murphy et al., and Epstein et al., however, did not find subtype differences *(67,78,97)*. Additional studies are needed to further explore the relationship between comorbidity and subtypes and neuropsychological task performance.

Studies also differed with respect to gender and representation of ethnic groups. Because of the issue of small sample size, few studies explored the role of these variables in task performance. The few adult studies that examined gender differences were contradictory in findings. Medication usage was an additional variable that may have influenced the results and interpretation of several studies. Some studies, for example, included only participants who were taking stimulant medications *(68)*, whereas others excluded participants who were taking medication *(79,86)* and still others included both participants who were and who were not taking medication *(85,89)*. Although efforts were sometimes made to explore whether individuals taking medication differed in performance from those not taking medication, studies were not able to assess potential differential effects of type or dose of medication. Furthermore, comparisons of those taking and not taking medication reveals nothing about task performance had the individuals not been medicated.

A related issue is that most adults participating in the studies self-referred and tended to come from higher socioeconomic status (SES) and higher levels of education. This adult ADHD profile is inconsistent with follow-up studies that suggest adults with ADHD attain lower levels of formal education, are more likely to have employment difficulties, and are at greater risk for legal problems *(5,6)*. Perhaps self-referred adults with ADHD have milder neuropsychological impairments than most adults with ADHD.

10.2. Design Issues

With regard to research design, many adult ADHD studies use between-subject, cross-sectional designs; consequently, these investigations do not provide information about the neuropsychological course of ADHD. In addition, by using cross-sectional designs it is impossible to determine whether null findings are the result of attenuation of symptoms or whether neuropsychological deficits were absent earlier in life. Some have suggested that disinhibition deficits of children with ADHD attenuate with age but inattention and cognitive restlessness persist *(9,79)*. Weyandt et al. recently found that young adults with ADHD reported significantly higher levels of internal restlessness; however, this study also found that internal restlessness ratings did not correlate significantly with executive function performance as measured by a CPT *(98)*.

Although purely speculative, it is possible that lack of significant findings on neuropsychological tasks may be partially explained by early treatment interventions. Research with adult depression, for example, has found that adults who are treated with antidepressants or a combination of antidepressants are more likely to reach remission than those who are not treated with antidepressants *(114)*. Stahl has suggested that untreated depression may have irreversible neuropathological effects on the brain, which likely leads to recurrent relapse and worsening of symptoms in adulthood *(114)*. With regard to ADHD, recent ADHD outcome studies have found that children who are treated with stimulant medications often fair better later in life than children with ADHD who have received stimulant treatment *(113)*. Perhaps at a physiological level, early treatment prevents further degradation of the systems responsible for ADHD symptomology; therefore, fewer neuropsychological deficits are observed in adulthood relative to childhood. This idea is conjectural but warrants further investigation. To resolve the issue of the types of neuropsychological deficits that may or may not persist into adulthood, longitudinal studies are sorely needed.

Another problematic issue is that most of the studies adopt an exploratory approach and few are theory-driven. In other words, rather than designing a study to test a neuropsychological theory of ADHD *(99,100)*, most studies use a battery of neuropsychological tests and examine whether groups perform differently on these tests. This approach is inductive rather than deductive and tends to result in the use of multiple dependent variables. The use of multiple dependent variables can be informative but, when accompanied by small sample sizes (as is characteristic of most studies reviewed), statistical power is encumbered and Type I error rate is increased. A related issue is that effect sizes are rarely reported that would assist in the interpretation of the findings. Some studies, however, have reported modest to large effect sizes (0.08–0.18) on executive function response inhibition measures and very small effect sizes on verbally mediated executive function tasks (0.00–0.01) *(74)*. More research is needed in this area to better understand and interpret the meaning of between-group differences.

10.3. Neuropsychological Task Issues

Perhaps the greatest limitation in interpreting the meaning of the adult ADHD studies concerns the psychometric properties of the neuropsychological tasks. Many of the measures lack age-appropriate norms and may have floor and ceiling effects. For example, Seidman et al. investigated the performance of adults with and without ADHD and used the same executive function battery that they had previously used with children *(63)*. Although Seidman et al. found that adults with ADHD performed more poorly than controls on several executive function measures, they also found that groups did not differ on the ROCF, WCST, and SNST. Perhaps these null findings were an accurate reflection of the executive functioning of these groups or perhaps, as Rapport suggested about the WCST, the tests were too easy for adults *(74)*.

In addition, some of the neuropsychological tasks used in the studies have questionable reliability and validity. For example, with regard to the construct validity of executive function tasks, many of the tasks are heterogenous and have not been validated as executive function measures. Moreover, executive function is a simply a construct, broad in scope, and it has been interpreted and described differently across disciplines. Definitions have varied from vague to more explicit *(40,101)*. Factor analysis studies suggest that executive function may be characterized by three dimensions (verbal working memory, cognitive flexibility, and motor inhibition) in child clinical and nonclinical populations *(102)*. Denckla, Barkley, Borkowski and Burke, and others have advanced additional models of executive function *(80,99,100)*. Future research is needed to clarify the number and nature of the components of executive functions, especially with the adult clinical and nonclinical adult populations.

An additional factor that likely contributes to the inconsistent findings among adult ADHD studies is that many of the neuropsychological tasks used in the studies reviewed involve multiple executive function processes, as well as nonexecutive function processes. Because of their lack of precision, neuropsychological tasks have been criticized for lacking sensitivity and specificity. Sensitivity refers to the number of individuals with ADHD who perform in the impaired range on a neuropsychological instrument, whereas specificity refers to the number of individuals who do not have ADHD but perform in the impaired range on the same instrument. As noted by Alexander and Stuss, "even modern frontal tasks have both sensitivity and specificity problems" *(103)*. Research with ADHD and other clinical populations indicates that executive function tasks do not reliably detect executive function deficits, and executive function deficits may be influenced by multiple brain regions. For example, individuals with documented frontal lobe damage do not always perform poorly on measures of executive function and those without localized frontal lobe damage may perform poorly on measures of executive function *(104)*. This is problematic in general, but with regard to ADHD in adults, normal scores on executive function measures do not necessarily indicate an absence of ADHD. Furthermore, studies often do not report specificity and sensitivity rates of the neuropsychological tasks. Of those that have addressed this issue, the overall findings are unimpressive *(68,74)*. Epstein et al., for example, found that nearly half the ADHD subjects would not have been classified as having ADHD based on their CPT performance *(97)*. Overall, these findings are consistent with the children's literature that has found many neuropsychological tasks to have fair positive predictive power in accurately identifying children with ADHD, but poor negative predictive power *(105–108)*.

Another problem in the literature is an apparent confirmation bias. In other words, in most studies there is a tendency to focus on significant findings and largely disregard null findings. Even when null findings emerge more frequently than significant findings within a study, the results are typically interpreted as supporting executive function and frontal theories of ADHD. For example, Kovner et al. included 38 neuropsychological dependent measures with a sample size of 29, and found significant differences on only a set of three variables *(109)*. The main conclusion of the study, however, was that adults with ADHD may have circumscribed neuropsychological deficits, and little attention was given to the implications of the nonsignificant measures. Other studies included in this chapter have also focused on significant findings and paid scant attention nonsignificant results. One of the most frequently cited explanations for null findings in the adult ADHD literature is poor statistical power because of small sample sizes. One approach to help make sense of null (and significant) findings is to examine studies that did have adequate statistical power *(110)*. Murphy et al. conducted the largest study reviewed, with 105 adults with ADHD and 64 control subjects *(78)*. To maximize statistical power, the 105 ADHD subjects were not divided into subtypes and served as one group. After controlling for IQ, results revealed that adults with ADHD performed more poorly than controls on six of 14 dependent measures and no differences were found on the remaining eight neuropsychological tasks. Although effect sizes were not provided in this study, previous research that has found moderate to small effects on executive function tasks *(74)* therefore with adequate statistical power group differences should have been detected had they existed on the eight executive function tasks that were nonsignificant.

The issue of small sample size is difficult to address on a practical level. Most of the studies reviewed in this chapter including ADHD groups composed of 20–30 subjects, which suggests that this number is achievable, whereas larger numbers may be unattainable for most researchers. Ideally investigators would estimate the anticipated effect size for the neuropsychological variables, select an appropriate α-level given the number of dependent variables, and then calculate the necessary sample size needed for adequate statistical power *(111)*. Unfortunately, given the large number of dependent variables typically used in adult ADHD studies, large sample sizes are generally required. Perhaps what would enhance the quality of the studies and results is an increase in multisite collaboration using standard diagnostic protocols for inclusionary criteria, methods, and procedures. This approach would enhance sample size, power, interpretation, and generalizability of the findings. Gender, subtypes, and ethnicity issues could be adequately addressed as well.

Whether adults with ADHD retain extensive or select executive function deficits remains unresolved. Taylor and Miller, Lovejoy et al., Woods et al., and Murphy et al. *(67–69,78)* interpreted their findings as evidence of broad executive function deficits, whereas others reported impaired performance on only a few neuropsychological tasks *(63,70,74,85)*. To enhance the diagnostic sensitivity of neuropsychological tests, Woods et al. advocate for a discrepancy analysis approach using IQ and executive function scores *(69)*. Of course, it is possible that the executive function tests measure vastly different aspects of neuropsychological functioning and therefore select differences emerge depending on the tasks included in the study *(62)*. Piatt et al. for example, found that verbal fluency performance was unrelated to other executive function measures in a group of healthy, elderly subjects *(112)*. The authors interpreted their findings as evidence that some tasks of executive function measure different cognitive processes. Clearly more research is needed to better understand the relationship among neuropsychological tasks. If large sample sizes were possible, multivariate statistical procedures, such as principal components analysis and factor analysis would be useful in elucidating the relationship among neuropsychological tasks.

It is important to note that impairments in executive function are not unique to ADHD and have been found in other clinical samples such as autism, Tourette's syndrome, learning disabilities, schizophrenia, Alzheimer's disease, Parkinsion's disease, and phenylketonuria *(51,54,55,116)*. The majority of these research studies have compared a clinical group to a control group. Future research would benefit from double-dissociation designs using an adult ADHD group, one to several clinical groups, and a control group. In this manner, the issue of whether specific types of executive function deficits are characteristic of many or few disorders could be addressed. A few studies that have compared child clinical groups and executive task performance suggest that executive function performance may differ within and across clinical groups *(51,106)*. Pennington and Ozonoff, for example, concluded that executive function deficits are found in both children with ADHD and children with autism but not in children with Tourette's syndrome or conduct disorder *(51)*. Pennington and Ozonoff also suggested that impairments in motor inhibition are more characteristic of ADHD than autism, although impairments in working memory are more characteristic of autism than ADHD. Such interpretations of the adult studies are tenuous at best. Several investigators have posited that adults with ADHD demonstrate neuropsychological deficits in response inhibition, sustained attention, and working memory relative to control subjects, however these deficits have not been demonstrated consistently across studies. Only a handful of studies have compared the performance of adults with ADHD to a clinical group and those that have suggest that, overall, neuropsychological tasks have poor ability to discriminate clinical groups. For example, Katz et al. used a large battery of neuropsychological tasks and found that a reduced set of tasks discriminated between adults with ADHD and adults with depression with 81% accuracy *(72)*. On further analysis, however, it was revealed that although most ADHD subjects were correctly classified, 60% of those with depression were inaccurately classified into the ADHD group. Walker et al. compared the performance of adults with ADHD, a psychiatric group, and a control group and found no significant differences between the ADHD and psychiatric groups on any of the 18 neuropsychological variables *(79)*. In a recent review article, Woods et al. reported that the majority of studies investigating neuropsychological functioning of adults with ADHD found differences between adults with ADHD and controls on at least one executive function measure, but concluded that these tests have limited predictive validity *(115)*. Despite findings such as these, neuropsychological tests continue to be recommended in the assessment of ADHD in adulthood *(107)*.

11. CONCLUSION

Overall, research indicates that adults with ADHD do not exhibit a unique neuropsychological profile. Rather, the studies collectively suggest that adults with ADHD may exhibit mild neuropsychological deficits on some tasks, particularly executive function tasks that measure response inhibition and working memory. These findings do not appear to be accounted for by comorbidity but may be influenced by intelligence. Importantly, neuropsychological impairments have not been consistently found across measures or across studies. Furthermore, neuropsychological tasks do not appear to have diagnostic utility as they do not reliably discriminate adults with ADHD from other clinical groups. Additional research is needed to further investigate the construct of executive function, the validity and reliability of executive function tasks, the role of task parameters, gender, ethnicity, comorbidity, and subtypes on neuropsychological task performance. To enhance the interpretation and generalizability of adult ADHD findings, research would benefit from studies that are theory derived and methodologically robust. The study of adult ADHD is in its infancy, and future studies will likely reveal the complexities that characterize neuropsychological functioning in adults with ADHD. Ultimately these complexities will be best understood when they are considered in conjunction with neurobiological models of ADHD, neurophysiological, and neuroimaging findings.

REFERENCES

1. American Psychiatric Association. Diagnostic and statistical manual of mental disorders (4th ed., revised). Washington DC: American Psychiatric Association 2000.
2. Wender PH, Wolf LE, Wasserstein J. Adults with ADHD: an overview. Ann NY Acad Sci 2001;931:1–16.
3. Biederman J, Mick E, Faraone SV. Age dependent decline of ADHD symptoms revisited: impact of remission definition and symptom subtype. Am J Psychiatry 2000;157:816–118.
4. Fischer M, Barkley RA. Childhood ADHD and later antisocial behavior and drug use. The ADHD Report 2003;11:6–111.
5. Mannuzza S, Klein, RG, Bessler A, Malloy P, LaPadula M. Adult outcome of hyperactive boys: educational achievement, occupational rank, and psychiatric status. Arch Gen Psychiatry 1993;50:565–576.
6. Mannuzza S, Klein RG, Moulton III JL. Young adult outcome of children with "situational" hyperactivity: a prospective, controlled follow-up study. J Abnorm Child Psychol 2002;30:191–198.
7. Murphy K, Barkley R. Prevalence of DSM-IV symptoms of ADHD in adult licensed drivers: implications for clinical diagnosis. J Attention Disord 1996; 1:147–161.
8. Hill J, Schoener E. Age-dependent decline of attention deficit hyperativity disorder. Am J Psychiatry 1996;153:1143–1146.
9. Barkley RA. Age dependent decline in ADHD: true recovery or statistical illusion. The ADHD Report 1997;5:1–5.
10. Barkley RA. International consensus statement on ADHD. Clin Child Fam Psychol Rev 2002;5:89–111.
11. Faraone SV, Biederman J, Spencer T, Wilens T, Seidman LJ, Mick E, Doyle AE. Attention-deficit/hyperactivity disorder in adults: an overview. Biol Psychiatry 2000;48:9–20.
12. Robins E, Guze SB. Establishment of diagnostic validity in psychiatric illness: its application to schizophrenia. Am J Psychiatry 1970;126:983–987.
13. Sherman DK, Iacono, WG, McGue MK. Attention-deficit hyperactivity disorder dimensions: a twin study of inattention and impulsivity-hyperactivity. J Am Acad Child Adolesc Psychiatry 1997;36:745–753.
14. Willcutt EG, Pennington BF, DeFries JC. Etiology of inattention and hyperactivity/impulsivity in a community sample of twins with learning difficulties. J Abnorm Child Psychol 2000;28:149–159.
15. Faraone SV, Biederman J. Neurobiology of attention-deficit hyperactivity disorder. Biol Psychiatry 1998;44:951–958.
16. Burt AS, Krueger RF, McGue M, Iacono W. Sources of covariation among attention-deficit/hyperactivity disorder, oppositional defiant disorder, and conduct disorder: the importance of shared environment. J Abnorm Psychol 2001;110;516–525.
17. Mostofsky SH, Reiss AL, Lockhart P, Denckla MB. Evaluation of cerebellar size in attention-deficit hyperactivity disroder. J Child Neurol 1998;9:434–439.
18. Castellanos FX, Giedd JN, Marsh WL, et al. Quantitative brain magnetic resonance imaging in attention-deficit hyperactivity disorder. Arch Gen Psychiatry 1996;53:607–616.
19. Castellanos FX, Lee PP, Sharp W, et al. Developmental trajectories of brain volume abnormalities in children and adolescents with attention-deficit/hyperactivity disorder. JAMA 2002;288:1740–1748.
20. Giedd JN, Castellanos FX, Casey BJ, et al. Quantitative morphology of corpus callosum in attention deficit hyperactivity disorder. Am J Psychiatry 1994; 151:665–669.

21. Hynd GW, Semrud-Clikeman M, Lorys AR, Novey ES, Eliopulos D, Lyytinen H. Corpus callosum morphology in attention deficit-hyperactivity disorder. J Learn Dis 1991;24:141–146.
22. Lyoo KI, Noam GG, Lee CK, Lee HK, Kennedy BP, Renshaw PF. The corpus callosum and lateral ventricles in children with attention-deficit hyperactivity disorder: a brain magnetic resonance imaging study. Biol Psychiatry 1996;40:1060–1063.
23. Halperin J, Newcorn JH, Kopstein I, et al. Serotonin, aggression, and parental psychopathology in children with attention-deficit/hyperactivity disorder. J Am Acad Child and Adolesc Psychiatry 1997;36:1391–1398.
24. Lou HC, Henrikson L, Bruhn P. Focal cerebral hypoperfusion in children with dysphasia and/or attention deficit disorder. Arch Neurol 1984;41:825–829.
25. Zametkin AJ, Nordahl ET, Gross M, et al. Cerebral glucose metabolism in adults with hyperactivity of childhood onset. N Engl J Med 1990; 323:1361–1366.
26. Yeo RA, Hill DE, Campbell RA, et al. Proton magnetic resonance spectroscopy investigation of the right frontal lobe in children with attention-deficit/hyperactivity disorder. J Am Acad Child Adolesc Psychiatry 2003;42:303–310.
27. Teicher MH, Anderson CM, Glod CA, Maas LC, Renshaw PF. Functional deficits in basal ganglia of children with attention-deficit/hyperactivity disorder shown with functional magnetic resonance imaging relaxomety. Nat Med 2000;6:470–474.
28. Teeter PA, Semrud-Clikeman M. Integrating neurobiological, psychosocial, and behavioral paradigms: a transactional model for the study of ADHD. Arch Clin Neuropsychol 1995;10:433–461.
29. Stefanatos GA, Wasserstein J. Attention deficit/hyperactivity disorder as a right hemisphere syndrome: selective literature review and detailed neuropsychological case studies. Ann NY Acad Sci 2001;931:172–195.
30. Berquin PC, Giedd JN, Jacobsen LK et al. Cerebellum in attention-deficit hyperactivity disorder: a morphometric MRI study. Neurology 1998;50:1087–1093.
31. LaHoste GJ, Swanson JM, Wigal SB, et al. Dopamine D4 receptor gene polymorphism is associated with attention deficit hyperactivity disorder. Mol Psychiatry 1996;1:121–124.
32. Lou HC. Etiology and pathogenesis of attention-deficit hyperactivity disorder (ADHD): significance of prematurity and perinatal hypoxic-haemodynamic encephalopahthy. Acta Pediatrics 1996;85:1266–1271.
33. Swanson J, Castellanos FX, Murias M, LaHoste G, Kennedy J. Cognitive neuroscience of attention deficit hyperactivity disorder and hyperkinetic disorder. Curr Opin Neurobiol 1998;8:263–271.
34. Stuss DT. Biological and psychological development of executive functions. Brain Cogn 1992;20:3–8.
35. Fletcher JM. Executive functions in children: introduction to the special series. Dev Neuropsychol 1996;12:1–3.
36. Pliszka SR. Attention-deficit/hyperactivity disorder. In: Steven R. Pliszka's Neuroscience for the mental health clinician. New York: Guilford Press, 2003:143–144.
37. Wender PH. Minimal brain dysfunction in children. New York: Wiley-Interscience, 1971.
38. Satterfield JH, Dawson ME. Electrodermal correlates of hyperactivity in children. Psychophysiology 1971;8:191–197.
39. Mattes J. The role of frontal lobe dysfunction in childhood hyperkinesis. Compr Psychiatry 1980;5:358–369.
40. Bianchi L. The mechanism of the brain and the function of the frontal lobes. Edinburgh: Livingstone, 1922.
41. Luria A. Hiher cortical functions in man. New York: Basic Books, 1966.
42. Goldman-Rakic P. Development of cortical circuitry and cognitive function. Child Dev 1987;58:601–622.
43. Cohen JD, Forman SD, Braver TS, et al. Activation of the prefrontal cortex in nonspatial working memory task with functional MRI. Human Brain Mapping 1994;1:293–304.

44. Carter CS, Braver TS, Barch DM, Botvinic MM, Noll D, Cohen JD. Anterior cingulate cortex, error detection, and online monitoring of performance. Science 1998;280:747–749.
45. Lou HC, Henrikson L, Bruhn P. Focal cerebral dysfunction in developmental learning disabilities. Lancet 1990;335:8–11.
46. Amen DG, Paldi JH, Thisted RA. Brain SPECT imaging. J Am Acad Child Adolesc Psychiatry 1993;32:1080–1081.
47. Rubia K, Overmeyer S, Taylor E, et al. Hypofrontality in attention deficit hyperactivity disorder during higher-order motor control: a study with functional MRI. Am J Psychiatry 1999;156:891–896.
48. Vaidya CJ, Austin G, Kirkorian Ridlehuber HW, Desmond JE, Glover GH, Gabrieli JDE. Selective effects of methylphenidate in attention deficit hyperactivity disorder: a functional magnetic resonance study. Proc Natl Acad Sci USA 1998;95:14,494–14,499.
49. Welsh MC, Pennington BF, Groisser, BB. A normative-developmental study of executive function: a window on prefrontal function in children. Dev Neuropsychol 1991;7:131–149.
50. Christ SE, White DA, Brunstrom JE, Abrams RA. Inhibitory control following perinatal brain injury. Neuropsychol 2003;17:171–178.
51. Pennington BF, Ozonoff S. Executive functions and developmental psychopathology. J Child Psychol Psychiat 1996;37:51–87.
52. Channon S, Pratt P, Robertson MM. Executive function, memory, and learning in Tourette's syndrome. Neuropsychol 2003;17:247–254.
53. Klorman R, Hael-Fernandez GA, Shaywitz SE, et al. Executive functioning deficits in attention deficit hyperactivity disorder are independent of oppositional defiant or reading disorder. J Am Acad Child Adolesc Psychiatry 1999;38:1148–1155.
54. Koss E, Weiffenback JM, Haxby JV, Friedland RP. Olfactory detection and identification performance are dissociated in early alzheimer's disease. Neurology 1988;38:1288–1232.
55. Arnett PA, Rao S, Grafman J, et al. Executive functions in multiple sclerosis: an analysis of temporal ordering, semantic encoding, and planning abilities. Neuropsychol 1997;11:535–544.
56. Dery M, Toupin J, Pauze R, Mercier H, Fortin L. Neuropsychological characteristics of adolescents with conduct disorder: association with attention-deficit-hyperactivity and aggression. J Abnorm Child Psychol 1999;27:225–236.
56a. Weyandt LL. Executive function in children, adolescents, and adults with ADHD: introduction to the special issue. Dev Neuropsychol 2004;27;in press.
57. Fischer M, Barkley RA, Edelbrock CS, Smallish L. The adolescent outcome of hyperactive children diagnosed by research criteria: II. academic, attentional, and neuropsychological status. J Consult Clin Psychol 1990;5:580–588.
58. Seidman LJ, Biederman J, Faraone SV, Weber W, and Ouellette C. Toward defining a neuropsychology of attention deficit-hyperactivity disorder: Performance of children and adolescents from a large clinically referred sample. Consult Clini Psychol, 1997;65:150–160.
59. Doyle AE, Biederman J, Seidman LJ, Weber W, Faraone SV. Diagnostic efficiency of neuropsychological test sc0ores for discriminating boys with and without attention deficit-hyperactivity disorder. J Consult Clin Psychol 2000;68:477–488.
60. Hinshaw SP, Carte ET, Sami N, Treuting JJ, Zupan BA. Preadolescent girls with attention-deficit/hyperactivity disorder: II. neuropsychological performance in relation to subtypes and individual classification. J Consult Clin Psychol 2000;70:1099–1011.
61. Barkley RA, Grodzinsky G, DuPaul GJ. Frontal lobe functions in attention deficit disorder with and without hyperactivity: a review and research report. J Abnorm Child Psychol 1992;20:163–188.
62. Tremont G, Halpert S, Javorsky DJ, Stern RA. Differential impact of executive dysfunction on verbal list learning and story recall. Clin Neuropsychol 2000;14:295–302.
63. Seidman LJ, Biederman J, Weber W, Hatch M, Faraone SV. Neuropsychological function in adults with attention-deficit hyperactivity disorder. Biol Psychiatry 1998;44:260–268.
64. Tannock R. Cognitive correlates of ADHD. In: Jensen, PS, Cooper JR, eds. Attention deficit hyperactivity disorder: state of the science, best practices, 8–1 to 8–27. NJ: Civic Research Institute.

65. Holdnack JA, Moberg PJ, Arnold SE, Ruben C, Gur RC, Gur RE. Speed of processing and verbal learning deficits in adults diagnosed with attention deficit disorder. Neuropsychiatr, Neuropsychol, Behav Neurol 1995;8:282–292.
66. Biederman J, Faraone SV, Spencer T, et al. Patterns of psychiatric comorbidity, cognition, and psychosocial functioning in adults with attention deficit hyperactivity disorder. Am J Psychiat 1993;150:1792–1798.
67. Taylor CJ, Miller, DC. Neuropsychological assessment of attention in ADHD adults. J Attention Disord 1997;2:77–88.
68. Lovejoy DW, Ball JD, Keats M, et al. Neuropsychological performance of adults with attention deficit hyperactivity disorder (ADHD): diagnostic classification estimates for measures of frontal lobe/executive functioning. J Intern Neuropsychol Society 1999;5:222–233.
69. Woods SP, Lovejoy DW, Stutts M, Ball JD, Fals-Stewart W. Comparative efficiency of discrepancy analysis for the classification of attention-deficit/hyperactivity disorder in adults. Arch Clin Neuropsychol 2002;17:351–369.
70. Gansler DA, Fucetola R, Krengel M, Stetson S, Zimering R, Makary C. Are there cognitive subtypes in adult attention deficit/hyperactivity disorder? J Nerv Ment Dis 1998;186:776–781.
71. Jenkins M, Cohen R, Malloy P, et al. Neuropsychological measures which discriminate among adults with residual symptoms of attention deficit disorder and other attentional complaints. Clin Neuropsychol 1998;12:74–83.
72. Katz LJ, Wood DS, Goldstein G, Auchenbach RC, Geckle M. The utility of neuropsychological tests in evaluation of attention deficit/hyperactivity disorder (ADHD) versus depression in adults. Assessment 1998;5:45–51.
73. Weyandt LL, Mitzlaff L, Thomas L. The relationship between intelligence and performance on the test of variables of attention (TOVA). J Learn Dis 2002;35:114–120.
74. Rapport LJ, Voorhis AV, Tzelepis A, Friedman SR. Executive functioning in adult attention-deficit hyperactivity disorder. Clin Neuropsychol 2001;15:479–491.
75. Silverstein SM, Como PG, Palumbo DR, West LL, Osborn LM. Multiple sources of attentional dysfunction in adults with Tourette's syndrome: comparison with attention deficit-hyperactivity disorder. Neuropsychol 1995;9:157–164.
76. Johnson DE, Epstein JN, Waid R, Latham PK, Voronin KE, Anton RF. Neuropsychological performance deficits in adults with attention deficit/hyperactivity disorder. Arch Neuropsychol 2001;16:587–604.
77. Klee S, Garfinkel BD, Beauchesne RN. Attention deficits in adults. Psychiatr Ann 1986;16:52–56.
78. Murphy KR, Barkley RA, Bush T. Executive functioning and olfactory identification in young adults with attention deficit-hyperactivity disorder. Neuropsychol 2001;15:211–220.
79. Walker AJ, Shores EA, Trollor JN, Lee T, Sachdev PS. Neuropsychological functioning of adults with attention deficit hyperactivity disorder. J Clin Exp Neuropsychol 2000;22:115–124.
80. Denckla MB. A theory and model of executive function: a neuropsychological perspective. In: Lyon RG, Krasnegor NA, eds. Attention, memory and executive function. Baltimore: Paul H. Brookes, 1996:263–278.
81. Gualtieri CT, Ondrusek MG, Finley C. Attention deficit disorders in adults. Clin Neuropharmacol 1985;8:343–356.
82. Murphy P. Cognitive functioning in adults with attention-deficit/hyperactivity disorder. J Attention Disord 2002;5:203–209.
83. Murphy P. Inhibitory control in adults with attention-deficit/hyperactivity disorder. J Attention Disord 2002;6:1–4.
84. Arcia E, Gualtieri CT. Neurobehavioural performance of adults with closed-head injury, adults with attention deficit, and controls. Brain Inj 1994;8:395–404.
85. Weyandt L, Rice JA, Linerman I, Mitzlaff L, Emert E. Neuropsychological performance of a sample of adults with ADHD, developmental reading disorder, and controls. Dev Neuropsychol 1998;14:643–656.
86. Himelstein J, Halperin JM. Neurocognitive functioning in adults with attention-deficit/hyperactivity disorder. CNS Spectrums 2000;5:58–64.

87. Roy-Byrne P, Scheele L, Brinkley J, et al. Adult attention-deficit hyperactivity disorder: assessment guidelines based on clinical presentation to a specialty clinic. Compr Psychiatry 1997;38:133–140.
88. Riccio CA, Reynolds CR, Lowe PA. Clinical applications of continuous performance tests: measuring attention and impulsive responding in children and adults. New York: John Wiley & Sons, 2001:233–257.
89. Dinn WM, Robbins NC, Harris CL. Adult attention-deficit/hyperactivity disorder: neuropsychological correlates and clinical presentation. Brain Cogn 2001;46:114–121.
90. Horton AM. Neuropsychological findings in adult attention deficit disorder: a pilot study. Appl Neuropsychol 1996;3:181–185.
91. Corbett B, Stanczak DE. Neuropsychological performance of adults evidencing attention-deficit hyperactivity disorder. Arch Clin Neuropsychol 1999;14:373–387.
92. Weyandt LL, Linterman I, Rice JA. Reported prevalence of attentional difficulties in a general sample of college students. J Psychopathol Behav Assessment 1995;17:293–304.
93. Demakis GJ. A meta-analytic review of the sensitivity of the wisconsin card sorting test to frontal and lateralized frontal brain damage. Neuropsychol 2003;17:255–264.
94. Schreiber HE, Javorsky DJ, Robinson JE, Stern RA. Rey-Osterreith complex figure performance in adults with attention deficit hyperactivity disorder: a validation study of the Boston qualitative scoring system. Clin Neuropsychol 1999;13:509–520.
95. Pennington BF, Bennetton L, McAleer O, Roberts RJ. Executive functions and working memory In: Lyon RG, Krasnegor NA, eds. Attention, memory and executive function. Baltimore: Paul H Brookes, 1996;327–348.
96. Downey KK, Stelson FW, Pomerleau OF, Giordani B. Adult attention deficit hyperactivity disorder: psychological test profiles in a clinical population. J Nerv Ment Dis 1997;185:32–38.
97. Epstein JN, Johnson DE, Varia IM, Conners CK. Neuropsychological assessment of response inhibition in adults with ADHD. J Clin Exp Neuropsychol 2001;23:362–371.
98. Weyandt LL, Iwaszuk W, Fulton K, et al. The internal restlessness scale: performance of college students with and without ADHD. J Learn Dis 2003;36:382–389.
99. Barkley RA. Behavioral inhibition, sustained attention, and executive functions: constructing a unifying theory of ADHD. Psychol Bull 1997;121:64–94.
100. Borkowski JG, Burke JE. Theories, models, and measurements of executive functioning: an information processing perspective. In: Lyon RG, Krasnegor NA, eds,. Attention, memory and executive function. Baltimore: Paul H Brookes, 1996;235–261.
101. Welsh MC and Pennington BF. Assessing frontal lobe functioning in children: views from developmental psychology. Dev Neuropsychol 1988;4:199–230.
102. Pennington BF. Dimensions of executive functions in normal and abnormal development. In: Krasnegor NA, Lyon RG, Goldman-Rakic PS, eds. Development of the prefrontal cortex: evolution, neurobiology, and behavior. Baltimore: Brookes 1997;265–281.
103. Alexander MP, Stuss DT. Disorders of frontal lobe functioning. Semin Neurol 2000;20:427–37.
104. Anderson SW, Damasio H, Jones RD, Tranel D. Wisconsin card sorting test performance as a measure of frontal lobe damage. J Clin Exper Neuropsychol 1991;13,909–922.
105. Grodzinsky GM, Barkley RA. The predictive power of frontal lobe tests in the diagnosis of attention deficit hyperactivity disorder. Clin Neuropsychol 1999;13:12–21.
106. Weyandt LL, Willis GW. Executive functions in school-aged children: potential efficacy of tasks in discriminating clinical groups. Dev Neuropsychol 1994;10:27–38.
107. Gallagher R, Blader J. The diagnosis and neuropsychological assessment of adult attention deficit/hyperactivity disorder: scientific study and practical guidelines. Ann NY Acad Sci 2001;931:148–171.
108. Perugini EM, Harvey WA, Lovejoy DW, Sandstrom K, Webb AH. The predicitve power of combined neuropsychological measures for attention-deficit/hyperactivity disorder in children. Child Neuropsychol 2000;6:101–114.
109. Kovner R, Budman C, Yitzchak F, Sison C, Lesser M, Halperin J. Neuropscychological testing in adult attention deficit hyperactivity disorder: a pilot study. Int J Neurosci 1998;96:225–235.

110. Rossi JS. Statistical power of psychological research: what have we gained in 20 years? J Consult Clin Psychol 1990;58:646–656.
111. Kraemer HC, Thiemann S. How many subjects: statistical power analysis in research. CA: Sage Publications, 1987, pp. 22–29.
112. Piatt AL, Fields JA, Paolo AM, Troster AI. Action (verbal naming) fluency as an executive function measure: convergent and divergent evidence of validity. Neuropsychologia 1999;37:1499–1503.
113. Barkley RA, Fischer M, Smallish L, Fletcher K. Does the treatment of attention-deficit/hyperactivity disorder contribute to drug use/abuse? A 13-year prospective study. Pediatrics 2003;111:97–109.
114. Stahl SM. Essential psychopharmacology of depression and bipolar disorder. New York: Cambridge University Press 2000.
115. Woods SP, Lovejoy DW, Ball JD. Neuropsychological characteristics of adults with ADHD: a comprehensive review of initial studies. Clin Neuropsychol 2002;16:12–34.
116. Heinrichs RW, Zakzanis K. Neurocognitive deficit in schizophrenia: a quantiative review of the evidence. Neuropsychol 1998;12:426–445.
117. Hopkins J, Perlman T, Hechtman L, Weiss G. Cognitive style in adults originally diagnosed as hyperactives. J Child Psychol Psychiatry 1979;20:209–216.

21

Psychostimulants in Attention Deficit Hyperactivity Disorder

Theoretical and Practical Issues for the Community Practitioner

Daniel F. Connor

1. INTRODUCTION

The clinical use of stimulants for behavioral disturbances in children and adolescents first began in 1937 at the Emma Pendleton Bradley Home for Children in Rhode Island. Charles Bradley, a psychiatrist, was working with brain-injured children who had received a pneumoencephalogram as part of a standard clinical diagnostic workup. This procedure commonly resulted in severe headache for the children. Bradley decided to use an amphetamine, Benzedrine, in an attempt to ameliorate the headache pain. When given amphetamine, the children demonstrated immediate improvements in their disruptive behaviors. Bradley also noted improved academic performance, better self-control, and improved attention to task. Bradley published his findings in 1950 after using amphetamines for two decades to treat hyperactivity, impulsivity, and moodiness in clinically referred children *(1)*.

In the 1960s the first double-blind placebo-controlled clinical trials of dextroamphetamine and methylphenidate were completed and confirmed Bradley's initial clinical impressions. Since then, more than 200 controlled trials of stimulants have been completed *(2)*. These studies demonstrate the efficacy of the stimulants in improving the core symptoms of attention deficit hyperactivity disorder (ADHD) and enhancing behavioral, academic, and social functioning in about 50% to 95% of children treated. Variability in response rates is largely because of the presence of comorbid psychiatric and developmental disorders *(3–5)*.

Historically, most of the individuals for whom stimulants were prescribed were school-aged children between 5 and 12 yr of age *(6)*. However, longitudinal studies in ADHD consistently demonstrate the persistence of symptoms and impairment across multiple domains of daily life functioning into adolescence and adulthood in the majority of children diagnosed with ADHD *(7,8)*. Increasingly, stimulants are being prescribed for adolescents and adults meeting criteria for ADHD *(9)*.

Despite the overwhelming amount of research documenting the efficacy of stimulants for the symptoms of ADHD, the stimulants should rarely be the only form of therapy provided to individuals with ADHD. For some cases of mild ADHD, enhanced organizational skills, cognitive behavioral therapies, education about the disorder, and/or school or occupational supports may be sufficient to lessen the impact of the disorder on daily life. However, it is

From: *Attention Deficit Hyperactivity Disorder: From Genes to Patients*
Edited by: D. Gozal and D. L. Molfese © Humana Press Inc., Totowa, NJ

important to recognize that stimulants are the only treatment modality to date that are known to normalize symptoms of inattention, impulsivity, and overactive behavior in individuals with ADHD *(10)*. Furthermore, the effect size of stimulants has been found to be greater than the effect size of psychosocial therapies for the core symptoms of ADHD, at least over periods of time up to 14 mo *(11)*.

The purpose of this chapter is to review recent advances in stimulant therapy for ADHD, review pharmacodynamic and pharmacokinetic actions of stimulants, and review safety and tolerability data for stimulant use. The emphasis in this chapter is clinical with the overall goal of enhancing the practitioner's safe and effective clinical use of stimulant medications, particularly in the treatment of ADHD.

2. STIMULANTS

Stimulants are referred to as such because of their ability to activate the level of activity, arousal, or alertness of the central nervous system (CNS). Stimulants in clinical use include racemic methylphenidate, dextromethylphenidate, dextroamphetamine, mixed amphetamine salts (a combination of D-amphetamine and amphetamine), and magnesium pemoline. Pemoline is rarely used because of elevated risk of liver toxicity and is considered a second-line agent for the treatment of ADHD; therefore, it will not be discussed further. Other CNS stimulants, such as caffeine and deanol, are not discussed here because they have not been found to be nearly as effective as the CNS stimulants, and cannot be recommended for clinical use.

2.1. *Indications for Use of Stimulant Medications*

2.1.1. *Established Indications*

Established indications for stimulants include ADHD in children, adolescents, and adults. Stimulants are helpful in treating age-inappropriate and impairing symptoms of inattention to task, impulsive behavior, and motor hyperactivity that are not owing to another cause, such as depression, bipolar disorder, anxiety disorders, or psychotic disorders, and are persistently severe enough to cause impaired functioning in school, work, home, or the community. All three subtypes of ADHD (combined, hyperactive-impulsive, and inattentive types) respond to stimulant therapy *(3)*. Narcolepsy is also an established indication for stimulant medications but will not be further discussed here.

2.1.2. *Probable Indications*

Probable indications for stimulants include the treatment of symptoms of ADHD in preschool children and children with comorbid conditions, such as mental retardation, autism spectrum disorders, head trauma, and seizure disorders *(12–21)*.

Seven out of eight randomized, controlled clinical trials demonstrate the efficacy of stimulants for symptoms of ADHD in 3- to 6-yr old children *(12)*. Compared with older ADHD children, the efficacy of stimulant treatment is more variable, and there is a higher rate of side effects, especially sadness, irritability, clinging behavior, insomnia, and anorexia *(22)*. Stimulant therapy for preschool children should be reserved for particularly severe cases of ADHD, and only after parent management training, family behavioral therapy, and preschool educational supports have been unsuccessful or are unavailable.

Stimulants may be effective for symptoms of ADHD in children with mental retardation. Recent studies support the use of stimulants in the treatment of ADHD symptoms in these youngsters, especially if the IQ is greater than 50 and the mental age is greater than 4.5 yr *(13–15)*. However, for youths with more severe mental retardation stimulant medications may not be well tolerated *(14,15)*.

According to the *Diagnostic and Statistical Manual of Mental Disorders*, 4th edition (DSM-IV) criteria, ADHD is excluded as an additional diagnosis when autism or pervasive developmental disorders are present. The symptoms of ADHD are then thought to be part of the autistic disorder and not thought to warrant an additional diagnosis of ADHD. However, the target symptoms of distractibility, impulsivity, and hyperactivity may respond to stimulants in children or adults with autism *(16)*. Careful clinical monitoring of autistic individuals on stimulants is indicated because adverse events may be hidden among all the other symptoms autistic patients may have and make medication side effects difficult to recognize.

Neurological injury may cause hyperactivity, distractibility, and/or impulsivity especially if the frontal cortex sustains injury. Randomized controlled studies suggest the efficacy of stimulant medications for brain-damaged children or adults with trauma-acquired symptoms of ADHD *(17)*.

Finally, attention deficit can be a frequent symptom of epilepsy in children, adolescents, and adults. It is unclear whether the symptoms of ADHD are caused by the epilepsy, are exacerbated by anticonvulsant medications, or are a separate, comorbid disease. A few controlled studies have investigated the safety and efficacy of methylphenidate in children with the dual diagnosis of ADHD and epilepsy *(18–21)*. These studies generally conclude that stimulant therapy is safe when epilepsy is stable on anticonvulsant therapy. No influence of methylphenidate on the plasma level of antiepileptic drugs is documented *(21)*. What remains unclear is the effect of stimulants on seizure thresholds in epileptic patients who are untreated or are poorly controlled on antiepileptic therapy. In such patients, there is evidence that methylphenidate may lower the seizure threshold and exacerbate the risk of seizures *(20)*.

2.2. *Pharmacoepidemiology of Stimulant Use*

Stimulant use among children and adolescents in the United States has grown substantially over the past 15 yr. Between 1987 and 1996 the prevalence of stimulant use among youths less than 18 yr old increased three- to sevenfold *(23)*. This growth also includes increased prescribing rates of stimulants for preschool children. Since 1990 there has been a threefold increase in stimulant prescriptions for 2- to 4-yr-old children *(24)*. This growth takes place within the context of a threefold overall increase in total psychoactive medication prescribing for youngsters across all classes of psychiatric medication since 1991 *(23)*.

Among stimulants, methylphenidate use ranked foremost among children and adolescents, accounting for 77–87% of all stimulant prescriptions since 1991. A dramatic increase in amphetamine prescribing occurred with the introduction of mixed amphetamine salts (Adderall®, Shire US, Inc., Florence, KY) in 1996. Over the past decade, a seven- to 14-fold increase in amphetamine prescriptions has been observed in both Medicaid and in health maintenance organizations *(23,25)*. Because of warnings about elevated risk of hepatic failure, pemoline use has declined in youngsters over this same time period *(26)*.

With growing recognition that ADHD persists into adulthood in the majority of children diagnosed in elementary school, physicians are beginning to use stimulants to treat ADHD across the lifespan *(2,27)*. To date, there have been no pharmacoepidemiological studies of stimulant use for ADHD in adulthood. However, with growing recognition of the ADHD diagnosis in adults, stimulant use in this population is expected to grow.

Stimulants are often combined with other psychiatric medications for the treatment of ADHD and comorbid conditions and the use of combined treatment is also increasing in the United States. In a national sample of physician office visits for youths less than 18 yr old, the rate of combined stimulant and antidepressant use increased from 4% in 1994 to 29% in 1997. This reflects a sevenfold increase over 3 yr *(28)*. On the basis of Medicaid claims data, it was reported that 30% of youths receiving a selective serotonin reuptake inhibitor (SSRI) antidepressant also had a stimulant prescription during the same year, strongly suggesting combined use *(29)*. A particularly common concomitant psychotropic medication combination for youths has been methylphenidate and clonidine. Estimates from a national pharmaceutical market source found that 41% of surveyed youths in 1994–1995 who were receiving methylphenidate were also receiving clonidine *(30)*. In clinical practice, stimulants are often combined with atypical antipsychotic medications in the treatment of the highly aggressive ADHD child. However, no data on the prevalence of this practice is presently available.

Although stimulants have been shown to be highly effective in the treatment of the core symptoms of ADHD *(11)*, their use is not without controversy. During the 1990s concerns were expressed over the increased prevalence of use among school-aged children, the uncertainty surrounding the implications of long-term use in children, and studies showing geographical variation in prevalence of use *(31)*. Particular concern was expressed about overmedication of children with stimulants *(32)*. However, pharmacoepidemiological research has reported both overprescribing and underprescribing of stimulants to youths in the United States *(25,32–35)*. Furthermore, marked geographic variation in stimulant prescribing rates has been reported, even after controlling for differences in predictors such as age and gender. Compared to children living in the western region of the United States, children living in the Midwest and South appear more likely to be prescribed a stimulant medication *(36)*. The reasons for geographic variation appear complex. Sources of variation may include differences in the populations studied by different pharmacoepidemiological researchers, differences in research methodology across studies, and differences in the way different specialty physicians identify and diagnose ADHD *(35,36)*.

2.3. *Basic Pharmacology of Stimulants*

Stimulants are structurally similar to the monoaminergic CNS neurotransmitters. There are two prevailing hypotheses regarding the underlying neurophysiology of ADHD that involve neural systems that are subserved by the catecholamines, dopamine and norepinephrine. The focus on dopamine was derived from the fact that stimulant medications are known to alter the transmission of dopaminergic neurons in the CNS. This hypothesis has been further substantiated by neuroimaging studies that have consistently identify alterations in the structure and functioning of dopamine-rich regions of the CNS, such as the prefrontal cortex, striatum, basal ganglia, and cerebellum, in children and adults meeting clinical criteria for the ADHD phenotype *(37,38)*. However, stimulants also affect noradrenergic neurotransmission and an alternative noradrenergic model has been proposed to explain the effects of stimulants in ADHD. This model focuses on the inhibitory influences of frontal cortical circuits, which are predominantly noradrenergic, acting on striatal structures to indirectly alter dopaminergic activity *(39)*. This model is further supported by the presence of an anterior CNS attentional system in the prefrontal cortex, and a posterior CNS attentional system located in prefrontal, posterior, and parietal-locus ceruleus neuronal networks, both of which involve noradrenergic transmission *(40)*.

2.3.1. Mechanism of Action

The primary mode of action of stimulants is to enhance catecholamine activity in the CNS, probably by increasing the availability of norepinephrine and dopamine at the synaptic cleft *(41)*. Preclinical studies have shown that methylphenidate and amphetamine block the reuptake of dopamine and norepinephrine into the presynaptic neuron *(1,3,39,42)*. The stimulants largely exert their action by reversibly binding to the presynaptic transporter protein with resultant inhibition of catecholamine reuptake into the presynaptic neuron, increasing concentrations of catecholamines in the extraneuronal space, and thus presumably enhancing postsynaptic CNS catecholaminergic neurotransmission *(43)*. Amphetamine also increases the release of dopamine from presynaptic cytoplasmic storage vesicles and blocks the uptake of dopamine into neuronal cytoplasmic storage vesicles, making dopamine more available in the presynaptic cytoplasm for release into the synaptic cleft. These slightly differing mechanisms of action of amphetamine and methylphenidate suggest that they are not identical and that both types of stimulants should be tried if a patient does not have a satisfactory response to an initial stimulant trial *(44)*. A meta-analysis of 141 subjects showed that 40% of the patients responded equally well to either methylphenidate or D-amphetamine, but 26% responded better to methylphenidate, and 35% had a superior response to D-amphetamine *(45)*.

Thus, it appears that alterations in both dopaminergic and noradrenergic function occur and may be necessary for clinical efficacy of the stimulants in treating ADHD *(39,46,47)*.

2.3.2. Absorption and Metabolism

In clinical practice, stimulants are given orally. Absorption is rapid and complete from the gastrointestinal tract. Stimulants reach their maximal clinical effect during the absorption phase of the kinetic curve, approx 2 h after ingestion *(48)*. Stimulants cross the blood–brain barrier and are taken up into the CNS. The absorption phase parallels the acute release of neurotransmitters into CNS synaptic clefts, supporting theories of stimulant mechanism of action on CNS catecholamines in ADHD *(46)*. Methylphenidate slow release has a more variable and less complete absorption, which may explain its diminished efficacy compared to more rapidly and completely absorbed stimulants *(49,50)*. Methylphenidate and amphetamine are metabolized in the body by different mechanisms. After absorption, methylphenidate undergoes extensive first-pass hepatic metabolism predominately by hydrolysis. The predominant route of metabolism is de-esterification to inactive ritalinic acid, which is readily excreted and accounts for 80% of the dose. The remaining 20% of the drug is oxidized by a hepatic mixed-function oxidase *(51)*.

Amphetamine is metabolized by side-chain oxidative deamination and ring hydroxylation in the liver *(46,51,52)*. The majority of amphetamine is excreted unchanged in the urine (~80%), along with benzoic acid, hippuric acid, and hydroxyamphetamine catabolites *(52)*. Because amphetamine is a highly basic compound, urinary excretion is dependent on urinary pH. Urine acidification (i.e., by ingestion of ascorbic acid or orange juice) results in a shortened plasma half-life and increased amphetamine clearance. Acidification of the urine is useful to facilitate amphetamine clearance in overdose and subsequent toxicity *(51)*. Patients receiving amphetamines for ADHD who note decreasing clinical efficacy should be monitored for vitamin C (ascorbic acid) consumption *(46)*.

2.3.3. Pharmacokinetics and Preparations

There are two theories that relate pharmacokinetics to stimulant efficacy in ADHD. The first theory is called the ramp effect. It has been theorized that the more rapidly the brain concentration of stimulants increases, the greater the effect on improved vigilance or reduction of hyperactivity. In this model, stimulant efficacy with regards to the symptoms of ADHD are proportional to the rate of stimulant absorption into the CNS *(53)*. This model argues that stimulants with a rapid rate of absorption will be more effective than stimulants with a slower rate of absorption. The second theory relates the maximal plasma concentration of stimulant to efficacy in ADHD. This theory is called the "threshold model" *(54)*. In this model, stimulant efficacy is proportional to peak stimulant brain concentrations. At present, it is unclear whether the rate of absorption (ramp effect) or the peak plasma or brain concentration of stimulants (threshold effect) accounts for stimulant efficacy in ADHD.

Table 1 shows the varying durations of action of the available stimulant formulations.

2.3.3.1. Immediate-Release Preparations

Immediate-release stimulants include both methylphenidate and amphetamine compounds. Methylphenidate has a rapid onset of action within 20–60 min and a peak plasma concentration within 1–2 h post ingestion, with an elimination half-life of 3–6 h *(46,51)*. Its plasma half-life is 1–3 h, but concentrations in the CNS exceed those in plasma *(51)*. Dextromethylphenidate is the optically pure stereoisomer of racemic methylphenidate and has pharmacokinetic parameters similar to D,L-methylphenidate *(55)*. Amphetamine compounds include D-amphetamine and mixed amphetamine salts. These agents have a rapid onset of action with peak clinical effects occurring within 1–2 h. They have a serum half-life and a behavioral half-life of 4–6 h, slightly longer than methylphenidate preparations.

2.3.3.2. Intermediate-Acting Preparations

Methylphenidate is available in intermediate-acting preparations. These compounds are designed to last longer than immediate-release preparations and have a somewhat slower onset of action. Newer formulations such as Metadate® CD and Ritalin-LA® have a bimodal clinical effect designed to mimic the actions of immediate release methylphenidate given twice daily *(56)*.

2.3.3.3. Once-Daily Preparations

Once-daily stimulant formulations are available as Concerta® and Adderall XR®. Concerta encapsulates methylphenidate in an oral osmotic-release drug delivery system (OROS) that is similar to immediate release methylphenidate given three times daily. The duration of action of Concerta is 10–14 h *(57)*. Concerta demonstrates an ascending methylphenidate plasma concentration curve throughout the day. Research has shown that rising methylphenidate plasma levels are necessary for stimulants to retain their efficacy over the course of the day. In contrast, flat methylphenidate dosing regimens (indicative of older slow release methylphenidate preparations) lose about 40% of their efficacy by the afternoon. This is owing to the phenomenon of tachyphylaxis, or acute tolerance, to methylphenidate that can develop under multiple daily dosing conditions. An ascending dose curve overcomes this acute tolerance and maintains methylphenidate efficacy throughout the day *(46,58,59)*. Adderall XR contains a bead technology consisting of 50% immediate release and 50% slow release XR beads *(60)*. The immediate release beads release stimulant medication immediately after ingestion, whereas the XR beads release 4 h later. The 50/50 ratio of immediate release to XR beads allows for therapeutic effects to begin within a time frame comparable to shorter-acting formulations, with ascending stimulant plasma levels facilitating ADHD

Table 1
Actions of Available Stimulant Medications[a]

	Brand name	Onset of action (min)	Peak clinical effect (h)	Serum half-life (h)	Duration of behavioral action (h)	Required number of daily doses
Immediate-release preparations						
Methylphenidate	Ritalin®, Methylin®, Metadate®	20–60	2 (range: 0.3–4)	3–6	3–6	2–3
Dextromethylphenidate	Focalin®	20–60	2 (range: 0.3–4)	2.2	4	2–3
Dextroamphetamine	Dextrostat®, Dexedrine®	20–60	1–2	12	4–6	2–3
Mixed amphetamine salts	Adderall®	30–60	1–2	12	4–6	2
Intermediate-release preparations						
Methylphenidate	Ritalin-SR®, Metadate®ER, Methylin®ER	60–90	~5 (range: 1.3–8.2)	NR	4–8	2
Methylphenidate	Metadate®CD, Ritalin-LA®	30–120	Bimodal pattern[b]	1.5–6.8	6–8	1–2
Dextroamphetamine	Dexedrine Spansule®	60–90	8	12	6–8	1–2
Extended-release preparations						
Methylphenidate	Concerta®	30–120	Bimodal pattern[b]	6–8	12	1
Mixed amphetamine Salts extended-release	Adderall®XR	60–120	Bimodal pattern[b]	9–11	10–12	1

NR, not reported; XR, slow releases
[a]Use of pemoline has been associated with rare but life-threatening hepatic failure. It is not considered first-line therapy for ADHD and is not included in this table.
[b]These medications display a bimodal release pattern of stimulant, representing early and late release of stimulant medication.

symptom relief over an extended time period *(61,62)*. Adderall XR is designed to mimic the actions of immediate release Adderall given twice daily *(62)*.

2.3.3.4. TRANSDERMAL PATCHES

Not included in Table 1 is a methylphenidate transdermal skin patch system under development called MethyPatch® (Noven Pharmaceuticals) *(63)*. This is an embedded drug adhesive transdermal patch, worn on the hip, in which methylphenidate is solubilized in a silicone and acrylic adhesive diffusion technology. Each patch provides duration of ADHD treatment for up to 12 h.

2.3.3.5. STIMULANT ENANTIOMERS

Numerous psychotropic drugs exist as a mixture of two mirror-image stereoisomers of each other; each is called an enantiomer (e.g., dextro [D] and levo [L]) and the mixture is called a racemate. Enantiomers are new drugs made by removing one mirror-image stereoisomer from a mixture of two contained in the original drug. Often the drug can be improved when only one of the enantiomers is clinically administered. Improvements may include lessened side effects, reduced drug–drug interactions, and better efficacy including a better relationship between efficacy and a reduced drug dose *(64)*.

Methylphenidate contains a 50/50 racemic mixture of the D-*threo* and L-*threo* isomers of methylphenidate. Research shows that D-*threo*-methylphenidate is the pharmacologically active enantiomer *(65)*. Recent advances in stereo-specific manufacturing allow commercial preparations of optically pure D-*threo*-methylphenidate (D-methylphenidate, dexmethylphenidate), and a preparation containing only this enantiomer could provide a better therapeutic index in ADHD than a racemic mixture. An immediate release enantiomer of methylphenidate called Focalin® (dextromethylphenidate) has been released by Novartis *(66)*. Compared with placebo, Focalin is effective for the symptoms of ADHD. However, its advantages over other immediate release stimulant preparations are presently not clear.

2.3.4. Clinical Effects of Stimulants

More than 200 randomized, controlled studies exist on the effects of the stimulants on the core symptoms of ADHD *(2,10,46,67)*. Most of these studies have been conducted with methylphenidate. The vast majority of research reports on studies of 6–12-yr-old ADHD children. However, preschool children, adolescents and adults have been shown to respond to stimulants as well *(12,46,68,69)*.

In general, studies indicate that between 73 and 77% of ADHD children initially treated with a stimulant are described as improved in their symptoms *(3,67)*. Between 25 and 30% of ADHD children do not respond or do not tolerate initial stimulant medication. If a second stimulant is clinically tried, response rates increase *(44,70)*. As stated previously, both a methylphenidate and an amphetamine preparation should be tried before other classes of agents are considered. Research has identified a group of ADHD children with preferential responses to methylphenidate, another group who responds to amphetamine, and a third group that responds to both stimulants *(45)*. It is important to note that placebo response rates in ADHD are generally low. Controlled efficacy studies of stimulants examining differences between stimulants and placebo in ADHD report placebo responses ranging from 2 to 39% *(67,71)*. In the recent large multimodal treatment study of children with ADHD, placebo response rates of about 13% were reported *(11)*.

2.3.4.1. Effects on Behavior

Impulsive aggressive and hyperactive behavior commonly accompanies ADHD in childhood and adolescence and may have large consequences for the affected individual *(72)*. Explosive outbursts of temper to common everyday frustrations are often difficult for families of ADHD youths to cope with and mange and often lead to a deterioration in familial functioning. In adolescence, impulsive and hyperactive behaviors contribute to social functioning problems, higher risk for antisocial behavior, increased risk of cigarette smoking, and automobile driving accidents *(73–76)*. In adulthood, impulsivity and poor judgment contribute to higher mortality rates from automobile accidents, vulnerability to antisocial behaviors, and increased risk for substance abuse *(76–79)*.

Stimulants have robust effects on these age inappropriate behaviors that commonly cause impairment on a daily basis for individuals with ADHD. These behaviors often include impulsivity, disruptiveness, noncompliance, talking out of turn and out-of-seat behaviors, restlessness, and impulsive displays of aggression *(80–82)*. Stimulant dose effects are generally linear and positive on core behavioral problems in ADHD, such that higher doses might be more effective than lower doses *(82)*. However, dose must be individualized for each ADHD patient. A meta-analysis of stimulant effects on aggressive behavior in ADHD, separate from effects on the core symptoms of inattention, impulsivity, and hyperactivity, found large effect sizes for stimulant treatment on symptoms of overt and covert aggression *(83)*. This suggests that ADHD may amplify or increase conduct problem behaviors in some children, and that treatment of ADHD symptoms with stimulants may reduce vulnerability to antisocial and aggressive behaviors *(84)*.

2.3.4.2. Effects on Cognition, Learning, and Academic Performance

Numerous studies have found that stimulants enhance performance on measures of vigilance, impulse control, fine motor coordination, and reaction time *(3,10,85–87)*. Higher stimulant doses tend to be associated with more robust responses, and clinicians should beware of underdosing. Positive drug effects have been obtained on measures of short-term memory and learning of paired verbal or nonverbal material *(88,89)*. Performance on both simple and complex learning paradigms appears to be enhanced, and perceptual efficiency and speed of symbolic and verbal information retrieval is facilitated *(90,91)*. Stimulant therapy improves school-based academic productivity and accuracy in treated ADHD children *(3,92–94)*. Studies support positive dose response relationships on cognitive measures associated with learning in the classroom *(95)*. ADHD laboratory school-based data suggest that positive medication effects in the classroom enhancing vigilance, attention focus, and impulse control do not adversely affect children's spontaneous play activities at recess *(46)*.

Despite beneficial effects on learning in ADHD children, stimulants do not enhance functioning on more traditional measures of cognitive potential and academic ability such as intelligence tests *(67)*. In general, stimulants seem particularly salient in school situations that require children to inhibit their behavior and focus on assigned tasks. It remains to be determined if these acute effects of stimulants on cognition, learning, and academic performance translate into enhanced academic success for ADHD children over the long term *(3,10)*.

2.3.4.3. Effects on Interpersonal and Social Relationships

Treatment with stimulant medication has been found to improve the quality of social interactions between children with ADHD and their parents, teachers, and peers *(10)*. In young

ADHD youths, stimulants increase children's compliance with parental commands, decrease hostile and negative responses, and enhance the ADHD child's responsiveness to the interactions of others *(22,96,97)*. Beneficial effects of stimulant treatment have also been documented in the interactions between ADHD children and their teachers *(98)*. Stimulant medications not only directly alter the behavior of children with ADHD but also indirectly affect the behaviors of important adults and peers toward the ADHD child. When these relationships improve, they may contribute further to a positive treatment response in the child.

Improvements in interpersonal and social relationships with stimulant treatment of the adolescent with ADHD and adult have not been studied as thoroughly as in children with ADHD. However, improvements in social judgment and interpersonal relationships with clinical treatment of the adolescent with ADHD and adult are beginning to be documented *(2,7,9,27,79,99,100)*.

3. LIFE-SPAN AND ADHD SYMPTOMS

3.1. Preschool ADHD Children

Because current diagnostic criteria require an early age of onset (<7 yr old) for a diagnosis of ADHD, children in the preschool age range (3–6 yr old) may come to clinical attention for accurate diagnosis and treatment. For example, in one study of 300 children consecutively referred to an ADHD clinic, mothers reported 202 children (67%) as having an age-of-onset of ADHD symptoms that interfered with daily functioning at age 4 yr or younger *(101)*. Thus, the physician who treats children with ADHD will be asked to evaluate and treat preschool children for ADHD.

Stimulants should not be the first line treatment for the symptoms of ADHD in the very young child. Parent-management behavioral methods using a compliance training model meet criteria for evidenced-based treatment for childhood ADHD, disruptive behavior, noncompliance, and oppositional–defiant behavior, and should always be tried first *(12,102,103)*. However, for the severely hyperactive youngster, or the ADHD preschool child for whom parent-management training methods have been tried and failed, stimulant therapy is sometimes considered.

Currently, nine controlled clinical trials of stimulants in ADHD preschool children 3–6 yr old are reported in the clinical literature. These studies appear in Table 2.

Eight controlled studies evaluate preschool ADHD children with normal cognition and one study evaluates ADHD in preschool children with developmental disabilities *(104)*. Random assignment to treatment occurred in 78% of these studies, and 89% (8 of 9) of studies support efficacy of stimulants for the symptoms of ADHD in the preschool age range. Only methylphenidate has been studied in preschool ADHD. Doses are generally low, ranging between 2.5 and 30 mg/d. Studies generally support linear dosing effects in the preschool age range, with higher doses improving inattention, impulsivity, and academic productivity compared with lower doses *(105)*. Children less than 3 yr old have not been studied. Side effects of stimulants are generally reported as elevated in the preschool ADHD child compared with treated older ADHD children *(106)*. Response rates may be more variable in this population compared with older children receiving stimulants *(12)*.

Rising rates of prescriptions for psychotropic medications given to US children aged 2–5 yr have raised concerns that not enough is known about the safety and efficacy of these agents in preschoolers *(24,107)*. The majority of these prescriptions are stimulants used for the

Table 2
Stimulant Efficacy for Preschool Minimal Brain Dysfunction, Hyperactivity, or ADHD

Study (ref.)	No. of subjects	Age in yr mean/range	Study design	Random assignment	Duration (wk)	Mean MPH dose/range	Response
Schleifer *(215)*	26	4.1/3.4–4.10	B-PC-CO	+	9	10 mg/d 2.5–30 mg/d	Mixed, many side effects reported. No improvements seen on direct obs or lab tests
Conners *(216)*	59	4.8/3–6	B-PC-PG	+	6	12 mg/d 0.7 mg/kg/d	Improvement in behavioral domains. High variability in individual response noted
Cunningham *(217)*	12	–/4–6	B-PC-CO	+	Four sessions	0.15–0.50 mg/kg/d	Improvement in cognitive, behavioral, and interpersonal domains
Barkley *(218)*	18	–/4–5.11	B-PC-CO	+	3	0.3–1 mg/kg/d	Improvement in interpersonal domain
Barkley *(22)*	27	–/2.5–5	B-PC-CO	+	3	0.3–1 mg/kg/d	Improvement in interpersonal domain
Mayes *(219)*	14	–/1.8–5	B-PC-ABA	–	3	7.5–30 mg/d	Improvement in behavioral domain
Monteiro-Musten *(220)*	31	–/4.0–5.8	B-PC-CO	+	3	0.6–1 mg/kg/d	Improvement in cognitive, behavioral, and interpersonal domains
Byrne *(221)*	8	5.2/–	B-CC	–	20	15–30 mg/d	Improvement in cognitive, behavioral, and interpersonal domains
Handen *(104)*	11	4.9/4–5.11	B-PC-CO	+	4	0.3 or 0.6 mg/kg/d	All with developmental delay. IQs ranged between 40 and 78. 73% responders. Increased rate of side effects
TOTAL *(9)*	206	1.8–6	Nine controlled	Seven/nine studies (78%)	3–20	0.15–1 mg/kg/d 2.5–30 mg/d	Eight/nine studies (89%) support efficacy in preschool ADHD. More side effects in those with dev delay

B-PC-CO, blind, placebo-controlled crossover design; B-PC-PG, blind, placebo-controlled, parallel-group design; B-PC-ABA, blind, placebo-controlled, off-on-off treatment reversal design; B-CC; blind, case-control design.

treatment of very early onset ADHD *(25)*. In response to these concerns, the National Institute for Mental Health is currently funding the Preschool ADHD Study, a multisite clinical trial now under way to determine the safety and efficacy of methylphenidate in preschoolers with ADHD *(107)*.

3.2. Adolescents With ADHD

In the past many clinicians believed that stimulant treatment lost its therapeutic effects after puberty. This view contributed to a common clinical practice of discontinuing stimulants at puberty. Current research demonstrates that stimulants continue to have efficacy for ADHD symptoms in adolescence, and that their effects are equivalent to the stimulant benefits seen in younger children with ADHD *(108,109)*. The current standard of care is to continue to treat ADHD with stimulants in the postpubertal years.

Although more is presently known about stimulant efficacy in ADHD adolescents, less research has been completed in this age group compared to research in the school age population. Seven controlled trials of stimulants for ADHD in adolescents are described in Table 3.

The majority of controlled studies (six of seven studies, 85.7%) support the continued efficacy of stimulants in the treatment of adolescents with ADHD. Most of these studies investigate methylphenidate preparations. Linear dosing effects are described in some studies of adolescents *(110,111)*, but not in other studies *(112,113)*. Currently, it remains unclear if adolescents with ADHD respond better to low or to high stimulant doses. Therefore, treatment must be individualized. Overall, studies show a stimulant response rate of about 60–75%, indicating that medication is effective in teenagers with ADHD *(46)*. In these studies no abuse or tolerance to stimulants were noted *(2)*.

3.3. Adults With ADHD

ADHD in adults is poorly recognized in most clinical settings and is a frequently missed clinical diagnosis. Comorbid psychiatric diagnoses, such as depression, substance abuse, anxiety, or antisocial behaviors frequently cloud the clinical picture and contribute to missing the diagnosis of ADHD in referred adults *(114)*. Current research indicates that between 30 and 70% of children with ADHD will continue to have symptoms of ADHD in adulthood *(115)*. The estimated prevalence of ADHD in all adults is 4.5% *(9)*. Unlike ADHD in children, in adults with ADHD outward signs of hyperactivity/impulsivity are replaced by a subjective sense of inner restlessness accompanied by cognitive disorganization, inattention to task, distractibility, forgetfulness, and impulsive decision-making *(79,116)*. This makes the task of clinical diagnosis more difficult for the clinician treating ADHD in adults. However, ADHD is important to recognize and treat in adulthood as continuing symptoms may impair adult functioning across a variety of domains *(117)*.

The role of stimulant medications in treating adults with ADHD is no different than it is with children and adolescents. Adults with ADHD respond to stimulants with improved attention span, decreased distractibility, diminished restlessness, and lessened impulsivity, in a similar fashion to younger patients with ADHD *(69)*. Controlled studies of stimulants in adults with ADHD are listed in Table 4.

In comparison with the large database that exists on the efficacy of stimulants for ADHD in children, only nine controlled stimulant trials have been reported in adult ADHD. These trials have examined methylphenidate, dextroamphetamine, and pemoline. In contrast to the robust and consistent 70% response rates reported for children with ADHD, controlled studies

Table 3
Controlled Stimulant Studies for Adolescent ADHD

Study (ref.)	No. of subjects	Age in yr mean/range	Study design	Random assignment	Duration (wk)	Mean stimulant dose/range	Response
Varley *(71)*	22	14.2/13–18	B-PC-CO	+	3	15.2–30.9 mg/kg/d	73% response rate
Klorman and Coons *(110,111)*	19	14.8/12–19	B-PC-CO	+	3	40 mg/d	Improvement: behavior and information processing parents > teachers
Brown *(222)*	11	13.7/12–15	B-PC-CO	+	8	5.8–25.9 mg/d	75% of measures showed improvement on drug
Barkley *(223)*	35	14.0/12–17	B-PC-CO	+	5	MPH: 5–10 mg/d MAS: 5–10 mg/d	No improvement
Smith *(113)*	46	13.8/12–17	B-PC-CO	+	8	25–75 mg/d	Improvement: no linear effects of dose on improvement
Bostic *(224)*	21	14.1/12–17	B-PC-CO	+	10	PEM 150 mg/d 93–225 mg/d	60% response rate compared to 11% placebo response rate
Greenhill *(68)*	177	13–18	B-PC-PG	+	2	OROS MPH 18, 36, 54, or 72 mg/d	Improvement on all measures compared with placebo
TOTAL *(7)*	331	12–19	Seven controlled	Seven randomized	3–10	MPH 5–75 mg/d PEM 93–225 mg/d MAS 5–10 mg/d	6/7 (85.7%) of studies support efficacy

MPH, methylphenidate; MAS, mixed amphetamine salts (Adderall®); OROS MPH, Concerta®; B-PC-CO, blind, placebo-controlled crossover design; B-PC-PG, blind, placebo-controlled parallel group design.

Note: medication is methylphenidate in this table unless otherwise stated.

Table 4
Controlled Stimulant Studies for Adult ADHD

Study (ref.)	No. of subjects	Age in yr mean/range	Study design	Random assignment	Duration (wk)	Mean stimulant dose/range	Response
Wood *(118)*	11	28 ± 4.5	B-PC-CO	–	4	23.5 mg/d 20–60 mg/d (MPH)	53% response rate
Wender *(119)*	51	28/21–45	B-PC-PG	+	6	65 mg/d 18–150 mg/d (PEM)	50% response rate
Mattes *(122)*	26	32/18–45	B-PC-CO	+	6	48 mg/d 10–60 mg/d (MPH)	25% response rate
Wender *(120)*	37	31 ± 6.7	B-PC-CO	+	5	48 mg/d 10–80 mg/d	57% response rate
Gualtieri *(225)*	22	27.5/18–38	B-PC-CO	+	2	0.5–2.0 mg/kg/d (MPH)	Moderate response rates
Spencer *(27)*	23	40/19–56	B-PC-CO	+	7	1.0 mg/kg/d (MPH)	78% response on drug 4% response to placebo
Wilens *(226)*	35	40.7/23–60	B-PC-CO	+	10	2.2 mg/kg/d 86–200 mg/d (PEM)	50% responders. 17% placebo responders
Paterson *(227)*	45	35.5/19–57	B-PC-PG	+	6	5–35 mg/d (DEX)	58% responders. 10% placebo responders
Schubiner *(228)*	48	38.3/18–55	B-PC-PG	+	12	26.2 ± 6.5 mg/d (MPH)	77% responders, 21% placebo responders. Comorbid cocaine abusers
TOTAL *(9)*	298	19–60	9 controlled	8 randomized	2–12	MPH 10–80 mg/d DEX 5–35 mg/d PEM 18.75–200 mg/d	Lower response rates than children

B-PC-CO, blind, placebo-controlled crossover design; MPH, methylphenidate; DEX, D amphetamine; PEM, pemoline; B-PC-PG, blind, placebo-controlled parallel group design.

in adults report more equivocal response rates. With the exception of the Spencer et al. *(27)* study, response rates in adults range between 25 and 58%.

Variability in adult ADHD response rates may be related to several factors. These include difficulty recognizing the adult ADHD phenotype with subsequent enrollment of heterogeneous subjects into clinical trials *(118–120)*, high rates of comorbidity in adults with ADHD *(9,121)*, and the low doses of stimulants used in many clinical trials of ADHD adults. For example, in controlled studies limiting methylphenidate to doses less than 0.7 mg/d, response rates range from 25 to 57% *(118,120,122)*. However, Spencer and colleagues report a much higher response rate of 78% when higher doses of methylphenidate are used, up to 1 mg/kg/d *(27)*. For adults with ADHD, response rates may become more robust when higher stimulant doses are used.

4. TREATMENT OF ADHD IN THE PRESENCE OF COMORBID PSYCHIATRIC DISORDERS

In children and adolescents with ADHD, higher rates of comorbid oppositional defiant disorder (ODD), conduct disorder (CD), major depressive disorder (MDD), and anxiety disorders are found compared with control youths without ADHD *(5,10,123,124)*. In adults with ADHD higher rates of antisocial personality disorder, substance abuse, bipolar disorder (BPD), MDD, and anxiety disorders are found compared to controls without ADHD *(79,125)*. This section reviews stimulant use for ADHD when the diagnosis is complicated by psychiatric comorbidity.

4.1. ADHD and ODD/CD

About 50% of ADHD children will meet criteria for either ODD or CD. The prevalence of the association between ADHD and ODD/CD will vary with the age of the child. Children under the age of 12 yr who meet criteria for ODD or CD will almost always meet criteria for ADHD *(126)*. In adolescent samples, pure CD is more common and only about 33% of teenage CD patients will also meet criteria for ADHD *(126)*.

Many studies have compared the response of ADHD + CD and ADHD-alone children to stimulant medications. When stimulant is compared with placebo in controlled clinical trials, ADHD + CD youths show an equally robust response to stimulant as do ADHD-without-CD children *(84,127,128)*. ADHD children with ODD/CD show the same reductions in inattention, impulsivity, and hyperactivity as do noncomorbid ADHD children. Thus childhood antisocial behavior does not seem to attenuate stimulant response for ADHD symptoms.

In ADHD youngsters with comorbid conduct disorder and aggression, stimulants appear to reduce antisocial behaviors in addition to their effects on the core symptoms of ADHD. In a meta-analysis of 28 controlled stimulant studies for ADHD, stimulants reduced symptoms of overt aggression (effect size = 0.84) and covert aggression (effect size = 0.69) *(83)*. Although it is not clear whether stimulants help impulsive aggression in children without ADHD, they can help decrease the frequency and intensity of aggressive outbursts in children with ADHD. The effects of stimulants on adults with ADHD and antisocial personality disorder have not been studied.

4.2. ADHD and Depression

It is not uncommon to encounter children who are demoralized or dysphoric about the consequences of their impulsive ADHD behaviors. Such children appear depressed, but the depression is short-lived and generally occurs only after a frustration or a disciplinary event. Thus brief episodes of depressed or irritable mood may be common in the ADHD child, occur many times a day, and do not necessarily meet the criteria for a major depressive disorder (MDD). This demoralization will get better as the ADHD is treated.

The syndrome of MDD, identified by a persistently depressed, sad, or irritable mood, different from the child's usual personality, lasting for days to weeks, and accompanied by guilt, anhedonia, social withdrawal, and suicidal thoughts, occurs in between 15 and 30% of ADHD children and adolescents *(123,124,129–131)*. True ADHD comorbidity with MDD requires treatment of both the ADHD and the depression.

No studies have compared stimulant response in a group of children with the diagnosis of ADHD and a group with the psychiatric diagnoses of ADHD + MDD. However, several studies have investigated stimulant response in ADHD accompanied by the symptoms of depression (internalizing psychopathology, not the psychiatric diagnosis of MDD). There are hints that symptoms of depression may reduce the clinical response to stimulants in ADHD. For example, DuPaul and colleagues studied 40 children with ADHD and divided the sample into three groups based on the severity of comorbid internalizing symptoms. Differential effects of three doses of methylphenidate (5, 10, and 15 mg) were evaluated in a controlled methodology using multiple outcome measures across home, school, and clinic settings. Results showed that ADHD children with comorbid internalizing symptoms were less likely to respond to methylphenidate than children without comorbid internalizing psychopathology *(132)*. In the large multimodal treatment studies for children with ADHD (MTA) study, ADHD children with anxiety/depression seemed to do best in the combined treatment arm (stimulants and behavioral therapy) rather than the stimulant arm alone *(133)*. In contrast, Gadow and colleagues found no diminished response rate to stimulants for the symptoms of ADHD when children had comorbid anxious and depressive psychopathology *(134)*.

The clinician treating patients with ADHD must be vigilant for comorbid depressive disorders. If present, both ADHD and depression should be treated. Stimulants have been safely combined with SSRIs, such as fluoxetine, in children, adolescents, and adults *(135,136)*.

4.3. *ADHD and Bipolar Disorder*

The prevalence of childhood bipolar disorder in children with ADHD is a topic of controversy and debate. This controversy arises out of a lack of consensus as to how to identify the bipolar child. Part of the problem is the high degree of symptom overlap between ADHD and bipolar symptoms (e.g., irritability, mood lability, aggression, hyperactivity/agitation, sleep disturbance). In primary care practice, the prevalence of childhood bipolar disorder is rare. Among ADHD children a few may have early onset bipolar disorder. For example, after screening many referrals Geller et al. identified 60 prepubertal children with bipolar mania. All had comorbid ADHD. Factors that most differentiated manic children from ADHD children were grandiosity, excessively elated mood, racing thoughts, hypersexuality, and decreased need for sleep *(137,138)*.

If the child is acutely manic as well as having ADHD, mood stabilization with lithium, divalproex sodium, and/or an atypical antipsychotic is indicated before treatment with a stimulant. Once the acute manic symptoms have stabilized, the clinician should reassess the patient for ADHD. If ADHD symptoms continue to be problematic, stimulants may be added to a mood stabilizer to treat continuing ADHD symptoms *(139)*.

4.4. *ADHD and Anxiety Disorders*

About 25–30% of children with ADHD will meet criteria for an anxiety disorder compared with 5–15% of comparison youths *(140,141)*. Initial studies suggested that the response of ADHD children to stimulant medications was less when comorbid anxiety disorders were present. For example, in a study of 43 ADHD children treated with methylphenidate under controlled conditions, more than 80% of the nonanxious ADHD children were stimulant responders, whereas only 30% of ADHD/anxiety children benefited from the medication *(142)*. In an unselected group of ADHD children, low anxiety ratings predicted a good response to stimulants *(143)*. These earlier studies suggested that anxiety disorders or symptoms could diminish ADHD stimulant response rates.

However, more recent studies have not supported diminished stimulant responses in anxious ADHD youths. In a short-term controlled trial, anxious and nonanxious ADHD children had equally robust responses to methylphenidate *(144)*. In the large MTA study, more than 100 children received a double-blind, placebo-controlled trial of methylphenidate, and more than one third of subjects had comorbid anxiety disorders. Anxiety did not predict a poorer response to stimulant medication *(11)*. However, in the MTA study anxious ADHD children seemed to benefit more from a combination of psychosocial treatment and medication than nonanxious ADHD children.

In clinical practice, the anxious ADHD child should be treated for ADHD first. Since the response to stimulant medication can be assessed quickly and anxious/ADHD children do not generally worsen on stimulant medications, a stimulant trial is the first intervention. Should anxiety continue to be a problem, a psychosocial intervention or a trial of an SSRI for anxiety could be implemented in addition to stimulant medication *(145)*.

4.5. ADHD and Tic Disorders

Tic disorders are common in non referred children assessed in the community. In large samples of children ascertained in the community the prevalence of motor tics is about 21% *(146)*. Motor tics appear more commonly than vocal tics. Tic prevalence appears to vary with gender and age of the child. Tics are more common in boys than girls, and are more common in preschool children than in older children *(147)*. For example, in a large nonclinical community study of more than 3000 children and adolescents, the prevalence of tic disorders in 3- to 5-yr-old children was six times the prevalence rate in 12- to 18-yr-old teenagers *(147)*. The prevalence of tic disorders may vary by the season of the year. One study of 553 children in kindergarten through sixth grade found that the incidence of motor tics increased in the winter months and diminished in the summer months *(148)*.

Controlled studies have demonstrated an association between tic disorders and ADHD that occurs at a rate greater than expected by chance alone *(146,147,149)*. In clinical samples of boys with tic disorders, Tourette's syndrome co-occurs with ADHD in between 21 and 54% of cases *(5,124,150)*. In samples of ADHD children tic disorders are found at a lesser rate. For example, in the MTA study of 579 ADHD children, 10.9% had a comorbid tic disorder *(11)*.

Methodologically controlled studies have shown that stimulant medications are highly effective for ADHD symptoms, aggression, and social skill deficits in children with Tourette's syndrome or chronic tic disorders *(147,151–155)*. These studies show that the rate of tic disorders in children with ADHD with preexisting tic disorders treated with stimulants are not different from rates of tics in placebo treated ADHD + tic children *(152,154,155)*.

However, numerous clinical observations have reported that stimulants exacerbate tic frequency and intensity in children with ADHD with preexisting tic disorders *(156)*. This has led clinicians to undertreat ADHD in children with tic disorders. There is now a much greater understanding that the consequences of untreated ADHD are much greater than the consequences of mild to moderate tic disorders on the child's social, behavioral, interpersonal, and academic development. Although stimulants may exacerbate a preexisting tic disorder, the frequency and intensity of tics generally return to baseline after several months of stimulant treatment. In children who develop severe tics with the use of stimulants, most tics will remit after the stimulant is discontinued *(46)*. There is little evidence that tic disorders are created *de novo* by the introduction of stimulants in children who are not already vulnerable to tic disorders (generally on a heritable basis).

The current standard of care has now evolved to a recommendation to treat moderate to severe ADHD in children with mild to moderate tic disorders. Careful informed consent with parents and close monitoring of tic frequency and severity are necessary aspects of treatment. Should tics become problematic controlled studies support the use of clonidine *(155)* or guanfacine *(157)* in the treatment of comorbid ADHD and tic disorders.

4.6. *ADHD and Learning Disabilities*

An overlap between ADHD and learning disabilities is frequently reported in both children and adults *(158,159)*. Learning disabilities include expressive and receptive language delays, auditory processing difficulties, and reading disabilities. A wide range of overlap was reported in some studies of between 10 and 92% of ADHD children also having learning disabilities *(160)*. More recent studies report a smaller overlap of ADHD and learning disabilities of between 20 and 25% *(150)*. The wide disparity in comorbidity is probably owing to different definitions of learning disabilities used in various studies.

Research supports independence of learning disabilities and ADHD as two separate disorders, although they may frequently co-occur. The two disorders are transmitted independently in families *(161)*. Neuropsychological testing supports different deficits in ADHD and learning disabilities *(158)*.

Stimulants are not a treatment for specific learning disabilities. These disabilities typically require specialized psychoeducational interventions. However, in ADHD children with comorbid learning disabilities, treatment of ADHD symptoms with stimulants can be helpful as part of an overall treatment plan.

4.7. *ADHD and Substance Use Disorders*

Despite stimulants' documented efficacy in the treatment of ADHD, there continues to be public concern that stimulant use in childhood and adolescence increases the risk for substance use disorders. Some lay groups such as the Church of Scientology's Citizens Commission on Human Rights have capitalized on public concerns to suggest that prescribing stimulants to ADHD children predisposes them to greater substance abuse risk in adolescence and young adulthood *(162)*.

There may be two reasons for this public concern. The first is that stimulants such as methylphenidate may be chemically similar to cocaine, and therefore may be highly addictive and abusable (like cocaine), especially when inhaled or injected intravenously. However, evidence shows that stimulants and cocaine possess distinctly different pharmacodynamic and pharmacokinetic properties. Methylphenidate enters and clears the brain much more slowly than does cocaine, eliciting a slow and steady dopamine release from dopamine-containing neurons. These characteristics are associated with clinical benefits and limit the abuse potential of stimulants. In contrast, cocaine enters the brain rapidly, clears the brain quickly, and elicits a large and fast release of dopamine from neurons. These characteristics are associated with the reinforcing properties of cocaine and contribute to its abuse potential *(43,163)*. The second reason for public concern comes from evidence that stimulants lead to increased sensitization to later stimulant exposure in preclinical animal models. Intermittent stimulant dosing in mammal models suggests that repeated stimulant exposure leads to subsequently greater craving and self-administration of stimulants in animals *(164)*.

However, the evidence to date on the actual risks of substance use and abuse in stimulant treated ADHD children is relatively weak. To date, there are 14 studies that address this issue (for review, *see* refs. *165* and *166*). Only one study found support for the sensitization hypothesis of increased risk for later substance abuse in stimulant-treated ADHD children *(167)*. This study did not control for comorbid conduct disorder in their ADHD sample, which is known to increase the risk of substance abuse independently of ADHD or stimulant treatment. Thirteen studies found no evidence that stimulant treatment increases risks for later substance abuse. Indeed, many studies find that stimulant treatment of ADHD actually reduces the risks for later substance abuse *(166,168,169)*. In a meta-analysis of six studies including 674 stimulant treated subjects and 360 unmedicated subjects followed for at least 4 yr, the pooled estimate of the odds ratio indicated a 1.9-fold reduction in risk for substance abuse in stimulant-treated ADHD youths *(166)*. Thus, it appears that stimulant treatment of ADHD actually reduces the risk of later substance use disorder.

A separate clinical challenge is the treatment of ADHD in an adolescent or young adult who is already a substance abuser. In uncontrolled environments active substance abuse is a relative contraindication to prescribing stimulant medications. Antidepressants with known efficacy for the treatment of ADHD and limited abuse potential, such as bupropion or atomoxetine, should be used *(170,171)*.

5. LONG-TERM TREATMENT

The vast majority of studies report on the short-term effects of stimulant medications. Clinical trials generally last 2 to 8 wk. There is a paucity of studies on the long-term (>4 mo) efficacy and safety of stimulants. Longer studies are important because ADHD is generally a chronic disorder, and it is important to know whether stimulants continue to be effective and safe over extended treatment periods.

Three controlled and one open-label study have examined the efficacy and safety of stimulants over 4- to 15-mo extended treatment durations *(11,93,172,173)*. All are studies of children with ADHD. Schachar and colleagues investigated methylphenidate in 91 children over a 4-mo clinical trial compared to placebo. ADHD children continued to demonstrate benefits to methylphenidate over the 16-wk trial. Lack of weight gain was a side effect documented in the treatment group *(172)*. The MTA study examined 579 children with ADHD and compared stimulant medication management with behavioral therapy, combined medication and behavioral therapy, or routine community care over 14 mo. Results showed children assigned to stimulant treatment (medication management and combined treatment) to have greater improvements than the other two groups (behavioral treatment alone and routine community care) *(11)*. Stimulant benefits were maintained over 14 mo. Gillberg and colleagues investigated amphetamine treatment on symptoms of ADHD in 62 children over 15 mo *(93)*. Amphetamine was clearly superior to placebo in reducing the core symptoms of ADHD over the 15 mo. The stimulant drug appeared well tolerated and side effects are reported as relatively few and mild *(93)*. In a 12-mo open-label study, Wilens and colleagues investigated the efficacy and tolerability of OROS (long-acting) methylphenidate (Concerta) in 289 children, aged 6–13 years, with

ADHD *(173)*. Stimulant effectiveness on the core symptoms of ADHD was maintained over the 12-mo clinical trial as assessed by teachers, parents, and clinicians. OROS methylphenidate was well tolerated over the year, with minimal impact on sleep quality, tics, blood pressure, pulse, or height. Only 2% of children reported weight loss as a significant side effect *(173)*.

These longer-term results include data from 1021 stimulant-treated children. Both methylphenidate and amphetamine preparations have been studied in these longer-duration clinical trials. The data are encouraging in that stimulants continue to be effective for the core symptoms of ADHD and appear well tolerated more than a 4–15-mo treatment duration. Future studies need to examine long-term tolerability and effectiveness of stimulants in ADHD adolescents and adults.

6. SIDE EFFECTS

6.1. Common, Short-Term, Acute Side Effects

Stimulant medications are generally well tolerated. Side effects do occur but are generally mild and can be managed by dose adjustment or changing the timing of medication intake. In a study of the prevalence of parent- and teacher-reported side effects to two doses (i.e., 0.3 and 0.5 mg/kg) of methylphenidate given twice daily in a sample of 82 children with ADHD more than half the sample exhibited decreased appetite, insomnia, anxiousness, irritability, and/or proneness to crying with both doses of methylphenidate. However, many of these apparent side effects were present during a placebo condition, and may actually represent characteristics of the disorder rather than its treatment *(174)*. Clinically, it is important to ascertain parent-reported medication side effects at baseline before the child is put on stimulant medication, and then again at full dose. Many of the reported medication side effects may actually be aspects of the disease and get better with treatment. Severe side effects were reported much less frequently than mild side effects. In this study, side effects were linearly related to dose, with higher doses associated with more reported side effects. Only 3.6% of children had side effects severe enough to warrant methylphenidate discontinuation *(174)*. Pooled side effect data from five pivotal clinical trials (four trials of methylphenidate and one trial of mixed amphetamine salts) are presented in Table 5.

In this table, side effects of subjects receiving active drug are compared to adverse events reported in subjects receiving placebo for six common acute stimulant side effects. Note that side effects are reported on placebo. For the clinician to obtain an accurate picture of stimulant treatment emergent side effects, a baseline evaluation before medication is initiated should be completed. Side effects are generally higher on active drug, but stimulants are generally well tolerated in these clinical trials.

In special populations there may be a higher incidence of stimulant-related side effects. Preschool ADHD children treated with stimulants may experience a higher rate of adverse effects than older ADHD children. This may especially be true of mood side effects and social withdrawal *(12)*. Children with developmental delay, such as autism or mental retardation, may experience elevated rates of stimulant side effects *(14,15)*. These populations require increased clinical attention to monitor stimulant-related side effects.

Stimulants are sympathomimetic drugs. Theoretically, they can raise blood pressure and pulse rate. This has led to concerns over their cardiovascular safety in children. However, the cardiovascular effects of stimulants in healthy children, adolescents, and adults are minimal and do not appear clinically significant *(175,176)*. Routine blood pressure and pulse checks

Table 5
Common Short-Term Stimulant Side Effects[a]

Side effect	Methylphenidate	Placebo	Mixed amp salts	Placebo
Body as a whole				
Abdominal Pain	11.3%	7%	14%	10%
Headache	13%	8.4%	—	—
Digestive system				
Anorexia	14%	6.4%	22%	2%
Vomiting	3.5%	3.2%	7%	4%
Nervous system				
Insomnia	7.8%	7.2%	17%	2%
Nervousness	13.4%	17.4%	6%	2%

[a]Pooled data from four methylphenidate clinical trials and one mixed amphetamine salts clinical trial *(56,59,66,229,230)*.

on healthy ADHD youths receiving stimulants are not indicated *(46)*. Studies of normotensive adults receiving stimulants report elevations of 4 mmHg of systolic and diastolic blood pressure and pulse increases of less than 10 beats per minute associated with treatment *(27)*. In adults at risk for hypertension higher increases in blood pressure might be noted. Given the high prevalence of hypertension in adults, blood pressure and pulse rate should be monitored in ADHD adults receiving stimulants.

Given the short half-life of many immediate-release stimulants, deterioration in behavior and ADHD symptom control can occur in the afternoon and evening following earlier administration of stimulant medication. The deterioration may exceed that expected from baseline ADHD symptoms. This phenomenon is referred to as rebound and has been described in previous stimulant research *(177)*. However, other studies of immediate-release stimulants have not found deterioration in evening ADHD symptoms over and above baseline *(178)*. Should rebound occur, the use of longer-acting stimulant preparations, or the addition of a small dose of immediate-release stimulant 1 h before the onset of symptom exacerbation, reduces rebound symptoms late in the day.

6.2. Rare, Acute Side Effects

6.2.1. Tics

As noted above, stimulants can exacerbate the frequency and intensity of motor and vocal tics in ADHD children with preexisting tic disorders. In a study of 1520 children diagnosed with attention deficit disorder and treated with methylphenidate, existing tics were exacerbated in six children (0.39%) and new tics developed in 14 cases (0.92%). After discontinuation of methylphenidate, all six of the tics that had worsened returned to their baseline intensity, and 13 of 14 new tics remitted completely *(179)*. Although there has been concern that stimulant-induced tic disorders may be severe and not remit with discontinuation of stimulant medication, these cases appear rare *(180)*. Most stimulant-induced tics are mild and transient. There are few subjects (about 0.1%) in whom tics do not diminish after stopping the medication *(179,181)*.

Concern has also been expressed that stimulant medications might cause the development of new tics de novo in ADHD children. Shapiro and Shapiro reviewed the relationship between treating attention deficit disorder with stimulants and the precipitation of new tics and

Tourette's syndrome in children *(182)*. They concluded that the evidence suggests that stimulants do not cause new tic disorders, although high doses of stimulants can cause or exacerbate tics in children already predisposed to tic disorder or Tourette's syndrome. This issue was further investigated in a longitudinal study comparing ADHD children treated with stimulants and ADHD children treated with placebo over the course of 1 yr. At the end of 1 yr 19.6% of stimulant-treated children and 16.7% of placebo treated children developed a new onset tic *(183)*. This was a nonsignificant difference and supports data suggesting that stimulants do not cause new tic disorders in children who are not already predisposed to develop a tic disorder. These data support the clinical recommendation to treat ADHD with stimulants when mild to moderate tic disorder comorbidity is present and after a careful risk-benefit discussion with the family. Close clinical monitoring of the tics during ongoing stimulant therapy is recommended.

6.2.2. *Psychosis*

Stimulants can cause psychosis in vulnerable individuals with a preexisting psychotic disorder such as schizophrenia or vulnerability to mania, and can cause psychosis as an acute manifestation of stimulant toxicity such as that occurring upon overdose of stimulant medications. Approximately 20 cases of stimulant-induced psychosis have been reported in the clinical literature *(184,185)*. Individuals with a psychotic reaction to stimulants should be clinically monitored for a recurrence or development of a psychotic illness.

6.3. *Long-Term, Chronic Adverse Events*

6.3.1. *Effects on Growth*

Stimulants routinely produce anorexia, appetite suppression, and weight loss. Weight loss is generally mild and is not permanent. When stimulants are discontinued, weight catches up to its usual developmental trajectory. Ultimate adult weight is generally unaffected by stimulant use. Weight should be monitored routinely during stimulant treatment. In the few children with more serious weight loss as a function of stimulant treatment, the clinician may have to alter the stimulant dose schedule or schedule a stimulant drug holiday to allow for catch-up weight gain. Another clinical strategy is to feed the child before bedtime, when the anorexic effects of stimulants are decreasing and the appetite may rebound.

Stimulant effects on height are less certain. Initial reports suggested that there was a persistent decrease in growth of height in stimulant-treated children *(186)*. However, other reports have failed to replicate this finding *(175,187–189)*. More recent studies conclude that ultimate height is unaffected by stimulant treatment during the developing years *(190)*.

Another possibility is that height differences between children with ADHD and control youths may be because of the disorder itself and not stimulant treatment. In a recent longitudinal study, data suggested that growth deficits in ADHD children may represent a temporary delay in the tempo of growth (e.g., dysmaturity of growth), but that final adult height is not to compromised *(189)*. This effect may be mediated by ADHD and not stimulant treatment *(46)*.

The issue of stimulant "medication holidays" to counteract the possible growth deficits associated with stimulant treatment remains unresolved. This practice rests on the premise that there exists a "growth rebound" during the time off stimulants *(191)*. For example, Klein and Mannuzza found a significant positive effect on height in stimulant treated ADHD children who did not receive stimulant medication over two summers *(191)*. However, not all studies support the possibility of "growth rebound" off stimulants. In a controlled trial of 58 ADHD children no major differences in growth were found in children receiving chronic stimulant treatment with and without summer drug holidays *(188)*. In considering a "medication holiday" clinicians and parents must balance the risks of being off stimulant medication with the slight risks to growth of continuing medication. Given the negative impact of untreated ADHD across multiple domains in the ADHD child's daily life, this decision must be made with care.

7. CLINICAL USE OF STIMULANTS

7.1. General Principles

Treatment with stimulant medications should always be part of an overall psychoeducational treatment plan for the child and adolescent with ADHD. Consideration should be given to all aspects of the youngster's and family's life. Stimulants are rarely the only treatment prescribed for the ADHD youth. Some adults with ADHD will receive medication as part of their treatment plan in the absence of other forms of treatment. However, even with the ADHD adult, education about the disease and its treatment should be given to both the patient and the immediate family or spouse. National organizations, such as Children and Adults with Attention-Deficit/Hyperactivity Disorder (www.chadd.org) are important sources of information for patients and families.

Treatment should always be preceded by a careful evaluation of the ADHD individual and his or her family. Evaluation should include attention to psychiatric, social, cognitive, and educational/occupational aspects of the patient. A recent screening physical examination should be available to rule out medical illness or sensory impairments, such as hearing loss that may contribute to symptoms or influence treatment decision-making. Special attention should focus on issues of comorbidity with learning disorders that may also contribute to educational or occupational underperformance. Comorbid learning disabilities are important to identify because they do not respond to stimulant medications and require supplemental educational remediation. Attention should also be given to issues of psychiatric comorbidity that may influence symptom presentation, treatment response, and prognosis. In the ADHD child, psychiatric comorbidity may include CD/ODD, anxiety disorders, and/or depression. In the ADHD adolescent additional attention should be paid to possible alcohol and substance use disorders and risk-taking behaviors. In the ADHD adult, these comorbidities, as well as interpersonal conflicts with spouses, children, and/or co-workers should also be inquired about. In those of driving age, it is recommended that a driving history be obtained, as ADHD can seriously impair judgment and performance related to operating a motor vehicle *(75)*.

In the evaluation of the families of children with ADHD attention must be paid to the possibility that a parent or sibling has ADHD. ADHD is a highly heritable disorder (heritability rates ~70%), and first-degree biological relatives of the identified patient frequently have ADHD *(192)*. The presence of parents or siblings with ADHD may complicate the family picture and must be taken into account during treatment planning. Another focus of evaluation is the question of possible substance use disorder in family members of the identified ADHD patient. In this case, stimulant medication should not be prescribed, as there exists a risk of its illicit use or sale. Nonstimulant medications to treat ADHD, such as bupropion or atomoxetine, can be considered in these cases.

Parental and child attitudes about pharmacotherapy must be evaluated. Some parents are simply not supportive of drug therapy for their child and alternative psychoeducational therapies for these ADHD children must be identified. Divorced parents may disagree about treating their child with stimulants. The clinician must be careful not to insist on stimulant therapy or coerce parents into agreeing to pharmacotherapy, as this may inadvertently undermine the efficacy and sustainability of the intervention. With older children and adolescents, it is important that the use of medication is discussed with them and its rationale in the treatment of ADHD be explained.

7.2. Goals of Stimulant Treatment for ADHD

Over the years, a change has occurred in the way ADHD is perceived by clinicians and researchers. Historically, ADHD was thought to be a disorder of childhood, confined to the 6- to 12-yr-old age range. Because hyperactivity generally diminishes at puberty, many clinicians thought ADHD disappeared at puberty as well. Stimulant treatment was confined to the elementary-school-aged child and stimulants were generally discontinued at puberty. In the past, the clinical goal of stimulant therapy was to help the disruptive, inattentive ADHD child during the school day. To meet this goal, stimulants were generally prescribed on a twice-daily basis *(10)*.

Over the past three decades, however, longitudinal research has demonstrated that ADHD is generally a lifelong disorder that continues in 30–70% of individuals meeting ADHD criteria in elementary school *(7,117,193–198)*. Although overt hyperactivity generally diminishes in adolescence, inner restlessness, impulsivity, inattention, distractibility, forgetfulness, cognitive disorganization, and fidgetiness may continue to impair functioning across the ADHD individual's lifespan *(193)*. Research has demonstrated that ADHD impairs not only academic performance, but also multiple social, interpersonal, school, occupational, family, leisure, cognitive, and behavioral domains in an affected individual's life, with a poor lifetime prognosis and much comorbid psychopathology across the life-span if untreated *(7,117,196,199)*.

This research has led clinicians to a better understanding of ADHD treatment. With this greater understanding, the clinical goal of stimulant therapy in the treatment of ADHD has evolved and changed. The two new goals are:

1. In the individual with continuing ADHD symptoms, treat ADHD throughout the life-span. Do not stop stimulant treatment just because an ADHD patient has achieved puberty and is less overtly hyperactive. Stimulants work for the adolescent and adult with ADHD in a similar manner as for the child with ADHD. Evaluate the patient for continuing cognitive signs of ADHD and continue to treat if necessary.
2. Stimulant coverage for ADHD now emphasizes extended treatment of symptoms throughout the day. The new clinical goal is to lessen the symptoms of ADHD in multiple areas of the patient's daily life. It is no longer sufficient to treat ADHD only during the school day or during work hours. Clinicians are now encouraged to reduce the overall daily burden of ADHD on the patient's life.

These treatment goals are more ambitious than historical treatment goals, and require broader ADHD coverage by stimulant medications. Consistent with these wider clinical goals, long-acting stimulant preparations are rapidly becoming the standard of care. When used, immediate release stimulants are now often prescribed three times a day, or are used to supplement the action of long-acting stimulants. To reduce the overall burden of ADHD on the child's development, stimulants are frequently prescribed 7 d a week, and often during the summer months.

7.3. Choice of Preparation

Table 6 shows the different stimulant preparations and dosing strengths. Immediate-release stimulants must be given at least twice daily, and preferably three times daily if ADHD coverage is to extend into the after-school hours. Intermediate-release stimulants are designed to mimic the action of immediate-release preparations given twice daily. They are

Table 6
Stimulant Preparations for ADHD

Preparation	Active agent	Dose availability	Dosing schedule
Immediate-release for 4- to 6-h coverage			
Adderall® tablets	Neutral sulfate salts of dextroamphetamine saccharate and D,L-amphetamine aspartate	5, 7.5, 10, 12.5, 15, 20, 30 mg	bid to tid
Desoxyn® tablets[a]	Methamphetamine HCl	5 mg	bid to tid
Dexedrine® tablets	Dextroamphetamine sulfate	5 mg	bid to tid
Dextrostat® tablets	Dextroamphetamine sulfate	5, 10 mg	bid to tid
Focalin™ tablets	Dexmethylphenidate HCl	2.5, 5, 10 mg	bid to tid
Ritalin® HCl tablets	Methylphenidate HCl	5, 10, 20 mg	bid to tid
Intermediate-acting for 8-h coverage			
Dexedrine® spansule	Dextroamphetamine sustained release	5, 10, 15 mg	bid
Metadate® CD	Methylphenidate HCl extended release	20 mg	bid
Metadate® ER	Methylphenidate HCl extended release	10, 20 mg	bid
Ritalin-slow release	Methylphenidate HCl sustained release	20 mg	bid
Long-acting for 10- to 12-h coverage			
Adderall XR® capsules	Neutral salts of dextroamphetamine and amphetamine with dextroamphetamine saccharate and D,L-amphetamine aspartate monohydrate extended release	5, 10, 15, 20, 25, 30 mg	Q AM
Concerta™ tablets	Methylphenidate HCl extended release	18, 27, 36, 54, 72 mg	Q AM

bid, twice a day; tid, three times a day, QAM, everyday before noon.
[a]High abuse potential.

useful for the ADHD youth who has difficulty in school, but not in after-school activities. Long-acting stimulants are designed to provide ADHD treatment throughout the day. They should be considered for the ADHD child with difficulty in and out of school. Intermediate and long-acting stimulant preparations can be supplemented with immediate-release formulations to sculpt the dose for break through ADHD symptoms.

Initiation of stimulant therapy with long-acting agents is now the accepted standard of care. Treatment may begin with either methylphenidate or amphetamine preparations as the first choice. Prior to initiation of stimulants, baseline measures of ADHD symptoms and potential medication side effects should be obtained and repeated when the child is on the drug. Objective data regarding the efficacy of stimulants for the individual's ADHD symptoms should always be collected across several different doses, given variability in each individual's responses to stimulant medications *(200)*. Stimulants are introduced in low dose and titrated weekly to achieve optimum clinical response and tolerability. In our clinic we tell parents that a stimulant trial to determine the child's most effective and well-tolerated dose will last about 1 mo. Although body weight has not been shown to be related to stimulant drug response, using it as a rough guideline for determining a starting dose continues to be recommended *(3)*. For the individual child, titrate the stimulant (for methylphenidate preparations) through low (0.3–0.5 mg/kg/dose), intermediate (0.6–0.8 mg/kg/dose), and high (0.9–1.2 mg/kg/dose) doses on a weekly basis and monitor efficacy, tolerability, and side effects. Amphetamine preparations are twice as potent as methylphenidate preparations and so are given in half the dose range (i.e., 0.2–0.6 mg/kg/dose). Determine the best final dose for each individual with ADHD. Immediate-release stimulants may be used as supplements to target break through ADHD symptoms.

Once an effective and well-tolerated stimulant dose is achieved, routine monitoring is recommended. In the large MTA study, children with ADHD assigned to the stimulant treatment arm were seen in monthly follow-up visits. Even though most of the ADHD children assigned to community treatment as usual also received stimulants, their clinicians saw them much less frequently. The children followed monthly by their physicians did better, suggesting that regular follow-up of stimulant-treated ADHD children is clinically helpful *(11)*. Routine clinical monitoring should inquire about continuing stimulant efficacy and side effects. Height and weight should be ascertained twice yearly. In the healthy child, routine monitoring of pulse and blood pressure is not indicated during stimulant therapy. Monitoring of the electrocardiogram is not necessary for the ADHD child on stimulants. Routine blood work, such as chemistry, liver function tests, and hematological indices are not indicated for routine stimulant use in the healthy child. The clinician and family should think about stimulant therapy in "school year units." That is, once a stable dose of stimulant has been achieved, treatment should continue for the duration of the school year. At the end of the school year clinical assessment and consultation with the family should determine whether the child continues stimulants over the summer or discontinues them until the start of the next school year.

7.4. Management of Stimulant-Induced Side Effects

As noted earlier, common clinical side effects of stimulants include insomnia, anorexia, nausea, abdominal pain, headache, mood lability, irritability, sadness, moodiness, and weight loss. In the face of a satisfactory clinical response to stimulants, it is important to attempt to manage side effects clinically, without having to discontinue stimulant medication. Many of these treatment emergent side effects occur early in the course of stimulant treatment and decline in intensity with time. It is important to distinguish between true stimulant side effects and or returning ADHD symptoms late in the day, when stimulant medications are wearing off. The time course of reported side effects may be helpful. Treatment-emergent side effects developing 1–2 h post-stimulant administration may represent true medication adverse events. Side effects reported as developing late in the day may represent ADHD rebound phenomena, and occur as stimulant efficacy is diminishing. If symptoms represent ADHD rebound, giving a small supplemental dose of stimulant late in the afternoon may help. Suggestions for the management of common stimulant side effects are included in the following Subheadings.

7.4.1. Gastrointestinal Symptoms

Administering the medication with meals can help anorexia, nausea, and abdominal pain that sometimes may occur with taking stimulants. For persistent distress despite administering medication with meals, it may be necessary to change stimulant preparations.

7.4.2. Weight Loss

Appetite may rebound in the evening when stimulants are wearing off. Offering a high-caloric snack before the child's bedtime may be helpful. Do not force the child to eat. If routine growth monitoring reveals more than 25th percentile decrement on standardized growth curves in weight for age since the start of stimulant medication, a medication holiday may be indicated.

7.4.3. Insomnia

It is important to determine if sleep difficulties are a true stimulant side effect or are actually a part of ADHD. It is well-known that children with ADHD have more sleep difficulties compared with controls regardless of stimulant treatment *(201)*. If insomnia represents a true side effect, give stimulant medication earlier in the day or switch to a shorter-acting preparation. Discontinue late afternoon or evening doses of stimulants. Consider supplementing stimulants with clonidine, imipramine, or mirtazapine to help induce sleep in the evening *(202)*.

7.4.4. Dizziness

It is important to monitor blood pressure to help rule out cardiovascular causes of dizziness. Reducing stimulant dose or switching to a long-acting formulation may be helpful.

7.4.5. Rebound Phenomena

Overlapping stimulant doses at least 1 h before rebound appears may be useful. Changing to a long-acting formulation may diminish the intensity of rebound symptoms. Consider changing to a longer-acting non stimulant ADHD medication, such as atomoxetine or bupropion, with or without concurrent stimulant supplementation.

7.4.6. Irritability and Mood Lability

Determine whether these symptoms are truly stimulant adverse events (occur 1–2 h after administration) or represent ADHD rebound symptoms (occur late in the day when stimulant efficacy is wearing off). A co-occurring mood disorder needs to be assessed if these symptoms are persistent and severe. If symptoms are a stimulant adverse event, consider changing to a different agent (i.e., methylphenidate to amphetamine) or a nonstimulant, such as atomoxetine or bupropion.

7.4.7. Growth Impairment

Consider a medication holiday. Consider switching to a nonstimulant medication.

7.4.8. Stimulant Tolerance

It remains unclear whether behavioral tolerance develops with chronic administration of stimulants. Research indicates that failure to maintain a clinical response at a given dose is more likely to occur at higher stimulant doses and with chronic use (i.e., more than 6 mo of continuous use) *(3)*. When parents call to complain about ineffective doses that were formerly effective, physicians should first evaluate whether new stressful family events are occurring. If no stressful precipitating event is found to account for the loss of stimulant efficacy, consider a dose increase or changing the stimulant formulation. If a stimulant effect on ADHD symptoms is truly lost, consider changing to a nonstimulant medication, such as bupropion or atomoxetine.

7.4.9. Emergence of Tics

If a successfully stimulant-treated ADHD child demonstrates onset of a tic disorder, the clinician should first assess the persistence of tics. After a period of time, tics may subside to a baseline frequency and severity. An informed-consent discussion should take place with the patient and family to assess whether the benefits of stimulant treatment remain worth the risk of possible tic exacerbation. If tics continue to be problematic, the addition of an α-adrenergic agent, such as clonidine *(155)* or guanfacine *(157)* may be added to ongoing stimulant treatment. Alternatively, the stimulant can be discontinued and treatment with clonidine, guanfacine, desipramine, nortriptyline, or atomoxetine can be initiated *(155,157,170,203,204)*. These alternative medications are effective in ADHD and do not exacerbate tic disorders.

7.5. Contraindications to Stimulant Use

Known hypersensitivity to stimulants is a contraindication. Stimulants can exacerbate narrow-angle glaucoma and should not be used in this condition. In vulnerable individuals or in overdose (toxicity) stimulants can cause psychotic symptoms. Stimulants are relatively contraindicated in children and adolescents with schizophrenia or other psychotic disorders because they may worsen these conditions in some cases. Severe tic or Tourette's disorder remains a relative contraindication to the use of stimulants. However, as noted above, stimulants may be used in more mild cases of tics when accompanied by impairing symptoms of ADHD. ADHD patients with unstable hypertension should not receive stimulants until their high blood pressure is treated and controlled. Stimulants have the potential to be abused. They should not be prescribed to patients with active substance abuse or when there is likelihood that family members or friends will abuse the medication. Stimulants have the potential to precipitate hypertensive crises when used with monoamine oxidase inhibitors (MAOIs). They should not be prescribed concurrently with a MAOI or within 14 d after a MAOI has been discontinued.

7.6. Management of Stimulant Overdose

Between 1993 and 1999 the American Association of Poison Control Centers Toxic Exposure Surveillance System identified 759 cases of stimulant overdose and abuse in youths aged 10 through 19 yr *(205)*. The majority concerned methylphenidate. Rising rates of methylphenidate abuse were noted comparing rates in 1999 with rates in 1993. The majority of cases who required health care facility management experienced clinical toxicity. Only seven cases of severe toxicity were identified. These cases occurred in adolescents with polydrug overdoses (i.e., stimulants plus other drugs/alcohol). For cases involving stimulants alone, the majority of symptoms included cardiovascular (tachycardia, hypertension) and/or CNS (agitation, irritability) toxicity. There were no deaths reported.

Signs and symptoms of acute overdose result from overstimulation of the central nervous system and from excessive sympathomimetic effects. Symptoms of stimulant toxicity include vomiting, agitation, tremor, convulsion, confusion, hallucinations, hyperpyrexia, tachycardia, arrhythmias, hypertension, paranoid delusions, and delirium. Treatment consists of prompt medical referral and appropriate supportive measures. The patient must be protected from self-injury and from environmental overstimulation that would aggravate heightened sympathomimetic arousal. Chlorpromazine has been reported to be useful in decreasing CNS stimulation and drug-induced sympathomimetic effects. If the patient is alert and conscious, gastric contents may be evacuated by induction of emesis or gastric lavage. For intoxication with amphetamine, acidification of the urine will increase amphetamine excretion. For severe overdose, intensive care must be provided to maintain adequate cardiopulmonary function and treat hyperpyrexia. The efficacy of peritoneal dialysis or extracorporeal hemodialysis for stimulant toxicity has not been established.

7.7. Stimulant Drug Combinations

In clinical practice stimulants are increasingly combined with other psychiatric medications for the treatment of comorbid psychiatric conditions, such as anxiety or depression, the management of side effects, such as insomnia or stimulant rebound, and to bolster a partial therapeutic response to stimulant monotherapy. Few controlled studies are presently available to assess the safety and efficacy of stimulant combinations, and scientific data to guide the clinician in this practice remain sparse.

7.7.1. Combined Stimulant/Antidepressant Therapy

Stimulants have been combined safely with SSRI antidepressants, such as fluoxetine, in the treatment of ADHD and depression *(136)*. Combinations of tricyclic antidepressants and stimulants have been evaluated. In a study of the separate and combined effects of desipramine and methylphenidate on ADHD symptoms and comorbid affective disorders, both medications alone produced reductions in ADHD symptoms and the combination produced positive effects on learning over and above the efficacy of each single agent *(206)*. The combination was associated with more side effects than either medicine alone, yet there was no evidence that the combination was associated with any unique or serious treatment emergent side effects *(207)*. Because little data from controlled studies are available on the combination of antidepressants and stimulants, close clinical monitoring is recommended in these cases.

7.7.2. Combined Stimulant/α-Adrenergic Agents

Clonidine and guanfacine are presynaptic α-adrenergic agents that downregulate endogenous norepinephrine outflow from the brain. They are frequently combined with stimulants in off-label use to manage severe hyperactive and aggressive symptoms or comorbid tic or Tourette's syndrome, or to help treat insomnia associated with stimulant therapy or ADHD *(155,208,209)*. Adrenergic antagonists do not improve attention span as dramatically as stimulants, but may be helpful in decreasing overarousal that contributes to behavior problems in these children. Clonidine is more sedating than guanfacine. Both may lower blood pressure and pulse; monitoring the vital signs is important when these agents are used with stimulants.

The clinical practice of combining stimulants with clonidine has been the subject of some controversy. In July 1995 National Public Radio reported that sudden death had occurred in three children taking the combination of methylphenidate and clonidine. Subsequent reviews and commentary in the scientific literature concluded that there was no convincing evidence of an adverse methylphenidate–clonidine interaction in any of these cases and that other factors were more proximally related to these three deaths *(210,211)*. Subsequent controlled studies have not reported increased serious adverse events with this combination compared with clonidine or methylphenidate alone *(155,209)*. Currently, the combination is considered usually safe and the available clinical literature does not support discontinuation of such combined therapy in patients experiencing significant clinical benefit *(212)*. However, clonidine may cause a withdrawal syndrome and rebound hypertension if discontinued abruptly without tapering the dose. In overdose clonidine can cause bradycardia and hypotension. Thus, careful clinical monitoring is important when this combination is used *(212)*.

7.8. Non-First Line or Ineffective Stimulants

7.8.1. Magnesium Pemoline (Cylert®)

Pemoline has been associated with life-threatening hepatic failure. Since it was first marketed in 1975, 15 cases of acute hepatic failure have been reported to the Food and Drug Administration. Twelve of these cases resulted in death or liver transplantation secondary to massive hepatic necrosis. This is four to 17 times the base rate expected in the general population *(213)*. Although the Food and Drug Administration allows use of pemoline, it is not a first-line drug and has a black box warning of potential acute liver failure. Liver function tests are required biweekly. With newer and safer long-acting stimulant formulations readily available, it is doubtful whether any ADHD patient should currently be treated with pemoline.

7.8.2. Caffeine

Caffeine is a weak stimulant drug. A review of the literature had concluded that caffeine is not a therapeutically useful drug in the clinical treatment of ADHD *(214)*.

8. SUMMARY

This survey of the clinical effects and side effects of stimulant medications suggests the following conclusions.

1. Up to 70–80% of children with carefully diagnosed ADHD appear to demonstrate a positive response to stimulants. Effects can be expected on improvement of attention span and the reduction of impulsive behavior including aggression. Social interactions and compliance with authority figure commands may improve. Academic improvements in work productivity and accuracy may occur. Stimulant dose should be individualized. Long-acting preparations are now the accepted standard of care.
2. Adolescents and adults with ADHD also respond to stimulant therapy. Stimulants should not be discontinued at puberty in an adolescent with ADHD with continuing impairment. Treatment can continue into the teenage years. Adults can respond to stimulants. The lower response rate to stimulant medications in adults with ADHD may be resulting from relative underdosing.
3. Stimulants do not cure ADHD. Rather, they are an intervention that must be used in conjunction with other psychoeducational interventions as part of an overall treatment plan.
4. Stimulant side effects are generally mild and the medication is well tolerated. A baseline, before medication, evaluation of potential stimulant side effects is recommended before stimulant treatment begins. Side effects attributed by parents to the stimulant may actually be part of ADHD.
5. Stimulants do not cause increased risk of substance abuse. Rather, the risk of substance abuse is conferred by ADHD. Appropriate treatment of ADHD, including use of stimulants, may actually decrease the risk of future substance use disorders.

6. In the treatment of ADHD it is important for the prescribing clinician to be aware of the high comorbidity rate between ADHD and depression, anxiety, learning disabilities, tic disorder, and conduct/oppositional disorders. The possibility of comorbid conditions needs to be considered in treatment planning for the ADHD individual.

In conclusion, the stimulants are first-line agents of choice for ADHD given their efficacy, safety, and tolerability. The treatment of ADHD should emphasize the clinical goals of diminishing the overall burden of ADHD on the individual's daily life and continued treatment of ADHD where necessary across the life-span.

REFERENCES

1. Pliszka SR. Neuroscience for the mental health clinician. New York: Guilford Press, 2003;279.
2. Spencer T, Biederman J, Wilens T, Harding M, O'Donnell D, Griffin S. Pharmacotherapy of attention-deficit hyperactivity disorder across the life cycle. J Am Acad Child Adolesc Psychiatry 1996;35:409–432.
3. Barkley RA, DuPaul GJ, Connor DF. Stimulants. In: Werry JS, Aman MG, eds. Practitioner's guide to psychoactive drugs for children and adolescents. New York: Plenum Medical Book Company, 1999;213–247.
4. Spencer T, Biederman J, Wilens T. Attention-deficit/hyperactivity disorder and comorbidity. Pediatr Clin North Am 1999;46:915–927.
5. Pliszka SR, Carlson CL, Swanson JM. ADHD with comorbid disorders: clinical assessment and management. New York: Guilford Press, 1999.
6. Barkley RA, Murphy KR. Attention deficit hyperactivity disorder: a clinical workbook. New York: Guilford Press, 1998;133.
7. Hechtman L, Weiss G, Perlman T. Young adult outcome of hyperactive children who received long-term stimulant treatment. J Am Acad Child Adolesc Psychiatry 1984;23:261–269.
8. Mannuzza S, Gittleman-Klein R, Bessler A, Malloy P, LaPadula M. Young adult outcome of hyperactive boys almost grown up: Educational achievement, occupational rank, and psychiatric status. Arch Gen Psychiatry 1993;50:565–576.
9. Faraone SV, Biederman J, Spencer T, et al. Attention-deficit/hyperactivity disorder in adults: an overview. Biol Psychiatry 2000;48:9–20.
10. Barkley RA. Attention-deficit hyperactivity disorder. Sci Am 1998;279:66–71.
11. Multimodal Treatment of ADHD Group. Moderators and mediators of treatment response for children with attention-deficit/hyperactivity disorder: the Multimodal Treatment Study of children with attention-deficit/hyperactivity disorder. Arch Gen Psychiatry 1999;56:1088–1096.
12. Connor DF. Preschool attention deficit hyperactivity disorder: A review of prevalence, diagnosis, neurobiology, and stimulant treatment. Dev Behav Pediatrics 2002;23:S1–S9.
13. Pearson DA, Santos CW, Roache JD, et al. Treatment effects of methylphenidate on behavioral adjustment in children with mental retardation and ADHD. J Am Acad Child Adolesc Psychiatry 2003;42:209–216.
14. Handen BL, Breaux AM, Janosky J, McAuliffe S, Feldman H, Gosling A. Effects and noneffects of methylphenidate in children with mental retardation and ADHD. J Am Acad Child Adolesc Psychiatry 1992;31:455–461.
15. Aman MG, Marks RE, Turbott SH, Wilsher CP, Merry SN. Clinical effects of methylphenidate and thioridazine in intellectually subaverage children. J Am Acad Child Adolesc Psychiatry 1991;30:246–256.
16. Handen BL, Johnson CR, Lubetsky M. Efficacy of methylphenidate among children with autism and symptoms of attention-deficit hyperactivity disorder. J Autism Dev Dis 2000;30:245–255.
17. Mahalick DM, Carmel PW, Greenberg JP, et al. Psychopharmacologic treatment of acquired attention disorders in children with brain injury. Pediatr Neurosurg 1998;29:121–126.
18. Feldman H, Crumrine P, Handen R, Alvin R, Teodori J. Methylphenidate in children with seizures and attention-deficit disorder. Am J Dis Child 1989;143:1081–1086.

19. McBride MC, Wang DD, Torres CF. Methylphenidate in therapeutic doses does not lower seizure threshold. Ann Neurol 1986;20:428.
20. Hemmer SA, Pasternak JF, Zecker SG, Trommer BL. Stimulant therapy and seizure risk in children with ADHD. Pediatr Neurol 2001;24:99–102.
21. Weber P, Lutschg J. Methylphenidate treatment. Pediatr Neurol 2002;26:261–266.
22. Barkley RA. The effects of methylphenidate on the interactions of preschool ADHD children with their mothers. J Am Acad Child Adolesc Psychiatry 1988;27:336–341.
23. Zito JM, Safer DJ, dosReis S, et al. Psychotropic practice patterns for youth: a 10-year perspective. Arch Pediatr Adolesc Med 2003;157:17–25.
24. Zito JM, Safer DJ, dosReis S, Gardner JF, Boles M, Lynch F. Trends in the prescribing of psychotropic medications to preschoolers. JAMA 2000; 283:1025–1030.
25. Zito JM, Safer DJ, dosReis S, Magder LS, Gardner JF, Zarin DA. Psychotherapeutic medication patterns for youths with attention deficit/hyperactivity disorder. Arch Pediatr Adolesc Med 1999;153:1257–1263.
26. Willy ME, Manda B, Shatin D, Drinkard CR, Graham DJ. A study of compliance with FDA recommendations for pemoline (Cylert). J Am Acad Child Adolesc Psychiatry 2002;41:785–790.
27. Spencer T, Wilens T, Biederman J, Faraone SV, Ablon JS, Lapey K. A double-blind, crossover comparison of methylphenidate and placebo in adults with childhood-onset attention-deficit hyperactivity disorder. Arch Gen Psychiatry 1995;52:434–443.
28. Bhatara VS, Feil M, Hoagwood K, Vitiello B, Zima BT. Concomitant pharmacotherapy in youths receiving antidepressants or stimulants. Abstracts of Posters Presented at the 47th Annual Meeting of the American Academy of Child and Adolescent Psychiatry, Washington, DC, 2000.
29. Rushton JL, Whitmire JT. Pediatric stimulant and SSRI prescription trends: 1992–1998. Arch Pediatr Adolesc Med 2001;155:560–565.
30. Swanson JM, Connor D, Cantwell D. Combining methylphenidate and clonidine: Ill-advised. J Am Acad Child Adolesc Psychiatry 1999;38:617–619.
31. Safer DJ, Zito JM, Fine EM. Increased methylphenidate usage for attention deficit disorder in the 1990s. Pediatrics 1996;98:1084–1088.
32. Angold A, Erkanli A, Egger HL, Costello EJ. Stimulant treatment for children: a community perspective. J Am Acad Child Adolesc Psychiatry 2000;39:975–984.
33. Jensen P, Kettle L, Roper MT, et al. Are stimulants overprescribed? J Am Acad Child Adolesc Psychiatry 1999;38:797–804.
34. Jensen PS, Bhatara VS, Vitiello B, Hoagwood K, Feil M, Burke LB. Psychoactive medication prescribing practices for U.S. children: gaps between research and clinical practice. J Am Acad Child Adolesc Psychiatry 1999;38:557–565.
35. Wolraich ML, Lindgren S, Stromquist A, Milich R, Davis C, Watson D. Stimulant medication use by primary care physicians in the treatment of attention deficit hyperactivity disorder. Pediatrics 1990;86:95–101.
36. Cox ER, Motheral BR, Henderson RR, Mager D. Geographic variation in the prevalence of stimulant medication use among children 5 to 14 years old: Results from a commercially insured US sample. Pediatrics 2003;111:237–243.
37. Jensen PS. ADHD: Current concepts on etiology, pathophysiology, and neurobiology. Child Adolesc Psychiatr Clin N Am 2000;9:557–572.
38. Levy F. The dopamine theory of attention deficit hyperactivity disorder (ADHD). Aus N Zea J Psychiatry 1991;25:277–283.
39. Zametkin A, Liotta W. The neurobiology of attention-deficit/hyperactivity disorder. J Clin Psychiatry 1998;59:17–23.
40. Posner MI, Raichle ME. Images of mind (revised). Washington, DC: Scientific American Books, 1996.
41. Solanto MV. Neuropsychopharmacological mechanisms of stimulant drug action in attention-deficit hyperactivity disorder: a review and integration. Behav Brain Res 1998;94:127–152.

42. Faraone SV, Biederman J. Neurobiology of attention-deficit hyperactivity disorder. Biol Psychiatry 1998;44:951–958.
43. Volkow ND, Wang GJ, Fowler JS, et al. Relationship between blockade of dopamine transporters by oral methylphenidate and the increases in extracellular dopamine: Therapeutic implications. Synapse 2002;43:181–187.
44. Elia J, Borcherding B, Rapoport J, Keysor C. Methylphenidate and dextroamphetamine treatments of hyperactivity: are there true non-responders? Psychiatry Res 1991;36:141–155.
45. Greenhill LL, Abikoff H, Arnold LE, et al. Medication treatment strategies in the MTA study: relevance to clinicians and researchers. J Am Acad Child Adolesc Psychiatry 1996;35:1304–1313.
46. Wilens TE, Spencer TJ. The stimulants revisited. Child Adolesc Psychiatr Clin N Am 2000;9:573–603.
47. Pliszka SR, McCracken JT, Maas JW. Catecholamines in attention-deficit hyperactivity disorder: current perspectives. J Am Acad Child Adolesc Psychiatry 1996;35:264–272.
48. Diener RM. Toxicology of ritalin. In: Greenhill LL, Osman BB, eds. Ritalin theory and patient management. New York: Mary Ann Liebert, Inc., 1991:35–43.
49. Pelham WE, Jr., Sturges J, Hoza J, et al. Sustained release and standard methylphenidate effects on cognitive and social behavior in children with attention deficit disorder. Pediatrics 1987;80:491–501.
50. Pelham WE, Jr, Swanson JM, Furman MB, Schwindt H. Pemoline effects on children with ADHD: a time-response by dose-response analysis on classroom measures. J Am Acad Child Adolesc Psychiatry 1995;34:1504–1513.
51. Hoffman BB, Lefkowitz RJ. Catecholamines, sympathomimetic drugs, and adrenergic receptor antagonists. In: Hardman JG, Limbird LE, Molinoff PB, Ruddon RW, Gilman AG, eds. The pharmacological basis of therapeutics. New York: McGraw-Hill, 1996:199–248.
52. Caldwell J, Sever PS. The biochemical pharmacology of abused drugs. Clin Pharmacol Ther 1974;16:625–638.
53. Greenhill LL. Attention deficit hyperactivity disorder: the stimulants. Child Adolesc Psychiatr Clin N Am 1995;4:123–168.
54. Birmaher B, Greenhill LL, Cooper TB, Fried J, Maminski B. Sustained release methylphenidate: pharmacokinetic studies in ADDH males. J Am Acad Child Adolesc Psychiatry 1989;28:768–772.
55. Ding YS, Fowler JS, Volkow ND, et al. Chiral drugs: Comparison of the pharmacokinetics of [11C]d-threo and l-threo-methylphenidate in the human and baboon brain. Psychopharmacol 1997;131:71–78.
56. Novartis Pharmaceuticals. Ritalin LA product monograph. East Hanover, NJ: Novartis Pharmaceuticals, 2002.
57. Pelham WE, Gnagy EM, Burrows-Maclean L, et al. Once-a-day Concerta methylphenidate versus three-times-daily methylphenidate in laboratory and natural settings. Pediatrics 2001;107:1–15.
58. Swanson JM, Gupta S, Guinta D, et al. Acute tolerance to methylphenidate in the treatment of attention deficit hyperactivity disorder in children. Clin Pharmacol Ther 1999; 66:295–305.
59. McNeil Pharmaceuticals. Concerta product monograph. 2001:2–28.
60. Grcevich S. SLI381: a long-acting psychostimulant preparation for the treatment of attention-deficit hyperactivity disorder. Expert Opin Investig Drugs 2001;10:2003–2011.
61. Michaels MA, Weston IE, Zhang Y, Tulloch SJ. Pharmacokinetics of SLI381, a two-component extended-release formulation of mixed amphetamine salts, administered in fasted and fed states, and sprinkled on food. New Drug Clinical Evaluation Unit, Phoenix, AZ, May 29, 2001.
62. Shire Pharmaceuticals. Adderall XR data on file. Shire US, Inc., 2001.
63. Greenhill LL, Pelham WE, Lopez FE, et al. Once-daily transdermal methylphenidate improves teacher, parent, and CGI-I ratings. 49th Annual Meeting of the American Academy of Child and Adolescent Psychiatry, San Francisco, CA, 2002.
64. Stahl SM. Mirror, mirror on the wall, which enantiomer is fairest of them all? J Clin Psychiatry 2002;63:656–657.
65. Eckerman DA, Moy SS, Perkins AN, Patrick KS, Breese GR. Enantioselective behavioral effects of threo-methylphenidate in rats. Pharmacol Biochem Behav 1991;40:875–880.

66. Novartis Pharmaceuticals. Focalin product monograph. 2002:5–19.
67. Barkley RA. A review of stimulant drug research with hyperactive children. J Child Psychol Psychiatry 1977;18:137–165.
68. Greenhill LL, Group AS. Efficacy and safety of OROS MPH in adolescents with ADHD. 49th Annual Meeting of the American Academy of Child and Adolescent Psychiatry, San Francisco, CA, 2002.
69. Wilens TE, Biederman J, Spencer TJ, Prince J. Pharmacotherapy of adult attention deficit/hyperactivity disorder: a review. J Clin Psychopharmacol 1995;15:270–279.
70. Elia J, Rapoport J. Ritalin versus dextroamphetamine in ADHD: both should be tried. In: Greenhill LL, Osman BB, eds. Ritalin: theory and patient management. New York: Mary Ann Liebert Publishers, 1991:69–74.
71. Varley CK. Effects of methylphenidate in adolescents with attention deficit disorder. J Am Acad Child Adolesc Psychiatry 1983;22:351–354.
72. Goldman L, Genel M, Bezman R, Slanetz PJ. Diagnosis and treatment of attention-deficit/hyperactivity disorder in children and adolescents. JAMA 1998;279:1100–1107.
73. Milberger S, Biederman J, Faraone SV, Chen L, Jones J. Further evidence of an association between attention-deficit/hyperactivity disorder and cigarette smoking. Findings from a high-risk sample of siblings. Am J Addict 1997;6:205–217.
74. Milberger S, Biederman J, Faraone SV, Chen L, Jones J. ADHD is associated with early initiation of cigarette smoking in children and adolescents. J Am Acad Child Adolesc Psychiatry 1997;36:37–44.
75. Barkley RA, Guevremont DC, Anastopoulos AD, DuPaul GJ, Shelton TL. Driving-related risks and outcomes of attention deficit hyperactivity disorder in adolescents and young adults: a 3- to 5-year follow-up survey. Pediatrics 1993;92:212–218.
76. Barkley RA, Murphy KR, Kwasnik D. Motor vehicle driving competencies and risks in teens and young adults with attention deficit hyperactivity disorder. Pediatrics 1996;98:1089–1095.
77. Milberger S, Biederman J, Faraone SV, Wilens T, Chu MP. Associations between ADHD and psychoactive substance use disorders. Findings from a longitudinal study of high-risk siblings of ADHD children. Am J Addict 1997;6:318–329.
78. O'Donnell D, Biederman J, Jones J, et al. Informativeness of child and parent reports on substance use disorders in a sample of ADHD probands, control probands, and their siblings. J Am Acad Child Adolesc Psychiatry 1998;37:752–758.
79. Murphy K, Barkley RA. Attention deficit hyperactivity disorder adults: comorbidities and adaptive impairments. Compr Psychiatry 1996;37:393–401.
80. Whalen CK, Henker B, Granger DA. Social judgment processes in hyperactive boys: effects of methylphenidate and comparisons with normal peers. J Abnorm Child Psychol 1990;18:297–316.
81. Swanson JM, Granger D, Kliewer W. Natural social behaviors in hyperactive children: dose effects of methylphenidate. J Consult Clin Psychol 1987;55:187–193.
82. Rapport MD, Stoner G, DuPaul GJ, et al. Attention deficit disorder and methylphenidate: A multilevel analysis of dose-response effects on children's impulsivity across settings. J Am Acad Child Adolesc Psychiatry 1988;27:60–69.
83. Connor DF, Glatt SJ, Lopez ID, Jackson D, Melloni RH Jr. Psychopharmacology and aggression. I: A meta-analysis of stimulant effects on overt/covert aggression-related behaviors in ADHD. J Am Acad Child Adolesc Psychiatry 2002;41:253–261.
84. Klein RG, Abikoff H, Klass E, Ganeles D, Seese LM, Pollack S. Clinical efficacy of methylphenidate in conduct disorder with and without attention deficit hyperactivity disorder. Arch Gen Psychiatry 1997;54:1073–1080.
85. Rapport MD, Kelly KL. Psychostimulant effects on learning and cognitive function in children with attention deficit hyperactivity disorder: Findings and implications. In: Matson JL, ed. Hyperactivity in children: a handbook. New York: Pergamon, 1991.
86. Rapport MD, Quinn SO, DuPaul GJ, et al. Attention deficit disorder with hyperactivity and methylphenidate: the effects of dose and mastery level on children's learning performance. J Abnorm Child Psychol 1989;17:669–689.

87. Vyse SA, Rapport MD. The effects of methylphenidate on learning in children with ADDH: the stimulus-equivalence paradigm. J Consult Clin Psychol 1989;57:425–435.
88. Swanson JM, Kinsbourne M. The cognitive effects of stimulant drugs on hyperactive children. In: Hale GA, ed. Attention and cognitive development. New York: Plenum, 1978;249–274.
89. Bergman A, Winters L, Cornblatt B. Methylphenidate: effects on sustained attention. In: Greenhill LL, Osman BB, eds. Ritalin: theory and patient management. New York: Mary Ann Liebert, 1991;223–232.
90. Swanson JM. What do psychopharmacological studies tell us about information processing deficits in ADDH? In: Bloomingdale LM, Sergeant JA, eds. Attention deficit disorder: criteria, cognition, intervention. New York: Pergamon Press, 1988, pp. 97–116.
91. Sergeant JA, van der Meere J. Ritalin effects and information processing in hyperactivity. In: Greenhill LL, Osman BB, eds. Ritalin: theory and patient management. New York: Mary Ann Liebert, 1991, pp. 1–13.
92. Schachar R, Tannock R. Childhood hyperactivity and psychostimulants: a review of extended treatment studies. J Child Adolesc Psychopharmacol 1993:81–97.
93. Gillberg C, Melander H, von Knorring AL, et al. Long-term stimulant treatment of children with attention-deficit hyperactivity disorder symptoms. A randomized, double-blind, placebo-controlled trial. Arch Gen Psychiatry 1997;54:857–864.
94. Famularo R, Fenton T. The effect of methylphenidate on school grades in children with attention deficit disorder without hyperactivity: a preliminary study. J Clin Psychiatry 1987;48:112–114.
95. Rapport MD, Jones JT, DuPaul GJ, et. al. Attention deficit disorder and methylphenidate: group and single-subject analyses of dose effects on attention in clinic and classroom settings. J Clin Child Psychol 1987;16:329–338.
96. Barkley RA. The use of psychopharmacology to study reciprocal influences in parent-child interaction. J Abnorm Child Psychol 1981;9:303–310.
97. Barkley RA. Hyperactive girls and boys: stimulant drug effects on mother-child interactions. J Child Psychol Psychiatry 1989;30:379–390.
98. Whalen CK, Henker B, Dotemoto S. Methylphenidate and hyperactivity: Effects on teacher behaviors. Science 1980;208:1280–1282.
99. Barkley RA, Anastopoulos AD, Guevremont DC, Fletcher KE. Adolescents with attention deficit hyperactivity disorder: mother-adolescent interactions, family beliefs and conflicts, and maternal psychopathology. J Abnorm Child Psychol 1992;20:263–288.
100. Seidman LJ, Biederman J, Weber W, Hatch M, Faraone SV. Neuropsychological function in adults with attention-deficit hyperactivity disorder. Biol Psychiatry 1998;44:260–268.
101. Connor DF, Edwards G, Fletcher KE, Baird J, Barkley RA, Steingard RJ. Correlates of comorbid psychopathology in children with ADHD. J Am Acad Child Adolesc Psychiatry 2003;42:193–200.
102. Pisterman S, McGrath P, Firestone P, et al. Outcome of parent-mediated treatment of preschoolers with attention deficit disorder. J Consult Clin Psychol 1989;57:628–635.
103. Forehand R, McMahon RJ. Helping the noncompliant child: a clinician's guide to parent training. New York: Guilford Press, 1981.
104. Handen BL, Feldman HM, Lurier A, et al. Efficacy of methylphenidate among preschool children with developmental disabilities and ADHD. J Am Acad Child Adolesc Psychiatry 1999;38:805–812.
105. Musten LM, Firestone P, Pisterman S, et al. Effects of methylphenidate on preschool children with ADHD: cognitive and behavioral functions. J Am Acad Child Adolesc Psychiatry 1997;36:1407–1415.
106. Firestone P, Monteiro-Musten L, Pisterman S, et. al. Short-term side effects of stimulant medication are increased in preschool children with attention-deficit/hyperactivity disorder: a double-blind placebo-controlled study. J Child Adolesc Psychopharmacol 1998;8:13–25.
107. Greenhill LL, Jensen P, Abikoff H, et al. Developing strategies for psychopharmacological studies in preschool children. J Am Acad Child Adolesc Psychiatry 2003;42:406–414.

108. Pelham WE, Vodde-Hamilton M, Murphy DA, Greenstein JJ, Vallano G. The effects of methylphenidate on ADHD adolescents in recreational, peer group, and classroom settings. J Clin Child Psychol 1991;20:293–300.
109. Smith BH, Pelham WE, Gnagy E, Yudell RS. Equivalent effects of stimulant treatment for attention-deficit hyperactivity disorder during childhood and adolescence. J Am Acad Child Adolesc Psychiatry 1998;37:314–321.
110. Coons HW, Klorman R, Borgstedt AD. Effects of methylphenidate on adolescents with a childhood history of attention deficit disorder: II. Information processing. J Am Acad Child Adolesc Psychiatry 1987;26:368–374.
111. Klorman R, Coons HW, Borgstedt AD. Effects of methylphenidate on adolescents with a childhood history of attention deficit disorder: I. Clinical findings. J Am Acad Child Adolesc Psychiatry 1987;26:363–367.
112. Evans SW, Pelham WE, Smith BH, et al. Dose-response effects of methylphenidate on ecologically valid measures of academic performance and classroom behavior in adolescents with ADHD. Exp Clin Psychopharmacol 2001;9:163–175.
113. Smith BH, Pelham WE, Evans S, et al. Dosage effects of methylphenidate on the social behavior of adolescents diagnosed with attention-deficit hyperactivity disorder. Exp Clin Psychopharmacol 19986:187–204.
114. Spencer T, Biederman J, Wilens TE, Faraone SV. Adults with attention-deficit/hyperactivity disorder: a controversial diagnosis. J Clin Psychiatry 1998;59:59–68.
115. Silver LB. Attention-deficit/hyperactivity disorder in adult life. Child Adolesc Psychiatr Clin N Am 2000;9:511–523.
116. Faraone SV, Biederman J, Mick E. Symptom reports by adults with attention deficit hyperactivity disorder: are they influenced by attention deficit hyperactivity disorder in their children? J Nerv Ment Dis 1997;185:583–584.
117. Fischer M, Barkley RA, Smallish L, Fletcher K. Young adult follow-up of hyperactive children: self-reported psychiatric disorders, comorbidity, and the role of childhood conduct problems and teen CD. J Abnorm Child Psychol 2002;30:463–475.
118. Wood DR, Reimherr FW, Wender PH, Johnson GE. Diagnosis and treatment of minimal brain dysfunction in adults. Arch Gen Psychiatry 1976;33:1453–1460.
119. Wender PH, Reimherr FW, Wood DR. Attention deficit disorder (minimal brain dysfunction) in adults. Arch Gen Psychiatry 1981;38:449–456.
120. Wender PH, Reimherr FW, Wood DR, Ward M. A controlled study of methylphenidate in the treatment of attention deficit disorder, residual type, in adults. Am J Psychiatry 1985;142:547–552.
121. Faraone SV, Biederman J, Chen WJ, Milberger S, Warburton R, Tsuang MT. Genetic heterogeneity in attention-deficit hyperactivity disorder (ADHD): gender, psychiatric comorbidity, and maternal ADHD. J Abnorm Psychol 1995;104:334–345.
122. Mattes JA, Boswell L, Oliver H. Methylphenidate effects on symptoms of attention deficit disorder in adults. Arch Gen Psychiatry 1984;41:1059–1063.
123. Brown TE. Attention-deficit disorders and comorbidities in children, adolescents, and adults. Washington, DC: American Psychiatric Press, 2000.
124. Biederman J, Newcorn J, Sprich S. Comorbidity of attention deficit hyperactivity disorder with conduct, depressive, anxiety, and other disorders. Am J Psychiatry 1991;148:564–577.
125. Biederman J, Faraone S, Spencer T, et al. Patterns of psychiatric comorbidity, cognition, and psychosocial functioning in adults with attention deficit/hyperactivity disorder. Am J Psychiatry 1993;150:1792–1798.
126. Szatmari P, Boyle M, Offord DR. ADDH and conduct disorder: degree of diagnostic overlap and differences among correlates. J Am Acad Child Adolesc Psychiatry 1989;28:865–872.
127. Barkley RA, McMurray MB, Edelbrock CS, Robbins K. The response of aggressive and nonaggressive ADHD children to two doses of methylphenidate. J Am Acad Child Adolesc Psychiatry 1989;28:873–881.

128. Klorman R, Brumaghim JT, Salzman LF, et al. Effects of methylphenidate on attention-deficit hyperactivity disorder with and without aggressive/noncompliant features. J Abnorm Psychol 1988;97:413–422.
129. Spencer T, Wilens T, Biederman J, Wozniak J, Harding-Crawford M. Attention-deficit/hyperactivity disorder with mood disorders. In: Brown TE, ed. Attention deficit disorders and comorbidities in children, adolescents, and adults. Washington, DC: American Psychiatric Press, 2000:79–124.
130. Biederman J, Lapey KA, Milberger S, Faraone SV, Reed ED, Seidman LJ. Motor preference, major depression and psychosocial dysfunction among children with attention deficit hyperactivity disorder. J Psychiatr Res 1994;28:171–184.
131. Biederman J, Mick E, Faraone SV. Depression in attention deficit hyperactivity disorder (ADHD) children: "true" depression or demoralization? J Affect Disord 1998;47:113–122.
132. DuPaul GJ, Barkley RA, McMurray MB. Response of children with ADHD to methylphenidate: interaction with internalizing symptoms. J Am Acad Child Adolesc Psychiatry 1994;33:894–903.
133. Jensen P, Hinshaw SP, Swanson JM, et al. Findings from the NIMH multimodal treatment study of ADHD (MTA): implications and applications for primary care providers. J Dev Behav Pediatr 2001;22:60–73.
134. Gadow KD, Nolan EE, Sverd J, Sprafkin J, Schwartz J. Anxiety and depressive symptoms and response to methylphenidate in children with attention-deficit/hyperactivity disorder and tic disorder. J Clin Psychopharmacol 2002;22:267–274.
135. Findling RL. Open-label treatment of comorbid depression and attentional disorders with co-administration of serotonin reuptake inhibitors and psychostimulants in children, adolescents, and adults: a case series. J Child Adolesc Psychopharmacol 1996;6:165–175.
136. Gammon GD, Brown TE. Fluoxetine and methylphenidate in combination for treatment of attention deficit disorder and comorbid depressive disorder. J Child Adolesc Psychopharmacol 1991;3:1–10.
137. Geller B, Zimerman B, Williams M, DelBello MP, Frazier J, Beringer L. Phenomenology of prepubertal and early adolescent bipolar disorder: examples of elated mood, grandiose behaviors, decreased need for sleep, racing thoughts, and hypersexuality. J Child Adolesc Psychopharmacol 2002;12:3–9.
138. Geller B, Zimerman B, Williams M, et al. DSM-IV mania symptoms in a prepubertal and early adolescent bipolar disorder phenotype compared to attention-deficit hyperactive and normal controls. J Child Adolesc Psychopharmacol 2002;12:11–25.
139. Scheffer RE. Combination pharmacotherapy in pediatric bipolars-treating comorbid ADHD. Presented at the 49th Annual Meeting of the American Academy of Child and Adolescent Psychiatry, San Francisco, CA, October 2002;22–27.
140. Cohen P, Cohen J, Kasen S, et al. An epidemiological study of disorders in late childhood and adolescence: I. age and gender specific pattern. J Child Psychol Psychiatry 1993;34:851–867.
141. Bird HR, Gould MS, Staghezza BM. Patterns of diagnostic comorbidity in a community sample of children aged 9 through 16 years. J Am Acad Child Adolesc Psychiatry 1993;32:361–368.
142. Pliszka SR. Effect of anxiety on cognition, behavior, and stimulant response in ADHD. J Am Acad Child Adolesc Psychiatry 1989;28:882–887.
143. Buitelaar JK, van der Gaag RJ, Swaab-Barneveld H, et. al. Prediction of clinical response to methylphenidate in children with attention-deficit hyperactivity disorder. J Am Acad Child Adolesc Psychiatry 1995;34:1025–1032.
144. Diamond IR, Tannock R, Schachar R. Response to methylphenidate in children with ADHD and comorbid anxiety. J Am Acad Child Adolesc Psychiatry 1999:402–409.
145. Research Units on Pediatric Psychopharmacology (RUPP) Group. Fluvoxamine for the treatment of anxiety disorders in children and adolescents. N Engl J Med 2001;344:1279–1285.
146. Kurlan R, Como PG, Miller B, et al. The behavioral spectrum of tic disorders: a community-based study. Neurology 2002;59:414–420.

147. Gadow KD, Nolan EE, Sprafkin J, Schwartz J. Tics and psychiatric comorbidity in children and adolescents. Dev Med Child Neurol 2002;44:330–338.
148. Snider LA, Seligman LD, Ketchen BR, et al. Tics and problem behaviors in school children: prevalence, characterization, and associations. Pediatrics 2002;110:331–336.
149. Sukhodolsky DG, Scahill L, Zhang H, et al. Disruptive behavior in children with Tourette's syndrome: association with ADHD comorbidity, tic severity, and functional impairment. J Am Acad Child Adolesc Psychiatry 2003;41:98–105.
150. Pliszka SR. Comorbidity of attention-deficit/hyperactivity disorder with psychiatric disorder: an overview. J Clin Psychiatry 1998;59:50–58.
151. Castellanos FX, Giedd JN, Elia J, et al. Controlled stimulant treatment of ADHD and comorbid Tourette's syndrome: effects of stimulants and dose. J Am Acad Child Adolesc Psychiatry 1997;36:1–8.
152. Gadow KD, Nolan EE, Sverd J. Methylphenidate in hyperactive boys with comorbid tic disorder: II. Short-term behavioral effect in school settings. J Am Acad Child Adolesc Psychiatry 1992;31:462–471.
153. Gadow KD, Nolan EE, Sverd J, Sprafkin J, Paolicelli L. Methylphenidate in aggressive-hyperactive boys: I. Effects on peer aggression in public school settings. J Am Acad Child Adolesc Psychiatry 1990;29:710–718.
154. Gadow KD, Sverd J, Sprafkin J, et al. Efficacy of methylphenidate for attention-deficit hyperactivity disorder in children with tic disorder. Arch Gen Psychiatry 1995;52:444–455.
155. Tourette's Study Group. Treatment of ADHD in children with tics: a randomized controlled trial. Neurology 2002;58:527–536.
156. Riddle MA, Lynch KA, Scahill L, DeVries A, Cohen DJ, Leckman JF. Methylphenidate discontinuation and reinitiation during long-term treatment of children with Tourette's disorder and attention-deficit hyperactivity disorder: a pilot study. J Child Adolesc Psychopharmacol 1995;3:191–205.
157. Scahill L, Chappell PB, Kim YS, et al. A placebo-controlled study of guanfacine in the treatment of children with tic disorders and attention deficit hyperactivity disorder. Am J Psychiatry 2001;158:1067–1074.
158. Purvis KL, Tannock R. Language abilities in children with attention deficit hyperactivity disorder, reading disabilities, and normal controls. J Abnorm Child Psychol 1997;25:133–144.
159. Murphy KR, Barkley RA, Bush T. Young adults with attention deficit hyperactivity disorder: subtype differences in comorbidity, educational, and clinical history. J Nerv Men Dis 2002;190:147–157.
160. Semrud-Clikeman M, Biederman J, Sprich-Buckminster S, Lehman BK, Faraone SV, Norman D. Comorbidity between ADDH and learning disability: a review and report in a clinically referred sample. J Am Acad Child Adolesc Psychiatry 1992;31:439–448.
161. Faraone SV, Biederman J, Lehman BK, et al. Evidence for the independent familial transmission of attention deficit hyperactivity disorder and learning disabilities: results from a family genetic study. Am J Psychiatry 1993;150:891–895.
162. Citizens Commission on Human Rights (CCHR). Ritalin: a warning to parents. Los Angeles, CA: Church of Scientology, 1987.
163. Volkow ND, Ding YS, Fowler JS, et al. Is methylphenidate like cocaine? Studies on their pharmacokinetics and distribution in the human brain. Arch Gen Psychiatry 1995;52:456–463.
164. Robinson TE, Berridge KC. The neural basis of drug craving: an incentive-sensitization theory of addiction. Brain Behav Rev 1993; 18:247–291.
165. Barkley RA, Fischer M, Smallish L, Fletcher K. Does the treatment of attention-deficit/hyperactivity disorder with stimulants contribute to drug use/abuse? A 13-year prospective study. Pediatrics 2003;111:97–109.
166. Wilens TE, Faraone SV, Biederman J, Gunawardene S. Does stimulant therapy of attention-deficit/hyperactivity disorder begat later substance abuse? A meta-analytic review of the literature. Pediatrics 2003;111:179–185.
167. Lambert NM, Hartsough CS. Prospective study of tobacco smoking and substance dependencies among samples of ADHD and non-ADHD participants. J Learn Disabil 1998;31:533–544.

168. Biederman J, Wilens T, Mick E, et al. Is ADHD a risk factor for psychoactive substance use disorders? Findings from a four-year prospective follow-up study. J Am Acad Child Adolesc Psychiatry 1997;36:21–29.
169. Biederman J, Wilens T, Mick E, Spencer T, Faraone SV. Pharmacotherapy of attention-deficit/hyperactivity disorder reduces risk for substance use disorder. Pediatrics 1999;104:e20.
170. Michelson D, Faries D, Wernicke J, et al. Atomoxetine in the treatment of children and adolescents with attention-deficit/hyperactivity disorder: a randomized, placebo-controlled, dose-response study. Pediatrics 2001;108:e83.
171. Riggs PD. Clinical approach to treatment of ADHD in adolescents with substance use disorders and conduct disorder. J Am Acad Child Adolesc Psychiatry 1998;37:331–332.
172. Schachar RJ, Tannock R, Cunningham CE, Corkum PV. Behavioral, situational, and temporal effects of treatment of ADHD with methylphenidate. J Am Acad Child Adolesc Psychiatry 1997;36:754–763.
173. Wilens T, Pelham WE, Stein MT, et al. ADHD treatment with once-daily OROS methylphenidate: interim 12-month results from a long-term open-label study. J Am Acad Child Adolesc Psychiatry 2003;42:424–433.
174. Barkley RA, McMurray MB, Edelbrock CS, Robbins K. Side effects of methylphenidate in children with attention deficit hyperactivity disorder: a systemic, placebo-controlled evaluation. Pediatrics 1990;86:184–192.
175. Rapport MD, Moffitt C. Attention deficit/hyperactivity disorder and methylphenidate. A review of height/weight, cardiovascular, and somatic complaint side effects. Clin Psychol Rev 2002;22:1107–1131.
176. Brown RT, Wynne ME, Slimmer LW. Attention deficit disorder and the effect of methylphenidate on attention, behavioral, and cardiovascular functioning. J Clin Psychiatry 1984;45:473–476.
177. Rapoport J, Buchsbaum MS, Zahn TP, et al. Dextroamphetamine: cognitive and behavioral effects in normal prepubertal boys. Science 1978;199:560–562.
178. Johnston C, Pelham WE, Hoza J, et al. Psychostimulant rebound in attention deficit disordered boys. J Am Acad Child Adolesc Psychiatry 1988;27:806–810.
179. Denckla MB, Bemporad JR, MacKay MC. Tics following methylphenidate administration: a report of 20 cases. JAMA 1976;235:1349–1351.
180. Bremness AB, Sverd J. Methylphenidate-induced Tourette syndrome: case report. Am J Psychiatry 1979;136:1334–1335.
181. Lipkin P, Goldstein I, Adesman A. Tics and dyskinesias associated with stimulant treatment in attention-deficit hyperactivity disorder. Arch Pediatr Adolesc Med 1994;148:859–861.
182. Shapiro AK, Shapiro E. Do stimulants provoke, cause, or exacerbate tics and Tourette syndrome? Compr Psychiatry 1981;22:265–273.
183. Law SF, Schachar R. Do typical clinical doses of methylphenidate cause tics in children treated for attention-deficit hyperactivity disorder? J Am Acad Child Adolesc Psychiatry 1999;38:44–51.
184. Koehler-Troy C, Strober M, Malenbaum R. Methylphenidate induced mania in a prepubertal child. J Clin Psychiatry 1986;47:566–567.
185. Bloom AS, L.J. R, Weisskopf B, et al. Methylphenidate-induced delusional disorder in a child with attention deficit disorder with hyperactivity. J Am Acad Child Adolesc Psychiatry 1988;27:88–89.
186. Safer DJ, Allen R, Barr E. Depression of growth in hyperactive children on stimulant drugs. N Engl J Med 1972;287:217–220.
187. Gross M. Growth of hyperkinetic children taking methylphenidate, dextroamphetamine, or imipramine/desipramine. Pediatrics 1976;58:423–431.
188. Satterfield JH, Cantwell DP, Schell A, et al. Growth of hyperactive children treated with methylphenidate. Arch Gen Psychiatry 1979;36:212–217.
189. Spencer TJ, Biederman J, Harding M, O'Donnell D, Faraone SV, Wilens TE. Growth deficits in ADHD children revisited: evidence for disorder-associated growth delays? J Am Acad Child Adolesc Psychiatry 1996;35:1460–1469.

190. Gittelman R, Mannuzza S. Hyperactive boys almost grown up: III. Methylphenidate effects on ultimate height. Arch Gen Psychiatry 1988;45:1131–1134.
191. Klein RG, Mannuzza S. Hyperactive boys almost grown up: III. Methylphenidate effects on ultimate height. Arch Gen Psychiatry 1988;45:1131–1134.
192. Biederman J, Faraone SV, Mick E, et al. High risk for attention deficit hyperactivity disorder among children of parents with childhood onset of the disorder: a pilot study. Am J Psychiatry 1995;152:431–435.
193. Biederman J. Attention-deficit/hyperactivity disorder: a life-span perspective. J Clin Psychiatry 1998;59:4–16.
194. Biederman J, Faraone S, Milberger S, et al. A prospective 4-year follow-up study of attention-deficit hyperactivity and related disorders. Arch Gen Psychiatry 1996;53:437–446.
195. Faraone SV, Biederman J, Mennin D, Gershon J, Tsuang MT. A prospective four-year follow-up study of children at risk for ADHD: psychiatric, neuropsychological, and psychosocial outcome. J Am Acad Child Adolesc Psychiatry 1996;35:1449–1459.
196. Fischer M, Barkley RA, Edelbrock CS, Smallish L. The adolescent outcome of hyperactive children diagnosed by research criteria: II. Academic, attentional, and neuropsychological status. J Consult Clin Psychol 1990;58:580–588.
197. Fischer M, Barkley RA, Fletcher KE, Smallish L. The stability of dimensions of behavior in ADHD and normal children over an 8-year follow-up. J Abnorm Child Psychol 1993;21:315–337.
198. Mannuzza S, Klein RG, Addalli KA. Young adult mental status of hyperactive boys and their brothers: a prospective follow-up study. J Am Acad Child Adolesc Psychiatry 1991;30:743–751.
199. Fischer M, Barkley RA, Fletcher KE, Smallish L. The adolescent outcome of hyperactive children: predictors of psychiatric, academic, social, and emotional adjustment [see comments]. J Am Acad Child Adolesc Psychiatry 1993;32:324–332.
200. Barkley RA, DuPaul GJ, McMurray MB. Attention deficit disorder with and without hyperactivity: clinical response to three dose levels of methylphenidate. Pediatrics 1991;87:519–531.
201. Chatoor I, Wells KC, Conners CK, Seidel WT, Shaw D. The effects of nocturnally administered stimulant medication on EEG sleep and behavior in hyperactive children. J Am Acad Child Adolesc Psychiatry 1983;22:337–342.
202. Wilens TE, Biederman J, Prince J, et al. Six-week, double-blind, placebo-controlled study of desipramine for adult attention deficit hyperactivity disorder. Am J Psychiatry 1996;153:1147–1153.
203. Spencer T, Biederman J, Kerman K, Steingard R, Wilens T. Desipramine treatment of children with attention-deficit hyperactivity disorder and tic disorder or Tourette's syndrome. J Am Acad Child Adolesc Psychiatry 1993;32:354–360.
204. Spencer T, Biederman J, Wilens T, Steingard R, Geist D. Nortriptyline treatment of children with attention-deficit hyperactivity disorder and tic disorder or Tourette's syndrome. J Am Acad Child Adolesc Psychiatry 1993;32:205–210.
205. Klein-Schwartz W, McGrath J. Poison centers' experience with methylphenidate abuse in preteens and adolescents. J Am Acad Child Adolesc Psychiatry 2003;42:288–294.
206. Rapport MD, Carlson GA, Kelly K, Pataki CS. Methylphenidate and desipramine in hospitalized children: I. Separate and combined effects on cognitive function. J Am Acad Child Adolesc Psychiatry 1993;32:333–342.
207. Pataki CS, Carlson GA, Kelly K, Rapport MD, Biancaniello T. Side effects of methylphenidate and desipramine alone and in combination in children. Am J Psychiatry 1993;32:1065–1072.
208. Prince JB, Wilens TE, Biederman J, Spencer TJ, Wozniak JR. Clonidine for sleep disturbances associated with attention-deficit hyperactivity disorder: a systematic chart review of 62 cases. J Am Acad Child Adolesc Psychiatry 1996;35:599–605.
209. Connor DF, Barkley RA, Davis HT. A pilot study of methylphenidate, clonidine, or the combination in ADHD comorbid with aggressive oppositional defiant or conduct disorder. Clin Pediatr (Phila) 2000;39:15–25.
210. Popper CW. Combining methylphenidate and clonidine: Pharmacologic questions and news reports about sudden death. J Child Adolesc Psychopharmacol 1995;5:157–166.

211. Fenichel RR. Combining methylphenidate and clonidine: the role of post-marketing surveillance. J Child Adolesc Psychopharmacol 1995;5:155–156.
212. Swanson JM, Flockhart D, Udrea D, Cantwell D, Connor D, Williams L. Clonidine in the treatment of ADHD: questions about safety and efficacy (letter). J Child Adolesc Psychopharmacol 1995;5:301–304.
213. Shevell M, Schreiber R. Pemoline-associated hepatic failure: A critical analysis of the literature. Pediatr Neurol 1997;16:14–16.
214. Klein RG. Pharmacotherapy of childhood hyperactivity: an update. In: Meltzer HY, ed. Psychopharmacology: the third generation of progress. New York: Raven Press, 1987:1215–1224.
215. Schleifer M, Weiss G, Cohen N, et al. Hyperactivity in preschoolers and the effect of methylphenidate. Am J Orthopsychiatry 1975;45:38–50.
216. Conners CK. Controlled trial of methylphenidate in preschool children with minimal brain dysfunction. Int J Ment Health 1975;4:61–74.
217. Cunningham CE, Siegel LS, Offord DR. A developmental dose-response analysis of the effects of methylphenidate on the peer interactions of attention deficit disordered boys. J Child Psychol Psychiatry 1985;26:955–971.
218. Barkley RA, Karlsson J, Strzelecki E, Murphy JV. Effects of age and Ritalin dosage on the mother-child interactions of hyperactive children. J Consult Clin Psychol 1984;52:750–758.
219. Mayes SD, Crites DL, Bixler EO, et al. Methylphenidate and ADHD: influence of age, IQ, and neurodevelopmental status. Dev Med Child Neurol 1994; 36:1099–1107.
220. Monteiro-Musten L, Firestone P, Pisterman S, et al. Effects of methylphenidate on preschool children with ADHD: cognitive and behavioral functions. J Am Acad Child Adolesc Psychiatry 1997;36:1407–1415.
221. Byrne JM, Bawden HN, DeWolfe NA, et al. Clinical assessment of psychopharmacological treatment of preschoolers with ADHD. J Clin Exp Neuropsychol 1998;20:613–627.
222. Brown RT, Sexson SB. A controlled trial of methylphenidate in black adolescents. Clin Pediatr 1987;27:74–81.
223. Barkley RA, Connor DF, Kwasnik D. Challenges to determining adolescent medication response in an outpatient clinical setting: Comparing Adderall and methylphenidate for ADHD. J Atten Dis 2000;4:102–113.
224. Bostic JQ, Biederman J, Spencer TJ, et al. Pemoline treatment of adolescents with attention deficit hyperactivity disorder: a short-term controlled trial. J Child Adolesc Psychopharmacol 2000;10:205–216.
225. Gualtieri CT, Ondrusek MG, Finley C. Attention deficit disorders in adults. Clin Neuropharmacol 1985;8:343–356.
226. Wilens TE, Biederman J, Spencer TJ, et al. Controlled trial of high doses of pemoline for adults with attention-deficit/hyperactivity disorder. J Clin Psychopharmacol 1999;19:257–264.
227. Paterson R, Douglas C, Hallmayer J, Hagan M, Krupenia Z. A randomized, double-blind, placebo-controlled trial of dexamphetamine in adults with attention deficit hyperactivity disorder. Aus NZ J Psychiatry 1999;33:494–502.
228. Schubiner H, Saules KK, Arfken CL, et al. Double-blind placebo-controlled trial of methylphenidate in the treatment of adult ADHD patients with comorbid cocaine dependence. Exp Clin Psychopharmacol 2002;10:286–294.
229. Greenhill LL, Findling RL, Swanson JM, et al. A double-blind, placebo-controlled study of modified-release methylphenidate in children with attention-deficit/hyperactivity disorder. Pediatrics 2002;109:e39.
230. Biederman J, Lopez F, Boellner S, Chandler M. A randomized, double-blind, placebo-controlled, parallel-group study of SLI381 (Adderall XR) in children with attention-deficit/hyperactivity disorder. Pediatrics 2002;110:258–266.

22

Pharmacokinetic and Pharmacodynamic Drug Interactions

Methylphenidate, Amphetamine, or Atomoxetine in ADHD

John S. Markowitz and Kennerly S. Patrick

1. INTRODUCTION

Attention deficit hyperactivity disorder (ADHD) is the most commonly diagnosed neurobehavioral disorder and one of the most prevalent chronic health problems afflicting school-aged children in the United States *(1)*. ADHD has a prevalence rate estimated to range from 4 to 9% of children and adolescents *(1–3)*. Multimodal treatment approaches—those that combine medication treatment with psychotherapeutic, environmental, educational, and school-based interventions—are generally recommended to treat the disorder. Pharmacotherapy is established as both a common and an effective intervention *(2,4,5)*. Although recently published practice guidelines, algorithms, and consensus statements support the judicious use of medication as a fundamental treatment for ADHD *(2,6,7)*, pharmacotherapy is not universal. A recent survey performed by the US Centers for Disease Control and Prevention reported that only approx 54% of children 6–11 yr of age diagnosed with ADHD receive prescription medication, with this number increasing to 61% among children with ADHD *and* a learning disorder *(8)*. Other data have suggested that these estimates may be conservative.

ADHD cases account for as many as 30–50% of all mental health services referrals for children. Once thought to be a disorder largely limited to childhood, and self-resolving on reaching adolescence, it now appears that up to 75% of children or adolescents diagnosed with ADHD have symptoms persisting into adulthood *(9)*. For a significant number of individuals, ADHD represents a lifelong disorder that requires treatment, often with pharmacotherapy, well into adult life *(9,10)*.

Drug–drug interactions are a considerable source of concern in all medical disciplines and subspecialties owing to their association with therapeutic failure, potential toxicity, and increased morbidity and mortality. Additionally, adverse drug reactions and interactions are not infrequently a source of litigation. A number of factors suggest that patients with ADHD are highly likely to receive more than a single therapeutic agent during the course of their treatment, potentially placing them at risk for drug–drug interactions. These factors include frequent comorbid psychiatric illnesses *(11)*, and the recent recognition that a substantial number of patients continue to have symptoms of the disorder into adulthood. The latter factor results in the concomitant use of ADHD medications with a variety of drugs typically associ-

From: *Attention Deficit Hyperactivity Disorder: From Genes to Patients*
Edited by: D. Gozal and D. L. Molfese © Humana Press Inc., Totowa, NJ

ated with adult patient populations rather than children or adolescents. Examples of such medications include maintenance pharmacotherapy for diabetes, hyperlipidemia, and hypertension.

Individuals with ADHD are at a greater risk for a variety of comorbid psychiatric disorders including oppositional defiant disorder, conduct disorder, depression, anxiety disorders, and bipolar disorder, many of which are also amenable to treatment with psychotherapeutic agents *(12,13)*. Over the last decade there has been an increasing trend in the use of combination pharmacotherapy with psychopharmacologic agents in child, adolescent and adult clinical psychiatric practice *(14,15)*. Recent reports and survey data, as well as analyses of health maintenance organization and prescription drug databases, suggest that 14–90% of children and adolescents are concurrently treated with a psychostimulant such as methylphenidate (MPH) or amphetamine (AMP) and one or more other psychotropic medication *(11,16–19)*. Additionally, some recently published guidelines recommend the use of combination drug therapy in patients with ADHD and other comorbid conditions, such as tic disorder or intermittent explosive disorder *(20)*. It has also been noted that greater risks of tobacco and substance abuse are present relative to non-ADHD peers *(21,22)*. Use of these substances may also lead to significant drug–drug interactions. Finally, recent studies indicate that overall health care utilization and costs for children and adolescents with ADHD are significantly higher than in those without the disorder that further suggests the potential for increased utilization of other medications *(23,24)*. Together, the recognized persistence of ADHD, the frequent occurrence of comorbid psychiatric conditions treated with medications, and the overall increased likelihood of clinic or hospital visits for other medical reasons suggests that the use of combinations of prescription and/or over-the-counter (OTC) medication(s) with ADHD pharmacotherapy on an acute or chronic basis is highly likely. The present chapter seeks to provide a comprehensive review of the drug interaction potential of medications used to treat ADHD with other therapeutic agents. While the list of potential drug–drug interactions with medications utilized in the treatment of ADHD appears quite lengthy on consultation of product information inserts or texts such as the *Physicians' Desk Reference*, systematic reviews of the pertinent biomedical literature finds the majority of these precautions to be without firm support, and essentially, few that have been verified through formal study *(25,26)*. A discussion of only those interactions that appear to have a firm foundation from a clinical or theoretical perspective will be discussed in this chapter.

2. POTENTIAL TYPES AND MECHANISMS OF DRUG–DRUG INTERACTIONS

Drug interactions are generally viewed as falling into one of three main categories: pharmaceutic, pharmacodynamic, and pharmacokinetic. Pharmaceutic drug interactions typically involve problems of incompatibility of medications in parenteral products, such as intravenous fluids, and are generally governed by the physiochemical properties of the various drugs, nutritional additives, and/or diluents, and may involve such processes as drug complexation or precepitation. These types of interactions are rarely of clinical concern with regard to the medications utilized to treat ADHD.

2.1. Pharmacodynamic Drug–Drug Interactions

Pharmacodynamic interactions are those that alter the pharmacological activity of therapeutic agents resulting in antagonistic, additive, or potentially synergistic effects upon one or more interacting medication. Because these interactions are not associated with an alteration in plasma, urine, or tissue concentration of drugs, they are often suspected on the basis of diminished (if antagonistic), exaggerated, or toxic (if additive or synergistic) effects in a patient previously maintained satisfactorily on a given medication regimen. Evidence of a pharmacodynamic interaction, as in ethanol given with diazepam, relies primarily on clinical observations and objective measures of drug pharmacological effects (e.g., respiratory depression owing to additive central nervous system [CNS] effects).

2.2. *Pharmacokinetic Drug–Drug Interactions*

Pharmacokinetic interactions may alter one or more of the aspects affecting drug absorption and disposition (distribution, metabolism or biotransformation, and elimination). Changes in absorption may occur when some medications are administered with high-fat meals or antacid formulations. Changes in distribution, which typically result from protein-binding displacement reactions, increase the amount of one or both medications' free or bioavailable form and were once widely thought to substantially contribute to changes in drug disposition. Protein-binding interactions are now seen as significant for only a few psychotropic medications *(27)*. It appears that the most important aspect governing clinically relevant drug–drug interactions is that of metabolic interactions *(28)*. The inclusion of information on metabolic interactions in both package inserts and new drug applications (NDAs) to the US Food and Drug Administration (FDA) has increased dramatically in the last decade, with the largest percentage of clinical drug interaction studies involving neuropharmacologic agents *(29)*.

Drug metabolic pathways are generally subdivided into two phases. Phase I (functionalization) reactions result in products containing new or modified functional groups. Oxidative pathways dominate phase I processes—for instance, the metabolism of AMP to *p*-hydroxyAMP (*see* Fig. 1). Reductive pathways are also included in phase I reactions as illustrated by the metabolic reduction of the ketone in the structure of the antidepressant (and third-line ADHD medication) bupropion. This biotransformation pathway yields one of the corresponding active affecting drug metabolism alcohol metabolites of bupropion. Phase I metabolism also includes hydrolysis reactions, such as the de-esterification of MPH to an amino acid (*see* Fig. 2). The majority of marketed medications are metabolized to varying extents by the cytochrome P450 (CYP) mixed-function oxidase system. The CYP enzyme system is a supergene family with more than a dozen prominent enzymes *(30)*. The primary isoforms of interest in human drug metabolism include *CYP1A2, CYP2C9, CYP2C19, CYP2D6, CYP2E1*, and *CYP3A4*. The majority of these enzymes may be induced or inhibited to varying degrees by different medications, dietary compounds, and environmental factors. Expression of CYPs are known to differ during fetal, newborn, and neonatal developmental stages, although few major age-related differences have been reported after reaching early childhood *(31)*. The recognition of genetic polymorphisms influencing the CYP system, as well as other metabolic enzymes that can significantly affect the disposition of, and response to, different medications has led to the development of specific programmatic research in pharmacotherapy, such as pharmacogenetics/pharmacogenomics *(32)*.

Phase II metabolism (conjugation) involves those processes generating addition products of drugs with biochemical substrates. The prototype conjugation reaction is glucuronidation involving the coupling of endogenous glucuronic acid with a drug, and/or drug phase I metabolite(s), to yield a glucuronide adduct. Unlike phase I products, the phase II conjugates only rarely contribute to the overall pharmacodynamic response to an administered drug. The highly CNS-active morphine-6-glucuronide represents a notable exception. Both phase I and II metabolic reactions usually result in more polar, highly water-soluble metabolites. The

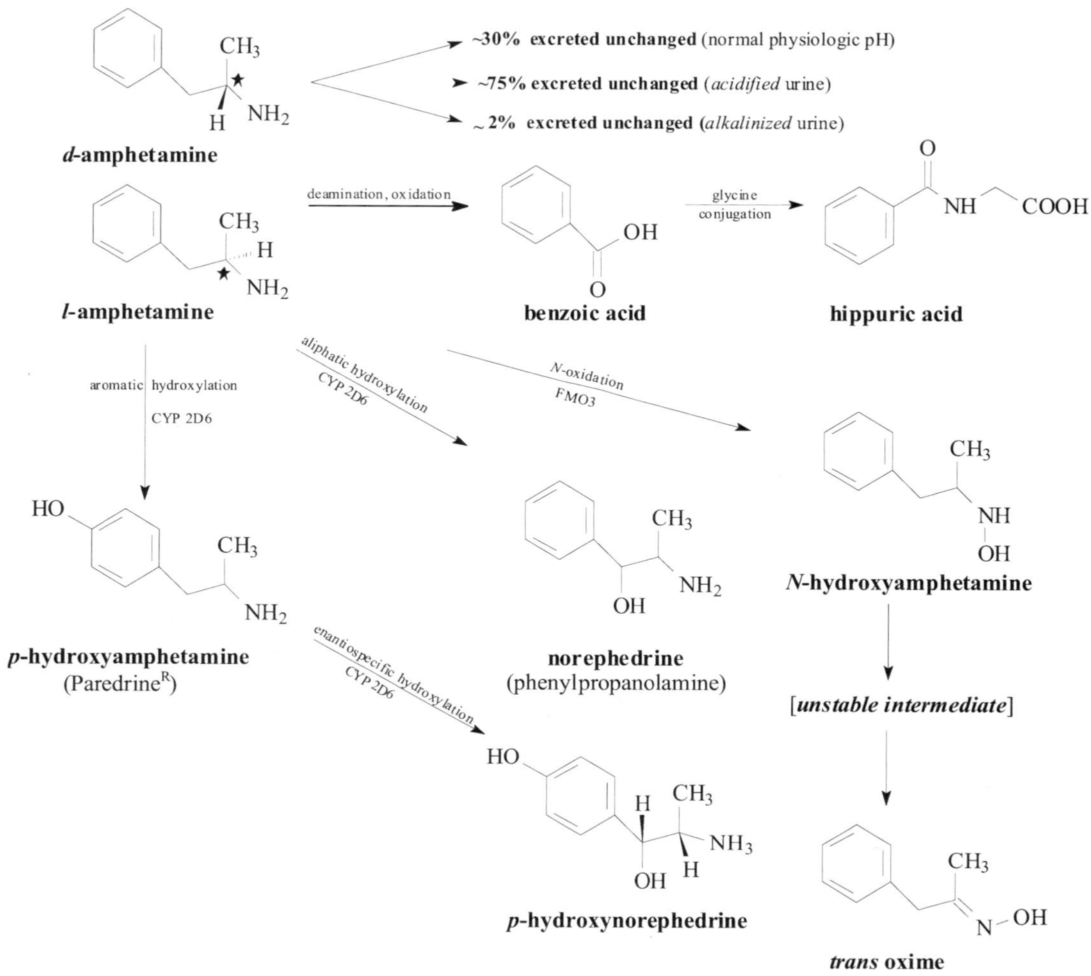

Fig. 1. Metabolic pathways of amphetamine in humans.

enzymes involved are frequently subject to either metabolic induction or inhibition by these other substrates or by genetic and environmental factors *(33)*. As with the CYP450 system, a number of genetic polymorphisms in the expression of specific phase II conjugative enzymes have been identified that are relevant to psychotherapeutic agents *(33)*.

Phase III drug interactions are transporter-mediated and have been the recent subject of intense study due to the potential of one drug to profoundly influence the bioavailability, tissue distribution, and elimination rate of another drug. Drug efflux transport proteins intercalated in cellular membranes influence gut uptake, biliary and renal secretion, as well as transport across the blood–brain barrier. Prominent among these is the ATP-binding cassette (ABC) transporter, P-glycoprotein *(34)*. As with most other metabolic processes, genetic polymorphisms are in evidence.

This chapter examines the clinical pharmacokinetics of the most commonly used ADHD medications in the context of dispositional and pharmacodynamic interactions associated with polytherapy. Documented, as well as theoretically possible, interactions are discussed and recommendations for avoidance or management of such interactions offered.

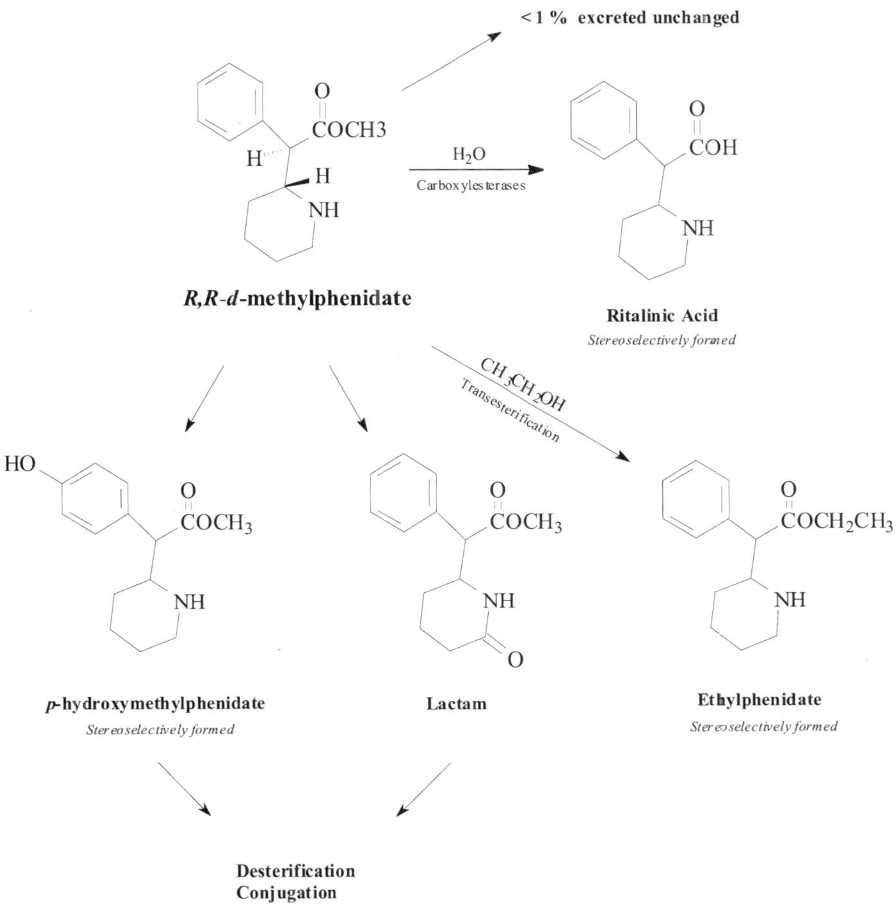

Fig. 2. Metabolic pathways of methylphenidate in humans.

3. PHARMACOTHERAPY OF ADHD

The primary pharmacotherapies utilized to treat ADHD are the psychostimulants MPH, *d*-AMP *(35)*, and mixed isomers of AMP *(36–38)* (containing 75% *d*-AMP and 25% *l*-AMP *[39,40]*, Adderall®). These agents account for approx 90% of ADHD drug treatment. The various formulations of MPH account for 70% of drug therapy. Interestingly, of the "new" FDA-approved medications introduced into US clinical practice over the past decade, approx 90% represent reformulations of MPH or AMP, agents that have been in clinical use for nearly 50 and 80 yr, respectively.

Atomoxetine (AMX), the most recently FDA-approved medication for ADHD, and the only nonstimulant approved for this indication, has emerged as an alternative to traditional stimulant therapy. Accordingly, AMX, in addition to the psychostimulants, will receive primary attention in this pharmacological review. Among the traditional psychostimulants, i.e., MPH and AMP formulations, recently established practice guidelines, algorithms, and consensus statements on the pharmacotherapy of ADHD have not identified an agent of first choice *(6,7,20,41)*, and no major guidelines have been set forth or published since the clinical availability of AMX.

4. METHYLPHENIDATE

4.1. MPH Pharmacodynamics

MPH is widely viewed as the "gold standard" treatment, as indicated by its choice as a comparator agent in numerous clinical trials of other medications for ADHD, including pivotal trials involving AMX, and its selection for the MTA study *(5)*. The beneficial behavioral effects of MPH appear to be elicited primarily through an inhibition of the presynaptic dopamine (DA) transporter *(43–45)*, with a minor influence on the norepinephrine (NE) transporter. This blockade amplifies neurotransmission *(46–48)* by increasing synaptic cleft residence time of impulse-released DA *(48–50)*. An opposing action of MPH on DA tone may relate to dopamine reuptake inhibition increasing the stimulation of presynaptic inhibitory autoreceptors *(48,50,51)*. The phenethylamine pharmacophore, common to the structures of MPH, DA, and NE, provides for transporter receptor docking recognition as MPH competes with DA *(52,53)*. MPH binds with the DA transporter, but does not possess the intrinsic activity required to induce the conformational change for translocation of the substrate, and binding site, to the cytoplasm. Thus, unlike AMP *(53,54)*, MPH cannot drive the release of cytoplasmic dopamine into the synaptic cleft as the transporter returns to its former conformation. MPH appears to only block DA synaptic clearance *(49)*.

Until the recent introduction of enantiopure the *d*-MPH product (*threo-R,R-d*-MPH, dexmethylphenidate, Focalin™), all marketed MPH formulations contained a racemic (50:50) mixture of *threo-R,R-d*-MPH (Fig. 2) and its mirror image *threo-S,S-l*-MPH. The ADHD psychotherapeutic effects *(55,56)*, and unfortunately, the cardiovascular *(53,57,58)* and anorexic side effects *(59,60)*, reside primarily in the *d*-enantiomer. However, the *l*-MPH isomer of racemic formulations may not necessarily represent a passive component in view of recent efforts to develop *l*-MPH as an antidepressant *(61)*. High-dose toxicity studies in rats found the racemate to be approximately half as toxic as *d*-MPH *(62)*.

A MPH *enantiomer–enantiomer interaction* has been associated with the neuropharmacology of racemic MPH. Davids and associates *(63)* assessed the activity of the separate MPH enantiomers in a rat model of ADHD and found that *d*-MPH was more than three times more active in reducing motor activity than was racemic MPH. A twofold reduction would be predicted if *l*-MPH were merely an inactive component. Additionally, pretreatment of the rats with *l*-MPH attenuated the motor activity response *d*-MPH. Comparative behavioral effects of *l*-MPH and *d*-MPH in rats revealed that females were more sensitive than males to some effects of the *l*-isomer, and more sensitive to both isomers in other elements of an observational battery *(63)*.

4.2. MPH Pharmacokinetics

The facile deesterification of MPH to the inactive *(65)* metabolite ritalinic acid *(67–69)* (Fig. 2) limits the absolute bioavailability to 11–53% *(69)*. Plasma concentrations of ritalinic acid far exceed those of the parent drug *(70–73)* and urinary elimination of ritalinic acid accounts for 60–80% of the dose *(67–69)*. This hydrolysis pathway appears primarily mediated by the carboxyesterase-1 isoform CES1A1*(74)*. The deesterification is an enantioselective process resulting in higher plasma concentrations and a longer $t_{1/2}$ for *d*-MPH. With few exceptions *(75)*, therapeutic drug monitoring studies of MPH have been limited to nonenantiospecific analytical approaches, i.e., reporting only pooled *d*- and *l*-MPH concentrations

(52). This lack of enantiospecific analyses may be of little clinical relevance in view of the much lower relative peripheral concentration of *l*-MPH in plasma and in dopaminergic regions of the human brain *(45)*. The area under the plasma concentration-time curve $(AUC)_{inf}$ value for the (*l*)-isomer has been reported to reach only 1% that of *d*-MPH *(72)*. However, radiolabeled *l*-MPH (or metabolite) has recently been reported to be taken up into the brain more readily than *d*-MPH after oral administration in rats or baboons *(76)*. Other minor urinary elimination products of MPH include the pharmacologically inactive lactam (<1%) *(67)*, the deesterified lactam (5–12% of dose) *(66)*, the active, yet minor metabolite *p*-hydroxy-MPH*(77)* (Fig. 2), and the unchanged parent drug (<1%) *(66–68)*.

The pharmacokinetics of MPH have not been found to differ significantly between children, adolescents, or adults, although a recent study evaluating normal adults indicated that the absolute bioavailability of MPH was greater in men than in women *(78)*. There is little evidence that variability in the bioavailability within a single subject is of the magnitude seen between subjects *(78,79)*. The *extent* of absorption of essentially all MPH dosage forms is unaffected by food intake, although consumption of a high-fat meal may result in a delay in the time to reach peak plasma concentration (T_{max}). Actual peak plasma concentration (C_{max}) may also be either increased or decreased after a high-fat meal, so inconsistent responses in some patients may be related to dietary fat intake. MPH is formulated as the highly water-soluble hydrochloride salt. In solution, MPH is rapidly and extensively absorbed from the intestine to the colon *(67,81)*. The governing factor controlling MPH absorption from immediate-release (IR) dosage forms is most likely gastric emptying time; for the various extended-release dosage forms, it is the programmed drug release and dissolution pattern. Because of extensive first-pass metabolism, the systemic exposure of unchanged drug (i.e., the absolute bioavailability) after oral dosing is low and variable *(82)*.

MPH is rapidly distributed to the various tissues with a steady-state volume of distribution (Vd) of approx 2 L/kg *(79)*. Oral clearance (Cl_O) of MPH is also rapid with little or no accumulation of the drug from day to day, even with the extended-release formulations *(71)*. At higher doses there is some evidence of nonlinearity, which may be related to saturation of the first pass metabolism. The $t_{1/2}$ of MPH is reported to range from approx 2–6 h, with most studies reporting an average of 2–3 h. With regard to the pharmacokinetics of the single-isomer formulation, *d*-MPH, clinical development and study doses utilized 50% that of racemic MPH. There were no significant differences observed in measured parameters such as C_{max}, T_{max}, and $t_{1/2}$ *(83,84)*.

4.3. MPH Drug Interactions

Package insert materials for all MPH-containing formulations suggest at least the potential for numerous drug–drug interactions, primarily of the pharmacokinetic type. These precautions largely reflect various case reports, early research abstracts reporting results of limited in vitro studies, and rodent studies that have accumulated following approximately half a century's clinical use of the drug. Little formal assessment in the way of drug interaction potential was required prior to the initial marketing of MPH (or AMP) formulations. However, a systematic review of the available MPH literature finds that very few of the case reports present convincing data, and essentially none have been verified when formal clinical studies were conducted with the medication in question in normal research subjects *(25,26)*.

4.3.1. MPH Pharmacodynamic Drug Interactions

MPH prescribing information carries a labeled contraindication regarding the initiation of MPH within 14 d of the use of a monoamine oxidase inhibitor (MAOI). Stimulant–MAOI combinations were employed in the past largely in an effort to obtain a therapeutic response in treatment-resistant depression in an era in which fewer therapeutic options were available. Contraindications between MAOIs and MPH are not surprising given the predisposition toward a hypertensive crisis when combining sympathomimetic agents. At least one published case report has documented symptoms consistent with a hypertensive crisis (e.g., occipital headache, hyperventilation) following the combination of MPH with the MAOI tranylcypromine, although blood pressure (BP) measurements were not reported *(85)*. The concomitant use of MPH and MAOIs, such as tranylcypromine or phenelzine, should be regarded as one of the few strict contraindications with MPH *(26)*.

The α_2-adrenergic agonist antihypertensive agent clonidine is known to be useful in the treatment of some symptoms of ADHD as well as a number of conditions known to frequently co-occur with ADHD *(86)*. As a consequence, clonidine is frequently coadministered with psychostimulants such as MPH. In the mid-1990s a series of cases came to light involving adverse cardiovascular effects experienced in children prescribed MPH-clonidine combinations and questions regarding the safety of this combination arose *(87)*. However, a review of the available cases contained within the FDA MedWatch database indicated that three of the four reported cases that resulted in fatalities were complicated by extenuating circumstances, whereas the fourth case may have been attributable to clonidine alone *(26)*. Two recent trials assessing the safety and efficacy of the MPH–clonidine combination in the treatment of comorbid Tourette's syndrome *(88)* and oppositional defiant disorder *(89)* revealed no significant adverse effects associated with this combination. Nevertheless, the seriousness of the suspected reaction and/or outcome, as well as the relatively limited number of patients studied in drug combination trials, suggests that some degree of vigilance should be maintained when using this combination. The hypotensive effects of the antihypertensive ganglionic-blocking agent guanethidine have been found to be attenuated or abolished by MPH administration. Although such an interaction could have clinical significance in select patients, guanethidine is rarely used in the management of hypertension today, and the likelihood of coadministration with MPH appears to be fairly remote *(26)*. A double-blind study conducted in ADHD subjects suggests that the antipsychotic (i.e., antidopaminergic) medication haloperidol may diminish the positive cognitive effects of psychostimulants *(90)*. The implications for general clinical use of these two therapeutic classes together are not clear but suggest the possibility of mutually antagonistic effects depending on the dosage of the respective agent.

Although the use of psychostimulant combinations (e.g., MPH + AMP) is not advocated in even recalcitrant cases of ADHD, or in any published ADHD treatment recommendations or algorithms, antecdotal reports suggest that the practice is sometimes undertaken. With this in mind, known pharmacodynamic interactions based on early clinical pharmacology studies follow.

Both enantiomers of AMP found in the mixed salt formulations (Adderall®) produce approximately equal elevation in BP, whereas the *d*-isomer increases heart rate to a greater degree than *l*-AMP *(91)*. The pressor effects of MPH reside almost exclusively in the *d*-isomer *(53)*. Based on imaging studies in humans *(92)*, physiological mechanisms underlying cardiovascular side effects of MPH are associated with alterations in both brain DA and circulating NE. In intravenous dosing experiments with dogs, the hypertensive effect of AMP subsides abruptly after MPH administration, and pretreatment with MPH blocks the pressor response of AMP altogether *(93–95)*. Related observations have been reported regarding the antagonism of tyramine induced hypertension by cocaine *(96)*. (*Note*: cocaine acts at the DA transporter in a fashion mechanistically indistinguishable to that of MPH [44,52,54]). This oppositional action of MPH to the pressor response to AMP supports the pharmacodynamic model outlined above, i.e., MPH blocks the transporter without serving as an uptake substrate, unlike AMP, which requires transport preceding DA release. It follows that AMP requires a functional transporter that MPH decommissions. The intravenous route of administration and the rapid time course of responses largely avoids pharmacokinetic considerations in interpreting the basis of this preclinical AMP–MPH drug interaction.

4.3.2. MPH Pharmacokinetic Drug Interactions

Though the majority of MPH is hydrolyzed by esterases, biotransformation to the lactam occurs through oxidative metabolism. The specific isoform(s) mediating this pathway has not been identified. A pilot clinical study (n = 6), utilizing the prototypic CYP2D6 inhibitor quinidine did not support a role for 2D6 *(97)*. Additionally, this quinidine study provides an indication that MPH may not be a substrate of the drug efflux transporter P-glycoprotein, as quinidine is a known inhibitor of P-glycoprotein *(98)*; this study found no differences in MPH pharmacokinetic parameters at baseline versus after quinidine coadministration. It is noted that the 50-mg quinidine dose used was modest *(97)*.

Early literature reports of pharmacokinetic drug interactions of MPH have generally only suggested an influence of MPH on the disposition of other drugs, rather than an influence of other drugs on MPH pharmacokinetics *(25,26)*. Relatively few clinically significant pharmacokinetic interactions with MPH have been confirmed through formal clinical study despite extensive precautions in MPH package labeling *(25,26)*. Although package labeling states that MPH should be used cautiously in patients treated with tricyclic antidepressants, a review of published case reports reveal that there is essentially no firm evidence supporting a pharmacokinetic interaction with desipramine and any purported effects on imipramine are highly questionable *(25,26)*. Surveillance studies do not indicate that coadministration of MPH and the anticonvulsants carbamazepine, valproic acid, ethosuximide, vigabatrin, phenytoin, or phenobarbital result in any peturbations in the anticonvulsant concentrations *(26)*. However, it is unclear whether these and/or other anticonvulsants may influence the disposition of MPH. Although MPH does not appear to be a significant substrate of any CYP isoform, its role as a potential inhibitor of one or more metabolic enzymes is less clear. The potential for racemic MPH, and its major metabolite ritalinic acid, to inhibit CYP enzymes was explored in an in vitro study utilizing human microsomes and pointed to a modest inhibition of CYP2D6 and 2B6 by racemic MPH, but not of 1A2, 2C19, 2E1, or 3A *(99)*. In the same study, ritalinic acid exhibited minimal effects on all enzymes assessed.

In contrast, another more recent in vitro study found that neither *d*-, *l*-, nor racemic MPH were likely to inhibit CYP1A2, 2C9, 2C19, 3A4, or 2D6 *(100)*. Likewise the prescribing information for *d*-MPH indicates that it was not found to be an inhibitor of any major CYP enzymes *(84)*. A study conducted in Swiss Webster mice (a nontransgenic model) found significantly decreased hepatic CYP3A, 1A, and 2E1 activity following large intraperitoneal (ip) doses of MPH designed to model MPH abuse. With lower oral doses, more consistent with "therapeutic" amounts were administered, only the activity of CYP1A was significantly diminished *(101)*. The ability to generalize these findings to that likely to occur in human subjects is limited.

A drug interaction between MPH and ethyl alcohol has recently been reported and involves the formation of an active metabolite, ethylphenidate (Fig. 2), identified initially in individuals who intentionally overdosed on MPH and ethanol *(102)*. Subsequently, the novel metabolite was identified in healthy volunteers who were systematically dosed with MPH and alcohol *(103)*. It is theorized that ethylphenidate is formed through an esterase-mediated transesterification pathway analogous to that known to be involved in the formation of cocaethylene following ethanol and cocaine co-ingestion. The possible pharmacodynamic significance of ethylphenidate formation is presently under investigation. As with the most predominant metabolic pathway of MPH (i.e., deesterification of MPH to ritalinic acid), the transesterification of MPH to ethylphenidate appears to occur with enantioselectively, favoring the *l*-MPH isomer as a substrate *(104)*. Further, the relative importance of polymorphism and expression of esterases *(105)*, as well as the potential for competitive inhibition of MPH deesterification by other ester-containing drugs (e.g., enalapril, meperidine), or by ethanol *(106)*, have not been explored. A number of broad metabolic inducers such as phenobarbital and rifampin appear to also be capable of inducing carboxylesterase enzymes *(105)* and their potential to increase the clearance of MPH via metabolic induction cannot be excluded.

5. AMPHETAMINE

5.1. AMP Pharmacodynamics

Both AMP and MPH provide therapeutic effects at the level of the dopamine transporter but are believed to differ in the specific mechanism. Current theory holds that MPH only inhibits synaptic clearance of DA by blocking the access of DA to the transporter binding site. Conversely, AMP serves as an actual substrate for transport into the presynaptic terminal *(49)*. Membrane transporters, while being gated, do not possess the architecture of membrane pores or channels, i.e., DA does not have direct access to both sides of the membrane simultaneously. Two sodium ions and one chloride ion serve as cosubstrates with DA and supply the transport energy based on their transmembrane concentration gradients. AMP and sodium ions dock within the 12 membrane spanning regions of the transporter, as envisioned in a pocketlike model where this receptacle first faces the extraneuronal biophase, and then, upon chloride binding, a protein conformational change translocates the binding regions to face the intraneuronal biophase. Subsequent unloading of AMP, and the cosubstrates, from the transporter exposes the vacant DA binding site that then binds cytoplasmic DA. Return of the transporter to its former conformation state ultimately releases DA into the synaptic cleft *(107)*.

5.2. AMP Pharmacokinetics

Both isomers of amphetamine are well absorbed orally and there appears to be little effect of food on the extent of absorption of at least *d*-AMP in either IR *(108)* or sustained-release (SR) formulations *(109)*. Plasma protein binding is at approx 16% and the Vd is similar for both isomers *(110)*. The T_{max} of AMP generally occurs within 2–3 h, though substantial intersubject variability has been reported. The T_{max} is 3–6 h for the SR formulation *(109)*. The mean C_{max} after 0.25 or 0.5 mg/kg doses of AMP are approx 40 and 70 ng/mL, respectively *(108)*. A $t_{1/2}$ of 7 h is typical *(111)*. The $t_{1/2}$ of *d*-AMP appears to be slightly shorter than that for *l*-AMP, and it has been postulated that stereoselective differences in metabolic deamination account for this difference *(110)*. Although both enantiomers accumulate in the brain, *d*-AMP may attain higher concentrations *(112)*.

AMP is eliminated primarily as benzoic acid and its corresponding glycine conjugate, hippuric acid (Fig. 1). Metabolism of AMP proceeds primarily through oxidative deamination forming the intermediate phenylpropanone, part of which is eliminated as a sulfate conjugate *(113)*. Aromatic hydroxylation appears to be medicated by CYP2D6 *(26)*. Rodent studies in which animals were pretreated with quinidine have suggested that inhibition of CYP2D6 may result in doubling of AMP plasma AUCs *(26)*. However, no systematic studies have been performed in humans evaluating the potential for CYP2D6 inhibitors or other agents to elevate circulating AMP concentrations. Approximately one third of a dose is excreted unchanged at an unadjusted urinary pH. Less than 10% of an oral dose is converted into the pharmacologically active metabolites, *p*-hydroxyamphetamine and phenylpropanolamine (Fig. 1) *(114)*. Although *p*-hydroxylation is not a major metabolic pathway in man, there is evidence that *d*-AMP, but not *l*-AMP, may be metabolized to *p*-hydroxynorepinephrine. This metabolite has been implicated in the depletion of CNS NE and post-AMP treatment clinical depression *(115)*.

5.3. AMP Drug Interactions

5.3.1. AMP Pharmacodynamic Interactions

As with MPH, coadministration of AMP formulations with MAOIs probably represents one of the few absolute contraindications—and, indeed, fatalities secondary to adverse cardiovascular effects have been documented with these combinations *(25,26)*. There is some evidence that AMP may antagonize the intended hypotensive effects of some centrally acting antihypertensive agents *(26)*. A pharmacokinetic component to the interaction of MAOIs with AMP is based on the reduced metabolic clearance of AMP resulting from inhibition of the AMP deamination pathway by MAOIs.

5.3.2. AMP Pharmacokinetic Interactions

Urinary acidifying agents, e.g., ascorbic acid or ammonium chloride, dramatically increase AMP urinary excretion and reduce $t_{1/2}$. Conversely, urinary alkalinizing agents, such as acetazolamide facilitate renal tubular reabsorption and extend $t_{1/2}$ *(116)*.

AMP has only recently undergone formal in vitro study assessing its potential inhibitory activity on a battery of CYP isoforms. DeVane and associates *(100)* assessed *d*-, *l*-, and racemic AMP for their inhibitory capacity utilizing human liver microsomes. Neither individual isomer, nor the racemic mixture, produced significant inhibitory effects on the activities of the enzymes studied: CYP1A2, 2C9, 2C19, 2D6, or 3A4 *(100)*. Although this study suggests that AMP is unlikely to produce clinically relevant interactions medicated by these major drug metabolism isoforms, clinical studies assessing the potential for AMP to inhibit metabolism have not been performed to date. AMP formulations are commonly coadministered with selective serotonin reuptake inhibitors (SSRIs) to patients with comorbid conditions and several case reports suggest the combinations may be well-tolerated. However, several animal studies suggest that the disposition of AMP, a compound at least partially metabolized through the CYP2D6 pathway, may be influenced (i.e., brain concentrations are increased) by the coadministration of SSRIs such as fluoxetine that are moderate to potent inhibitors of this enzyme *(26)*. No study has been performed in human subjects to assess the potential for such an interaction.

Table 1
Comparison of Atomoxetine Pharmacokinetic Parameters Between Extensive and Poor Metabolizers of CYP2D6

Parameter	Extensive metabolizer	Poor metabolizer
Atomoxetine (parent compound)		
Bioavailability	94%	63%
T_{max}	1–2 h	3–4 h
$t_{1/2}$	~5 h	~22 h
Principal metabolites		
4-hydroxyatomoxetine		
$t_{1/2}$	6–8 h	35–40 h
AUC (μg[a] h/mL)[a]	2.74 (13.6)	0.935 (17)
Percent of circulating atomoxetine concentration	1%	0.1%
N-desmethylatomoxetine		
$t_{1/2}$	6–8 h	34–40 h
AUC (μg[a] h/mL)[a]	0.618 (86.4)	2.82 (41.2)
Percent of circulating atomoxetine concentration	5%	45%

[a]Based on values determined after multiple 20-mg doses of Atomoxetine administered twice daily.

6. ATOMOXETINE

6.1. AMX Pharmacodynamics

Atomoxetine (AMX) exhibits high NE transporter inhibitory activity and relatively minor DA transporter activity. It was initially developed as an antidepressant *(117)*. AMX was recently introduced as the first nonstimulant agent to gain Food and Drug Administration approval for the treatment of ADHD and was the first agent of any class to carry a labeled indication for adult ADHD. The drug was originally known generically as tomoxetine during earlier development as a selective noradrenergic antidepressant, but this designation was later modified to avoid potential prescribing and dispensing errors due to confusion with other agents of sound-alike names, primarily tamoxifen.

The exact mechanism of action of AMX in the treatment of ADHD is unknown. However, unlike traditional stimulant agents currently approved for the treatment of ADHD in children that are thought to exert therapeutic effects via inhibition of DA uptake in the neural synapse *(52,107)*, the therapeutic action of AMX appears to result from the selective inhibition of the presynaptic NE transporter, thereby elevating levels of impulse released NE *(117,118)*. There appears to be little affinity for cholinergic, histaminergic, serotonergic, or α-adrenergic neurotransmitter receptors.

6.2. AMX Pharmacokinetics

AMX is rapidly and extensively absorbed from the gastrointestinal tract following oral administration. Significant differences are noted in the disposition of AMX and its principal metabolites between genetically extensive metabolizers (EM) of CYP2D6 substrates vs genetically poor metabolizers (PM). These are outlined in Table 1. For instance, the absolute bioavailability of AMX in EMs is 63 vs 94% in PMs *(119)*. In single- and multidose studies, the C_{max} of AMX was reached in 1–2 h after dosing in EM subjects and approx 3–4 h in PM subjects *(120,121)*. The absolute bioavailability of AMX is not significantly affected by food. Although the administration of AMX following the ingestion of a standardized high-fat meal did not affect the extent of absorption, it did decrease the rate of absorption *(1)* and resulted in a 37% lower C_{max} and a delayed T_{max} of approx 3 h *(119)*. In PMs, the steady state concentration of AMX in the plasma is three fold higher after multiple doses compared to a single dose *(121)*. In pharmacokinetic studies comparing both single dosing and multiple twice-daily dosing in EMs, the steady-state plasma concentration (Css) profiles of patients administered twice-daily dosing were similar to those who received once-daily dosing, suggesting that the C_{max} is unaffected following multiple daily dosing *(122)*. The distribution of AMX is primarily into total body water with a Vd of 0.85 L/kg. AMX is 98% protein-bound, whereas the principal and active metabolite, 4-hydroxyatomoxetine, is approx 67% protein-bound *(122)*. The 4-hydroxyatomoxetine metabolite is equipotent to the parent compound in terms of NE reuptake inhibition but low circulating concentrations found in pediatric patients (e.g., 1% and 0.1% in EMs and PMs, respectively) indicate that its effects are unlikely to be of clinical significance *(121)*.

AMX is predominantly metabolized in the liver via the CYP enzyme system—primarily the CYP2D6 isoform. The degree of CYP2D6 metabolism in pediatric patients compared with adults is similar *(121,123)*, suggesting little difference in CYP2D6 activity in 7–14-yr-olds vs adults. Based on single- and multiple-dose pharmacokinetic studies in EMs, it appears that the primary mechanism of clearance (Cl) is by oxidative metabolism followed by conjugation (i.e., glucuronidation) *(121,123)*. Studies performed in healthy adults have also shown that AMX's pharmacokinetics are influenced by the genetic polymorphism of CYP2D6 *(123)*.

AMX undergoes three major phase I metabolic pathways: aromatic ring hydroxylation, benzylic oxidation, and *N*-demethylation (Fig. 3) *(120,122)*. The primary phase I metabolite, 4-hydroxyatomoxetine, is conjugated to 4-hydroxyatomoxetine-*O*-glucoronide. The formation of another phase I metabolite, *N*-desmethylatomoxetine, appears to be mediated by the CYP 2C19 pathway. The *N*-desmethyl metabolite is considerably less active pharmacologically than 4-hydroxyatomoxetine (Fig. 3) *(122)*. Low plasma concentrations of the demethylated metabolite were detected in EM patients, possibly as a result of further oxidative metabolism to *N*-desmethyl-4-hydroxyatomoxetine and its corresponding glucuronide (Fig. 3) *(122)*. Pharmacokinetic studies have indicated that individuals who are PMs display a significantly higher Css of both AMX and *N*-desmethylatomoxetine than EMs *(121)*. In a single-dose pharmacokinetic study conducted in EMs in which the dose of AMX was 10 mg, the plasma concentrations and AUC values of the metabolites were much lower than the AMX concentration. Though the concentration of 4-hydroxyatomoxetine was measurable in plasma, it was still more than 25 times less than the concentration of the parent compound *(121)*. In a multidose pharmacokinetic study conducted in EMs in which the dose was 20 to 40 mg twice daily, the degree of accumulation of AMX or its metabolites at Css was low, as the $t_{1/2}$, Cl, and Vd were similar to single-dose pharmacokinetic parameters *(121)*. The plasma concentration of 4-hydroxyatomoxetine was 35 times lower than the concentration of AMX. If the rate of hydroxylation via CYP2D6 is inhibited, the elimination pathway is believed to be "shunted" through the *N*-demethylation pathway, resulting in accumulation of *N*-desmethylatomoxetine *(119,123)*.

The mean elimination $t_{1/2}$ of AMX following oral administration is 5.2 h. In PMs, the mean $t_{1/2}$ is significantly increased to approx 22 h as a result of reduced Cl. This results in an

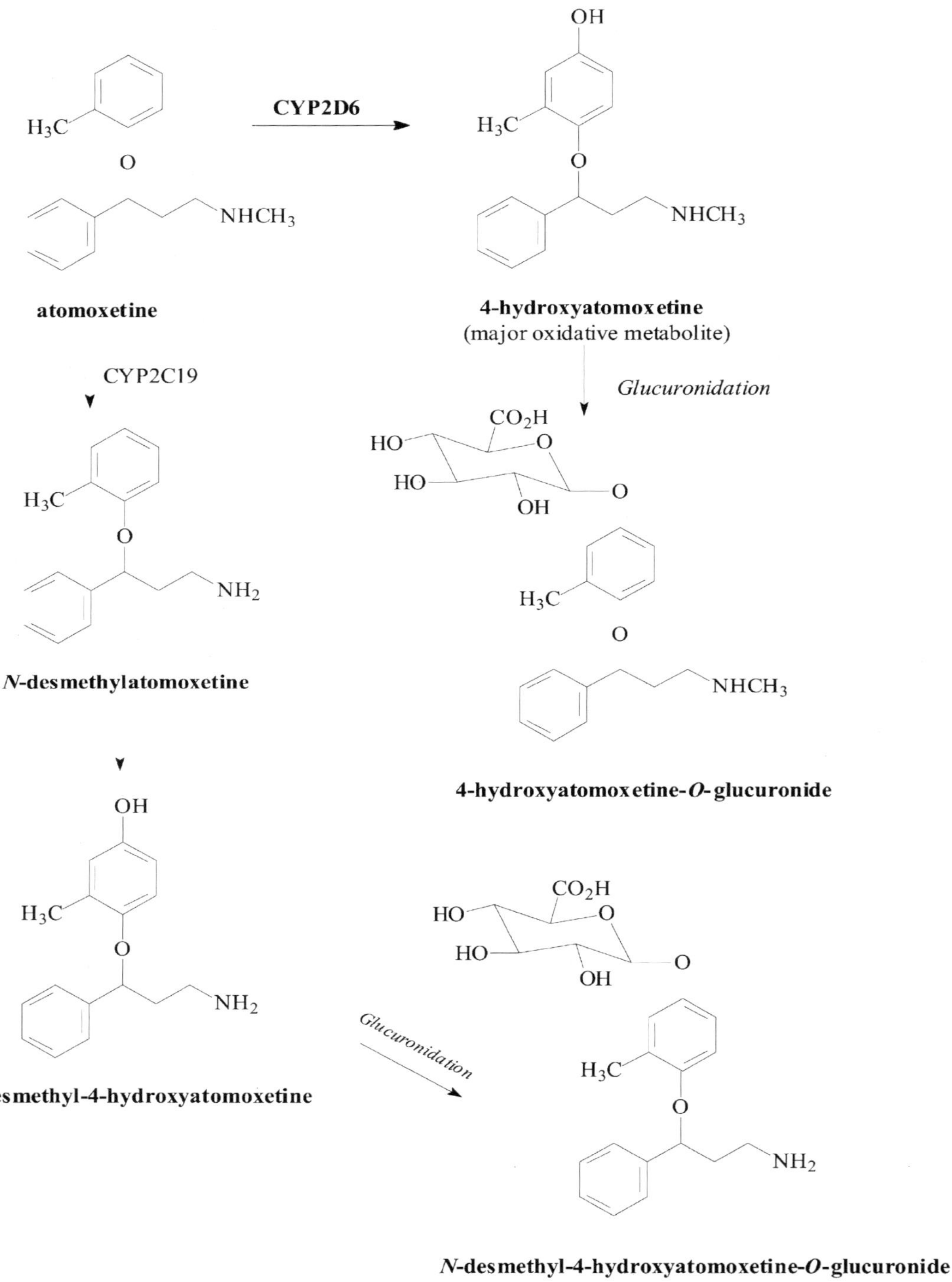

Fig. 3. Metabolic pathways of atomoxetine in humans.

AUC that is approx 10-fold greater than that of EMs. The elimination $t_{1/2}$ of the metabolites 4-hydroxyatomoxetine and *N*-desmethylatomoxetine is similar, ranging from 6 to 8 h in EMs and 34 to 40 h in PMs. More than 80% of the dose of AMX is excreted in the urine as

Table 2
Clinically Relevant Medications Known to Inhibit CYP2D6

Amiodarone	Doxorubicin
Bupropion	Fluoxetine (norfluoxetine)
Celecoxib	Methadone
Chlorpheniramine	Paroxetine
Chlorpromazine	Quinidine
Cimetidine	Ritonavir
Clomipramine	Terbinafine
Diphenhydramine	Thioridazine

4-hydroxyatomoxetine-*O*-glucuronide, whereas approx 17% of the total dose is excreted via the feces. Less than 3% of the dose is excreted unchanged, demonstrating extensive biotransformation *(119)*.

It should be noted that although AMX is highly dependent on CYP2D6 for its metabolism and elimination, in vitro studies suggest it is not a significant inhibitor of this or any other major CYP isoform *(119)*.

6.3. AMX Drug Interactions

6.3.1. AMX Pharmacodynamic Interactions

The clinical experience with AMX is limited because of its recent introduction into general clinical use. Package labeling indicates that several interactions may be relevant when considering combination therapies. MAOIs are considered to be contraindicated with the use of AMX resulting from the potential for serious, and potentially fatal, reactions to result when noradrenergic agents are coadministered with MAOIs. Additionally, there is a general labeling precaution regarding the potentially additive effects on BP that AMX may exert on persons already maintained on unspecified "pressor" agents. The administration of albuterol or other β_2-agonists via the oral or intravenous route should be undertaken with some degree of caution in AMX-treated patients owing to the possibility for potentiated effects on the cardiovascular system *(119)*. Finally, at least one pharmacokinetic study assessing the potential for an interaction between the SSRI antidepressant and known CYP2D6 inhibitor, paroxetine, and atomoxetine in normal volunteers found higher standing pulse rate and orthostatic changes compared to the administration of either agent alone *(124)*. It was speculated that this was because of a pharmacodyanamic mechanism rather than an observed pharmacokinetic interaction as the change in cardiovascular parameters was greater than that experienced by PMs in earlier studies whom had comparable AMX plasma concentrations *(124)*.

6.3.2. AMX Pharmacokinetic Interactions

As previously indicated, AMX, though a substrate of CYP2D6, does not appear to inhibit this or any other major CYP isoform to any appreciable degree *(119)*. Nevertheless, a number of clinically used medications can inhibit CYP2D6 activity significantly (Table 2), and may effectively produce a "phenocopy" mimicking the PM status, resulting in higher-than-expected plasma concentrations of AMX and its principal metabolites. A formal study conducted in normal volunteers ($n = 22$) who were EMs has indicated that clinically relevant doses (20 mg) of the antidepressant paroxetine, a potent CYP2D6 inhibitor, result in marked changes in AMX pharmacokinetics. For example, paroxetine administration resulted in a 3.5-fold increase in the $C_{ss,max}$, a 6.5-fold increase in the AUC_{0-12h}, and more than doubling of the AMX $t_{1/2}$. Additionally, following paroxetine administration, *N*-desmethylatomoxetine concentrations were increased, whereas 4-hydroxyatomoxetine concentrations *declined (124)*. An additional finding of this study was that AMX had no significant effects on paroxetine concentrations.

It has also been reported that another common SSRI antidepressant and CYP2D6 inhibitor, fluoxetine, will also elevate AMX concentrations. The degree of metabolic inhibition was not reported *(124)*. Taken together, these results suggest the potential for the concomitant use of known CYP2D6 inhibitors, such as those presented in Table 2, to result in elevated AMX concentrations and potentially greater dose-dependent side effects.

7. CONCLUSIONS

Pharmacotherapy of ADHD remains the foundational intervention for this disorder. Drug use in ADHD is increasing dramatically. Emerging surveillance data indicate that the traditional psychostimulants MPH and AMP, as well as the newer agent AMX, are often used in combination with a variety of other medications from diverse therapeutic classes. Relatively few absolute contraindications exist with these agents, with the exception of MAOIs. Most in vitro data indicate that neither MPH nor AMP significantly inhibits any of the major CYP isoforms.

Accordingly, this eliminates the dominant metabolic bases for most clinically significant drug–drug interactions. However, limited animal studies suggest that AMP metabolism may be reduced to a limited degree by inhibitors of CYP2D6. No clinical studies have been performed to investigate any relevance of CYP2D6 to drug interactions with AMP. The potential for known inhibitors or inducers of metabolic enzymes to influence the disposition of drugs used in ADHD therapy remains largely unexplored. There are few case reports available in this realm and therapeutic drug monitoring studies that might detect such interactions have only rarely been performed with psychostimulants. In the case of the nonstimulant AMX, circulating concentrations can be expected to elevate following exposure to inhibitors of CYP2D6, such as paroxetine or fluoxetine.

MPH appears to be largely unaffected by oxidative CYP enzymes owing to its facile hydrolytic metabolism. The role of concomitant medications competing for carboxylesterase(s), and thereby inhibiting MPH metabolic clearance, has not been explored. The role of phase II enzymes and drug transporters, conspicuously P-glycoprotein, are other potential sources of variability in drug disposition and response that have not been systematically explored. The existing biomedical literature yields few substantive reports of significant drug–drug interactions with MPH, AMP, or AMX, as consistent with the generally favorable safety profile of these agents.

REFERENCES

1. Goldman LS, Genel M, Bezman RJ, Slanetz PJ. Diagnosis and treatment of attention-deficit/hyperactivity disorder in children and adolescents. JAMA 1998;279:1100–7.
2. Swanson JM, Seargent JA, Taylor E, Sonuga-Barke EJS, Jensen PS, Cantwell DP. Attention deficit disorder and hyperkinetic disorder. Lancet 1998;351:429–33.
3. Dulcan M, the Work Group on Quality Issues. Practice parameters for the assessment and treatment of children, adolescents, and adults with attention-deficit/hyperactivity disorder. J Am Acad Child Adolesc Psychiatry 1997;36:85S–121S.
4. Homer CJ, Baltz RD, Hickson GB, et al. Clinical practice guideline: diagnosis and evaluation of the child with attention-deficit/hyperactivity disorder. Pediatrics 2000;105:1158–70.
5. The MTA Cooperative Group. A 14-month randomized clinical trial of treatment strategies for attention-deficit/hyperactivity disorder. Arch Gen Psychiatry 1999;56:1073–86.

6. Zametkin AJ, Ernst M. Problems in the management of attention-deficit-hyperactivity disorder. N Eng J Med 1999;340:40–6.
7. American Academy of Pediatrics Subcommittee on Attention-Deficit/Hyperactivity Disorder Committee on Quality Improvement. Clinical practice guideline: treatment of the school-aged child with attention-deficit/hyperactivity disorder. Pediatrics 2001;108:1033–44.
8. Attention deficit disorder and learning disability: United States, 1997–98. Centers for Disease Control, Vital and Health Statistics, Series 10, No. 206, May 2002.
9. Wilens TE, Biederman J, Spencer TJ. Attention deficit/hyperactivity disorder across the lifespan. Annu Rev Med 2002;53:113–31.
10. Weiss M, Murray C. Assessment and management of attention-deficit hyperactivity disorder in adults. Can Med Assoc J 2003;168:715–22.
11. Safer DJ, Zito JM, dosReis S. Concomitant psychotropic medication for youths. Am J Psychiatry 2003;160:438–49.
12. Spencer T, Biederman J, Wilens T. Attention-deficit/hyperactivity disorder and comorbidity. Pediatr Clin North Am 1999;46:915–27.
13. Kowatch RA, Sethuraman G, Hume JH, Kromelis M, Weinberg WA. Combination pharmacotherapy in children and adolescents with bipolar disorder. Biol Psychiatry 2003;53:978–84.
14. Wilens TE, Spencer T, Biederman J, Wozniak J, Connor D. Combined pharmacotherapy: an emerging trend in pediatric psychopharmacology. J Am Acad Child Adolesc Psychiatry 1995; 34:110–2.
15. Connor DF, Ozbayrak KR, Kusiak KA, Caponi AB, Melloni RH Jr. Combined pharmacotherapy in children and adolescents in a residential treatment center. J Am Acad Child Adolesc Psychiatry 1997;36:248–54.
16. Rushton JL, Whitmire JT. Pediatric stimulant and selective serotonin reuptake inhibitor prescription trends. 1992 to 1998. Arch Pediatr Adolesc Med 2001;155:560–5.
17. Guevara J, Lozano P, Wickizer T, Mell L, Gephart H. Psychotropic medication use in a population of children who have attention-deficit/hyperactivity disorder. Pediatrics 2002;109:733–9.
18. Zito JM, Safer DJ, dosReis S, Magder LS, Gardner JF, Zarin DA. Psychotherapeutic medication patterns for youths with attention-deficit/hyperactivity disorder. Arch Pediatr Adolesc Med 1999;153:1257–63.
19. Olfson M, Gameroff MJ, Marcus SC, Jensen PS. National trends in the treatment of attention deficit hyperactivity disorder. Am J Psychiatry 2003;160:1071–7.
20. Pliszka SR, Greenhill LL, Crismon ML, et al. The Texas children's medication algorithm project: Report of the Texas consensus conference panel on medication treatment of childhood attention-deficit/hyperactivity disorder. Part I. Attention-deficit/hyperactivity disorder. J Am Acad Child Adolesc Psychiatry 2000;39:908–19.
21. Milberger S, Biederman J, Faraone SV, Chen L, Jones J. ADHD is associated with early initiation of cigarette smoking in children and adolescents. Am Acad Child Adolesc Psychiatry 1997;36:37–44.
22. Biederman J, Wilens T, Mick E, Spencer T, Faraone SV. Pharmacotherapy of attention deficit/hyperactivity disorder reduces risk for substance use disorder. Pediatrics 1999;104:e20-e4.
23. Leibson CL, Katusic SK, Barbaresi WJ, Ransom J, O'Brien PC. Use and costs of medical care for children and adolescents with and without attention-deficit/hyperactivity disorder. JAMA 2001;285:60–6.
24. Chan E, Zhan CL, Homer CJ. Health care use costs for children with attention-deficit/hyperactivity disorder: national estimates from the medical expenditure panel survey. Arch Pediatr Adolesc Med 2002;156:504–11.
25. Markowitz JS, Morrison SD, DeVane CL. Drug interactions with psychostimulants. Int Clin Psychopharmacol 1999;14:1–18.
26. Markowitz JS, Patrick KS. Pharmacokinetic and pharmacodynamic drug interactions in the treatment of attention-deficit hyperactivity disorder. Clin Pharmacokinet 2001;40:753–72.
27. DeVane CL. Clinical significance of drug binding, protein binding, and binding displacement drug interactions. Psychopharmacol Bull 2002;36:5–21.

28. Balian JD, Rahman A. Metabolic drug-drug interactions: Perspective from FDA medical and clinical pharmacology reviewers. Adv Pharmacol 1997;43:231–8.
29. Alfaro CL. Emerging role of drug interaction studies in drug development: the good, the bad, and the unknown. Psychopharmacol Bull 2001;35:80–93.
30. Michalets EL. Update: clinically significant cytochrome P-450 drug interactions. Pharmacother 1998;18:84–112.
31. Oesterheld JR. A review of developmental aspects of cytochrome P450. J Child Adolesc Psychopharmacol 1998;8:161–74.
32. Evans WE, McLeod HL. Pharmacogenomics—drug disposition, drug targets, and side effects. N Eng J Med 2003;348:538–49.
33. Liston H, Markowitz JS, DeVane CL. Glucuronidation: Implications in psychopharmacology. J Clin Psychopharmacol 2001;21:500–15.
34. Borst P, Elferink RO. Mammalian ABC transporters in health and disease. Annu Rev Biochem 2002;71:537–92.
35. James RS, Sharp WS, Bastain TM, et al. Double-blind, placebo-controlled study of single-dose amphetamine formulations in ADHD. J Am Acad Child Adolesc Psychiatry 2001;40:1268–76.
36. Manos MJ, Short EJ, Findling RL. Differential effectiveness of methylphenidate and Adderall in school-age youths with attention-deficit/hyperactivity disorder. J Am Acad Child Adolesc Psychiatry 1999;38:813–89.
37. Pliszka SR, Brown R, Olvera RL, Wynne SK. A double-blind, placebo-controlled study of Adderall and methylphenidate in the treatment of attention-deficit/hyperactivity disorder. J Am Acad Child Adolesc Psychiatry 2000;39:619–26.
38. Faraone SV, Biederman J, Roe C. Comparative efficacy of Adderall and methylphenidate in attention deficit/hyperactivity disorder: a meta-analysis. J Clin Psychopharmacol 2002;22:468–73.
39. Zabik JE, Levin RM, Maickel RP. Drug interaction with brain biogenic amines and the effects of amphetamine isomers on locomotor activity. Pharmacol Biochem Behav 1978;8:429–35.
40. Arnold LE, Huestis RD, Smeltzer DJ, Scheib J, Wemmer D, Colner G. Levamphetamine vs. dextroamphetamine in minimal brain dysfuction. Arch Gen Psychiatry 1976;33:292–301.
41. Greenhill LL, Pliszka S, Dulcan MK, and the Work Group on Quality Issues: AACAP. Practice parameters for the use of stimulant medications in the treatment of children, adolescents, and adults. J Am Acad Child Adolesc Psychiatry 2002;41(2 Suppl):26S-49S.
42. NIH Consensus Development Program. Diagnosis and treatment of attention deficit hyperactivity disorder. NIH Consensus Statement 1998 Nov 16–18;16(2):1–37. Available from http://odp.od.nih.gov/consensus/cons/110/110_statement.htm. Accessed March 25, 2003.
43. Volkow ND, Wang GJ, Fowler JS, et al. Dopamine transporter occupancies in the human brain induced by therapeutic doses of oral methylphenidate. Am J Psychiatry 1998;155:1325–31.
44. Volkow ND, Wang G-J, Fowler JS, et al. Methylphenidate and cocaine have a similar in vivo potency to block dopamine transporters in the human brain. Life Sci 1999;65:PL7–12.
45. Volkow ND, Wang G-J, Fowler JS, et al. Relationship between blockade of dopamine transporters by oral methylphenidate and the increases in extracellular dopamine: therapeutic implications. Synapse 2002;43:181–7.
46. Ruskin DN, Berstrom DA, Shenker A, Freeman LE, Back D, Walters JR. Drugs used in the treatment of attention-deficit/hyperactive disorder affect postsynaptic firing rate and oscillation without preferential dopamine autoreceptor action. Biol Psychiatry 2001;49:340–50.
47. Volkow ND, Wang G-J, Fowler JS, et al. "Nonhedonic" food motivation in humans involves dopamine in the dorsal striatum and methylphenidate amplifies this effect. Synapse 2002;44:175–80.
48. Seeman P, Madras BK. Anti-hyperactivity medication: methylphenidate and amphetamine. Mol Psychiatry 1998;3:386–96.
49. Hitri A, Hurd YL, Wyatt RJ, Deutsch SI. Molecular, functional and biochemical characteristics of the dopamine transporter: regional differences and clinical relevance. J Clin Neuropharmacol 1994;17:1–22.

50. Solanto MV. Neuropsychopharmacological mechanisms of stimulant drug action in attention-deficit hyperactivity disorder: a review and integration. Behav Brain Res 1998;94:127–52.
51. Seeman P, Madras B. Methylphenidate elevates resting dopamine which lowers the impulse-triggered release of dopamine: a hypothesis. Behav Brain Res 2002;130:79–83.
52. Patrick KS and Markowitz JS. Pharmacology of methylphenidate, amphetamine enantiomers and pemoline in attention-deficit hyperactivity disorder: a review. Hum Psychopharmacol 1997;12:527–46.
53. Patrick KS, Caldwell RW, Ferris RM, Breese GR. Pharmacology of the enantiomers of *threo*-methylphenidate. J Pharmacol Exp Ther 1987;241:152–8.
54. Heron C, Costentin J, Bonnet J-J. Evidence that pure uptake inhibitors including cocaine interact slowly with the dopamine neuronal carrier. Eur J Pharmacol 1994;264:391–8.
55. Srinivas NR, Hubbard JW, Quinn D, et al. Enantioselective pharmacokinetics and pharmacodynamics of dl-*threo*-methylphenidate in children with attention deficit hyperactivity disorder. Clin Pharmacol Ther 1992;52:561–8.
56. Aoyama T, Sasaki T, Kotaki J. Pharmacokinetics and pharmacodynamics of (+)-*threo*-methylphenidate enantiomer in patients with hypersomnia. Clin Pharmacol Ther 1994;55: 270–6.
57. Findling RL, Short E, Manos MJ. Short-term cardiovascular effects of methylphenidate and Adderall. J Am Acad Child Adolesc Psychiatry 2001;40:525–9.
58. Stowe CD, Gardner SF, Gist CC, Schulz EG, Wells TG. 24-hour ambulatory blood pressure monitoring in male children receiving stimulant therapy. Pediatrics 2002;36:1142–9.
59. Efron D, Jarman F, Barker M. Side effects of methylphenidate and dexamphetamine in children with attention deficit disorder: A double-blind, crossover trial. Pediatrics 1997;100:662–6.
60. Eckerman DA, Moy SS, Perkins AN, Patrick KS, Breese GR. Enantioselective behavioral effects of *threo* methylphenidate in rats. Pharmacol Biochem Behav 40;875–80.
61. Rouhi AM. Chirality at work. Chem Engin News 2003; May 4:56–61.
62. Teo S, Stirling D, Thomas S, Hoberman A, Kiopes A, Khetani V. A 90-day oral gavage toxicity study of d-methylphenidate and d,l-methylphenidate in Sprague-Dawley rats. Toxicology 2002;179:183–96.
63. Davids E, Zhang K, Tarazi FI, Baldessarini RJ. Stereoselective effects of methylphenidate on motor hyperactivity in juvenile rats induced by neonatal 6-hydroxydopamine lesioning. Psychopharmacology 2002;160:92–8.
64. Teo SK, Stirling DI, Thomas SD, Khetani VD. Neurobehavioral effects of racemic *threo*-methylphenidate and its D and L enantiomers in rats. Pharmacol Biochem Behav 2003;74:747–54.
65. Patrick KS, Kilts CD, Breese GR. Synthesis and pharmacology of hydroxylated metabolites of methylphenidate. J Med Chem 1981;29:1237–40.
66. Bartlett MF, Egger HP. Disposition an metabolism of methylphenidate in dog and man. Fed Proc 1972;31:537.
67. Faraj BA, Israili ZH, Perel JM, et al. Metabolism and disposition of methylphenidate-^{14}C: studies in man and animals. J Pharmacol Exp Ther 1974;191:535–47.
68. Redalieu E, Bartlett MF, Waldes LM, Darrow WR, Egger H, Wagner WE. A study of methylphenidate in man with respect to its major metabolite. Drug Metab Dispos 1982;10: 708–9.
69. Chan Y-P, Swanson JM, Soldin SS, Thiessen JJ, Macleod SM, Logan W. Methylphenidate hydrochloride given with or before breakfast: II. Effects on plasma concentration of methylphenidate and ritalinic acid. Pediatrics 1983;72:56–9.
70. Wargin W, Patrick K, Kilts C, et al. Pharmacokinetics of methylphenidate in man, rat and monkey. J Pharmacol Exp Ther 1983;226:382–6.
71. Modi NB, Lindemulder G, Gupta SK. Single- and multiple-dose pharmacokinetics of oral once-a-day osmotic controlled-release OROS™ (methylphenidate HCl) formulation. J Clin Pharmacol 2000;40:379–88.

72. Modi NB, Wang B, Hu WT, Gupta SK. Effect of food on the pharmacokinetics of osmotic controlled-release methylphenidate HCl in healthy subjects. Biopharm Drug Dispos 2000;21:23–31.
73. Modi NB, Wang B, Noveck RJ, Gupta SK. Dose-proportional and stereospecific pharmacokinetics of methylphenidate delivered using an osmotic controlled-release oral delivery system. J Clin Pharmacol 2000;40:1141–9.
74. Sun Z, Murry DJ, Sanghani SP, Davis WI, Kedishvili NY, Zou Q, Hurley TD, Bosron WF. Methylphenidate is stereoselectively hydrolyzed by human carboxylesterase CES1A1. J Pharmacol Exp Ther 2004;310: 469–76.
75. Jonkman LM, Verbaten MN, deBoer D, et al. Differences in plasma concentrations of the D- and L-*threo* methylphenidate enantiomers in responding and non-responding children with attention-deficit hyperactivity disorder. Psychiatry Res 1998;78:115–8.
76. Ding Y-S, Fowler JS, Volkow ND. Is the *l-threo* enantiomer of methylphenidate (Ritalin) inactive in the brain when given orally [abstr] Am Col Neuropsychopharmacol 2002;Dec 8–12:255.
77. Patrick KS, Ellington KR, Breese GR, Kilts CD. Gas chromatographic-mass spectrometric analysis of methylphenidate and *p*-hydroxymethylphenidate using deuterated internal standards. J Chromatogr B Biomed Appl 1985;343:329–38.
78. Markowitz JS, Straughn AB, Patrick KS. Advances in the pharmacotherapy of attention-deficit hyperactivity disorder: Focus on methylphenidate formulations. Pharmacotherapy 2003;23:(10):1281-99.
79. Meyer MC, Straughn AB, Jarvi EJ, et al. Bioequivalence of methylphenidate immediate-release tablets using a replicated study design to characterize intrasubject variability. Pharm Res 2000;17:381–4.
80. Shader RI, Harmatz JS, Osterheld JR, Parmalee DX, Sallee FR, Greenblatt DJ. Population pharmacokinetics of methylphenidate in children with attention-deficit hyperactivity disorder. J Clin Pharmacol 1999;39:775–85.
81. Concerta (methylphenidate HCI) Extended-Release Tablets. Company: Alza Corporation. Application No. 21–121. Available from http://www.fda.gov/cder/approval/index. Accessed April 15, 2003.
82. Chan Y-PM, Soldin SJ, Swanson JM, Deber CM, Thiessen JJ, Macleod S. Gas chromatographic/mass spectrometric analysis of methylphenidate (Ritalin) in serum. Clin Biochem 1980;13:266–72.
83. Keating GM, Figgitt DP. Dexmethylphenidate. Drugs 2002;62:1899–904.
84. Novartis Pharmaceuticals Corporation. Focalin™ (dexmethylphenidate HCl) package insert. East Hanover, NJ, 2001.
85. Sherman M, Hauser GC, Glover BH. Toxic reactions to tranylcypromine. Am J Psychiatry 1964; 120:1019–21.
86. Newcorn JH, Schulz K, Harrison M, DeBellis MD, Udarbe JK, Halperin JM. α_2-adrenergic agonists: neurochemistry, efficacy, and clinical guidelines for use in children. Pediatr Clin North Am 1998;45:1099–122.
87. Swanson JM, Flockhart D, Udrea D, et al. Clonidine in the treatment of ADHD: questions about safety and efficacy. J Child Adolesc Psychiatry 1995;5:301–4.
88. The Tourette's Syndrome Study Group. Treatment of ADHD in children with tics—a randomized controlled trial. Neurology 2002;58:527–36.
89. Connor DF, Barkley RA, Davis HT. A pilot study of methylphenidate, clonidine, or the combination in ADHD comorbid with aggressive oppositional defiant or conduct disorder. Clin Pediatr 2000;39:15–25.
90. Levy F, Hobbes G. Does haloperidol block methylphenidate? Psychopharmacology 1996;126: 70–4.
91. Janowski DS, Davis JM. Methylphenidate, dextroamphetamine and levamphetamine. Arch Gen Psychiatry 1976;33:304–8.

92. Volkow ND, Wang G-J, Fowler JS, et al. Cardiovascular effects of methylphenidate in humans are associated with increases of dopamine in brain and of epinephrine in plasma. Psychopharmacology 2003;166:264–70.
93. Maxwell RA, Plummer AJ, Ross SD, Paytas JJ, Dennis AD. Antihypertensive effects of the central nervous stimulant, methylphenidate. Arch Int Pharmacodyn Ther 1957;CXII:26–35.
94. Maxwell RA, Plummer AJ, Ross SD, Daniel AL. Studies concerning the cardiovascular actions of the central nervous stimulant methylphenidate. J Pharmacol Exp Ther 1958;123:22–7.
95. Povalshi HJ, Goldsmith ED. Effect of methylphenidate on cardiovascular actions of pressor amines. Proc Soc Exp Biol Med 1959;101:717–21.
96. Tainter ML, Chang DK. The antagonism of the pressor action of tyramine by cocaine. J Pharmacol Exp Ther 1927;30:193–207.
97. DeVane CL, Markowitz JS, Carson SW, et al. Single dose methylphenidate pharmacokinetics in CYP 2D6 extensive and poor metabolizers. J Clin Psychopharmacol 2000;20:347–9.
98. Lin JH, Yamazaki M. Role of P-glycoprotein in pharmacokinetics: clinical implications. Clin Pharmacokinet 2003;42:59–98.
99. Remich SA, Desta Z, Soukhova NV, Flockhart DA. In vitro inhibition of cytochrome P450s by ephedrine, methylphenidate and its main metabolite ritalinic acid [abstr]. Clin Pharmacol Ther 2002;P60.
100. DeVane CL, Wang J-S, Pennick M, et al. Effects of amphetamine and methylphenidate on cytochrome P450 activity. Poster presentation; American Psychiatric Association 156th Annual Meeting, May 19, 2003, San Francisco, CA.
101. Le Nedelec MJ, Rosengren RJ. Methylphenidate inhibits cytochrome P450 in the Swiss Webster mouse. Hum Exp Toxicol 2002;21:273–80.
102. Markowitz JS, Logan BK, Diamond F, Patrick KS. Detection of the novel metabolite ethylphenidate following methylphenidate overdose with alcohol co-ingestion. J Clin Psychopharmacol 1999;19:362–6.
103. Markowitz JS, DeVane CL, Boulton DW, et al. Ethylphenidate formation in human subjects after the administration of a single dose of methylphenidate and alcohol. Drug Metab Dispos 2000;28:620–4.
104. Thomson MR, Dowd JJ, Markowitz JS, DeVane CL, Patrick KS. Enantioselective transesterification of methylphenidate to ethylphenidate after coadministration with ethanol [abstr]. J Clin Pharmacol 2002;42:1069.
105. Satoh T, Hosokawa M. The mammalian carboxyesterases: From molecules to function. Annu Rev Pharmacol Toxicol 1998;38:257–88.
106. Roberts SM, Harbison RD, James RC. Inhibition by ethanol of the metabolism of cocaine to benzoylecgonine and ecgonine methyl ester in mouse and human liver. Drug Metab Dispos 1993;21:537–41.
107. Schenk JO. The functioning of neuronal transporter for dopamine: kinetic mechanisms and effects of amphetamine, cocaine and methylphenidate. Prog Drug Res 2002;59:111–37.
108. Angrist B, Corwin J, Bartlik B, Cooper T. Early pharmacokinetics and clinical effects of oral d-amphetamine in normal subjects. Biol Psychiatry 1987;22:1357–68.
109. Brown GL, Ebert MH, Mikkelsen RJ, Hunt RD. Behavior and motor activity response in hyperactive children and plasma amphetamine levels following a sustained release preparation. J Am Acad Child Psychiatry 1980;19:225–39.
110. Wan SH, Martin SB, Azarnoff DL. Kinetics, salivary excretion of amphetamine isomers and effect of urinary pH. Clin Pharmacol Ther 1978;23:585–90.
111. Brown GL, Hunt RD, Ebert MH, Bunney WH, Kopin IJ. Plasma levels of d-amphetamine in hyperative children. Serial behavior and motor response. Psychopharmacology 1979;62:133–40.
112. Goldstein M, Anagnoste B. The conversion in vivo of D-amphetamine to (+)-p-hydroxynorephedrine. Biochim Biophys Acta 1965;107:166–8.
113. Smith RL, Dring LJ. Patterns of metabolism of b-phenethylamines in man and other species. In: Costa E, Garattini S, eds. Amphetamines and related compounds. New York: Raven Press, 1970:121–39.

114. Caldwell J, Dring LG, Williams RT. Norephedrines as metabolites of [14C] amphetamine in urine in man. Biochem J 1972;129:23–4.
115. Van Kammen DP, Ninan PT, Hommer D. Amphetamine enantiomers: psychopharmacological effects. In: Smith DF, ed. CRC handbook of stereoisomers: drugs in psychopharmacology. Boca Raton, FL: CRC, 1984:297–315.
116. Beckett AH, Rowland M, Turner P. Influence of urinary pH on excretion of amphetamine. Lancet 1965;I:303.
117. Chouinard G, Annable L, Bardwejn J. An early phase II clinical trial of tomoxetine (LY139603) in the treatment of newly admitted depressed patients. Psychopharmacology 1984;83:126–8.
118. Bymaster FP, Katner JS, Nelson DL, et al. Atomoxetine increases extracellular levels of norepinephrine and dopamine in prefrontal cortex of rat: A potential mechanism for efficacy in attention deficit/hyperactivity disorder. Neuropsychopharmacology 2002;27:699–711.
119. Strattera™ (atomoxetine), Package Insert. Eli Lilly and Company: Indianapolis, IN, 2002.
120. Chalon SA, Desager JP, DeSante KA, et al. Effect of hepatic impairment on the pharmacokinetics of atomoxetine and metabolites. Clin Pharmacol Ther 2003;73:178–91.
121. Witcher JW, Long A, Smith B, et al. Atomoxetine pharmacokinetics in children and adolescents with attention deficit hyperactivity disorder. J Child Adol Psychopharmacol 2003;1:53–63.
122. Sauer JM, Ponsler GD, Mattiuz EL, et al. Disposition and metabolic fate of atomoxetine hydrochloride: the role of CYP2D6 in human disposition and metabolism. Drug Metab Dispos 2003;31:98–107.
123. Farid NA, Bergstrom RF, Ziege EA, Parli CJ, Lemberger L. Single-dose and steady-state pharmacokinetics of tomoxetine in normal subjects. J Clin Pharmacol 1985;25:296–301.
124. Belle DJ, Ernest CS, Sauer J-M, Smith BP, Thomasson HR, Witcher JW. Effect of potent CYP2D6 inhibition by paroxetine on atomoxetine pharmacokinetics. J Clin Pharmacol 2002;42:1219–27.

INDEX